MW00561024

MORE ADVANCE ACCLAIM FOR
Pediatric Psychopharmacology: Fast Facts

"The field of child and adolescent psychopharmacology is rapidly changing. *Pediatric Psychopharmacology: Fast Facts* thoughtfully considers this very important topic. It addresses those areas of pediatric psychopharmacology that are most often encountered in clinical practice. This up-to-date and useful book covers its multiple topics well. It is both concise and practical. It also succinctly puts key facts about various aspects of child and adolescent psychopharmacology at the reader's fingertips."

—Robert L. Findling, M.D.,
Professor of Psychiatry and Pediatrics,
Case Western Reserve University,
and Director of Child and Adolescent Psychiatry,
University Hospitals of Cleveland

PEDIATRIC PSYCHOPHARMACOLOGY
FAST FACTS

PEDIATRIC PSYCHOPHARMACOLOGY
FAST FACTS

Daniel F. Connor, M.D.
Bruce M. Meltzer, M.D.

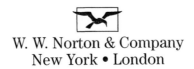

W. W. Norton & Company
New York • London

For information about permission to
reproduce selections from this book, write to
Permissions, W. W. Norton & Company, Inc.,
500 Fifth Avenue, New York, NY 10110

Production Manager Leeann Graham
Manufacturing by Courier Westford

Library of Congress Cataloging-in-Publication Data

Connor, Daniel F.
   Pediatric psychopharmacology : fast facts / Daniel F. Connor, Bruce M. Meltzer.
      p.   ;   cm.
"A Norton professional book."
Includes bibliographical references and index.
ISBN: 978-0-393-70461-7
1. Pediatric psychopharmacology. I. Meltzer, Bruce M. II. Title.
[DNLM: 1. Psychotropic Drugs—therapeutic use—Adolescent. 2. Psychotropic
Drugs—therapeutic use—Child. 3. Affective Symptoms—drug therapy—
Adolescent. 4. Affective Symptoms—drug therapy—Child. 5. Child Behavior
Disorders—drug therapy. 6. Psychopharmacology—methods. QV 77.2 C752 2005]
RJ504.7.C66 2005
615'.78'083—dc22   2005051284

W. W. Norton & Company, Inc., 500 Fifth Avenue, New York, N.Y. 10110
www.wwnorton.com

W. W. Norton & Company Ltd., Castle House, 75/76 Wells St., London W1T 3QT

1   3   5   7   9   0   8   6   4   2

DEDICATION

Dedicated to our young patients and their families,
who have taught us so much over the years

Contents

CONTENTS

PART III: THE DISORDERS AND THEIR TREATMENT

Preface

Pediatric psychopharmacology came of age in the 1970s. Since then, the use of psychiatric medications to treat neuropsychiatric disorders of childhood and adolescence has become much more widely accepted by clinicians, physicians, teachers, and parents. Indeed, recent studies have shown a dramatic increase over the last decade in the use of pharmacological agents to treat neuropsychiatric disorders of behavior and emotion in children and adolescents. This increase corresponds to (1) a dramatic advance in scientific knowledge about disorders of emotion and behavior in youngsters, and (2) the beginnings of more sophisticated clinical medication treatment trials using rigorous methodology in this age group.

Although some psychopharmacological treatment of juveniles involves mental health professionals such as child and adolescent psychiatrists, primary care physicians such as family practice doctors and pediatricians provide the largest amount of treatment. Clinical nurse specialists in pediatric mental health increasingly prescribe psychiatric medications in a wide variety of clinical settings. Specialists such as pediatric neurologists often care for children and adolescents with neuropsychiatric disorders. Medical students and graduate medical residents training in pediatrics, primary care, pediatric neurology, psychiatry, and child and adolescent psychiatry require an increasingly wide empirical knowledge base in pediatric psychopharmacology. Clinical psychologists are increasingly confronted with medication issues if and when they evaluate and treat youngsters with mental health problems. At the time of this writing, psychologists have been granted psychiatric medication prescribing rights in New Mexico and Louisiana. Given the continuing national shortage of child and adolescent psychiatrists, the number of states granting prescriptive rights to psychologists may very well increase in the future. Often treatment involves a collaborative effort between the prescribing clinician, the primary care provider, and a number of other adults who may be responsible for the welfare of the child, including parents, guardians, the courts, nurses, teachers, counselors, therapists, and clergy. Providing a mechanism for broadly sharing state-of-the-art knowledge about psychopharmacological treatment of children and adolescents is very timely and important. There exists a great need for accurate, up-to-date information provided in an easy-to-read and highly organized reference book that is accessible to both the clinician and layperson alike.

This book meets that need by providing the reader with an overview of the use of psychiatric medication to treat emotional and behavioral disorders of childhood and adolescence. Organized into three parts, Pediatric Psychopharmacology Fast Facts first reviews general introductory topics, including principles of psychopharmacology and general assessment issues in pediatric psychopharmacology. The psychiatric medications are introduced next and discussed by drug class. Finally, a review of psychiatric disorders is provided to give the reader a firm grounding in current diagnostic topics. This book provides (1) guidelines regarding general principles of care for the practice of pediatric psychopharmacology, (2) a review of the most common neuropsychiatric disorders encountered in this age group, (3) a review of the literature regarding the pharmacological treatment of these disorders, and (4) specific recommendations and guidelines for treatment. Several appendices provide useful pediatric psychopharmacological tools for the practicing clinician. Pediatric Psychopharmacology Fast Facts offers empirically based, state-of-the-art knowledge for child mental health practitioners as well as basic knowledge for clinical nurse practitioners in mental health, pediatricians, pediatric neurologists, and family medicine physicians, in particular, and for other concerned adults, family members, and teachers.

This book is meant to be used as a practical clinical guide. Although the book may be read cover to cover, we anticipate that it will be used more as a reference, with chapters read out of context as the need for specific clinical information arises in the course of daily clinical care. As such, there is a certain amount of repetition in the chapters as practical information is repeated in multiple areas of the book. The chapters are not heavily referenced in the text. All information used is cited in the bibliography at the end of the book, organized by chapter.

We wish to thank a number of people who supported our efforts in this endeavor. Jean Foran, Barbara Buchanan, and Sorcha O'Sullivan Murphy at the University of Massachusetts Medical School provided much needed administrative support and cheerful encouragement. Ronald J. Steingard, M.D., helped us create a structure for the book. Paul C. Marshall, M.D., Chief of Pediatric Neurology at the University of Massachusetts Memorial Health Care, provided much needed suggestions on several chapters. Richard H. Melloni, Jr., M.A., Ph.D. Associate Professor of Psychology and Assistant Director of Behavioral Neuroscience at Northeastern University, Boston, MA, provided many useful comments on information to include in the book. Andrea Costella, assistant editor at Norton Books, provided invaluable assistance. We especially thank A. Deborah Malmud, director of Professional Books at W. W. Norton, for commissioning this project. Without her support and encouragement, we would not have succeeded.

Daniel F. Connor, M.D.
Bruce M. Meltzer, M.D.
Worcester, MA

PEDIATRIC PSYCHOPHARMACOLOGY
FAST FACTS

Part I
Introduction

1. Introduction to Pediatric Psychopharmacology

Compared to most medical specialties, pediatric psychopharmacology is a relatively new field. Although medications in various forms as well as home-grown "potions and remedies" have been given to soothe sleepless, fretful, and fearful children for many decades, the modern practice of pediatric psychopharmacology, with its emphasis on empirically derived data to establish the efficacy, safety, and tolerability of psychiatric medications for the treatment of neuropsychiatric disorders in children and adolescents, is really only about three decades old. In that time the field has seen vigorous growth in the number of clinical studies investigating psychiatric medications in children and adolescents. There are now scientific journals dedicated to pediatric psychopharmacology, child and adolescent psychiatry, pediatric neurology, developmental and behavioral pediatrics, and developmental neurobiology. Several fine pediatric psychopharmacology textbooks are presently available. In 1997, federal legislative passage of the Food and Drug Administration Modernization Act (FDAMA) encouraged pediatric drug development and testing by giving the pharmaceutical industry an incentive in the form of additional marketing exclusivity if pediatric data were obtained on already patented and new drugs. Since then, there has been a rapid increase in the number of methodologically controlled medication trials in children and adolescents, including early-onset psychiatric disorders. There is an ever-expanding knowledge base in pediatric psychopharmacology that is increasingly informed by scientific advances in molecular genetics, cell biology, noninvasive neuroimaging of the central nervous system, developmental psychology, and methodologically sound clinical drug trials in children and adolescents. Although not without its share of social and scientific issues and controversies, pediatric psychopharmacology is on a much firmer scientific footing now than it was 30 years ago. This chapter introduces the practicing clinician to the growing field of pediatric psychopharmacology.

A BRIEF HISTORY OF THE FIELD

The beginnings of pediatric psychopharmacology occurred in the 1930s in Providence, Rhode Island, where Charles Bradley worked with behaviorally disturbed children at the Emma Pendleton Bradley Hospital. Racemic amphetamine (Benzedrine®) had only recently been synthesized, and there was great medicinal interest in the drug. Bradley administered amphetamine to his young patients and observed that the drug calmed and settled hyperactive, impulsive, and behaviorally disturbed youngsters. The 1937 publication by Charles Bradley of "The Behavior of Children Receiving Benzedrine" in the *American Journal of Orthopsychiatry* marked the formal scientific beginning of the field of pediatric psychopharmacology.

With World War II and the years thereafter came growing enthusiasm for the field of psychoanalytic psychiatry. Psychoanalysis seemed to offer hope for understanding and treating emotional and psychiatric problems. Although this hope ultimately proved false, Bradley's beginnings in pediatric psychopharmacology became obscured.

In the 1950s, searching for better anesthetic drugs, the first of the modern psychiatric medications, chlorpromazine, was accidentally discovered. In that decade lithium and the tricyclic antidepressants were synthesized. In the following decade, the benzodiazepines, including diazepam and chlordiazepoxide, were introduced into clinical psychiatry. Methylphenidate for "hyperkinetic behavior" was synthesized. Still later, in the late 1980s and early 1990s, the serotonin reuptake inhibiting (SSRI) antidepressants were introduced and proved effective for anxiety, obsessive–compulsive disorder, and depression, and were safer than the older tricyclic antidepressants. Second-generation atypical antipsychotics possessed less risk of neurological side effects and replaced older neuroleptics for the treatment of schizophrenia, psychotic disorders, and mania. With the introduction of aripiprazole in 2003, a third generation of antipsychotic medication (partial agonist–antagonist dopamine modulators) is possibly on its way. Anticonvulsant medications such as valproic acid and carbamazepine were found effective as mood stabilizers in psychiatric patients. Still later, lamotrigene was found useful for both the depressive as well as manic phases of adult bipolar illness. Extended-release methylphenidate and mixed amphetamine salts compounds were introduced into pediatric psychopharmacology in the early 21st century. These longer-acting stimulant drugs changed the standard of care in the treatment of attention-deficit/hyperactivity disorder (ADHD). In 2003, atomoxetine became the first nonstimulant medication to receive Food and Drug Administration (FDA) labeling for ADHD in children, adolescents, and adults. In 2004, a combination capsule of olanzapine and fluoxetine became the first FDA-approved medication labeled for use in adult bipolar depression. In 2005 extended release carbamazepine was approved for adult bipolor disorder. The fields of psychopharmacology and pediatric psychopharmacology are rapidly growing, and the clinician can expect that further advances will continue in the near future.

Lacking a robust scientific database, early pediatric psychopharmacology was initially highly dependent on developments in adult psychopharmacology.

From the 1950s through the mid-1980s the main influences on medication treatments for youngsters "trickled down" from adult psychiatry and were largely derived from adult psychiatric medication developments. In the 1970s the field began to stir once more, largely under the influence of behavioral scientists and academic psychologists who introduced better scientific assessment methods, more rigorous experimental designs, and better research methodology into the field of pediatric psychopharmacology. Although largely preoccupied in the past with only one disorder, ADHD, for which stimulants proved very effective, pediatric psychopharmacology began to expand its boundaries into the search for effective and safe medications in the treatment of a variety of other early-onset neuropsychiatric disorders.

Beginning in the 1980s and continuing to the present, a variety of studies have been conducted to investigate psychiatric medications in children and adolescents with disorders other than ADHD. These disorders include behavioral disturbances in persons with developmental delay and autistic spectrum disorders, schizophrenia and early-onset psychotic disorders, depression and pediatric bipolar illness, obsessive–compulsive disorder, other anxiety disorders, and conduct disorders. Aided by advances in developmental neurobiology, molecular pharmacology, developmental psychology, and clinical child and adolescent psychiatry, the pace of research quickened. With legislative passage of the FDAMA (Food and Drug Administration Modernization Act) in 1997, the way was open for the pharmaceutical industry to use its huge resources to encourage and finance large methodologically sound clinical trials of psychiatric medications in early-onset neuropsychiatric disorders. By the mid-to-late 1990s pediatric psychopharmacology had emerged as a medical discipline in its own right.

At the beginning of the new century pediatric psychopharmacology faces a number of continuing and new challenges. First, there is the continuing challenge of testing the efficacy, safety, and tolerability of existing psychiatric medications used in children and adolescents who have early-onset neuropsychiatric disorders. After all, children are not just "little adults," and what works for adults with psychiatric disorders may or may not work in children and adolescents with the same disorders.

Next is the question of developing new medicines for children and adolescents. Although existing medications work well for some early-onset psychiatric disorders, such as ADHD and obsessive–compulsive disorder, they may not prove as effective in children as compared to adults for other disorders, such as depression.

Third, as clinicians we need to know more about how to integrate pediatric psychopharmacological interventions with psychosocial therapies in order to provide the most effective treatment plan for a specific child or adolescent. Medications should never be given as the only treatment to a youngster, and treatment plans for an individual should never be dichotomized between a psychosocial treatment and a psychopharmacological intervention. Both treatments should be used as needed.

Finally, there is a huge unknown in pediatric psychopharmacology: the question of the possible long-range effects of perturbing developmental neurobiological systems with pharmacological agents while these systems are still developing in childhood and adolescence, and the effects downstream on the fully formed adult central nervous system (CNS). If the developing brain is exposed to medications for a period of time during development, are there permanent effects that emerge later in life? If so, some of these effects may be therapeutic. For example, if we intervene for depression in childhood with antidepressant medications, do we alter the neurobiological systems that go awry in depression in such a way that depression is less frequent and/or severe later in life? If so, that would be a good thing. On the other hand, if we change some of these CNS neurobiological systems with medications before they are fully developed and complete, do we inadvertently cause harm to the person that only emerges later in life? If so, that would be bad. The pathway to the answer(s) lies in preclinical and clinical scientific research investigating the longitudinal effects of pediatric pharmacological agents on the CNS throughout the lifespan. Clinically, we do not presently believe that intervening with psychiatric medications in childhood is unwarranted. After all, untreated childhood neuropsychiatric illness is far more damaging to the individual across his or her lifespan than the presently known side effects of psychiatric medications. However, as clinicians we need to be cautious, keep scientifically informed, prescribe psychiatric medications to children and adolescents thoughtfully and only after a systematic and thorough clinical assessment, consider other nonpharmacological treatments for an individual child, if indicated, systematically and rigorously assess benefits and side effects of the prescribed medication(s), and be guided by the moral principle of the dictum *Primum non nocere* (first do no harm).

EPIDEMIOLOGICAL TRENDS IN PEDIATRIC PSYCHOPHARMACOLOGY

Epidemiological research has reported that up to 21% of children between the ages of 9 and 17 has a diagnosable mental health or addictive disorder (Shaffer et al., 1996), and as many as 10% of these children and adolescents may have a medication-responsive psychiatric disorder (Riddle et al., 1998). In the past 15 years there has been a dramatic increase in the use of psychiatric medications to treat early-onset neuropsychiatric disorders in children and adolescents. Although substantial regional, professional, and demographic variations exist in prescribing practices, the increase in prescribing rates of psychiatric medications to children and adolescents appears to have occurred at all pediatric ages, in both genders, and in many different geographic areas of the United States.

Stimulants and SSRI antidepressants are the medication classes most often prescribed to youngsters. Prescribing rates for these medications have increased substantially over the past 15 years (Hoagwood et al., 2000; Safa et al., 2003; Zito & Safa, 2005). Clonidine prescription rates and the combination of clonidine and a stimulant in the treatment of ADHD have also risen dramatically. In addition, antipsychotic use is rising in the pediatric population, although more slowly than medications used to treat ADHD, depression, and anxiety disorders (Jensen et al., 1999).

Combined pharmacotherapy, defined as treatment with multiple concurrent medications, is also rising in the pediatric population, despite a paucity of research supporting its use (Safa et al., 2003). Combined pharmacotherapy (CPT) rates vary by the population sampled. In inpatient units and residential treatment facilities that treat the most seriously disturbed children, rates of CPT up to 60% have been reported (Connor et al., 1998). In these children, antipsychotics are most often combined with other agents (Connor et al., 1997). Lower rates of CPT are described in ambulatory samples, where stimulants and antidepressants are often combined with other agents.

Prescribing rates vary by physician specialty. Previously, psychiatrists prescribed the majority of stimulant medications to children and adolescents. The most recent prescribing data suggest a change. Now it appears that pediatricians prescribe the majority of stimulants to youth in the United States (Jensen et al., 2003). Although psychiatrists still prescribe antidepressants most commonly, the number of pediatricians, child neurologists, and family practitioners who prescribe SSRIs to children and adolescents is rising rapidly. Child and adolescent psychiatrists (and adult psychiatrists) prescribe the most antipsychotic, neuroleptic, tricyclic antidepressant, lithium, and mood stabilizer medications to youngsters.

PRESCRIBING ALGORITHMS

In an effort to reduce heterogeneity in clinical medication use and facilitate a more systematic approach to prescribing psychoactive medications for children and adolescents, prescribing algorithms are being introduced into pediatric psychopharmacology. These algorithms are based on psychiatric diagnosis and attempt to define initial and follow-up steps for the prescription of medications in specific disorders. The clinician moves through the algorithm in a stepwise fashion. Medication prescribing algorithms have been introduced for the medication treatment of ADHD, obsessive–compulsive disorder (OCD), bipolar disorder, and depression in pediatric psychopharmacology. Preliminary research suggests better outcomes when prescribing algorithms are used in clinical practice, as compared to clinical treatment as usual in the community. These prescribing algorithms are presented in the pertinent chapters describing the treatment of these specific disorders.

PSYCHIATRIC MEDICATION USE IN PRESCHOOL CHILDREN

The increase in prescribing rates for psychiatric medications is also being seen in very young preschool children. Studies examining health insurance database records report stimulant use has increased 3-fold between 1991 and 1995 in preschool children 2–4 years old. During this same time period, clonidine use increased 28-fold, and use of SSRIs increased 3-fold among preschoolers.

There is evidence that stimulants are effective and well tolerated for severe early-onset ADHD in preschool children. Since 1970, 10 methodologically controlled studies investigating stimulants in 3- to 6-year-old children with ADHD have been completed. Nine of 10 studies (90%) report benefits and safety of stimulants for early-onset ADHD in preschoolers (Connor, 2002). Presently there is a multisite federally funded study investigating the efficacy and safety of stimulants in preschool ADHD, the Preschool ADHD Treatment Study (PATS)(Greenhill et al. 2003), so more information will be available in the future. All studies note that family behavioral therapy treatment should be attempted first in preschoolers with ADHD. Only when psychosocial treatments fail and ADHD symptoms are severe and impairing to the child, should stimulant medications be considered in this age range. Use of stimulants in children less than 3 years old is not recommended, because so little information is available about the developing brain in very young toddlers.

Psychiatric medications other than stimulants have not yet been studied in preschoolers, so clinicians have no scientific evidence on which to base treatment decisions in this age group. Thus the clinical prescription of a variety of psychiatric medications to preschoolers presently outstrips the scientific evidence to support their clinical use. It is recommended that family parent management, and psychosocial therapies always be attempted as a first-line treatment intervention in very young children with early-onset neuropsychiatric disorders. *Prescription of psychiatric medications to children younger than 3 years old is not recommended.*

REGULATORY ISSUES IN PEDIATRIC PSYCHOPHARMACOLOGY

Off-Label Prescribing

The FDA is charged with labeling medications for manufacturers' advertising. Labeling occurs for a particular drug in the treatment of a specific disease when adequate information is available from methodologically sound clinical trials about safety, side effects, effectiveness for symptoms of the particular disease, and dosing range. Once this information is available for a medication, and the medication is found effective and safe for a specific disease in a particular age of patient (i.e., child, adolescent, or adult) the drug is "labeled" by the FDA for advertising by the manufacturer as treatment for the specific disease in a specific age range.

Presently the scientific evidence base in pediatric psychopharmacology is inadequate to support the level of clinical prescribing in this area. Although many psychiatric medications are labeled as safe and effective for use in adults, there simply have not been enough completed controlled clinical studies of psychiatric medications in children and adolescents to allow a scientific determination of the efficacy, safety, and tolerability in the pediatric age range. Most psychiatric medications are prescribed to children and adolescents "off-label." The reader should note that the FDA does not regulate physician-prescribing practices, only manufacturer advertising for medications. If the clinician has a medically accepted reason and a sound rationale for prescribing a drug to a child, the FDA does not prohibit "off-label" use. Thus the clinician may prescribe FDA-approved drugs for non-FDA-approved indications. An example is the use of atypical antipsychotics to treat aggression, hyperactivity, and conduct problems in youth with conduct disorder. The physician may also prescribe FDA-approved drugs for approved indications in children below the age limit for which the drugs are approved. An example is the use of citalopram to treat pediatric depression. Because off-label prescribing may increase the potential for liability, the clinician must assess the risk–benefit ratio for prescribing a medication for a non-FDA-approved indication and be careful to document in the medical record a scientifically reasonable rationale for choosing a particular mediation over other possible treatment interventions.

The Regulatory Process of Drug Development

The FDA has regulatory authority over the development and marketing of new pharmaceutical agents. There is a stepwise process by which new drugs are tested and undergo approval that is mandated by the FDA.

- *Preclinical testing:* Testing a new drug in animal models always precedes testing in humans. At least two animal species are exposed to a wide range of doses of the new drug for varying periods of time. Assessments include observation for abnormal signs, blood chemistry testing, vital signs, electrocardiograms, and both gross anatomical and histopathological evaluations. If the new drug is found suitable for human testing, findings from early animal studies are used to determine the dose range for later human trials and the identification of specific organ systems to be selected for safety monitoring.
- *Investigational new drug application:* Once enough preclinical testing has been done to identify the new drug as suitable for human trials, an investigational new drug (IND) application is submitted to the FDA. If approved, the IND application allows the initiation of human testing.
- *Phase 1 trials:* Human testing of the new drug begins in Phase 1 clinical trials. These tests focus on human pharmacology, pharmacokinetics, and tolerability, generally in normal volunteer adults. The goal of these early trials is to find a range of tolerable doses and to determine safety at each dose and over varying durations of drug treatment. Plasma samples are evaluated to ascertain plasma drug concentration–adverse event relationships.
- *Phase 2 trials:* During this phase patients with the disease or disorder in question are first exposed to the new drug. The goals of Phase 2 clinical trials are to evaluate the efficacy of the drug in patients with the disease of interest, and to determine the most common short-term adverse events associated with the new drug.
- *Phase 3 trials:* These trials are the pivotal clinical trials that provide the FDA with adequate scientific evidence of the new drug's efficacy for the claimed intervention. Safety monitoring occurs during Phase 3 trials, but is often less intense than safety monitoring during the earlier trials. Often Phase 3 clinical trials are accompanied by a long-duration open-label extension phase designed to gather information about safety and tolerability of the new drug over long periods of time, often 6 months to 2 years.

- *New drug application:* Once a pharmaceutical company has completed its drug development program for a new agent, it submits a new drug application (NDA) to the FDA to gain federal approval for advertising and marketing.
- *Post-marketing surveillance:* If the FDA approves a new drug as safe and effective for a specific disorder, the drug is labeled for that condition. This labeling allows the manufacturer to advertise the drug for that disease. The government requires a commitment from the pharmaceutical company to conduct postmarketing Phase 4 studies to follow up on certain outstanding concerns about the new drug if additional questions arise. In addition, all drugs are subject to postmarketing surveillance through the FDA's Medwatch reporting system. This system depends on physicians to voluntarily report adverse events to the FDA as more experience with the drug emerges in real-world clinical practice.

FDA Initiatives to Promote Pediatric Drug Development

Because all types of medications are clinically prescribed to children and adolescents, and because previous FDA drug labeling did not specifically require scientific data in youth, the FDA has taken action to encourage pharmaceutical companies to conduct scientific clinical trials in youngsters. A brief history of these efforts includes the following.

- *FDA 1979:* The Pediatric Use subsection under the Precautions section of labeling: This rule affirmed the need for substantial evidence from adequate and methodologically controlled clinical trials in support of any new pediatric indications. In the absence of such data, the rule called for the standard disclaimer in drug labeling; "safety and effectiveness in children and adolescents have not been established."
- *FDA 1994:* A second FDA initiative was launched in the early 1990s to propose an alternative approach to obtaining substantial evidence of drug effectiveness in pediatric populations. It was noted that in certain circumstances pediatric indications and use information in labeling could be based on adequate and well-controlled studies in adults. If the FDA could conclude that the course of the disease and the drug's effects were sufficiently similar in the child and adult populations, the agency would permit extrapolation from the adult efficacy data to pediatric patients. Supplementary pharmacokinetic data for childhood dosing and additional pediatric safety information would be required. This FDA initiative required voluntary efforts on the part of the pharmaceutical industry, was difficult to enforce, and ultimately had very little impact on pediatric drug research.
- *FDA 1997:* The Food and Drug Administration Modernization Act (FDAMA): The FDAMA encouraged the pharmaceutical industry to voluntarily conduct pediatric drug testing by providing manufacturers with the possibility of gaining an additional 6 months of marketing exclusivity (i.e., no generic competitors allowed) either for new drugs or for drugs already FDA approved and marketed if the extant patent had not already lapsed. For this incentive, the FDA must specifically request such information, and the

pharmaceutical company would have to establish that information relating to the use of the active drug moiety in some pediatric population had the potential for producing health benefits in that population. This is a voluntary program designed to provide incentives to sponsors to develop and scientifically test new drugs or new indications for existing drugs for pediatric patients.

• *FDA 1998:* The Pediatric Rule: The Pediatric Rule gives the FDA authority to require pediatric studies for certain new and marketed drug and biological products in child and adolescent populations. Thus the process of providing pediatric drug information became not entirely voluntary on the part of the pharmaceutical industry. Several different types of pharmaceutical development programs, including a new drug indication, a new dosage form, a new dosing regimen, or a new route of drug administration, can trigger the Pediatric Rule. For any of these situations, it is first necessary for the pharmaceutical manufacturer to establish that the drug and its indications may provide a meaningful therapeutic benefit or that there may be substantial use of the drug in the pediatric population. For drug development programs that trigger the Pediatric Rule, pediatric studies are to be completed at the time the NDA or supplement is submitted.

• *FDA 2002:* The Best Pharmaceuticals for Children Act: This law renews the pediatric exclusivity provision provided by FDAMA.

Some psychiatric medications are FDA labeled for use in children and adolescents with mental health disorders. Current FDA-approved labeling for psychiatric medications in children and adolescents is given below.

Table 1.1 FDA Labeling and Pediatric Psychiatric Medications

Drug	Pediatric Label Indication
Methylphenidate	ADHD
Amphetamines	ADHD
Pemoline	ADHD
Atomoxetine	ADHD
Clomipramine	OCD
Fluvoxamine	OCD
Sertraline	OCD
Fluoxetine	MDD, OCD
Lithium	Mania ≥ 12 years old
Pimozide	Tourette's syndrome ≥ 8 years old
Haloperidol	Tourette's syndrome
Imipramine	Enuresis
DDAVP	Enuresis ≥ 4 years old
Trifluoperazine	Psychosis 6–12 years old
Chlorpromazine	Severe behavioral problems 1–12 years old
Haloperidol	Severe behavioral problems 1–12 years old
Modafinil	Narcolepsy ≥ 16 years old

DDAVP = desmopressin; MDD = major depressive disorder; OCD = obsessive–compulsive disorder

ETHICAL ISSUES IN PEDIATRIC PSYCHOPHARMACOLOGY

The clinical practice of child and adolescent psychopharmacology must be guided by ethical principles. The doctrine of informed consent is the embodiment of ethical and clinical rules that serves to protect patient autonomy by ensuring that patients are informed of the diagnosis, treatment options, alternatives to treatment, and risks and benefits of those options. Consent to treatment must be given voluntarily and not be coerced in any way by the physician. Under law, to coerce a patient into treatment is to open the physician to a charge of battery: the intentional touching of another person without permission or legal privilege. In addition, the consenting person must be competent to understand his or her medical situation, have an appreciation of the seriousness of his or her condition, understand the consequences of accepting or rejecting treatment, be able to express a preference, and be capable of manipulating the provided medical information in a rational manner.

Children have a limited capacity to understand informed consent and medical treatment issues. They need their parents or legal guardians to act in their best interests. Because the law deems that all decisions concerning a child, including decisions about medical treatment, are deemed to fall within the province of the parent or the child's legal guardian, these adults must give informed consent to treat a child with psychiatric medication. Handling informed consent issues with parents includes a discussion of the following:

- The nature of the condition that requires treatment.
- The nature and purpose of the proposed treatment and the probability that it will succeed.
- The risks and consequences of the proposed course of treatment.
- Alternatives to the proposed treatment and their accompanying risks and consequences.
- Prognosis with and without the proposed treatment.
- The possibility of unknown risks to the use of medications in children, especially when using novel or new psychopharmacological agents or treatments in which the risks versus the benefits are uncertain.

It is widely recognized that children 7 years or older must provide their assent to treatment. *Assent* means a general agreement to undertake the treatment. The elements of child assent are:

- Helping the child achieve a developmentally appropriate awareness of the nature of his or her condition.
- Telling the child patient what to expect from tests and treatments.
- Making a clinical assessment of the child's understanding of the medical situation and the factors that are influencing his or her response.
- Soliciting a statement of the child's willingness to accept the recommended tests and/or treatment.

It is to be emphasized that informed consent and assent to treatment are ongoing processes, not single events to be completed and then forgotten as treatment proceeds. The physician must repeatedly inform patients as to the benefits and risks of interventions if these change or become clearer over time, and be available to answer patient questions as these arise in the course of treatment. A statement as to informed consent and child assent should be entered into the patient's medical record at the start of treatment.

DEVELOPMENTAL PHARMACOLOGY, NEUROBIOLOGY, AND PEDIATRIC PSYCHOPHARMACOLOGY

Children may respond to psychiatric medications differently from adults, and it cannot be assumed that medications behave in children and young adolescents like they behave in developmentally mature adults. For example, depression appears to be phenomenologically similar in children and adults, and about 60%–70% of adults with a major depressive disorder appears to respond to therapeutic interventions with tricyclic antidepressants. To date, a response to tricyclic antidepressants has yet to be found compared with responses to placebo in depressed children. Children and adolescents may require larger doses of a drug than adults to obtain equivalent plasma levels. For example, this need for a larger dose has been found for the neuroleptic chlorpromazine. There are a number of possible developmental and neurobiological reasons for these differences between children and adults, including developmental differences in drug pharmacokinetics, pharmacodynamics, and developmental neurobiology.

Pharmacokinetics is the science that explains the relationship between a drug dosing regimen and the concentration of the drug in the body. Essentially, pharmacokinetics is the study of what the body does to a drug. Drug concentration is related to drug dose, dosing frequency, absorption, distribution, drug metabolism, and excretion. The younger the child, the more rapid is drug metabolism in the liver and the greater is the renal glomerular filtration rate, compared with adults. Thus children and young adolescents may require larger doses of some psychoactive medications, per unit of body weight, than adults to attain similar serum levels and therapeutic efficacy.

Pharmacodynamics is the study of what the drug does to the body. Free drug binds to target receptors on end organs and initiates changes that result in benefits to lessen the impact of disease and treat symptoms, and also results in drug side effects. In the case of psychopharmacology, the end organ is the brain. Children may respond to drugs differently from adults because target receptors on the neural substrates that bind drugs may be different in neurobiologically immature children, compared to developmentally mature adults.

Finally, *developmental neurobiological* factors may explain some of the differences between children and adults in the response to psychopharmacological agents. Catecholamine systems in the CNS are not fully anatomically developed and operationally functional until adulthood. Serotonin neural networks continue to develop through the third decade of life. Since psychiatric medications act on these distributed neural systems, drug effects in children may be different from drug effects on neurobiologically mature adults.

2. Basic Pharmacology

A working knowledge of basic pharmacology is important for the clinical child and adolescent psychopharmacologist. Although not intended to be an in-depth review, this chapter briefly discusses how the body handles drugs (pharmacokinetics). Reported differences in pharmacokinetics between children and adults are examined. A discussion of pharmacodynamics is outside the scope of this chapter and can be found in Appendix 2. Finally, a discussion of drug metabolism via the cytochrome P450 superfamily of enzymes is presented. A knowledge of CYP 450 substrates, inducers, and inhibitors is important, given the growing prevalence of combined pharmacotherapy and the possibility of drug–drug interactions in children and adolescents treated with psychiatric medications.

PHARMACOKINETICS

There is a relationship between the action of a given drug and its concentration in the blood or at its end organ site of effect. The science that explains and predicts the relationship between a drug dosing regimen and drug concentration in blood and various body compartments is called pharmacokinetics. These drug relationships are determined by the interaction of several factors, including (1) the drug dosage regimen, (2) drug absorption, (3) drug distribution into various body tissues, and (4) metabolism and elimination of the drug. Absorption and distribution are primarily responsible for determining the speed of onset of drug effect. Metabolism and elimination terminate the action of the drug by removing it from the body. Taken together, these four processes determine how long the drug lasts in the body and its duration of action.

In real life, these pharmacokinetic processes are quite variable among patients and within a given patient, depending on patient age, disease state, diet, and concurrent drugs. Thus for many drugs the relationship between drug dose and the resulting therapeutic effect is unpredictable. The relationship between drug concentration in the body and drug effects is more robust. A better

15

approximation of the relationship between drug dose and drug effects is found with the use of plasma drug monitoring. This type of monitoring is available for only a few of the agents used in pediatric psychopharmacology, such as lithium, carbamazepine, valproic acid, and the tricyclic antidepressants.

Absorption

In order to produce desired pharmacological effects, an appropriate concentration of drug must be available at its target site of action. Absorption into the body varies according to the route of drug administration and the ease at which the drug molecule crosses cell membranes. With the exception of topical agents, all drugs must enter the bloodstream to be carried to their receptor sites. There are several routes for drug absorption:

- *Intravenous (IV) injection:* This is the most efficient route for drug administration, in that the entire dose is available for distribution by the bloodstream to its site of action. Few psychiatric medications are administered intravenously.
- *Intramuscular (IM) injection:* The IM route of drug delivery is very slow and incomplete, because it often results in some precipitation of the drug at the injection site. This precipitation may irritate the adjacent muscle and tissue. Some formulations, such as risperidone long-acting injection or fluphenazine decanoate, are especially formulated to provide a slow release of drug from intramuscular sites, providing a greatly prolonged effect over 2–4 weeks.
- *Rectal administration:* Much of the blood supply to the rectum bypasses the liver, thus avoiding first-pass hepatic metabolism and increasing bioavailability. Rectal administration has obvious advantages for the vomiting or unconscious patient. For example, diazepam suppositories are given rectally for children and adolescents in status epilepticus. Compazine suppositories are administered rectally to stop intractable vomiting.
- *Sublingual administration:* Sublingual routes of drug absorption are only suitable for a small amount of drug with rapid dissolution. Rapid entry into the bloodstream after sublingual administration affords rapid relief of symptoms. Psychiatric medications such as some benzodiazepines may be administered in sublingual preparations.
- *Respiratory administration:* The respiratory tract may also be used to absorb a drug into the body. Gaseous anesthetics and asthma inhalers are examples. These compounds are relatively nonpolar, highly lipid-soluble molecules that readily diffuse across alveolar membranes and rapidly enter the bloodstream.
- *Transdermal administration:* Transdermal preparations are suitable for small drug doses and usually employ a rate-controlling membrane that allows a small amount of drug to diffuse through the skin into the bloodstream. In psychiatry, clonidine is available in a transdermal patch preparation, and a transdermal methylphenidate system is in development.
- *Oral administration:* Oral administration is the most common method of delivery of psychiatric medications. Although very convenient, it is also very

unpredictable in both the extent and rate of absorption from the gastrointestinal tract into the bloodstream. Factors that determine the rate and extent of drug absorption are the dosage form (e.g., tablet, liquid, or capsule), the degree of tablet compaction, size of drug particles, crystal and salt forms of the drug, and presence of various inert binding and wetting agents (e.g., starch, lactose, sucrose, calcium sulfate). The pH of the stomach and small bowel may also affect the absorption rate of some drugs such as amphetamines.

Key Concepts

After absorption from the gut, orally administered drugs are carried by the portal blood supply to the liver, and after metabolism in the liver, are carried into the systemic circulation for distribution to end organ sites of action.

• *First-pass elimination:* The extensive drug extraction and metabolism in the liver immediately after being absorbed from the gut. First-pass elimination substantially reduces the amount of orally administered drug available to enter the systemic circulation.
• *Bioavailability:* The fraction of the drug that reaches the systemic circulation and is available to exert a biological effect on target tissues. Bioavailability is an important determinant of drug action.
• *Cmax:* The maximum plasma concentration of the drug. Drug concentration in the blood rises until the rate of drug absorption equals the rate at which the drug is removed from the body.
• *Tmax:* The time after ingestion to maximum plasma concentration of the drug. Tmax is determined in the individual patient by both absorption and elimination rates.

Distribution

After entering the bloodstream, a drug undergoes multiple processes of distribution that are affected by its lipid solubility, its rate of absorption from the gut, the pH of body fluids, the extent of blood protein and tissue receptor binding, and differences in regional blood flow. Organs that are richly perfused with blood, such as the heart, kidney, and liver, undergo rapid equilibration of drug concentration between plasma and tissue. In contrast, drug distribution to the brain may take much longer because a protective cellular sheath of glial cells that results in decreased permeability characteristics—the blood–brain barrier— surrounds the brain. To enter the central nervous system, drugs must be highly lipid soluble or subject to energy-dependent active transport mechanisms.

Drug binding to plasma proteins provides another source of individual variation in drug distribution. Most drugs exist in the blood in a dynamic equilibrium between a form that is free in the plasma and one that is bound to plasma proteins. This drug binding is reversible, with very fast rates of association and dissociation. There is increasing evidence indicating a better correlation between drug response and unbound drug concentration rather than total (bound and free) drug concentration.

B A S I C   P H A R M A C O L O G Y

- Albumin, the major plasma protein involved in drug binding, binds both acidic and basic drugs.
- alpha-1-acid glycoprotein (AAG), another protein that plays a major role in plasma binding of a number of basic drugs, is an acute-phase reactant protein whose concentrations increase under conditions of physiological stress, such as infectious disease, inflammatory disease, cancer, and tissue trauma.
- Elevated AAG levels are associated with increased binding of basic drugs such as imipramine and chlorpromazine, with reduced bioavailability of drug at tissue target sites of action.

Elimination

Drugs are eliminated from the body either as unchanged drug in the urine or feces, or by undergoing metabolic biotransformation to make metabolites that are more water-soluble than the parent compound and that are then excreted. Lithium is an example of a psychiatric drug that is eliminated by excretion in the urine, largely without undergoing biotransformation. Most psychiatric drugs are lipid-soluble and must undergo extensive metabolism and biotransformation to make them more water-soluble before excretion. The enzymatic reactions that biotransform drugs and make them more water-soluble for excretion are divided into two phases.

- *Phase I reactions:* Involve breaking off a part of the drug and inserting or uncovering a molecule (usually oxygen) to expose a functional group, such as a hydroxyl or amine group, so that the drug is in the appropriate chemical form for further modification by Phase II enzymatic reactions. The chemicals involved in Phase I processes, cytochrome enzymes, are primarily present in gut and liver cells but also present in kidney, brain, and other tissues. Other Phase I hydrolytic enzymes include (1) plasma esterases, which mediate the metabolism of psychostimulants; (2) microsomal epoxide hydrolases, which form carbamazepine 10,11 epoxide (an active metabolite of carbamazepine); and (3) flavin-containing monooxygenases, which are involved in the biotransformation of clozapine and olanzepine. The metabolic products of Phase I reactions may have pharmacological activity similar to the parent drug.
- *Phase II reactions:* Involve the formation of a link between the functional group on a drug and a conjugate via a transferase enzyme. The most common conjugate is glucuronic acid. Other Phase II systems involve N-acetyltransferases, which help to metabolize clonazepam, and sulfotransferases, which conjugate acetaminophen. Conjugates serve to make the drug metabolites more water-soluble for excretion. The biotransformed products of Phase II reactions rarely exhibit pharmacological activity.

Elimination Kinetics

Most psychotropic drugs follow first-order or linear elimination kinetics. First-order kinetics implies that a linear relationship exists between changes in drug dosage and changes in plasma concentration. Such a linear relationship allows for clinically relevant predictions of the impact of a dose change on plasma drug concentrations.

Some drugs, such as phenytoin, salicylate, and ethanol, do not follow this pattern; they follow zero-order or nonlinear elimination kinetics. Because the liver has a very limited number of metabolizing enzymes for these drugs, the enzyme sites quickly become saturated even at normal therapeutic drug concentrations. Once saturation is achieved, the plasma level rises disproportionately to any increase in drug dose. A constant amount of drug is then eliminated per unit time, regardless of the plasma concentration. Fluoxetine and nefazodone are antidepressant drugs that have been observed to demonstrate zero-order kinetics. At clinically relevant doses, the relationship between dose and plasma level is much less predictable for these drugs.

Elimination Half-Life

The elimination half-life of a drug is the time it takes for the blood concentration to fall by 50%. A drug's half-life is a useful parameter for the determination of a suitable dosage interval. When a drug is dosed at regular intervals, it is the plasma half-life that determines the plasma steady-state concentration. A steady-state concentration is reached after approximately 4–5 times the half-life of the drug (not doses of the drug). Upon discontinuing the drug, the half-life identifies the time required for a drug to totally clear the body. For drugs that follow first-order elimination kinetics:

- First half-life: 50% of drug eliminated and 50% remains in the body.
- Second half-life: 75% of drug eliminated and 25% remains in the body.
- Third half-life: 87.5% of drug eliminated and 12.5% remains in the body.
- Fourth half-life: 93.8% of drug eliminated and 6.25% remains in the body.
- Fifth half-life: 96.9% of drug eliminated and 3.12% remains in the body.

Pediatric Variations in Pharmacokinetics

Children and adolescents are not "little adults"; they handle drugs differently from developmentally mature adults. They do not necessarily require smaller doses of drugs, and in some cases may actually require larger doses of drugs compared to adults. Because of faster metabolic rates than adults, drug doses must be given at shorter intervals (more frequent dosing) in children than in adults. Some differences in pharmacokinetics between children and adults include the following.

- *Metabolic capacity:* Corrected for size, children and adolescents have greater metabolic capacity than adults and more rapidly eliminate drugs that utilize hepatic pathways. These drugs include neuroleptics, tricyclic antidepressants, pemoline, and methylphenidate. Because children eliminate drugs rapidly, more frequent daily doses may have to be used to prevent between-dose withdrawal effects.
- *Renal elimination:* Children and adolescents have more efficient renal elimination than adults and will excrete drugs that utilize renal pathways (e.g., lithium) more rapidly than adults.
- *Tissue differences:* Compared to adults, children have relatively less adipose tissue, which can cause differences in drug distribution and accumulation of

lipophilic agents and their metabolites in children compared with adults. For example, in children with less fat stores, we would expect to find a larger plasma concentration of lipophilic drugs than that found in adults after being given the same weight-adjusted dose.

- *Whole body water:* Compared to adults, children have a greater volume of extracellular water. For drugs that are primarily distributed in body water (e.g., lithium), at a given dose children will have a lower plasma concentration than adults, because the volume of water distribution is higher in children.

By age 15 or so, children begin to develop adult pharmacokinetic parameters. As metabolism slows to adult levels, the clinician should be alert to signs that the drug dose may have to be lowered to prevent toxicity. Dose schedules can become more adult-like in the mid-teenage years.

CYTOCHROME P450 ENZYMES

Cytochrome P450 enzymes are a superfamily of heme-containing enzymes that are very important in drug biotransformation during Phase I reactions. One group, found in mitochondria, is involved in synthesis or metabolism of endogenous compounds such as steroids, prostaglandins, and bile acids. The second CYP group, found in cellular endoplasmic reticulum, is involved in the biotransformation of exogenous compounds such as drugs in Phase I metabolic processes. There are presently 14 families of CYP enzymes identified in humans. Of these, 9 hepatic CYP groups are involved in human metabolism of exogenous agents. These include CYP1A2, CYP2A6, CYP2B6, CYP2C8, CYP2C9, CYP2C19, CYP2D6, CYP2E1, and CYP3A. CYP3A is the single most important hepatic CYP family, because it metabolizes more than 30–40% of drugs known to be metabolized by human CYP enzymes.

Most drugs are metabolized by more than one CYP enzyme. A specific drug may be a substrate of one or two CYP enzymes and an inhibitor of others. Because many psychiatric patients are prescribed more than one drug, complicated drug–drug interactions may occur at the level of the CYP enzyme system. The clinician needs a working understanding of these drug–drug interactions to prevent toxicity from occurring in patients taking multiple drugs. The following table presents substrates, inhibitors, and inducers of common human CYP 450 isoenzymes.

Genetic variations result in variable expressions of CYP proteins for many CYP isoenzymes, including CYP3A4, CYP2C19, and CYP2D6. For individuals with these variations, metabolic pathways served by these CYP enzyme systems either do not exist or are very slow. This defect leads to rising concentrations of drugs that are substrates of that CYP family and results in drug toxicity at usual clinical doses.

- *CYP2C19:* 20% of Asians, 19% of African-Americans, 8% of Africans, and 3–5% of Caucasians are genetically deficient in this enzyme system. Among other drugs, this may affect their metabolism of citalopram, diazepam, sertraline, and imipramine.

Table 2.1 Human CYP 450 Isoenzymes: Some Substrates, Inhibitors, and Inducers

Enzyme	Substrates	Inhibitors	Inducers	Genetic Polymorphism
CYP1A2	Amitryptiline, caffeine, clomipramine, clozapine, fluvoxamine, haloperidol, imipramine, olanzepine, phanacetin, propranolol, tacrine, theophylline, verapamil, R-warfarin	Cimetidine, fluvoxamine, grapefruit juice, viloxazine, fluoroquinolines, furafylline, fluvoxamine	Cigarette smoke, cabbage (etc.), barbecue meat, polycyclic aromatic hydrocarbons, carbamazepine, insulin, modafinil	Possible
CYP2C9	Diclofenac, fluoxetine, phenytoin, piroxicam, tenoxicam, tetrahydrocannabinol, ticrynafen, tienilic acid, tolbutamide, torsemide, S-warfain, valproate	Sulfaphenazole, phenytoin, sulfinpyrazone, ketoconazole, fluconazole, fluoxetine, sertraline, fluvoxamine, valproate	Rifampin, barbiturates	Possible
CYP2C19	Citalopram, clomipramine, cycloguanil, diazepam, hexobarbital, imipramine, lansoprazole, S-mephenytoin, mephobarbital, moclobemide, omeprazole, pentamidine, propranolol, sertraline	Tranylcypromine, sertraline, ketoconazole, moclobemide, cimetidine, fluoxetine, fluvoxamine, modafinil, topiramate	Rifampin, carbamazepine, prednisone	Yes
CYP2D6	Amitriptyline, atomoxetine, brofaromine, clomipramine, citalopram, codeine, debrisoquin, desipramine, dextromethorphan, encinide, flecainide, fluoxetine, fluvoxamine, haloperidol, imipramine, maprotiline, metoprolol, mirtazapine, mainserin, nefazodone, nortriptyline, paroxetine, perphenazine, propafenone, propranolol, remoxipride, risperidone, sparteini, thioridazine, trazodone, venlafaxine	Amitriptyline, chloroquine, chlorpromazine, cimetidine, clomipramine, desipramine, desmethylcitalopram, dextropropoxyphene, diphenhydramine, flecainide, fluoxetine, fluphenazine, haloperidol, imipramine, meclobemide, methotrimeprazine, metoclopramide, metoprolol, mexiletine, nicardipine, norfluoxetine, nortriptyline, paroxetine, phenylcyclopropylamine, pindolol, primaquine, propafenone, propranolol, quinidine, quinine, sertraline, thioridazine, timolol, trifluperidol	Carbamazepine, dexamethasone, phenobarbital, phenytoin, rifampin, ritonavir	Yes
CYP2E1	Acetaminophen, caffeine, ethanol, dapsone, halothane, chlorzoxazone, isoflurane, enflurane	Disulfiram, ethanol	Ethanol, isoniazid	Probable
CYP3A4	Alfentanil, alprazolam, amiodarone, amitriptyline, astemizole, carbamazepine, clomipramine, clonazepam, citalopram, cyclophosphamide, cyclosporine, dexamethasone, dextromethorphan, diazepam, triazolam, zaleplon, zolpidem, erythromycin, fluoxetine, trazodone, haloperidol, quetiapine, pimozide, risperidone, ziprasidone, felodipine, imipramine, lidocaine, lovastatin, midazolam, nefazodone, omeprazole, quinidine, retinoic acid, sertraline, terfenadine, triazolam, verapamil, vinblastine	Cimetidine, erythromycin, ethinylestradiol, fulconazole, fluoxetine, fluvoxamine, grapefruit juice, ketoconazole, nefazodone, paroxetine, progestins, sertraline, troleandromycin	Carbamazepine, dexamethasone, phenobarbital, phenytoin, rifampin, sulfamethazine, sulfinpyrazone,oxcarbazepine, St. John's wort, topiramate, modafinil, ethanol (chronic)	Possible

Adapted from Paxton WJ and Dragunow M. **Pharmacology.** In: Werry J and Aman M (Eds.), *Practitioner's Guide to Psychoactive Drugs* (2nd ed.). New York: Plenum Press. p. 33, 1999; and Osterheld JR and Flockhart DA, Pharmacokinetics II: Cytochrome P450-Mediated Drug Interactions. In: Martin A, Scahill L, Charney DS, Leckman JF (Eds.), *Pediatric Psychopharmacology Principles and Practice.* New York: Oxford University Press, pp. 61–62, 2003.

BASIC PHARMACOLOGY

- *CYP2D6:* 5–10% of Caucasians and 1% of Asians are genetically deficient in this enzyme system. This deficiency may affect their metabolism of atomoxetine, tricyclic antidepressants, citalopram, fluoxetine, fluvoxamine, haloperidol, mirtazapine, nefazodone, paroxetine, perphenazine, propranolol, risperidone, trazodone, and venlafaxine.
- *CYP3A4:* Lower activity has been reported in Indian/Bangladeshi subjects compared to Europeans.

SUMMARY

The body handles drugs in complicated ways that vary with the age of the patient, the drug, concomitant drugs, the patient's health, and the patient's genetic heritability. It should be clear that children handle drugs differently from adults. For clinical purposes, it can be assumed that children older than 1 year will generally inactivate and eliminate drugs somewhat faster than adults. Thus they may require a greater mg/kg dose than adults. Around mid-adolescence, pharmacokinetic parameters become more adult-like and dosage may need to be lowered and/or dose schedules may need to lengthen in order to prevent drug toxicity.

3. General Principles of Treatment

Several principles guide the clinical approach to pediatric psychopharmacology. The first is that children and adolescents are developmentally different from adults. This fact has implications for psychiatric diagnosis, evaluation of the patient, consent and assent issues, patient autonomy, as well as psychiatric medication choice, dosing, and schedule. Juveniles are immature and not yet fully formed. They continue to develop over time neurobiologically, cognitively, socially, behaviorally, and psychologically. Thus a developmental approach must inform the clinical practice of pediatric psychopharmacology. Second, children and adolescents are embedded in a family and neighborhood network involving parents or caretakers, siblings, friends, school, and other institutions. The child-patient may have different vulnerabilities, behaviors, and symptoms in different settings of his or her daily life. Thus psychiatric evaluation of child and adolescent mental disorders must incorporate information gathered from multiple informants, including parents, teachers, and others in the child's life, as well as the patient him- or herself.

Third, the current psychiatric diagnostic classification systems such as the *Diagnostic and Statistical Manual for Mental Disorders* (DSM, currently in the 4th edition) and the *International Classification of Disease* (ICD, currently in the 10th edition) have marked limitations in the assessment of child and adolescent mental health disorders due to the developmental trajectory of early-onset mental health disorders and to symptom overlap across psychiatric diagnoses. It remains difficult to empirically validate child and adolescent psychiatric diagnoses in the absence of biological markers of disease and thus to match evidence-based psychopharmacological treatments to specific psychiatric diagnoses. Evidence for the efficacy of medication treatment for some child psychiatric diagnoses has been established. For example, this is true for ADHD and stimulants, bupropion, or atomoxetine; and for OCD and SSRI antidepressants and clomipramine. However, for most conditions medication treatment should focus on target symptoms as well as psychiatric diagnosis. Specific pharmacological interventions should be grounded in empirical evidence that supports a match between identified target symptoms and the prescribed medication according to the likelihood that medication will improve the target symptom.

Fourth, clinical approaches to pediatric psychopharmacology must recognize the chronicity of most childhood neuropsychiatric disorders. This principle means that pediatric psychopharmacologists must remain clinically involved with their patients in an ongoing manner. Rarely are the psychiatric conditions for which medications prescribed, "cured." Ongoing clinical involvement, periodic reassessment, and treatment plan adjustment over the course of the child's development are the norm for pediatric psychopharmacology patients.

Next, psychiatric medications are usually adjunctive to an ongoing multidisciplinary psychoeducational treatment plan. Medications are rarely prescribed to a child alone, in the absence of other accompanying therapies. Finally, treatment of the child or adolescent with mental health disorders usually requires a treatment team approach. The team may involve parents, the prescribing physician, the primary care physician, psychosocial therapists, and school personnel. For clinical care, it is important that team members communicate with one another as the child's treatment evolves over time.

This chapter reviews principles of psychiatric evaluation, clinical information integration, and case formulation in pediatric psychopharmacology. Informed consent issues are described in Chapter 1. A discussion of medical decision making in pediatric psychopharmacology is presented. Finally, approaches to medication treatment and follow-up are discussed.

PSYCHIATRIC EVALUATION IN PEDIATRIC PSYCHOPHARMACOLOGY

Children and adolescents must have a complete psychiatric and medical evaluation before psychiatric medications are prescribed. The goals of the psychiatric evaluation are (1) to evaluate the youngster to determine if diagnostic criteria for a specific psychiatric disorder, or for multiple disorders, exist; (2) to ascertain medication target symptoms; and (3) to determine if the disorder(s) and target symptoms are responsive to psychiatric medication(s). The evaluation must be comprehensive and lead to treatment planning that considers other interventions (e.g., individual and/or family psychosocial therapies and/or psychoeducational interventions), if indicated, in addition to questions about psychopharmacology. Findings must be communicated to the child and parents in a manner that is free of medical and psychiatric jargon and at a level that they can understand. We recommend that a written report be generated and sent to the parents, and consent sought to communicate with, and send the report to, the child's primary care physician.

Sources of Information

Information from multiple sources must be integrated into the comprehensive psychiatric evaluation. Common sources of information are the youngster, the parents, and information from the classroom teacher. Child and adolescent patients should be interviewed directly about their symptoms. Children and adolescents are better at describing their internalizing symptoms, such as anxiety and depression or suicidal thoughts and feelings, than outside observers such as parents or teachers. Parents should be interviewed about their offspring. Outside observers are often better at describing externalizing behavior problems, such as ADHD, conduct problems, or oppositional defiant behavior, than the individual child, who may be tempted to minimize these symptoms.

Types of Information

In a comprehensive psychiatric evaluation it is important to gather information in different ways. Direct interview data are one type of information. Often the clinical interview is supplemented by the use of rating scales, which are a time-efficient way of gathering information from teachers and parents. Children with a third- to fourth-grade reading level can complete many self-report rating scales. It is important to use rating scales that have been shown to be both reliable and valid. Some validated rating scales of general psychopathology used in child and adolescent mental health are given in the table below.

Table 3.1 Reliable and Valid Rating Scales for Assessing General Psychopathology in Children and Adolescents

Rating Scale	Type of Scale	What Is Assessed?	Age Range (yrs)
Behavior Assessment System for Children (BASC)	Parent, teacher, and self-report	Behavioral functioning	4–18
Child Behavior Checklist (CBCL)	Parent and teacher report forms, self-report for children ≥ 11 years old	Psychopathology	4–18
Conners Rating Scales—Revised (CRS-R)	Parent and teacher report forms	Psychopathology	3–17
Devereux Scales of Mental Disorders (DSMD)	Parent and teacher report forms	Psychopathology	5–12, 13–18
Personality Inventory for Children—Revised (PIC-R)	Parent and child	Intellectual screening, psychopathology, achievement	9–18

These validated scales allow for a comparison of symptoms in patients with symptoms in nonreferred children of the same age and gender. This comparison allows the clinician to ascertain if the referred child's parents and teachers endorse more frequent and/or severe symptoms compared to same-age and same-sex peers in the non-mental-health-referred general population. It is important to note that categorical psychiatric diagnoses cannot be ascertained from rating scales, however. Psychiatric diagnoses are only made after a clinical evaluation has established that diagnostic criteria are met. Rating scales can supplement categorical diagnoses by providing information on symptom severity, compared to nonreferred children and adolescents.

The Psychiatric Interview

The initial psychiatric interview should include the child or adolescent and the parent(s)* and must obtain the following information.

- Chief complaint and what the child-patient and parent hope to obtain from the psychiatric evaluation
- History of symptoms, including type, age of onset, impairment caused by them, and longitudinal course
- Child's developmental history
- Family history, including family members, family structure, family functioning, and a history of familial mental disorders and stressors
- Current and past mental health treatment plan(s)—which treatments seemed effective and which did not?
- Current and past psychiatric medication history, including specifics about drug type, target symptom(s), effectiveness, side effects, highest dose achieved, and duration of each specific drug treatment
- School and educational history, including the presence of any associated learning disabilities
- Review of any previous psychological and academic testing reports, if available
- Medical history: All children and adolescents who are being considered for psychopharmacological treatment should have a complete medical history and physical examination completed within 1 year of the current psychopharmacological assessment.
  - Drug allergies should be noted.
  - Laboratory assessments are at the discretion of the child's primary care physician, depending on findings from the medical history and physical examination.
  - The type of psychiatric medication prescribed also determines laboratory assessments. For example, use of lithium requires baseline thyroid function tests, urinalysis and specific gravity, pregnancy testing in females, complete blood count, chemistry analysis, and possibly a baseline electrocardiogram.
  - Concomitant medications and any ongoing medical treatments should be noted.
  - Any medical consultants or specialists involved with the child or adolescent's care should be documented.

Mental Status Examination

A mental status examination (MSE) must be completed and documented on every referred child or adolescent. Essential elements of the MSE include the following.

- *General appearance:* Eye contact, appropriateness of dress, physical features and any evidence of physical anomalies or facial dysmorphic features

---

*We use the term *parent(s)* to include any person in a primary caregiving role with children.

suggestive of an underlying neurodevelopmental or genetic condition, presence of motor/vocal tics, or presence of any involuntary abnormal movements.

- *Behavior:* Activity level, restlessness, engagement with parents and the interviewer, attention span, physical signs of anxiety or behavioral inhibition.
- *Affect:* The patient's expressed affect and emotions should be characterized. These may include anxiety, depression, fear, boredom, or constricted affect.
- *Thought process and thought content:* Are the child's patterns of thinking consistent with his or her developmental age? The predominant themes and concerns that preoccupy the patient should be noted. An assessment of how the child's thoughts connect to one another in a logical and understandable manner should be documented. The presence of any hallucinations, delusions, or illogical thinking patterns should be noted.
- *Safety:* Any homicidal or suicidal thoughts, plans, availability of weapons, and means to carry out plans should be evaluated.
- *Social relatedness:* Nonverbal means of communication, eye contact, evidence of social reciprocity, symbolic thinking or play, capacity to empathize with others, and the reciprocal use of language should be observed.
- *Language and speech:* Expressive and receptive language abilities, articulation, spontaneity of speech, and prosody should be documented.
- *Estimation of cognitive functioning:* To estimate the child's age-appropriate intellectual abilities or to document any developmental delays, the examiner should use developmental norms.
- *Substance use:* In adolescents it is important to complete an illicit substance use history including cigarettes, drugs, and alcohol.

DIAGNOSTIC CASE FORMULATION

Because psychiatric diagnosis based on the current DSM or ICD taxonomies offers little help to the practicing clinician in integrating and understanding complicated child mental health data obtained from multiple sources, other tools are necessary. The diagnostic case formulation serves as a clinical tool for integrating complex problems and disparate information presented by the child and family into a clear focus that facilitates treatment planning. As such, the diagnostic case formulation should not be ignored in pediatric psychopharmacology.

The case formulation is designed to be a working, useful summary of the assessment that results in integration of information and assignment of clinical treatment priorities and generates clinical hypotheses to be examined. These then result in diagnosis, individualized case treatment targets and goals, and a rational treatment plan within the identified resources available for clinical care. The process is diagrammed below:

Information Gathering (Assessment) → Case Formulation →
Diagnosis → Treatment Goals and Priorities → Treatment Plan

In pediatric psychopharmacology the case formulation should answer the following questions:

GENERAL PRINCIPLES

- Why does this child with these symptoms in the context of this family system present for treatment at this particular point in time and development?
- What are the patient, family, and/or larger institutional/treatment system(s) requesting from the clinical psychopharmacology evaluation?
- Do there exist target symptoms or psychiatric diagnoses, based on the child's current clinical assessment, that are known from evidence-based treatment studies to be responsive to psychiatric medication?
- Will medication treatment of the child or adolescent's target symptoms or psychiatric diagnosis facilitate his or her optimal developmental trajectory?
- What is the most effective treatment plan that could be implemented, given the available resources to address the above questions? Should medication be part of the treatment plan?

As can be seen, the formulation in pediatric psychopharmacology has a focus that includes medications, target symptoms, and psychiatric diagnosis but is also much broader, with the overall objective of helping to develop a treatment plan that will optimize the developmental trajectory of the child or adolescent. In our opinion, current models of case formulation extrapolated from adult psychiatric are inadequate to capture the complexities of child and adolescent psychiatric assessment. As such, the biopsychosocial formulation model and the psychoanalytic model of psychotic → borderline → neurotic personality functioning are often talked about in the psychiatric literature but rarely used in actual clinical practice. Other formulation models that are more useful for developmental psychiatry and pediatric psychopharmacology are needed.

One such model (see Connor, 2002; Connor & Fisher, 1997) describes a transactional approach to child and adolescent psychiatric clinical case formulation that (1) emphasizes interactional patterns between the child and important others in his or her environment, (2) is dynamic rather than static, and (3) allows for developmental changes over time. Identifying just where psychopharmacological interventions fit into the model will help the clinician and family better understand the benefits and limitations of psychiatric medication interventions for the child within the context of an overall treatment plan.

The model of transactional case formulation shown in the figure below describes how the child interacts with parents, the family, and larger systems, and how these domains interact with the child in a reciprocal manner to influence either adaptive or maladaptive outcomes. The identification of transactional elements (the arrows in the figure) serves to focus specific treatment interventions on interrupting maladaptive interactions and strengthening adaptive interactions across domains. The overall goal of treatment is to restore the interactions among youngster, parents, family, and larger system domains to a more functional equilibrium.

The model emphasizes the concept of "goodness of fit" first articulated by Chess and Thomas in 1986. This refers to the idea that healthy functioning and optimal individual development occur when there is a good match between the individual youth's capacities and the demands and expectations of the environment, including parents and other family members. "Poorness of fit," in which there is a mismatch between the youth's intrinsic capabilities and the

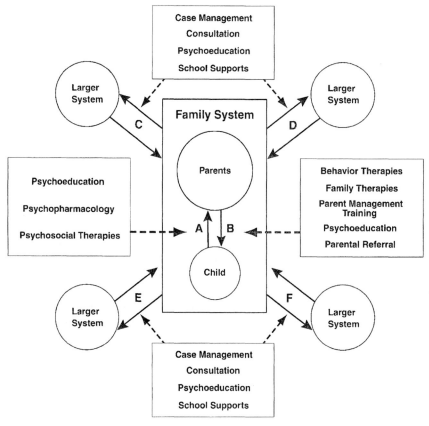

Figure 3.1 The Transactional Case Formulation Model.
Interactive elements (solid arrows) across the three domains of child,
parents/family, and larger systems serve to maintain clinical problems via
reciprocal interactions. These maladaptive interactions serve to define clinical
interventions (dashed arrows) designed to disrupt maladaptive transactions and
restore the system to a more functional equilibrium. Adapted from Connor DF.
*Aggression and Antisocial Behavior in Children and Adolescents: Research and
Treatment.* New York: Guilford Press, p. 312, 2002; and Connor DF and Fisher SG,
An interactional model of child and adolescent mental health clinical case
formulation. *J Clin Child Psychol Psychiatry* 2(3):353–368, 1997.

expectations of the environment, results in increased risk of psychopathology.
By identifying transactional elements (how the domains interact and recipro-
cally influence one another; i.e., the arrows in the figure) among the three
domains of functioning (child, parents and family, and larger systems), the case
formulation seeks to clarify the goodness or poorness of fit. The end product of
the case formulation is a description of the interactive elements across
domains that serve to maintain the clinical problems that caused the parents
and child to seek the current mental health referral.

GENERAL PRINCIPLES

This model of clinical case formulation implies that the goodness or poorness of fit is the result of bidirectional relationships (i.e., mutual influences) between the child and important others in his or her life. The notion of "fit" leads away from a focus on psychiatric diagnosis, psychopathology, and blame, and introduces a more normalizing framework. The formulation is broader in its focus than simply medicating a young patient for the target symptoms of a psychiatric diagnosis, and it makes manifest the idea that psychiatric medications are only one part of an overall comprehensive mental health treatment plan. As constructed, the model of transactional clinical case formulation allows for consideration of multiple types of treatments, not just psychopharmacology. Each treatment is introduced with the overall goal of (1) interrupting maladaptive interactions across domains that serve to perpetuate psychopathology, (2) improving the child's goodness of fit with his or her environment, and (3) helping to optimize individual development and quality of life.

So, where does pediatric psychopharmacology fit in this model? Ideally, two conditions must be met before a physician prescribes psychiatric medication to a child or adolescent with mental health problems:

1. Is there empirical evidence that psychoactive medication is effective for the youngster's particular psychiatric diagnosis or specific target symptoms?
2. If so, does the transactional clinical case formulation suggest that by improving the psychiatric diagnosis or target symptoms, the child's or adolescent's goodness of fit with parents, family, and larger systems will improve and become more adaptive, thus facilitating the youngster's overall development?

As conceptualized, the transactional clinical case formulation is much richer than the concept of psychiatric diagnosis or target symptoms in organizing a clinical approach to pediatric psychopharmacology. When using psychiatric target symptoms and diagnosis as the organizing principle, the goal of medication treatment becomes medical, to treat a psychiatric condition. In contrast, the case formulation allows the clinician to appreciate the developmental and interpersonal context in which the patient's diagnosis and symptoms occur. The goal of medication treatment when using the concept of an interactional clinical case formulation is not just to treat a psychiatric syndrome or symptoms, but also to enhance adaptive fit and promote optimal development by treating psychiatric diagnoses and target symptoms. The case formulation clarifies that this enhancement occurs in the context of a multidisciplinary treatment plan, and not by medications alone.

PSYCHIATRIC DIAGNOSIS, TARGET SYMPTOMS, AND TREATMENT PLANNING

The clinical case formulation is inclusive of, and does not replace, the identification of psychiatric diagnoses, medication target symptoms, and the development of a problem list. In making a clinical decision about which psychiatric medicine to prescribe, both diagnostic issues and medication target symptoms should be considered. Often these issues are interrelated. For example, sometimes the same medication is appropriate for both the target symptom and the psychiatric diagnosis. Inattention is a core symptom of ADHD, and stimulant medication can help both the targeted inattentiveness and the overall ADHD diagnosis. However, sometimes medication considerations for the target symptom are different from medication considerations for the psychiatric diagnosis. For example, inattention is also a symptom of psychotic disorders. In this case, giving stimulants for the target symptom of inattention would be inappropriate because stimulants may actually worsen symptoms of psychosis. Thus both target symptoms and the psychiatric diagnosis must be taken into account when considering medication therapy in pediatric psychopharmacology.

The initial treatment plan should identify (1) a hierarchical problem list that prioritizes symptoms for treatment; (2) medication-responsive target symptoms; (3) baseline impairment and symptom severity; preferably with the use of quantitative rating scales; and (4) principle psychiatric diagnosis and comorbid psychiatric diagnoses and conditions to be monitored and treated. Based on the clinical case formulation and problem list, other individual and family psychosocial therapies and educational supports can be recommended, as needed.

The proposed treatment plan should be presented to the child and family, as can psychoeducational teaching about the psychiatric disorder in question. They can be guided to access additional informational sources either in books or using the Internet. Medication and nonmedication therapies prescribed to address target symptoms should be discussed. Once the family and physician agree to treat the child with a psychiatric medication, the medication options to treat target symptoms should be described. Possible risks and benefits, use of medications, and possible medication side effects should be thoroughly explored. The therapeutic dose range of the medication, schedule for introducing the medication and dose titration, and the duration of treatment necessary to achieve an effect should be described. What to do in an emergency or if an adverse drug reaction occurs should be clarified to parents. Lastly, parents often want to know how long their child will be on the medication if initial target symptoms improve.

THE THREE PHASES OF PSYCHOPHARMACOLOGICAL TREATMENT

It is helpful to divide the process of pediatric psychopharmacology treatment into three phases: initiation, continuation, and maintenance.

- *Initiation phase:* The goals of the initiation phase are to (1) complete a comprehensive psychiatric evaluation, (2) identify a medication-responsive psychiatric diagnosis and target symptoms to treat, (3) quantify baseline target symptom severity, (4) form a treatment agreement with the child or adolescent and parents, (5) engage the child and parents in the informed consent and assent process and establish permission to treat, (6) choose a psychiatric medication, (7) initiate medication treatment, (8) titrate the medicine to the therapeutic dose range, and (9) monitor the patient for medication effectiveness, tolerability, and side effects. Depending on the psychiatric condition being treated and the type of psychiatric agent used, the initiation phase may take anywhere from 2 weeks to 3 months. At the end of the medication initiation phase a decision is reached with the patient and parents as to whether the medication treatment is effective and tolerable. If so, the patient proceeds to the continuation phase of medication treatment. If not, the patient discontinues the medication and a reevaluation takes place.

• *Continuation phase:* The goal of the continuation phase is to prevent relapse of the index psychiatric episode by not prematurely discontinuing effective medication treatment. The continuation phase is most important for episodic but time-limited psychiatric disorders such as major depressive episodes, manic episodes, or brief psychotic episodes. The continuation phase has less meaning for chronic psychiatric conditions such as ADHD or Tourette's syndrome. For example, in a major depressive episode that responds to psychiatric medication, the continuation phase of medication treatment may last between 6 and 9 months. Stopping medicine prematurely may result in a return of the original depressive episode.

• *Maintenance phase:* For chronic psychiatric disorders, maintenance medication treatment is often necessary to prevent the recurrence of disease. Although psychiatric medications do not cure psychiatric disorders, these medications, like insulin for diabetes or anticonvulsants for seizure disorders, are part of a treatment plan designed to minimize the overall burden of the disease on the patient's life and optimize individual functioning. For frequently chronic and disabling child and adolescent psychiatric disorders such as ADHD, OCD, bipolar disorder, recurrent episodes of major depressive disorder, or Tourette's syndrome, maintenance medication therapy is often required as part of a comprehensive treatment plan that may apply for years. It is incumbent on the prescribing physician to periodically monitor and document the need for continuing psychiatric medication treatment, its tolerability, and any possible side effects that occur.

MEDICATION INITIATION AND TITRATION

It is recommended that the prescribing physician initiate psychiatric medications at a low dose. This dose is often subtherapeutic but serves to minimize the frequency and severity of side effects as medication treatment begins. Depending on effectiveness and tolerability, the medication is titrated into the therapeutic dose range. If the patient does not respond to a medication titrated to a low effective dose for an adequate length of time, the treating physician should explore the moderate and high dose range of the medication for an adequate duration (depending on patient tolerability) before either adding medicines to the ongoing treatment or abandoning the initial medication as ineffective. Indeed, a common mistake made by inexperienced clinicians is to change medications in patients who are not responding to initial treatment, before moderate or high doses are explored, and to abandon a medicine as ineffective before allowing an adequate length of time on the drug to ascertain treatment benefits. For example, data from adults indicate that moderate to high doses of antidepressants are much more effective than low doses in depression treatment outcome and that antidepressants take anywhere from 2 to 12 weeks to exert their therapeutic effects. Changing treatment at low doses or after only several weeks on antidepressant therapy may interrupt a potential clinical response that might be obtained at higher antidepressant doses or after a slightly longer duration of treatment. The same argument may be made for stimulants in ADHD. Some patients respond to low doses, but others require high doses of stimulants to treat their symptoms. To fail to explore higher doses of medications in patients who are not responding to low doses is to potentially deprive them of a possibly effective treatment.

The number of times a medication is administered per day to a child is related to the pharmacokinetics of the drug. Younger children have a higher drug metabolism capacity than adults, which generally causes drugs to have shorter half-lives in children compared to adults, and usually requires more frequent daily administrations of the drug to maintain stable serum levels and prevent interdose withdrawal effects. Around age 15 years (Tanner Stage V of sexual maturity), adolescents physically develop and acquire adult metabolic rates. At this time, the drug dose may have to be lowered and/or drug dose schedules extended to prevent potential toxicity as the teenager matures into a more adult-like metabolism.

Changes in medication dose should be based on the clinical response of the patient and the presence of emergent medication-related side effects. The goal of psychopharmacological treatment is to achieve meaningful clinical benefits for the patient, with the fewest possible drug side effects.

CLINICAL MANAGEMENT AND THE EVALUATION OF OUTCOME

The chronicity of almost all child and adolescent psychiatric disorders mandates that the prescribing physician remain involved with the patient over time. The physician needs to follow up with the patient to evaluate the effectiveness of the medications and determine their tolerability and the presence of any side effects. Clinical management of the patient should (1) monitor target symptoms, (2) evaluate medication efficacy and the need for any additional interventions, (3) provide ongoing support to the child and family, (4) continue to educate the patient and family about the psychiatric condition in question, (5) evaluate the need for educational interventions and supports, and (6) evaluate the need for any additional case management services. When possible, it is important to use quantifiable rating scales in the evaluation of medication effectiveness and side effects. It is best to combine self-report data from the patient with observer reports from parents and teachers.

During follow-up visits, the physician has a chance to explore the meaning of the psychiatric illness with the patient and family. Often families are confused about the nature of the psychiatric disorder, may have had previous negative experiences with psychiatric medications or the mental health treatment system,

GENERAL PRINCIPLES

are worried about the use of medications whose primary site of action is the brain, and are misinformed about the child's psychiatric diagnosis and its treatment. Giving the patient and family written information and other sources to obtain further scientific information about the condition is often greatly appreciated. The wise clinician will understand that informed consent and assent are ongoing processes and therefore continue to discuss with the patient (1) the reason medications are being prescribed, (2) the goals of medication treatment, (3) the duration of medication treatment, (4) the common side effects that might occur, (5) the rare side effects that might emerge, (6) the activities, foods, drinks, and other medications that might result in drug–drug interactions or be contraindicated, and (7) what parents should do if there are medication side effects, how to communicate with the physician, and what should happen on weekends and holidays if parents need to speak with the physician.

COMPLIANCE

The issue of nonadherence to the clinical treatment plan is a serious problem in pediatric psychopharmacology. Indeed, the most common reason for a patient's lack of responsivity to treatment, unexpectedly poor clinical response to treatment, or increased variability in response to a prescribed medication is generally noncompliance with treatment. There are many reasons for patient noncompliance in pediatric psychopharmacology, including parents' fears about the medication and their withholding of the drug or changing the dose of a drug; parents' increasing of the dose of the drug (without informing the prescribing physician) when the child's symptoms or behaviors worsen, or parents' concerns about the medication's side effects. Children and teenagers may avoid taking the drug because of side effects or concerns that it makes them feel different from their friends and peers. Establishing a trusting clinician–patient–parent working alliance is crucial to the assessment of drug compliance in pediatric psychopharmacology. Explaining how the drug works in the body, the reasons for prescribing the medication, possible side effects, and the dangers of suddenly discontinuing the medication are important to explain to the child and parents. Assessing patient and parental concerns about the prescribed medication and evaluating treatment compliance at follow-up visits are important ongoing clinical processes.

MEDICAL RECORD DOCUMENTATION

Appropriate medical record documentation is increasingly important in medicine, including pediatric psychopharmacology. The medical record serves a plethora of purposes, including providing (1) a clinical treatment record, (2) medical health care insurers and payers with information that serves to justify monetary reimbursement for clinical services, (3) a legal document, and (4) written proof to reviewers that medical standards of care are followed in the clinical treatment of the patient. The medical record must be legible, up-to-date, and stored in a secure place that protects patient confidentiality.

At a minimum, the initial written pediatric psychopharmacology evaluation should include the following:

- Patient's name, date of birth, current age, medical record number, and date of evaluation
- Chief complaint and reason for referral
- History of present illness
- Current and past mental health treatments
- Current and past psychiatric medications
  - Reason prescribed: target symptoms and psychiatric diagnosis
  - Highest dose achieved and duration of treatment
  - Effectiveness and side effects
- School history
  - Current functioning and grades
  - School supports
- Family history
  - Family structure
  - Family functioning
  - Family psychiatric history
- Medical history
  - Known drug allergies
  - Medical/surgical conditions that are a current focus of treatment
  - Medications
  - Hearing and vision screen
- Child mental status examination
- Impression and case formulation
- Psychiatric diagnosis
- Problem list
- Treatment plan and informed consent/assent for the treatment plan

The written pediatric psychopharmacology follow-up note should contain the following information, at a minimum, for every visit:

- Patient's name, medical record number, length of visit, and date of service
- Medication name, dose, and administration schedule
- The psychiatric diagnosis and target symptoms for which the medication is prescribed
- Medication effectiveness and side effects (i.e., outcome evaluation)
- Examination results such as vital signs, lab results, height, and weight monitoring
- Quantifiable results from objective rating scales
- Treatment plan, including any dose changes, clinical rationale for any dose changes, prescriptions written, and recommendations for any consultation, psychosocial, or educational interventions
- Date of next follow-up visit

SUMMARY

Assessment, case formulation, medication decision making, and monitoring the patient for the effects of medications involve an approach that emphasizes the young patient's development, psychosocial and familial context, and the limitations of current psychiatric diagnosis to accurately predict response to psychiatric medications. Successful pediatric psychopharmacological treatment requires continuing efforts to educate the patient and parents about the nature of the psychiatric condition and treatment, and entails a close and ongoing collaboration with the family. Documentation in the medical record of the psychiatric evaluation and continuing treatment is an ongoing necessity.

Part II
The Medications

4. Stimulants

Stimulants are sympathomimetic agents and activate the level of activity, arousal, and alertness of the central nervous system (CNS). Stimulants in clinical use include various short-acting, intermediate-acting, and long-acting formulations of racemic methylphenidate, dextromethylphenidate, dextroamphetamine, mixed amphetamine salts (a combination of d-amphetamine and amphetamine), and magnesium pemoline. Pemoline is rarely used because of elevated risk of liver toxicity. If pemoline is to be used at all, it is considered a second- or third-line agent for the treatment of attention-deficit hyperactivity disorder (ADHD). This chapter generally focuses on the use of stimulants for ADHD.

STIMULANT DRUG SCHEDULES

- Stimulants are Schedule II drugs.
  - The federal Drug Enforcement Agency (DEA) determines "scheduling" based on potential abuse liability.
  - Prescribing of Schedule II drugs is closely regulated.
  - Different federal, state, and local laws regulate the prescription of Schedule II drugs.
  - Duplicate or triplicate prescriptions may be required by the state for Schedule II drugs.
  - Stimulant prescriptions are limited and must be filled either monthly or bimonthly, depending on the state.
    - Only a 30- or 60-day supply of drug provided; no refills are allowed on the prescription.
  - Written refill prescriptions are necessary; the prescribing physician may not telephone an order to refill a Schedule II drug into the pharmacist.
  - Refills may not be honored if the prescription is dated less than 30 days (or 60 days, depending on state laws) from the last Schedule II drug refill.
- Magnesium pemoline (Cylert®) is a Schedule IV drug.

INDICATIONS

• ADHD
• Narcolepsy

EFFICACY IN ADHD

Stimulant medications for the treatment of ADHD are one of the best-studied medications in medicine.

• Safety and efficacy have been studied in over 200 controlled studies of ADHD in school-age children.
  ○ Stimulants are effective in ~70% of ADHD children.
  ○ Placebo response rates in ADHD range between 4% and 20%.
• The safety and efficacy of stimulants have been studied in 10 controlled investigations of preschool children with ADHD, ages 3–6 years old.
  ○ Efficacy is reported in 9/10 (90%) studies.
  ○ There is an ongoing multisite study sponsored by the National Institute of Mental Health to assess safety, tolerability, and efficacy of stimulants in ADHD preschoolers who do not improve when first given family behavioral therapy: The Preschool ADHD Treatment Study (PATS).
• The safety and efficacy of stimulants have been studied in seven controlled investigations of ADHD adolescents.
  ○ Efficacy is reported in 6/7 (86%) studies.
• The safety and efficacy of stimulants have been studied in nine controlled investigations of ADHD adults.
  ○ Lower response rates are reported for ADHD adults given low to moderate stimulant doses (~60%).
  ○ Response rates > 70% are found in ADHD adults when high doses of stimulants are used (up to 1.0 mg/kg/day methylphenidate).

EFFICACY IN NARCOLEPSY

Stimulants are used in the treatment of sleep attacks and daytime sleepiness in narcolepsy.

• Narcolepsy rarely occurs in children younger than 12 years old.
• Narcolepsy is usually diagnosed in the second decade of life.
• Both methylphenidate and dextroamphetamine are effective in the sleep attacks of narcolepsy.
  ○ High doses may be required (20–200 mg/day in divided doses).
  ○ Tolerance may develop.
  ○ In the treatment of narcolepsy, the clinician should encourage drug holidays and brief daytime naps.
• Stimulants are not helpful for cataplexy or sleep paralysis that may be associated with the sleep attacks of narcolepsy.

PHARMACOEPIDEMIOLOGY

- Between 1987 and 2002 the prevalence of stimulant use among youth less than 18 years old increased three- to seven-fold.
- Among stimulants, methylphenidate use ranked foremost among children and adolescents, accounting for 77–87% of all stimulant prescriptions since 1991.
- Since 1990 there has been a three-fold increase in stimulant prescriptions for 2- to 4-year-old children.

CURRENTLY AVAILABLE STIMULANTS

- There are presently three types of stimulant formulations available for clinical use.
  - Immediate release preparations
    - Short-acting, must be given 2–4 times per day; duration of action is 2–4 hours.
  - Intermediate-acting
    - Given once daily; duration of action is 6–8 hours (i.e., the school day).
  - Long-acting
    - Given once daily; duration of action is 10–12 hours (i.e., the school day and after-school hours).

Table 4.1 Stimulant Preparations for ADHD

Brand Name	Active Agent	Manufacturer
IMMEDIATE-RELEASE (4–6-HOUR COVERAGE)		
Adderall® tablets	Neutral sulfate salts of dextroamphetamine saccharate and d,l-amphetamine aspartate	Shire, U.S.
Desoxyn® tablets[a]	Methamphetamine HCL	Abbott
Dextroamphetamine sulfate tablets	Dextroamphetamine sulfate	Mallinckrodt
Dexedrine® tablets	Dextroamphetamine sulfate	GlaxoSmithKline
Dextrostat® tablets	Dextroamphetamine sulfate	Shire, U.S.
Focalin™ tablets	Dexmethylphenidate HCL	Novartis
Ritalin® HCL tablets	Methylphenidate HCL	Novartis
Methylin tablets	Methylphenidate HCL	Mallinckrodt
Methylin® chewable tablets and elixir	Methylphenidate HCL	Alliant
Methylphenidate IR tablets	Methylphenidate HCL	Geneva
INTERMEDIATE-ACTING (8-HOUR COVERAGE)		
Dexedrine® spansule	Dextroamphetamine sustained release	GlaxoSmithKline
Metadate® CD	Methylphenidate HCL extended release	Celltech
Metadate® ER	Methylphenidate HCL extended release	Celltech
Ritalin® LA	Methylphenidate HCL extended release	Novartis
Ritalin-slow release	Methylphenidate HCL sustained release	Novartis
LONG-ACTING (10–12-HOUR COVERAGE)		
Adderall XR® capsules	Neutral salts of dextroamphetamine and amphetamine with dextroamphetamine saccharate and d,l-amphetamine aspartate monohydrate extended release	Shire, U.S.
Concerta™ tablets	Methylphenidate HCL extended release	McNeil Pharmaceuticals

[a] High abuse potential

• Adderall® and Adderall XR® are single-entity mixed amphetamine products

Mixed Amphetamine Salts: Tablet Composition

Dextroamphetamine saccharate	25%
Amphetamine aspartate	25%
Dextroamphetamine sulfate	25%
Amphetamine sulfate	25%

• Metadate® CD, Ritalin® LA, and Adderall XR® capsules may be opened and the contents sprinkled onto applesauce with no change in absorption, bioavailability, or pharmacokinetics.
• Methylin® is available as a chewable tablet or as an elixir (5 mg/5 ml and 10 mg/5 ml).
• Dextroamphetamine is available as an elixir (5 mg per 5 ml).
• Desoxyn® (methamphetamine) has a high-abuse potential.
• The release characteristics of intermediate-acting and long-acting preparations differ with varying amounts of drug available in each formulation for immediate-release and extended-release.

Table 4.2 Extended-Release Stimulant Formulations: Comparison of Release Characteristics

Stimulant Formulation (mg)	Immediate-Release (mg)	Extended-Release (mg)
Adderall-XR®	50%	50%
5	2.5	2.5
10	5	5
15	7.5	7.5
20	10	10
25	12.5	12.5
30	15	15
Concerta®	22%	78%
18	4	14
27	6	21
36	8	21
54	12	42
Metadate CD®	30%	70%
20	6	14
Ritalin® LA	50%	50%
20	10	10
30	15	15
40	20	20

PHARMACOLOGY

Stimulants are noncatecholamine sympathomimetic amines that have specific mechanisms of action in the CNS.

Pharmacodynamics

• Methylphenidate and dextroamphetamine block the reuptake of catecholamines (dopamine and norepinephrine) into presynaptic neurons, thereby:
  ○ Increasing the available concentration of catecholamines in the synaptic cleft.

○ Increasing the availability of catecholamines to interact with receptors on dopaminergic and noradrenergic postsynaptic neurons.
○ Presumably facilitating catecholaminergic neurotransmission in brain areas known to be involved with ADHD and the regulation of attention and impulse control, including:
  ▪ Frontal cortex
  ▪ Striatum (caudate and putamen)
  ▪ Cerebellum
• Dextroamphetamine also promotes the release of free and vesicular cytoplasmic catecholamines from neurons.
• There are two proposed theories that relate stimulant pharmacokinetics and stimulant pharmacodynamics to stimulant efficacy in ADHD; it is not yet proven which (or if both) is correct.
○ The ramp effect: The shorter the time to peak concentration (Tmax), the more effective the stimulant for the symptoms of ADHD.
○ The concentration effect: The higher the peak concentration of stimulant (Cmax), the more effective the stimulant for the symptoms of ADHD.

Pharmacokinetics

• Absorption
○ Methylphenidate and amphetamine preparations are rapidly absorbed.
  ▪ Stimulants reach their maximal clinical effect during the absorption phase of the kinetic curve, approximately 2 hours after ingestion.
  ▪ Stimulants cross the blood–brain barrier and are taken up into the CNS; the absorption phase parallels the acute release of neurotransmitters into CNS synaptic clefts.
○ The presence of food may delay absorption or delay the time to Tmax in some intermediate- and long-acting preparations; this does not appear to affect clinical efficacy.
○ After a high-fat breakfast, methylphenidate plasma concentrations may show less variability than amphetamine plasma concentrations; this does not appear to alter clinical efficacy.
○ Methylphenidate SR (slow-release) preparations have more variable and less complete absorption, which may explain their diminished efficacy compared to more rapidly and completely absorbed stimulants.
• Stimulant-release patterns
○ All intermediate-acting and long-acting stimulant formulations contain an immediate-release mechanism and an extended-release mechanism either in an overcoat formulation, such as Concerta®, or in a capsule containing both immediate-release and extended-release beads. These stimulant formulations all exhibit a bimodal stimulant-release pattern.
  ▪ Immediate-release stimulant overcoat or beads take advantage of the "ramp effect" for rapid onset of action.
  ▪ Extended-release preparations/beads also release stimulant about 4 hours after ingestion and take advantage of the "concentration effect" for longer duration stimulant efficacy.

Table 4.3 Stimulant Formulations: Pharmacokinetics

Drug	Dose (mg)	Cmax-1 (ng/ml)	Cmax-2 (ng/ml)	Tmax-1 (hrs; fasting state)	Tmax-2 (hrs; fasting state)	$AUC_{0 \to \infty}$ (ng · h/ml)	$T_{1/2}$ (hrs)
dextroamphetamine generic	5	36.6	——	1.5	——	NR	12
methylphenidate generic	5, 10, 20	10.2 ± 4.2	——	1.8	——	102.4 ± 54.6	2.5
dexmethylphenidate Focalin™	5	10.2 ± 4.2	——	1.5	——	102.4 ± 54.6	2.2
OROS methylphenidate Concerta®	18	2.0 ± 1.0	3.7 ± 1.0	1–2	6–8	41.8 ± 13.9	3.5
methylphenidate extended release Metadate® CD	20	8.6 ± 2.2	10.9 ± 3.9	1.5	4.5	63.0 ± 16.8	6.8
methylphenidate long-acting Ritalin® LA	20	10.3 ± 5.1	10.2 ± 5.9	1–3	6–11	86.6 ± 64.0	1.5–4
mixed amphetamine salts XR (d-amphetamine) Adderall XR®	10	——	28.8	——	6.4	431.9	11
mixed amphetamine salts XR (l-amphetamine) Adderall XR®	10	——	8.8	——	6.4	138.3	9

Cmax-1, first maximum stimulant plasma concentration; Cmax-2, second maximum stimulant plasma concentration; Tmax-1, time to first maximum stimulant plasma concentration; Tmax-2, time to second maximum stimulant concentration; AUC, area under the curve (extent of absorption); $T_{1/2}$, serum half-life of drug.
NR: Not reported.
——; ——. not applicable

- Metabolism and elimination
  - Amphetamine and methylphenidate are metabolized in the body by different mechanisms.
  - Amphetamine is metabolized partly by the liver and is partly excreted unchanged in the urine.
    - Amphetamine is metabolized by side-chain oxidative deamination and ring hydroxylation in the liver.
    - Amphetamine excretion is enhanced by acidification of the urine.
    - Amphetamine excretion is decreased by alkalinization of the urine.
  - Methylphenidate undergoes extensive first-pass hepatic metabolism predominately by hydrolysis to ritalinic acid.
    - No accumulation of drug is noted with multiple daily dosing.

STIMULANT FORMULATIONS AND DOSE

Because of their safety and efficacy, stimulants are considered the medications of first choice in the treatment of ADHD.

- Extended-release preparations are now the standard of care in ADHD.
- Use intermediate-acting preparations for the ADHD patient with mild to moderately severe symptoms who requires coverage only during the school (or work) day.
- Use long-acting preparations for the ADHD patient with moderate to severe-symptoms who requires coverage for the extended day (i.e., school and after-school hours)
- Use immediate-release preparations to supplement longer-acting stimulant formulations.

Clinical Efficacy

- Stimulants significantly reduce hyperactivity in children and adolescents with ADHD.
- Stimulants decrease distractibility and enhance vigilance in tasks requiring sustained attention in patients with ADHD.
- Stimulants have been shown to increase a child's responsiveness to, and compliance with, parental requests.
- Although stimulants do not normalize social behaviors, they enhance social behaviors in patients with ADHD.
- Stimulants do not increase a child's IQ but may enhance academic performance and efficacy in doing schoolwork.
- Stimulants may decrease associated oppositional defiant behavior and overt and covert aggression in children and adolescents with ADHD.

FDA Approval

- The FDA allows physicians off-label use of medication if compelling reasons exist.
- The FDA regulates drug manufacturers' advertising claims.

- Dextroamphetamine and Adderall® medications are FDA approved for manufacturers' advertising in children ≥ 3 years old with ADHD.
- Adderall XR® is FDA approved for manufacturer's advertising in adults with ADHD.
- Methylphenidate medications are FDA approved for manufacturer's advertising in children ≥6 years old with ADHD.

Pemoline

- Use of pemoline (Cylert®) is not recommended.
- Pemoline use is associated with hepatic toxicity and liver damage.
  - Since the marketing of pemoline in 1975, 15 cases of acute hepatic failure have been reported to the FDA.
    - 12 cases resulted in death or liver transplantation.
  - This rate of reporting represents between 4 and 17 times the rate of acute hepatic failure expected in the population.
  - The earliest reported onset of hepatic abnormalities occurred 6 months after initiation of pemoline.
    - Symptoms include dark urine, anorexia, malaise, and gastrointestinal symptoms.
    - Markedly elevated liver function tests (SGPT [ALT]) may occur with pemoline use.
- Pemoline is considered a second- or third-line therapy for ADHD. Use only if all other options have been tried and failed.
  - Serum SGPT (ALT) required at baseline and every 2 weeks.
  - Discontinue pemoline if serum SGPT (ALT) ≥2 times the upper limit of normal.
  - Discontinue pemoline if clinical symptoms of liver failure emerge.
  - Discontinue a clinical trial of pemoline if, after 3 weeks, no clinical benefit emerges.

Stimulant drug doses, recommended starting doses, titration, usual therapeutic doses, and usual dose schedules for ADHD are given in the following table.

STIMULANT SIDE EFFECTS

Stimulants are generally very safe medications. Severe side effects occur in 4–10% of children treated with stimulants and generally resolve when stimulants are discontinued.

In assessing stimulant side effects in the clinical setting, it is important to:

- Distinguish between symptoms of ADHD and side effects of the drug.
  - Often parents report a medication side effect that is actually part of ADHD.
    - Obtain baseline (before drug) rating of stimulant side effects.
    - Obtain on-drug rating of stimulant side effects.
    - Often parent reports of stimulant side effects decrease as ADHD symptoms improve.
  - Consider stimulant pharmacokinetics

Table 4.4 Stimulant Drug Doses

Generic Name	Trade Name	Available Doses (mg) (tablet/capsule color)	Scored Tablet?	Starting Dose (mg/day)	Titration (mg)	Usual Therapeutic Dose (mg/kg/dose) [Usual Daily Dose Range] (mg/kg/day)	Dose Schedule
		SHORT-ACTING (4–6-HOUR COVERAGE)					
mixed amphetamine salts	Adderall® tablets	5 (blue) 7.5 (blue) 10 (blue) 12.5 (orange) 15 (orange) 20 (orange) 30 (orange)	Yes Yes Yes Yes Yes Yes Yes	3–5 years old: 2.5 ≥ 6 years old: 5 once or twice daily	2.5 weekly 5 weekly	0.15–0.5 [0.3–1.5]	bid–tid
methamphetamine HCL	Desoxyn® tablets	5 (white)	No	≥ 6 years old: 5 once or twice daily	5 weekly	0.15–0.4 [0.15–0.8]	daily–bid
dextroamphetamine sulfate	Dexedrine® tablets	5 (orange)	Yes	3–5 years old: 2.5 ≥ 6 years old: 5 once or twice daily	2.5 weekly 5 weekly	0.15–0.5 [0.3–1.5]	bid–tid
dextroamphetamine sulfate	Dextrostat® tablets	5 (yellow) 10 (yellow)	Yes Yes	3–5 years old: 2.5 ≥ 6 years old: 5 once or twice daily	2.5 weekly 5 weekly	0.15–0.5 [0.3–1.5]	bid–tid
dexmethylphenidate	Focalin™ tablets	2.5 (blue) 5 (yellow) 10 (white)	No No No	≥ 6 years old: 2.5 once or twice daily	2.5–5 weekly	0.15–0.35 [0.3–1.0]	bid
methylphenidate HCL	Ritalin® HCL tablets	5 (yellow) 10 (green) 20 (yellow)	Yes Yes Yes	≥ 6 years old: 5 once or twice daily	5–10 weekly	0.3–0.7 [0.6–2.1]	bid–tid
	Methylin® chewable tablets	2.5 (white) 5 mg (cream) 10 mg (white to cream)	No No No				
	Methylin® oral elixir	5 mg/5 ml 10 mg/5 ml					

(Continued)

Table 4.4 *Stimulant Drug Doses* (Cont.)

Generic Name	Trade Name	Available Doses (mg) (tablet/capsule color)	Scored Tablet?	Starting Dose (mg/day)	Titration (mg)	Usual Therapeutic Dose (mg/kg/dose) [Usual Daily Dose Range] (mg/kg/day)	Dose Schedule
INTERMEDIATE-ACTING (8-HOUR COVERAGE)							
dextroamphetamine sulfate sustained release	Dexedrine® spansule capsules	5 (brown/clear) 10 (brown/clear) 15 (brown/clear)	No No No	≥ 6 years old: 5 once daily	5 weekly	0.15–0.5 [0.3–1.5]	daily–bid
methylphenidate HCL extended release	Metadate® CD capsules	10 (green/white) 20 (blue/white) 30 (reddish-brown/white)	No No No	≥ 6 years old: 20 once daily	20 weekly [0.6–2.1]	0.3–0.7	daily
methylphenidate HCL extended release	Metadate® ER tablets	10 (white) 20 (white)	No No	≥ 6 years old: 10 once daily	10 weekly	0.3–0.7 [0.6–2.1]	daily
methylphenidate HCL extended release	Ritalin® LA capsules	20 (white) 30 (yellow) 40 (light brown)	No No No	≥ 6 years old: 20 once daily	10 weekly	0.3–0.7 [0.6–2.1]	daily
methylphenidate HCL sustained release	Ritalin-SR® tablets	20 (white)	No	≥ 6 years old: titrate with immediate release 5: once or twice daily, then substitute SR	5–10 weekly	0.3–0.7 [0.6–2.1]	daily–bid
LONG-ACTING (8–12-HOUR COVERAGE)							
Mixed amphetamine salts	Adderall XR® capsules	5 (clear/blue) 10 (blue/blue) 15 (blue/white) 20 (orange/orange) 25 (orange/white) 30 (natural/orange)	No No No No No No	3–5 years old: No data ≥ 6 years old: 10 once daily	5–10 weekly	0.15–0.5 [0.3–1.5]	daily
methylphenidate extended release	Concerta® tablets	18 (yellow) 27 (gray) 36 (white) 54 (brownish-red)	No No No No	≥ 6 years old: 18 once daily	18 weekly	0.3–0.7 [0.6–2.1]	daily

- If a side effect is reported 1 to 2 hours postdosing, it probably represents a true stimulant side effect.
- If a side effect is reported at the end of the drug's half-life when stimulant plasma and brain levels are declining, it probably represents the reemergence of poorly controlled symptoms of ADHD, and not a true stimulant drug side effect.

Common acute stimulant side effects are presented in the following table. Decreased appetite, minor weight loss, sleep difficulties, and nervousness are the side effects most commonly reported in clinical trials of stimulants compared with placebo.

Table 4.5 Common, Acute Stimulant Side Effects[a]

Abdominal pain	Insomnia[b]
Anorexia	Mood lability
Diminished appetite[b]	Nausea
Headache	Nervousness[b]
	Vomiting

[a] Reported in various controlled clinical trials at rates ≥ 5% and numerically greater than placebo.
[b] Most commonly reported with stimulants.

In controlled stimulant trials for ADHD, few patients discontinue medication because of acute side effects. This suggests that stimulants are largely well tolerated by patients and generally effective for the symptoms of ADHD.

Table 4.6 Stimulant Discontinuation Rates in Controlled Clinical Trials

Discontinuation Rate of Stimulant Subjects	0.9–3.7%
Discontinuation Rate of Placebo Subjects	0–2.7%

Less common side effects that sometimes occur with stimulants are listed in the following table.

Table 4.7 Less Common Stimulant Side Effects

Psychosis (auditory/visual hallucinations)
Manic symptoms (euphoria, excitability)
Irritability
Depression/sadness/weeping
Dizziness
Lethargy/fatigue
Rash/hives
Formication
Nervous habits
Skin picking
Behavioral rebound
Growth retardation
Motor and/or vocal tics
Sudden death in patients with structural cardiac defects.

Stimulant Contraindications

- Stimulants, especially mixed amphetamine salts (Adderall® and Adderall XR®), have been associated with reports of sudden unexplained death (SUD) in children. SUD has been associated with amphetamine abuse and reported in children with underlying cardiac abnormalities taking therapeutic doses of mixed amphetamine salts and methylphenidate preparations. In addition, a very small number of cases of SUD have been reported in children without structural cardiac abnormalities while taking Adderall® and Adderall XR®.
  - Between 1999 through 2003 the FDA's Adverse Event Reporting System database identified 12 cases of sudden death in pediatric patients 1 to 18 years of age who were being treated for ADHD with mixed amphetamine salts (FDA Alert [02/09/05]: Sudden death in children). Five of the 12 pediatric sudden death cases described cardiac risk factors including undiagnosed cardiac defects (aberrant origin of coronary artery, bicuspid aortic valve, idiopathic hypertrophic subaortic stenosis). Seven of the cases occurred in children without such abnormalities, but were complicated by factors such as a family history of ventricular arrhythmia, other illness, and very rigorous exercise.
  - At the present time, the FDA does not conclude that mixed amphetamine salts cause SUD. However, as a precaution the FDA currently recommends that Adderall® and Adderall XR® not be used in children, adolescent, or adults with structural cardiac abnormalities.
  - Relative stimulant contraindications are given below.

Table 4.8 Relative Stimulant Contraindications

Psychotic disorders
Severe Tourette's disorder
Monoamine oxidase inhibitors (minimum 2-week washout interval)
Active substance abuse (in patient or family)
Unstable seizure disorder
Structural cardiac defects
Unstable hypertension
Unstable cardiovascular disorder
History of adverse reaction to stimulants
Pregnancy
Child age <3 years old

STIMULANT DRUG–DRUG INTERACTIONS

Important stimulant drug–drug interactions are outlined in the table below.

- Most stimulant drug–drug interactions are mild.
- There are two very important stimulant drug–drug interactions for the clinician to be aware of:
  - Stimulant use within 2 weeks of concomitant MAOI use can result in life-threatening hypertensive crisis.

- ∘ Stimulant use with furazolidone (a nitroheterocyclic compound used as an antibiotic against a variety of protozoan and anaerobic infections) can result in life-threatening hypertensive crisis.
- Potential stimulant–clonidine interaction.
  - ∘ Three cases of sudden death have been reported in children with ADHD on combination clonidine–methylphenidate therapy (Cantwell et al., 1997).
  - ∘ All cases were complex and other causes of death are probable; whether these medications played a role in the sudden deaths is presently unknown.
  - ∘ Close monitoring of vital signs is recommended if a clonidine-stimulant combination is used.

Table 4.9 Stimulant Drug–Drug Interactions

Stimulant Type	Drug	Interaction
AMP	Lithium	↓ Stimulatory effects of AMP
AMP	Acidifying agents (e.g., ascorbic acid, fruit juice, glutamic acid)	↓ Absorption of AMP
AMP	Alkalinizing agents	↑ AMP effects (preferred by drug abusers)
AMP	Antihistamines	↓ Sedative effects of antihistamines
AMP	Antihypertensives	May antagonize antihypertensives
AMP	Antipsychotics (chlorpromazine, haloperidol)	AMP may inhibit antipsychotic action
AMP	SSRI antidepressants	↑ Agitation, may augment antidepressant response
AMP	**Furazolidone**	**Hypertensive crisis**
AMP	Meperidine	↑ Analgesic action
AMP	Norepinephrine	↑ Pressor response
AMP	Phenobarbitol, phenytoin	↓ Absorption of anticonvulsant
AMP	Opiates	↑ Analgesic and anorectic effects of opiates
AMP	Sedative hypnotics	↓ Sedative and anxiolytic effects
MPH and AMP	**MAOIs**	**Hypertensive crisis (tranylcypromine is most dangerous)**
MPH and AMP	Sympathomimetic drugs	Potentiate action
MPH	Imipramine	↑ Imipramine level
MPH	Desipramine	↑ Adverse events
MPH	Guanethidine	Paradoxical hypotension
MPH	Tricyclic antidepressants	Inhibit TCA metabolism
MPH	Warfarin	↑ MPH levels
MPH	Anticonvulsants (phenytoin, diphenylhydantoin, primidone)	↑ Anticonvulsant plasma levels

Note: Bold-face type indicates most serious drug–drug interactions.

MANAGEMENT OF STIMULANT OVERDOSE

Between 1993 and 1999 the American Association of Poison Control Centers Toxic Exposure Surveillance System identified 759 cases of stimulant overdose and abuse in youth 10–19 years old (Klein-Schwartz & McGrath, 2003). The majority concerned methylphenidate. Rising rates of methylphenidate abuse were noted when 1999 rates were compared with rates in 1993. The majority of youth who required health care facility management experienced clinical toxicity. Only seven cases of severe toxicity were identified. These cases occurred in adolescents with polydrug overdoses (i.e., stimulants plus other drugs/alcohol).

For cases involving stimulants alone, the majority of symptoms included cardiovascular (tachycardia, hypertension) and/or CNS (agitation, irritability) toxicity. There were no deaths reported.

Signs and symptoms of acute overdose result from over stimulation of the CNS and from excessive sympathomimetic effects. Symptoms of stimulant toxicity include:

- Vomiting
- Agitation
- Tremor
- Convulsion
- Confusion
- Hallucinations
- Hyperpyrexia
- Tachycardia
- Arrhythmias
- Hypertension
- Paranoid delusions
- Delirium

Treatment consists of prompt medical referral and appropriate supportive measures. The patient must be protected from self-injury and environmental overstimulation that would aggravate heightened sympathomimetic arousal. Chlorpromazine has been reported to be useful in decreasing CNS stimulation and drug-induced sympathomimetic effects. If the patient is alert and conscious, gastric contents may be evacuated by induction of emesis or gastric lavage. For intoxication with amphetamine, acidification of the urine will increase amphetamine excretion. For severe overdose, intensive care must be provided to maintain adequate cardiopulmonary function and to treat hyperpyrexia. The efficacy of peritoneal dialysis or extracorporeal hemodialysis for stimulant toxicity has not been established.

5. Antidepressants

The antidepressants are a heterogeneous class of compounds that includes selective serotonin reuptake inhibitors (SSRIs), tricyclic antidepressants (TCAs), monoamine oxidase inhibitors (MAOIs), serotonin norepinephrine reuptake inhibitors (SNRIs) such as venlafaxine and duloxetine, and the atypical antidepressants bupropion, trazodone, nefazodone, and mirtazapine. SSRIs are now the most frequently prescribed antidepressants for children and adolescents because of the evidence base supporting their efficacy and their favorable side-effect profile. The clinical use of TCAs is declining because of concern over the cardiovascular side effects and toxicity of these agents. Little controlled research to date supports the use of SNRIs and atypical antidepressants in early-onset disorders of anxiety or depression. There is currently no place in pediatric psychopharmacology for the use of MAOIs because of the necessity for dietary restrictions to prevent hypertension in the use of these agents.

SSRIs are considered the agents of first choice in pediatric depression and anxiety disorders because they are less toxic in overdose than TCAs or MAOIs. To date, only fluoxetine has been shown to work convincingly in pediatric major depressive disorder (MDD), and it is presently the only FDA-approved agent for the treatment of MDD in children and adolescents. There are several randomized, controlled clinical trials suggesting that sertraline, citalopram, and possibly paroxetine may be effective for pediatric MDD, but there is no FDA approval for these three agents. There is no evidence of efficacy for the other classes of antidepressants in treating pediatric depression, including the TCAs, MAOIs, and SNRIs, or the atypical antidepressants trazodone, nefazodone, bupropion, or mirtazapine. Five SSRIs have been shown to be effective in the treatment of pediatric OCD, and three have FDA approval: fluoxetine, fluvoxamine, and sertraline. Clomipramine, a TCA, also has FDA approval in the treatment of pediatric OCD in children 10 years and older. Fluvoxamine, sertraline, fluoxetine, and paroxetine have been shown to be effective in the treatment of anxiety disorders.

In October 2004 the FDA issued a black box warning on all antidepressant use in the pediatric age group. The FDA completed an analysis of 24 controlled pediatric antidepressant studies involving over 4,400 children and adolescents treated with a variety of antidepressants for various disorders, including depression, OCD, GAD, and ADHD. The antidepressants investigated included fluoxetine, sertraline, paroxetine, citalopram, fluvoxamine, mirtazapine, venlafaxine, bupropion, and nefazodone. A black box warning was initiated after analysis revealed an increased rate of suicidal behaviors and suicidal thinking in children and adolescents randomized to active drug compared with placebo. There was a doubling of risk for suicidality on drug compared to placebo. It is important to emphasize that no child or adolescent died by suicide in these studies. Only 78 suicidal events were noted in these 4,400 children, suggesting that such events are uncommon. The FDA has not concluded from these studies that antidepressants cause suicidality in young people. Most likely, these events are due to a complex interaction between the disorder and the side effects of antidepressant medication in certain (not all) vulnerable children and adolescents. However, the FDA recommends increased physician monitoring of antidepressant side effects, especially in the first 2 months after antidepressant initiation and for 1 month after antidepressant discontinuation. In addition, careful screening of depressed youngsters for bipolar disorder prior to prescribing an antidepressant is advised. It is further recommended that prescribing physicians carefully discuss antidepressant risks and benefits with families before the initiation of antidepressant treatment.

This chapter discusses antidepressants in pediatric psychopharmacology with a particular emphasis on SSRIs. Additional antidepressants discussed include bupropion, mirtazapine, nefazodone, trazodone, and the tricyclic antidepressants. Less common agents such as MAOIs are only briefly mentioned. Available antidepressant medications and usual dose ranges in the treatment of depression and anxiety are presented in the following table. Atomoxetine is an antidepressant but is used primarily for ADHD; it is discussed in detail in Chapters 11 and 14.

Recent controlled studies of antidepressants in children and adolescents are presented in the next table.

SELECTIVE SEROTONIN REUPTAKE INHIBITORS

Fluoxetine

PHARMACOLOGY

Fluoxetine is a selective serotonin reuptake inhibitor (SSRI).

PHARMACODYNAMICS

The antidepressant, anti-obsessive–compulsive, and antibulimic actions of fluoxetine are presumed linked to the inhibition of CNS neuronal uptake of serotonin. Fluoxetine is a much more potent uptake inhibitor of serotonin than of norepinephrine. Reuptake inhibition is associated with enhanced serotonergic neurotransmission in the CNS, which is presumably related to the clinical effectiveness of fluoxetine in depressive and anxiety disorders.

Table 5.1 Available Antidepressant Medications

Drug	Dosage Forms (mg)	Usual Daily Dose (mg/day)	Extreme Dosage (mg/day)	Therapeutic Plasma Levels (ng/mL)
SELECTIVE SEROTONIN REUPTAKE INHIBITORS				
Citalopram (Celexa)	T: 10, 20, 40 LC: 5 mg/5 ml	20–40	10–60	
Fluoxetine (Prozac)	C: 10, 20 LC: 20 mg/5mL	20	10–80	
Fluvoxamine (Luvox)	T: 25, 50, 100	150–200	50–300	
Escitalopram (Lexapro)	T: 5, 10, 20 LC: 5 mg/5 ml	10–20	5–20	
Paroxetine (Paxil)	T: 10, 20, 30, 40 LC: 10 mg/5 ml CR: 12.5, 25, 37.5	20	10–50	
Sertraline (Zoloft)	T: 25, 50, 100 LC: 20 mg/1 ml	25–200	50–250	
CYCLIC COMPOUNDS				
Amitriptyline (Elavil and generics)	T: 10, 25, 50, 75, 100, 150 INJ: 10 mg/mL	50–150	50–300	>120[b]
Clomipramine (Anafranil)	C: 25, 50, 75	50–200	50–200	
Desipramine (Norpramin and generics)	T: 10, 25, 50, 75, 100, 150 C: 25, 50	25–150	50–150	>125
Imipramine (Trofranil and generics)	T: 10, 25, 50 C: 75, 100, 125, 150 INJ: 12.5 mg/1 mL	50–200	50–300	>225[a]
Nortriptyline (Pamelor and generics)	C: 10, 25, 50, 75 LC: 10 mg/5 mL	75–100	25–150	50–150
Doxepin (Adapin, Sinequan, and generics)	C: 10, 25, 50, 75, 100, 150 LC: 10 mg/mL	150–200	25–300	100–250
Trimipramine (Surmontil)	C: 25, 50, 100	150–200	50–300	
Protriptyline (Vivactil)	T: 5, 10	15–40	10–60	
Maprotiline (Ludiomil)	T: 25, 50, 75	100–150	50–200	
Amoxapine (Asendin)	T: 25, 50, 100, 150	150–200	50–300	
OTHER COMPOUNDS				
Bupropion (Wellbutrin)	T: 75, 100 SR: 100, 150, 200 XL: 150, 300	75–225	100–450	
Duloxetine (Cymbalta)	C: 20, 30, 60	40–60	40–60	
Mirtazapine (Remeron)	T: 15, 30, 45	15–45	7.5–45	
Nefazodone	T: 50, 100, 150, 200, 250	200–300	100–600	
Trazodone (Desyrel and generics)	T: 50, 100, 150, 300	100–300	100–600	
Venlafaxine (Effector)	T: 25, 37.5, 50, 75, 100 XR: 37.5, 75, 150	75–150	75–225	
MONOAMINE OXIDASE INHIBITORS				
Phenelzine (Nardil)	T: 15	45–60	15–90	
Tranylcypromine (Parnate)	T: 10	30–50	10–90	

C, capsules; INJ, injectable form; LC, liquid concentrate or solution; SR: slow release, T: tablets, XL, CR, and XR: extended release.
[a] Sum of imipramine plus desipramine.
[b] Sum of amitriptyline plus nortriptyline.

ANTIDEPRESSANTS

Table 5.2 Controlled Pharmacological Trials in Child and Adolescent Major Depressive Disorder

Study	N/Age in Years/ Duration	Treatment (Dose)	Study Design and Measures	% Responders (Endpoint Analysis): Drug vs. PBO
TRIALS WITH TRICYCLIC ANTIDEPRESSANTS				
Kramer and Feiguine (1981)	20/13–17/ 6 weeks	Amitriptyline (200 mg/day) vs. PBO	1- to 3-week washout; parallel, author's, improvement scale	80% vs. 60% (ns)
Geller et al. (1990)	31/12–17/ 8 weeks	Nortriptyline (45–140 mg/day) vs. PBO	2-week PBO washout; parallel CDRS, CGAS	8% vs. 21% (ns)
Kutcher et al. (1994)	42/15–19/ 6 weeks	Desipramine (200 mg/day) vs. PBO	1-week PBO washout; parallel HDRS, BDI, SCL-58	48% vs. 35% (ns)
Kye et al. (1996)	31/12–18/ 6 weeks	Amitriptyline (5 mg/kg/day) vs. PBO	2-week PBO washout, parallel CGI, HDRS, K-SADS-L	90% vs. 90% (ns)
Birmaher et al. (1998)	27/13–17/ 10 weeks	Amitriptyline (173 ± 56 mg/day) vs. PBO	Resistant depression; parallel HDRS, BDI, CGI	77% vs. 79% (ns)
Klein et al. (1998)	45/13–18/ 6 weeks	Desipramine (214 ± 87 mg/day) vs. PBO	2-week PBO washout; parallel CGI, HDRS, K-SADS-L	67% vs. 50% (ns)
TRIALS WITH SELECTIVE SEROTONIN REUPTAKE INHIBITORS				
Simeon et al. (1990)	30/13–18/ 7 weeks	Fluoxetine (20–60 mg/day) vs. PBO	1-week, PBO washout; parallel HDRS, CGI, SCL-58	66% vs. 66% (ns)
Emslie et al. (1997)	96/8–18/ 8 weeks	Fluoxetine (20 mg/day) vs. PBO	3-week washout; parallel CGI, CDRS ($p = 0.02$) but per protocol	ITT: 56% vs. 33% 74% vs. 58% (ns)
Milin et al. (1999)	286/13–19/ 12 weeks	Paroxetine (20–40 mg/day) vs. PBO	Parallel K-SADS-L, MADRS	74% vs. 71% (ns)

Study	N/age/duration	Treatment	Design/measures	Results
Keller et al. (2001)	275/13–17/ 8 weeks	Paroxetine (20–40 mg/day) vs. Imipramine (200–300 mg/day) vs. PBO	1 to 2-week washout; parallel CGI, HDRS, K-SADS-dep	ITT: 65.6% vs. 52.1 vs. 48.3% (p = 0.02)
Emslie et al. (2002)	219/8–18/ 8 weeks	Fluoxetine (20 mg/day) vs. PBO	3-week washout; parallel CGI, CDRS the CDRS-R score was more improved on active drug (p < 0.01)	ITT: 65% vs. 53% (ns)
Wagner et al. (2003)	366/6–17/ 10 weeks	Sertraline (50–200 mg/day) vs. PBO	2-week washout; parallel CDRS-R, CGI (p = 0.05)	ITT: 69% vs. 59%
Braconnier et al. (2003)	121/12–20/ 8 weeks	Paroxetine (20–40 mg/day) vs. clomipramine (75–150 mg/day)	2-week washout; parallel MADRS, CGI	ITT: 65.1% vs. 48.3% (ns)
Emslie et al. (2004)	40/8–18/ 32 weeks	Fluoxetine (20–60 mg/day) vs. PBO	32 week continuation CDRS-R, MADRS, CGI, CDI, BDI PBO 60%	% Relapse F 34%
Wagner et al. (2004)	174/7–17/ 8 weeks	Citalopram (20–40 mg/day)	parallel CDRS-R	ITT: 36% vs. 24% (p < 0.05)
TADS (2004)	439/12–17 12 weeks	Fluox+CBT vs. Fluox vs. CBT vs. PBO 10–40 mg/day	CDRS-R CGI	Response rates Fluox + CBT 71% PBO 34% Fluox 61%, CBT 43%

Scale; BDI = Beck depression inventory; CD = Children's Depression Inventory; CDRS = Children's Depression Rating Scale; CGAS = Children's Global Assessment CGI = Clinical Global Impression-Severity; HDRS = Hamilton Depression Rating Scale; ITT = intent-to-treat analysis; K-SADS-L = Schedule for Affective Disorders and Schizophrenia for Adolescents-Lifetime version, nine-item depression subscale; MADRS = Montgomery-Asberg Depression Rating Scale; PBO = placebo; SCL-58 = 58-item Hopkins Symptom Checklist; TADS = Treatment of Adolescent Depression Study.

Antagonism of muscarinic, histaminergic, and (alpha) 1-adrenergic receptors is thought to be associated with various anticholinergic, sedative, and cardiovascular effects of classical tricyclic antidepressant (TCA) drugs. Fluoxetine binds to these and other membrane receptors much less potently in vitro than the tricyclic drugs. Thus fluoxetine appears to have less treatment-emergent side effects than the TCAs.

PHARMACOKINETICS

Absorption
• Well absorbed from the GI tract.
• Absorption is delayed but not decreased in the presence of food.

Distribution
• 94.5% bound to albumin and alpha-1-glycoprotein.
• Peak serum levels of fluoxetine occur in 4–8 hours after ingestion.
• Peak serum levels of the long-acting active metabolite norfluoxetine occur in 76 hours.

Metabolism and excretion
• Metabolized primarily via N-demethylation to the active metabolite, norfluoxetine.
  ○ Norfluoxetine has similar pharmacological activity to the parent compound and exerts antidepressive and antianxiety effects.
• The elimination half-life of fluoxetine is
  ○ 2–3 days (after short-term administration)
  ○ 4–6 days after long-term administration
  ○ Up to 16 days for the active metabolite, norfluoxetine
• As a result of the long elimination half-lives of fluoxetine and its metabolites, changes in dose will not be fully reflected in plasma for several weeks, affecting both strategies for titration to final dose and withdrawal from treatment.
• Excreted in breast milk; *nursing while on fluoxetine is not recommended.*

INDICATIONS

• Indicated for the treatment of depression in children and adolescents ages 7–17 years and in adults.
  ○ Safety and effectiveness in pediatric patients younger than age 7 have not been established.
  ○ Indicated for the treatment of OCD in children and adolescents ages 7–17 years and in adults.

Possible indications
• Adult panic disorder; has not yet been evaluated in pediatric panic disorder.
• Adult bulimia nervosa; has not yet been evaluated in the treatment of adolescents with bulimia nervosa.

• Adult females with premenstrual dysphoric disorder; has not yet been evaluated in the treatment of adolescents with premenstrual dysphoric disorder.

DOSING AND DURATION OF TREATMENT

Available fluoxetine preparations
• Pulvule 10 mg, 20 mg, and 40 mg
• Liquid, oral solution 20 mg per 5 mL with mint flavor
• Tablets 10 mg
• Prozac ® Weekly™ capsules 90 mg

Before initiating treatment
• A routine pediatric examination, including height, weight, blood pressure, and heart rate, should be completed within the 6 months previous to medication initiation.
• Given recent concerns that antidepressants may exacerbate suicidal behaviors in some pediatric patients, a baseline assessment ascertaining any suicidal thoughts, means to carry out a suicide plan, and the severity of depression and/or anxiety is advised.

General dosing suggestions
• It is advisable to initiate fluoxetine at a low dose of 10 mg given once daily in the morning in pediatric patients. For young patients, the dose may be initiated at 5 mg/day. The dose may be titrated upward by 5–10 mg every 5–7 days, depending on effectiveness and patient tolerability. The effective dose range ranges between 10 and 80 mg/day.
  ○ Medication tolerability is enhanced and treatment-emergent adverse events are minimized by starting antidepressants at a low dose and titrating upward gradually.
• Patients should be advised that the therapeutic effects of fluoxetine, and all antidepressants, take between 2 and 12 weeks to occur. Therefore, a medication titration trial of 1–3 months is necessary in order to ascertain if the antidepressant is effective for an individual patient.
• In adult depression, more robust daily doses ≥ 30 mg/day are associated with greater antidepressant effectiveness than lower daily doses.
• For children with OCD, a full fluoxetine response may require up to 6 months on drug. Treatment of pediatric OCD may require higher doses than treatment of depression.
• Once-weekly fluoxetine formulation: Once weekly dosing of 90 mg enteric-coated capsules appears to be safe, effective, and well tolerated for the long-term treatment of adult depression. After responding to 20 mg daily for the acute treatment of depression, adult patients with depression were successfully treated with the once-weekly formulation. The weekly dosing should be initiated 7 days after the last daily dose of fluoxetine. It is unknown if weekly dosing provides the same protection from relapse as does daily dosing. Studies of the long-acting enteric fluoxetine formulation in pediatric depression are lacking. The following chart gives the conversion between the weekly

ANTIDEPRESSANTS

dose of the long-acting preparation and the daily fluoxetine dose equivalent for adults.

Weekly dose	Daily dose equivalent
90 mg	12.8 mg
180 mg	25.6 mg
270 mg	38.4 mg
360 mg	51.2 mg
540 mg	76.8 mg

Discontinuing fluoxetine treatment
- The most common adverse event associated with fluoxetine discontinuation in patients treated for MDD is anxiety (1%) or nervousness (1%).
- Patients who have received fluoxetine for 6 weeks or more should have their dose tapered gradually over at least a 2-week period.
- Due to accumulation of fluoxetine and its long-lasting active metabolites, patients who have received fluoxetine treatment for 6 months or more may continue to have measurable serum levels up to 6 months after discontinuation.
- Upon discontinuation, the patient should be carefully monitored for signs and symptoms of relapse and/or worsening suicidality.

DRUG CONTRAINDICATIONS

Absolute contraindications
- Hypersensitivity
- Thioridazine administration within a minimum of 5 weeks of fluoxetine administration (due to the potential of drug–drug interactions and thioridazine-induced lengthening of the EKG QTc interval).
- MAOI use.
- After fluoxetine is discontinued, at least 5 weeks must elapse before starting an MAOI.

Relative contraindications
- Hepatic disease (dose reduction may be required).
- History of seizures.
- Bipolar disorder.
- Activation of mania/hypomania may occur with fluoxetine use.
- May alter glycemic control; hypoglycemia may occur when fluoxetine is started.

DRUG INTERFERENCE WITH LABORATORY TESTING

Fluoxetine has not been found to interfere with any known laboratory tests.

Paroxetine

PHARMACOLOGY

Paroxetine is a selective serotonin reuptake inhibitor (SSRI).

Pharmacodynamics

Paroxetine is a phenylpiperidine antidepressant agent that selectively inhibits serotonin uptake. It is similar to other SSRIs and was developed as an alternative to tricyclic antidepressants that have effects on the reuptake of both serotonin and other neurotransmitters. More specific and more potent serotonin uptake inhibitors may result in more effective antidepressant therapy in the absence of adverse effects associated with norepinephrine uptake inhibition.

PHARMACOKINETICS

Absorption
- Completely absorbed after an oral dose.
- Food only slightly increases paroxetine absorption (6%), but the time to reach peak plasma concentration decreases from 6.4 hours postdosing to 4.9 hours.
- No adjustment needs to be made to dosing whether paroxetine is taken with food or without.

Distribution
- Distributed throughout the body, including the CNS, with only 1% remaining in the plasma.
- Approximately 95% is bound to plasma proteins.

Metabolism and excretion
- Because the relative potencies of its major metabolites are at most 2% of the parent compound, they are essentially inactive.
- Undergoes extensive first-pass metabolism after oral administration.
- Approximately 66% is excreted in the urine, with 2% as the parent compound and 62% as metabolites.
- Approximately 33% is excreted in the feces, mostly as metabolites and less than 1% as the parent compound.
- Increased plasma concentrations of paroxetine occur in patients with renal and hepatic impairment.

INDICATIONS

Paroxetine is not presently indicated for use in the pediatric population.

Paroxetine has received FDA approval for treating adult depression, GAD, OCD, panic disorder, and social anxiety disorder.

Possible indications
- Depression in the pediatric age group
- GAD in the pediatric age group
- OCD in the pediatric age group
- Panic disorder in the pediatric age group
- Posttraumatic stress disorder in the pediatric age group
- Social anxiety disorder in the pediatric age group
- Premenstrual dysphoric disorder in the adolescent age group

ANTIDEPRESSANTS

DOSING AND DURATION OF TREATMENT

Available drug preparations
• Tablets: 10 mg, 20 mg, 30 mg, and 40 mg
• Oral suspension: 10 mg/5 mL, orange-colored, orange-flavored
• Extended release tablet: 12.5 mg, 25 mg, 37.5 mg

Before initiating treatment
• Obtain a routine pediatric examination, including height, weight, blood pressure, and heart rate, completed within the 6 months previous to medication initiation.

General dosing suggestions
• Morning administration may reduce insomnia.
• May be administered with or without food.
• Do not chew or crush sustained-release form.
• The effective dose range is between 10 mg and 50 mg/day.

Pediatric major depression
• An initial single paroxetine dose of 10 mg is recommended.
• Full response may be delayed 2–12 weeks.
• Advise patient to continue on paroxetine for 1–3 months to ascertain response.
• Titrate by weekly increments of 10 mg/day to 20 mg/day.
• Some children may benefit from higher doses, up to a maximum daily dose of 50 mg.

Pediatric OCD
• An initial single dose of 10 mg is recommended.
• An initial response in OCD may be observed in 2–4 weeks.
• Full response in OCD may take up to 6 months to occur at full dose.
• Titrate by weekly increments of 10 mg/day to 20 mg/day.
• Some children may require higher doses, up to a maximum daily dose of 50 mg per day.

Discontinuing paroxetine treatment
Of all the SSRIs, the greatest care needs to be given to paroxetine discontinuation due to its very short half-life. Discontinuation of paroxetine, particularly when abrupt, has lead to spontaneous reports of the following: severe depression, dizziness, sensory disturbances (such as paresthesias and electric shock sensations), agitation, anxiety, nausea, and sweating. These events are generally self-limited.

• Incrementally decrease the daily dose by 10 mg/day at weekly intervals.
• When a daily dose of 10 mg/day is reached, patients should continue on this dose for 1 week before treatment is stopped.
• Some patients may require much smaller incremental decreases (2mg every other week) in the daily dose.
• This may require having a pharmacist compound 10 mg tablets into 2 mg caplets.

- Patients who have received paroxetine for 6 weeks or more should have their dose tapered gradually over at least a 2-week period.

DRUG CONTRAINDICATIONS

Absolute contraindications
- Concurrent use of MAOI.
- Concurrent use of thioridazine.
- Drug–drug metabolic interactions with paroxetine may increase serum levels of thioridazine and predispose to lengthening of the EKG QTc interval with increased risk for fatal cardiac arrhythmias.
- Hypersensitivity to paroxetine.

Relative contraindications
- Activation of mania/hypomania.
- Concurrent use of NSAIDs, aspirin, or other drugs that affect coagulation (associated risk of bleeding).
- Worsening depression or suicidality.
- History of seizures.
- Impaired platelet aggregation.

DRUG INTERFERENCE WITH LABORATORY TESTING

Paroxetine has not been found to interfere with any known laboratory tests.

Sertraline

PHARMACOLOGY

Sertraline is a selective serotonin reuptake inhibitor (SSRI).

PHARMACODYNAMICS

Sertraline is an antidepressant with selective inhibitory effects on presynaptic serotonin (5-HT) reuptake. It appears to have little effect on dopamine and norepinephrine metabolism.

It has a higher degree of potency and specificity for the serotonin receptor than any other agent studied, including clomipramine, fluoxetine, and fluvoxamine. Like most other antidepressants (except fluoxetine), sertraline also causes an indirect down-regulation of postsynaptic beta-adrenergic receptors, which may be at least partially responsible for its therapeutic effect and for its delay in clinical efficacy.

PHARMACOKINETICS

Absorption
- Absorption of the tablet and oral solution are approximately equal.
- Food increases the mean peak plasma concentration of sertraline by 25%, and it decreases the time to peak plasma concentrations from a mean of 8 hours to a mean of 5.5 hours postdose.

ANTIDEPRESSANTS

Distribution
• 99% bound to plasma proteins.
• A mean peak plasma sertraline concentration is observed at 4 hours after oral dosing.

Metabolism and excretion
• Undergoes extensive first-pass metabolism via N-demethylation in the liver to the weakly active metabolite, desmethylsertraline.
• About 40–45% of an oral dose is eliminated in urine.
• About 40–45% of an oral dose is eliminated in feces.
• Low plasma concentrations of sertraline and norsertraline were detected in 3 breast-fed infants whose mothers were taking sertraline 75–100 mg daily; none experienced an adverse event.

INDICATIONS

• Indicated for the treatment of pediatric OCD in children 6–17 years old.
• Effective in the treatment of adult depression, OCD, panic disorder, posttraumatic stress disorder (PTSD), premenstrual dysphoric disorder, and social anxiety disorder.

Possible indications in the pediatric age group
• Depression
• Panic disorder
• PTSD
• Social anxiety disorder
• Premenstrual dysphoric disorder
• GAD

DOSING AND DURATION OF TREATMENT

Available drug preparations
• Tablet 25 mg, 50 mg, and 100 mg
• Sertraline concentrated solution 20 mg /1 ml

Before initiating treatment
• Obtain a routine pediatric examination, including height, weight, blood pressure, and heart rate, completed within the 6 months previous to medication initiation.

General dosing suggestions
• Effective dose range is between 25 mg and 200 mg per day for children and between 25 mg and 250 mg per day for adolescents.
• Treatment may be initiated at 25 mg/day in children and 50 mg/day in adolescents.
• Doses are generally given in the morning; if sedation is a treatment-emergent side effect, may be given in the evening.
• Titrate by 25 mg weekly in young children or 50 mg weekly in older children and adolescents, until the therapeutic dose range is reached.

- Titration then occurs individually, based on patient tolerability and effectiveness of the medication.
- Generally prescribed on a bid dosing schedule for young children but may be given once daily in adolescents.

OCD dosing
- In children 6–12 years: 25 mg/day orally as a single dose in the morning or the evening; the dose may be increased at intervals of at least 1 week to a maximum dose of 200 mg/day, generally prescribed in two divided daily doses.
- In children 13–17 years: 50 mg/day orally as a single dose in the morning or the evening; the dose may be increased at intervals of at least 1 week to a maximum dose of 250 mg/day, generally prescribed in two divided daily doses.
- Treatment for OCD may require higher doses than are effective for the treatment of depression.
- Maximum response may not be clinically observed until up to 6 months on drug.
- Oral concentrate should be mixed with 4 ounces of water, ginger ale, lemon/lime soda, lemonade, or orange juice immediately before taking.

Discontinuing sertraline treatment
- Abrupt sertraline discontinuation may be associated with withdrawal symptoms and is not recommended.
- When discontinuing, taper the dose by 25% every 2–3 days to prevent withdrawal symptoms.

DRUG CONTRAINDICATIONS

Absolute contraindications
- Hypersensitivity to sertraline.
- Avoid concomitant use in patients taking MAOIs. Do not use sertraline within 2 weeks of discontinuing an MAOI. Do not use an MAOI for at least 2 weeks after stopping sertraline.
- Pimozide use.
- Drug–drug interactions with sertraline may lead to increased plasma pimozide levels and increased risk for QTc interval lengthening on EKG.
- Oral solution should not be used with disulfiram because it contains 12% alcohol.
- Oral solution should be used cautiously in patients with latex allergy because the dropper contains dry natural rubber.

Relative contraindications
- Use with caution in patients with history of seizures.
- History of mania/hypomania.

DRUG INTERFERENCE WITH LABORATORY TESTING

Sertraline has not been found to interfere with any known laboratory tests.

A
N
T
I
D
E
P
R
E
S
S
A
N
T
S

Citalopram

PHARMACOLOGY

Citalopram is a selective serotonin reuptake inhibitor (SSRI). The mechanism of action of citalopram is through enhancement of serotoninergic neurotransmission, similar to other 5-HT reuptake inhibitors.

Pharmacodynamics

Citalopram is a bicyclic phthalane derivative and is structurally unrelated to tricyclic antidepressants. Its selectivity for serotonin reuptake inhibition is greater than other antidepressants, including fluoxetine, paroxetine, and tricyclic agents. The drug essentially has no effect on norepinephrine or dopamine reuptake.

- Can reduce serotonin turnover rates secondary to reuptake inhibition.
- Does not inhibit monoamine oxidase.
- Has a low affinity for muscarinic acetylcholine receptors and has shown no significant effect on alpha- or beta-adrenergic receptors or dopamine-1, dopamine-2, histamine, 5HT1A, 5HT1B, gamma-aminobutyric acid, opioid, or benzodiazepine receptors.

PHARMACOKINETICS

Absorption
- 80% absorbed after oral administration.
- The tablet and oral solution are absorbed equally.
- Food does not affect absorption.

Distribution
- 80% protein bound.

Metabolism and excretion
- 20% metabolized by renal excretion.
- Approximately 12–13% of an oral dose is excreted unchanged in urine.
- 80% metabolized by the liver.
- The primary liver enzymes involved are CYP3A4 and CYP2C19.
- Inhibits the cytochrome P-450 enzyme CYP2D6, but is significantly less potent an inhibitor than fluoxetine, norfluoxetine, paroxetine, or sertraline.
- Has 3 active metabolites (desmethylcitalopram [primary metabolite], didesmethylcitalopram, citalopram-N-oxide), but its antidepressant effect appears related to the parent compound only.
- Serum half-life in adults is 33–37 hours.

INDICATIONS

Citalopram is labeled for use in adults with depression. It is not presently FDA approved for any pediatric disorder.

Possible indications
- OCD in children and adults.
- Anxiety disorders in children and adults.
- Depression in the pediatric age group.

DOSING AND DURATION OF TREATMENT

Available drug preparations
- Tablet 10 mg, 20 mg, 40 mg
- Citalopram solution 10 mg/5 ml

Before initiating treatment
- Obtain a routine pediatric examination, including height, weight, blood pressure, and heart rate, completed within the 6 months previous to medication initiation.

General dosing suggestions
- The effective dose range of citalopram is between 10 mg and 60 mg/day.
- Initiate citalopram as a single 10 mg dose either in the morning or evening.
- Titrate the dose by 10 mg weekly into the therapeutic dose range; the final dose will depend on individual patient tolerability.
- For depression, treatment response my take between 2 and 12 weeks to occur.
- For OCD, treatment response may require doses in the upper half of the dosing range; a full treatment response may not occur for up to 6 months.

Discontinuing citalopram treatment
- Abrupt withdrawal of citalopram is not advised.
- Taper the citalopram dose by 25% every 3 days until discontinued.

DRUG CONTRAINDICATIONS

Absolute contraindications
- Concomitant use of MAO inhibitors
- Hypersensitivity to citalopram

Relative contraindications
- History of mania/hypomania
- History of seizure disorders
- Hepatic or severe renal insufficiency

DRUG INTERFERENCE WITH LABORATORY TESTING

Citalopram has not been found to interfere with any known laboratory tests.

Escitalopram

PHARMACOLOGY

Escitalopram is a selective serotonin reuptake inhibitor (SSRI); it is the S(+)-enantiomer of citalopram and is used in the treatment of adult depression.

ANTIDEPRESSANTS

Research has shown that the S(+)-enantiomer of citalopram is the effective antidepressant agent in racemic mixtures of drug; citalopram is a racemic mixture. With the advent of cost-effective manufacturing techniques for optically pure drugs, it is hoped that treatment with the S(+)-enantiomer of citalopram may diminish adverse events associated with the racemate and enhance antidepressant treatment response. The mechanism of action is through enhancement of serotoninergic neurotransmission that is similar to other 5-HT reuptake inhibitors.

PHARMACODYNAMICS

Escitalopram appears responsible for most or all antidepressant activity of the racemic compound. In vitro, it is about twice as potent as racemic citalopram and 130 times as potent as R(-)-citalopram as an inhibitor of 5-HT reuptake. In addition, the R(-)-citalopram (Celexa®) but not escitalopram (Lexapro®) is associated with slightly more adverse events.

PHARMACOKINETICS

Absorption
• No data available.
• Absorption is not affected by food.

Distribution
• Peak plasma levels occur 3–6 hours after a single oral dose.
• 56% bound to serum protein.

Metabolism and excretion
• Elimination half-life is approximately 22–32 hours in adults; no data available in children and adolescents.
• Greater than 90% is metabolized by the liver via cytochrome P450 isoenzymes 2D6, 2C19, and 3A4.
• Has two very weak therapeutic metabolites, S(+)-desmethylcitalopram and S(+)-didesmethylcitalopram.
• Less than 10% of an oral dose appears unchanged in the urine.
• Specific data on escitalopram in relation to breastfeeding are lacking; however, citalopram appears in breast milk, and somnolence, weight loss, and decreased feeding have been reported in breastfeeding infants.

INDICATIONS

Escitalopram is indicated for the treatment of adult depression and generalized anxiety disorders. There presently exist no indications for use in the pediatric age group.

DOSING AND DURATION OF TREATMENT

Available drug preparations
• Tablet 5 mg, 10 mg, 20 mg (scored)
• Escitalopram solution 5 mg/5 ml

Before initiating treatment
• Obtain a routine pediatric examination including height, weight, blood pressure, and heart rate.

General dosing suggestions
• Effective dose range is 5–20 mg/day.
  ○ Escitalopram is twice as potent as citalopram; therefore, its dose is generally one-half that of citalopram.
• Little experience with escitalopram in the pediatric age group has accrued to date; dosing suggestions are generally extrapolated from the adult literature. *In adults*:
  ○ Depression: Initial dose 10 mg/day orally as a single dose in the morning or evening; maintenance dose 10–20 mg/day orally.
  ○ GAD: initial dose 10 mg/day orally as a single dose in the morning or evening; maintenance dose 10–20 mg/day orally.
  ○ Anxiety with depression: initial dose 10 mg/day orally as a single dose in the morning or evening; maintenance dose 10–20 mg/day orally.
• Escitalopram is dosed once daily.

Discontinuing escitalopram treatment
• Patients who have received escitalopram for 6 weeks or more should have their dose tapered gradually over at least a 2-week period.

DRUG CONTRAINDICATIONS

Absolute contraindications
• Concomitant use of MAO inhibitors within 14 days before or after escitalopram use.
• Hypersensitivity to escitalopram or citalopram products.

Relative contraindications
• Abnormal bleeding
  ○ Concurrent use of NSAIDs or aspirin may potentiate risk of upper GI bleeding.
• Hepatic function impairment (reduce dose).
• History of mania/hypomania.
• History of seizure disorder.

DRUG INTERFERENCE WITH LABORATORY TESTING

Escitalopram has not been found to affect any known laboratory tests.

Fluvoxamine

PHARMACOLOGY

Fluvoxamine is a selective serotonin reuptake inhibitor (SSRI). The mechanism of action of fluvoxamine is through enhancement of serotoninergic neurotransmission that is similar to other 5HT reuptake inhibitors.

ANTIDEPRESSANTS

PHARMACODYNAMICS

Fluvoxamine is a 2-aminoethyl oximethers of aralkylketones. The drug acts as an antidepressant and has no structural similarities to tricyclic antidepressants. Fluvoxamine

- Is a potent selective inhibitor of presynaptic serotonin.
- Does not have any significant noradrenergic neurotransmission, similar to other specific inhibitors of serotonin uptake.
- Does not have any significant monoamine oxidase inhibitor activity.
- Does not have any significant effects on central norepinephrine function, as determined by measurement of MHPG, VMA, NMN, and HVA in urine and NE in plasma.
- Demonstrates a very low affinity for alpha-1, alpha-2, beta-1, dopamine-2, histamine-1, serotonin-1, serotonin-2, and muscarinic receptors, unlike the tricyclic antidepressants.

PHARMACOKINETICS

Absorption
- 53% absorbed after oral administration.
- Time to peak concentration is 5–6 hours.
- Not significantly affected by food.

Distribution
- 77% protein bound.

Metabolism and excretion
- Metabolized via oxidation, demethylation, and deamination.
- Nine metabolites have been identified as accounting for the majority of drug recovered in the urine.
- Even though reports of adverse effects in breastfed infants are lacking, the American Academy of Pediatrics classifies fluvoxamine as a drug that may be of concern in infants.
- Excreted 94% in the urine as metabolites.
- Elimination half-life in adults is 15 hours.

INDICATIONS

OCD in children ≥ 8 years old, adolescents, and adults.

Possible indications
- Depression in children and adults.
- Obsessive–compulsive and anxiety symptoms in autistic disorder in children and adults.
- Panic disorder in children and adults.
- Social anxiety disorder in children and adults.

DOSING AND DURATION OF TREATMENT

Available drug preparations
• Tablets 25 mg, 50 mg, and 100 mg

Before initiating treatment
• Obtain a routine pediatric examination, including height, weight, blood pressure, and heart rate.

General dosing suggestions
• The effective dose range for pediatric OCD is between 50 mg and 300 mg a day.
• Total doses above 50 mg should be divided into two daily doses.
• Initiate fluvoxamine in children and adolescents at 25 mg at bedtime; titrate the dose upward by 25 mg every 4–7 days.
• Maximum dose
• In children, 200 mg/day
• In adolescents, 300 mg/day.

Discontinuing fluvoxamine treatment
• Gradual dose reduction by 25% every 3 days is recommended.
• Patients who have received fluvoxamine for 6 weeks or more should have their dose tapered gradually over at least a 2-week period.

DRUG CONTRAINDICATIONS

Absolute contraindications
• Coadministration of thioridazine, terfenadine, astemizole, pimozide, or cisapride increases risk for prolonged QTc interval and cardiac arrythmias.
• Hypersensitivity to fluvoxamine or its metabolites

Relative contraindications
• History of mania/hypomania.
• History of seizures.
• Hepatic disease (dose reductions may be required).
• Avoid concurrent use of fluvoxamine and MAOIs: Do not start an MAOI for 2 weeks after stopping fluvoxamine; do not start fluvoxamine for 2 weeks after stopping an MAOI.
• Concurrent administration of theophylline or warfarin with fluvoxamine requires careful monitoring of theophylline concentration and prothrombin time.

DRUG INTERFERENCE WITH LABORATORY TESTING

Fluvoxamine has not been found to interfere with any known laboratory test.

SSRI Side Effects

Mild side effects from SSRIs are common. More serious side effects require clinical attention and possible dose reduction or medication discontinuation.

ANTIDEPRESSANTS

SSRIs may be activating in children and adolescents and increase behavioral agitation and emotional disinhibition. In depressed children, these side effects may increase risk for suicidal thoughts or behaviors and require careful physician attention. Side effects of SSRIs are given in the following table.

Table 5.3 SSRI Side Effects

Common:
• Gastointestinal: nausea, vomiting, anorexia, dry mouth, dyspepsia
• CNS: headache, anxiety, nervousness, agitation, insomnia, nocturnal myoclonus, tremor
• Sexual: anorgasmia, decreased libido, erectile difficulties in males, abnormal ejaculation in males, impotence
• General: asthenia, increased sweating, weight loss
• Allergic: rash

Uncommon and potentially serious:
• Increased suicidality
• Hyponatremia
• Mania/hypomania

Drug–Drug Interactions

SSRIs have the potential to interfere with the metabolism and clearance of a variety of drugs. The long-acting metabolite of fluoxetine, norfluoxetine, is a potent inhibitor of CYP3A4. Fluoxetine and paroxetine are potent CYP2D6 inhibitors. Fluoxetine and fluvoxamine inhibit the CYP2C9 enzyme system, and fluvoxamine is also an inhibitor of the CYP1A2, CYP2C19, and CYP3A4 systems. The following table presents some SSRI drug–drug interactions.

Table 5.4 SSRI Drug-Drug Interactions

SSRI	Drug	Interaction
Fluoxetine	TCAs	↑ TCA levels and cardiac risk
Fluoxetine	Thioridazine	↑ Thioridazine levels and cardiac risk
Fluoxetine	Benzodiazepines	↑ Sedation
Fluoxetine	Carbamazepine	↑ Carbamazepine levels and toxicity
Fluoxetine, fluvoxamine	Phenytoin	↑ Phenytoin levels and toxicity
Fluoxetine, fluvoxamine	Warfarin	↑ Warfarin levels and toxicity
Fluoxetine, fluvoxamine, paroxetine, sertraline	Bupropion	↑ Bupropion levels and seizure risk
Fluvoxamine	Lithium	↑ Toxicity
Fluvoxamine	Melatonin	↑ Melatonin levels and sedation

Management of SSRI Overdose

Common signs and symptoms of overdose with SSRIs include CNS symptoms such as delirium and coma, cardiac arrhythmias, pyrexia, syncope, hypotension, and the serotonin syndrome. Fatalities in the pediatric age group have been reported with SSRI overdose alone and in combination with other agents.

Treatment of SSRI poisoning consists of the following.

• Institute usual supportive care.
• Monitor vital signs and mental status following overdose.
• Monitor cardiovascular functioning.

- Monitor fluid and electrolyte status in symptomatic patients.
  - Both hyponatremia and hypokalemia have been reported after overdoses.
- Serum levels are generally not clinically useful in guiding patient management.
- Administer activated charcoal, perform gastric lavage if large ingestion.
- Ipecac is contraindicated.
- Monitor for evidence of serotonin syndrome.
- There are no specific antidotes to SSRIs when poisoning occurs.

ATYPICAL ANTIDEPRESSANTS

Atypical antidepressants include bupropion, trazodone, mirtazapine, and nefazodone. Their chemical structures are unlike other classes of antidepressant agents.

Bupropion

Bupropion, an atypical antidepressant, has been shown to be pharmacologically and biochemically distinct from all other available antidepressants.

- Different in structure from tricyclic antidepressants, SSRIs, and MAOIs.
- Patients may be unusually susceptible to grand mal seizures on bupropion.
- In particular, bupropion should not to be used alone as treatment for bulimia.
  - Electrolyte abnormalities may exacerbate risk by lowering the seizure threshold in these patients.

PHARMACOLOGY

Bupropion is 2-tert-butylamino-3'chloropropionphenone in the aminoketone class of agents.

PHARMACODYNAMICS

Bupropion is a weak inhibitor of norepinephrine and of dopamine uptake. Additionally, its antidepressant activity has not been associated with alteration of postsynaptic beta-receptors. It lacks anticholinergic activity, is not sympathomimetic, and is at least 10-fold weaker as a cardiac depressant than the tricyclic antidepressants. Other studies have suggested an antidepressant mechanism involving effects on the dopaminergic systems in the brain.

PHARMACOKINETICS

Absorption
- Rapidly absorbed after oral administration.
- Undergoes extensive first-pass hepatic metabolism.
  - It appears that only a small proportion of the oral drug reaches the systemic circulation intact.
- Immediate-release, sustained-release, and extended-release products are bioequivalent.
- Food does not affect the bioavailability of bupropion.

Distribution
- Highly protein bound.
- Serum half-life in adults is 3–4 hours.
- Maximum plasma concentrations are achieved in 2 hours for the immediate-release preparation and 3 hours for the sustained-release formulation.

Metabolism and excretion
- Primarily metabolized by the CYP2B6 isoenzyme.
- Has three active metabolites:
  ◦ Hydroxybupropion is half as potent as bupropion.
  ◦ Threohydrobupropion and erythrohydrobupropion are about one-fifth as potent as the parent drug.
- The elimination half-life in adults is 14 hours.
  ◦ After chronic administration, the elimination half-life in adults is 21 hours.
  ◦ The elimination half-life in adolescents ages 13–18 years is 20 hours, higher than in adults.
- 87% excreted in urine and 10% in feces.
- Accumulates in human breast milk in concentrations much higher than in maternal plasma. Caution is advised in nursing mothers receiving bupropion.

INDICATIONS

Bupropion is indicated for the treatment of adult depression and in the management of smoking cessation. Safety and effectiveness in pediatric patients under 18 years old have not been established.

Possible indications
- ADHD in children, adolescents, and adults.
- Depression in the pediatric age group.

DOSING AND DURATION OF TREATMENT

Available drug preparations
- Tablets 75 mg, 100 mg, and 300 mg
- Sustained-release (SR) tablets 100 mg and 150 mg
- Extended-release (XL) tablets 150 mg and 300 mg

Before initiating treatment
- Obtain a routine pediatric examination, including height, weight, blood pressure, and heart rate.
- Screen the patient's medical history: *Patients with a history of seizures or eating disorders are not candidates for bupropion.*

General dosing suggestions
Little experience, to date, has been published about the use of bupropion for non-ADHD indications in the pediatric age range. The following suggestions are extrapolated from the adult literature and from clinical experience with this agent in pediatric ADHD.

- Effective dose range for depression in children is between 75 mg and 225 mg/day.
- Effective dose range for adolescents and adults is between 150 mg and 400 mg/day.
- Effective dose range for ADHD may be higher than the effective dose range for depression, between 300 mg and 450 mg/day in adolescents and adults.
- Risk of bupropion-induced seizures is about 4 per 1,000 at doses > 450 mg/day.
- Dose increases should be very gradual.
- In children, initiate bupropion at a dose between 37.5 mg and 75 mg once daily. Increase by 75 mg every week until the therapeutic dose range is reached.
  - To avoid peak plasma concentrations and increased risk of inducing seizures, give immediate-release bupropion in three or four daily divided doses to children.
  - Each single dose should not exceed 150 mg for immediate-release tablets.
- In adolescents, initiate bupropion at a dose of 75 mg and titrate upward by 75 mg weekly until the therapeutic dose range is reached.
  - Give immediate-release bupropion in two or three daily divided doses to adolescents.
  - Each single dose should not exceed 150 mg for immediate-release tablets.
- When using the bupropion SR preparation, twice daily dosing is recommended.
  - Initiate as 150 mg in the morning for 1 week; then increase to 150 mg two times a day.
  - The maximum daily dose of bupropion SR is 200 mg twice a day.
- When using the bupropion XL preparation, once daily dosing is recommended for children, adolescents, and adults.
  - Initiate as 150 mg once a day for 3 days; then increase to 300 mg once a day for several weeks.
  - Maximum daily dose of bupropion XL is 450 mg given as a single daily dose.
- When switching patients from immediate- or sustained-release tablets to extended-release (XL) tablets, give the same total daily dose when possible.

Discontinuing bupropion treatment
- Abrupt discontinuation of bupropion is not advised. Discontinue gradually (10–25% of the full dose) until stopped.

DRUG CONTRAINDICATIONS

Absolute contraindications
- Seizure disorders, either ongoing or by history
  - Bulimic patients may be unusually susceptible to grand mal seizures while on bupropion.
- Patients undergoing abrupt discontinuation of alcohol or sedatives (including benzodiazepines) may be at risk for bupropion-induced seizures.
- Prior or current diagnosis of bulimia or anorexia
- Concomitant MAO inhibitor
- Hypersensitivity to bupropion products

Relative contraindications

• Mania/hypomania (treating with an antidepressant alone may increase the likelihood of precipitation of a mixed/manic episode in patients at risk for bipolar disorder).
• Excessive alcohol or sedative use.
• Hepatic impairment (reduce the dose of bupropion).
• Medications or treatments that lower seizure threshold.

DRUG SIDE EFFECTS

Bupropion use is associated with many mild treatment-emergent side effects.

• Common bupropion side effects
   ◦ Agitation, anxiety, confusion
   ◦ Auditory disturbance, blurred vision
   ◦ Constipation, dry mouth, gustatory disturbance, nausea/vomiting
   ◦ Dizziness, headache, hostility
   ◦ Hypertension, tachycardia
   ◦ Impaired sleep quality, insomnia
   ◦ Menstrual complaints
   ◦ Pruritus, rash
   ◦ Sweating
   ◦ Weight change
   ◦ Tremor
• Uncommon but potentially serious bupropion side effects
   ◦ Activation of psychosis and/or mania
   ◦ Cardiac arrhythmias
   ◦ Hypertension
   ◦ Seizures (0.4%), especially in doses >450 mg/day
   ◦ Increasing suicidal ideation.

DRUG–DRUG INTERACTIONS

Bupropion is associated with several drug–drug interactions.

• Known to inhibit the action of CYP2D6.
• May increase the plasma concentration of type 1C antiarrhythmic agents such as propafenone and flecainide.
• Concomitant carbamazepine use may induce the metabolism of bupropion.

DRUG INTERFERENCE WITH LABORATORY TESTING

Bupropion has not been found to interfere with any known laboratory tests.

MANAGEMENT OF BUPROPION OVERDOSE

Tremors and seizures are the most likely effects in acute bupropion overdose, generally occurring within 1–4 hours following ingestion, with the exception of sustained-release preparations, which have been reported to result in delayed seizures. Sinus tachycardia is common in overdose. Toxicity may be delayed after ingestion of sustained-release bupropion. Seizures have been reported with bupropion doses of 600–900 mg. In 12 of 13 adults with bupropion overdoses, patients ingested 850–4200 mg and recovered without significant sequelae. Overdoses of 9 grams in adults have resulted in seizures but no reported fatalities. In the emergent treatment of bupropion poisoning, the following should be considered.

- Institute usual supportive care.
- Monitor vital signs and the patient's mental status.
  ○ Hypotension and bradycardia have been reported after bupropion overdose.
- Monitor EKG, LFTs, and the patient's fluid and electrolyte status.
  ○ Both hyponatremia and hypokalemia have been reported after bupropion overdose.
- Serum bupropion levels are generally not clinically useful in guiding patient management.
- Administer activated charcoal, perform gastric lavage if a large ingestion has occurred.
- Ipecac is contraindicated.
- There is no specific antidote to bupropion.

Trazodone

Trazodone is termed an "atypical" tetracyclic antidepressant because it has antidepressant and also anxiolytic and hypnotic activities. It is a powerful antagonist of 5HT2A receptors and has serotonin reuptake blockade action.

Despite a lack of empirical evidence, trazodone is used frequently as a sleep aid in children and adolescents with psychiatric disorders and in depressed adults. The main benefit of trazodone in adult antidepressant therapy is its short onset of action and low incidence of anticholinergic and cardiovascular effects. Trazodone appears to be equally effective in adult bipolar and unipolar depression. Data on the clinical use of trazodone in the pediatric age group for any disorder are scarce.

PHARMACOLOGY

Pharmacodynamics
Trazodone is a triazolopyridines. Structurally, it does not bear any similarity to SSRIs, SNRIs, tricyclic antidepressants, tetracyclic antidepressants, or MAO inhibitors. The antidepressant activity of trazodone appears to be due to its ability to selectively inhibit serotonin reuptake.

At low doses, trazodone appears to act as a serotonin antagonist and at higher doses as an agonist. Trazodone does not potentiate catecholamines. It does appear to have a sedative effect and slight muscle relaxant properties and for this reason it is often used as a sedative/hypnotic, although there is no empirical evidence that it is effective for sleep induction in any age group.

PHARMACOKINETICS

Absorption
- Trazodone is well absorbed after oral administration.
- Total drug absorption may be up to 20% higher when the drug is taken with food rather than on an empty stomach.

○ Therefore, trazodone should be given shortly after a meal or light snack.
• The risk of some side effects may increase under fasting conditions.

Distribution
• Very highly protein bound.
• Peak plasma concentrations are achieved in 0.5–2 hours.

Metabolism and excretion
• Extensively metabolized in the liver by cytochrome P-450 3A4 oxidation and hydroxylation.
  ○ One active metabolite, m-chlorophenylpiperazine
  ○ It appears that cytochrome P-450 2D6 is involved in the metabolism of this metabolite.
• Excreted in low concentrations in breast milk following single doses.
• Renal mechanisms account for 70–75% of excretion.
• 21% of a trazodone dose is excreted in the feces.
• The elimination half-life in adults is 7 hours.
• Despite the absence of reports of adverse effects in breastfed infants, the American Academy of Pediatrics classifies trazodone as a drug whose effect on nursing infants is unknown but may be of concern.

INDICATIONS

Safety and effectiveness in pediatric patients have not been established. In adults, trazodone is labeled for treatment of adult depression.

Possible indications
• Insomnia in adults and in the pediatric age group.
• Migraine headache in the pediatric age group.

DOSING AND DURATION OF TREATMENT

Available drug preparations
• Tablets 50 mg, 100 mg, 150 mg, and 300 mg

Before initiating treatment
• Obtain a routine pediatric examination, including height, weight, blood pressure, and heart rate.

General dosing suggestions
The data on trazodone dosing in the pediatric age group are very limited. The following suggestions are extrapolated from the adult literature.

• For the treatment of depression, the effective trazodone dose range is 100–400 mg/day.
  ○ Initiated at 50 mg at night for depressed adolescents and adults.
  ○ Increase dose every 5–7 days by 50 mg until the therapeutic dose range is achieved.

○ Gradual dose increases of 25–50 mg every 2 weeks may reduce drowsiness and dizziness associated with initiation of therapy.
○ Usually prescribed in two divided daily doses.
• For the treatment of initial insomnia, trazodone doses range between 25 mg and 100 mg qhs.

Discontinuing trazodone treatment
• Abrupt trazodone discontinuation may result in noradrenergic rebound.
○ The short half-life of this compound is involved in the development of these symptoms.
○ From a clinical point of view, it is suggested that trazodone be tapered off slowly at a rate of 10–25% of the full dose until discontinuation.

DRUG CONTRAINDICATIONS

Absolute contraindications
• Hypersensitivity to trazodone.
• Initial recovery phase of myocardial infarction.
• Trazodone is potentially arrhythmogenic.

Relative contraindications
• Cardiac disease; trazodone is potentially arrhythmogenic.
• Concomitant administration of antihypertensive drugs may require decreasing the dose of the antihypertensive drug because of the hypotensive effects of trazodone.
• In suicidal or seriously depressed patients, prescribe in limited quantities until significant remission occurs.
• May increase or decrease prothrombin time (PT) in patients taking warfarin.

DRUG SIDE EFFECTS

Trazodone use is associated with many potential side effects.
• Common trazodone side effects
○ Anorexia, constipation, dry mouth, nausea, vomiting, diarrhea
○ Blurred vision, sweating, weight changes
○ Dizziness, drowsiness, lethargy
○ Headache, insomnia, memory impairment
• Rare but potentially serious trazodone side effects
○ Cardiac arrhythmias
○ Hypertension or hypotension
○ Hemolytic anemia, leukocytosis
○ Priapism, at times requiring surgical intervention
○ Seizures

DRUG–DRUG INTERACTIONS

• Trazodone may increase phenytoin levels.
• Trazodone may elevate digoxin levels.

ANTIDEPRESSANTS

DRUG INTERFERENCE WITH LABORATORY TESTING

Trazodone has not been found to interfere with any known laboratory tests.

MANAGEMENT OF TRAZODONE OVERDOSE

The most common manifestation of trazodone overdose is CNS depression. Lethargy, drowsiness, and ataxia are the most frequent symptoms. Nausea and vomiting are also frequent. Coma is rare, but can be prolonged. Bradycardia and transient first-degree heart block have been the most frequently reported cardiovascular effects. Trazodone ingestion in adults of 2–3 g has produced respiratory arrest. Fatalities are rarely due solely to trazodone, but generally due to poisoning with multiple agents simultaneously.

The management of trazodone poisoning is similar to that for SSRIs and bupropion.

• Institute supportive care.
• Serum levels are generally not clinically useful in guiding patient management.
• There is no specific antidote to trazodone poisoning.

Nefazodone

PHARMACOLOGY

Nefazodone is an atypical antidepressant that is unlike any other compound in any other class of antidepressant, including the tricyclic antidepressants, SSRIs, SNRIs (serotonin norepinephrine reuptake inhibitors), and norepinephrine uptake inhibitors. Nefazodone offers potential advantages over other antidepressants.

• Minimal cardiovascular effects
• Fewer anticholinergic and noradrenergic effects
• Less sedation and activation
• Fewer sexual side effects

However, *elevated rates of hepatic toxicity limit its use in pediatric psychopharmacology.*

PHARMACODYNAMICS

Nefazodone is a phenylpiperazine agent that inhibits serotonin (5HT) reuptake and also has 5HT2 antagonist properties. At least two of its metabolites appear to be pharmacologically active and contribute to its overall antidepressant activity: hydroxynefazodone, which has properties similar to nefazodone and m-chlorophenylpiperazine (mCPP) and exhibits direct central serotoninergic agonist activity and possibly some degree of 5HT2 and 5HT3 antagonism. The relative contribution of the parent compound and its metabolites to antidepressant or adverse effects has not been determined. It is unclear if only one mechanism is required for clinical efficacy or if all mechanisms or a balance between them is responsible. Nefazodone also has weak alpha-1-adrenergic blocking activity but no significant affinity for alpha-2-adrenergic receptors. Nefazodone does not inhibit monoamine oxidase.

PHARMACOKINETICS

Absorption
• Absorption after oral dosing is rapid and complete.
• Due to extensive metabolism, systemic bioavailability is about 20%.
• Food delays absorption and decreases systemic bioavailability by about 20%.

Distribution
• Completely protein bound.

Metabolism and excretion
• Undergoes extensive first-pass metabolism to three metabolites:
  ○ Hydroxy-nefazodone
  ○ Desethyl-hydroxynefazodone
  ○ M-chlorophenylpiperazine (mCPP)
• Half-life of nefazodone and two of its metabolites appear to be shorter in children and adolescents than in adults.
• The metabolism of nefazodone and its metabolites shows high intra- and interpatient variability.
• Renal elimination accounts for 55% of excretion.
• Elimination through feces accounts for 20–30% of excretion.
• The elimination half-life of the nefazodone parent compound is 1.9–5.3 hours in adults.
• There is no information regarding excretion of nefazodone in breast milk.

INDICATIONS

Safety and effectiveness in individuals below 18 years of age have not been established. Nefazodone is indicated for the treatment of depression in adults.

DOSING AND DURATION OF TREATMENT

Available drug preparations
• Tablets 50 mg, 100 mg, 150 mg, 200 mg, and 250 mg

Before initiating treatment
• Obtain a routine pediatric examination, including height, weight, blood pressure, and heart rate.
• Because nefazodone is associated with elevated rates of hepatic toxicity, baseline LFTs are recommended before starting therapy.
  ○ Nefazodone should not be started in patients with elevated transaminases or active liver disease.

General dosing suggestions
There is little data available in pediatric psychopharmacology to guide the dosing of nefazodone. The following suggestions are extrapolated from the adult literature.

- The effective dose range for depression in adults is between 300 mg and 600 mg/day.
- Initiate nefazodone at a dose of 50 mg orally twice a day.
- The dose may be titrated upward by 50–100 mg/day in two divided doses at intervals of no less than 1 week.
- The maximum dose is 600 mg/day.

Medical monitoring
- The FDA has recently required that nefazodone add a black box warning to its labeling. Nefazodone is associated with liver abnormalities ranging from asymptomatic reversible serum transaminase increases to cases of hepatic failure, resulting in liver transplantation and/or death.
  - The reported rate in the United States is about one case of liver failure per 250,000–300,000 nefazodone patient-years.
  - Patients should be alert to the signs and symptoms of liver dysfunction, including anorexia, jaundice, gastrointestinal complaints, and malaise.
  - Should be discontinued if clinical signs or symptoms indicate liver failure.
  - Periodic testing of LFTs should be considered for patients on nefazodone.
    - If serum AST or ALT levels increase to three times or more above the normal upper limits, nefazodone should be discontinued.

Discontinuing nefazodone treatment
Nefazodone discontinuation can result in withdrawal symptoms and therefore needs to be tapered gradually. In adults acute discontinuation has been reported to cause nausea, vomiting, diarrhea, ataxia, insomnia, marked agitation, headache, and flu-like symptoms. Patients recover completely in 5–10 days. Those who have experienced discontinuation symptoms with other antidepressants in the past may be at increased risk.

- It is recommended that nefazodone be tapered gradually by 25% of the full dose every 2–4 days until discontinued.
- Patients who have received nefazodone for 6 weeks or more should have their dose tapered gradually over at least a 2-week period.

DRUG CONTRAINDICATIONS

Absolute contraindications
- Coadministration of nefazodone with terfenadine, astemizole, cisapride, pimozide, or carbamazepine, due to increased risk for cardiac arrhythmias.
- Due to increased plasma concentrations of triazolam, concurrent use of triazolam and nefazodone should be avoided.
- Hypersensitivity to nefazodone or other phenylpiperazine antidepressants.
- Patients previously withdrawn from nefazodone due to evidence of liver injury.
- Hepatic disease.

Relative contraindications
- Concurrent use of MAOI drugs. Do not use nefazodone within 2 weeks of discontinuing an MAOI; do not use an MAOI for at least 1 week after stopping nefazodone.
- Postural hypotension
- History of seizures
- History of mania/hypomania

DRUG SIDE EFFECTS

Nefazodone is generally well tolerated and has minimal associated sexual dysfunction.

- Common nefazodone side effects
  - Abnormal vision, increased cough
  - Asthenia, headache
  - Confusion, memory impairment, paresthesias
  - Constipation, dry mouth, dyspepsia, nausea
  - Dizziness, insomnia, somnolence, lightheadedness
  - Blurred vision
- Uncommon but potentially serious nefazodone side effects
  - Activation of mania/hypomania
  - Postural hypotension
  - Seizures
  - Liver failure

DRUG–DRUG INTERACTIONS

Nefazodone and its metabolites are inhibitors of the CYP3A4 and weak inhibitors of the CYP2D6 enzyme systems. Thus, nefazodone has the potential for several drug–drug interactions.

- Nefazodone elevates plasma levels of alprazolam and triazolam.
- Nefazodone used in combination with cisapride elevates risk for cardiac arrhythmias.
- Nefazodone elevates digoxin levels.
- Use with terfenadine, astemizole, pimozide, or carbamazepine may increase plasma levels of these agents and predispose to cardiac arrhythmias.

DRUG INTERFERENCE WITH LABORATORY TESTING

Nefazodone has not been found to affect any known laboratory tests.

Mirtazapine

PHARMACOLOGY

Mirtazapine is the 6-aza analogue of the antidepressant mianserin and belongs to the piperazine/azepine group of drugs. It has a tetracyclic chemical structure unrelated to other antidepressants in use.

ANTIDEPRESSANTS

PHARMACODYNAMICS

Mirtazapine appears to act as an antagonist at CNS presynaptic alpha-2-adrenergic inhibitory autoreceptors and heteroreceptors, resulting in an increase in central noradrenergic and serotonergic activity. Mirtazapine antagonizes 5HT2 and 5HT3 receptors but appears to have no significant affinity for 5HT1A or 5HT1B receptors. This agent is a potent inhibitor of histamine (H1) receptors, which may cause its prominent sedative effects. It also inhibits alpha-1-adrenergic receptors, which may cause hypotension. Mirtazapine's enantiomers have been shown to be stereoselective for alpha-2 antagonism, with the most activity attributed to the (+)-enantiomer. However, studies of CNS effects in healthy volunteers have suggested that both (−) and (+)−enantiomers possess antidepressant activity.

PHARMACOKINETICS

Absorption
• Tablets are rapidly and completely absorbed after oral administration.
• The low bioavailability of 50% is due largely to extensive hepatic first-pass metabolism.
• Food has minimal effects on the rate and extent of absorption.

Distribution
• Peak concentration in serum occurs in 1.5–2 hours after an oral dose.
• Women have higher plasma concentrations compared to men and young adults.
• Plasma mirtazapine levels are linearly dose-related, between 15 to 80 mg.
• Mirtazapine is highly bound to serum proteins.

Metabolism and excretion
• Mirtazapine is extensively metabolized via cytochrome 2D6, 1A2, and 3A and has four metabolites.
   ○ Demethylmirtazapine, active, contributing 5–10% of the antidepressant activity of the parent compound
   ○ 8-hydroxy, inactive
   ○ N-desmethyl, inactive
   ○ N-oxide mirtazapine, inactive
• The kidneys excrete 75% of a mirtazapine dose and 15% appears in feces.
• Little is known about the distribution of mirtazapine into breast milk.
• Mirtazapine metabolism is decreased by approximately 30% in hepatic disease and with moderate and severe renal impairment.
   ○ Mean oral clearance of mirtazapine was reduced by 30% and 50%, respectively.
• Females of all ages had significantly longer elimination half-lives than males.
   ○ The mean half-life for females was 37 hours, versus 26 hours for males.

INDICATIONS

Safety and effectiveness of mirtazapine in pediatric patients have not been established. Mirtazapine is indicated for the treatment of depression in adults.

Possible indications
• Depression in pediatric age group.
• Anxiety disorders in adults and pediatric age group.
• Insomnia associated with depression and anxiety in adults and pediatric age group.

There are presently no published controlled studies of mirtazapine in children and adolescents.

DOSING AND DURATION OF TREATMENT

Available drug preparations
• Coated tablet and orally disintegrating (SolTab®) 15 mg, 30 mg, and 45 mg.

Before initiating treatment
• Obtain a routine pediatric examination, including height, weight, blood pressure, and heart rate.

General dosing suggestions
Little experience with the clinical use of mirtazapine in pediatric psychopharmacology is available at present to guide practice. The following dose suggestions are extrapolated from the adult experience.

• Effective dose range of mirtazapine for adult depression is 15–45 mg/day.
• Initiate mirtazapine at 15 mg at bedtime.
  ◦ The dose may be titrated upward, depending on patient response and tolerability, by 15 mg every 1–2 weeks.
  ◦ More frequent changes in dose are not recommended because of its relatively long half-life.

Use of the orally disintegrating tablets (SolTab®)

• Open blister pack with dry hands and place the tablet on the tongue.
• Use tablet immediately after removal from package; once removed, it cannot be stored.
• Tablet will disintegrate rapidly on the tongue and can be swallowed with saliva; no water needed.
• Do not attempt to split the tablet.

Discontinuing mirtazapine treatment
• When discontinuing mirtazapine after more than 1 week of therapy, it is recommended that the dose be tapered.
• Patients who have received mirtazapine for 6 weeks or more should have their dose tapered gradually over at least a 2-week period.

DRUG CONTRAINDICATIONS

Absolute contraindications
• Hypersensitivity to mirtazapine
• MAOI therapy within 14 days

ANTIDEPRESSANTS

Relative contraindications
- Heart disease
- Hypersensitivity to other antidepressants
- Hypotension
- Liver impairment
- History of mania/hypomania
- Phenylketonuria (orally disintegrating tablets contain phenylalanine)
- Pregnancy
- Seizure

DRUG SIDE EFFECTS

Sedation and somnolence are the most common side effects associated with mirtazapine therapy.

- Common mirtazapine side effects
  - Abnormal dreams, abnormal thinking, somnolence, dizziness
  - Mild ALT (SGPT) elevations
  - Asthenia
  - Constipation.
  - Increased appetite, weight gain
  - Nonfasting cholesterol increases and nonfasting triglyceride increases
- Uncommon but potentially serious mirtazapine side effects
  - Agranulocytopenia, neutropenia
  - Mania
  - Seizures

DRUG–DRUG INTERACTIONS

Because mirtazapine does not induce or inhibit any of the cytochrome enzyme systems, few drug–drug interactions occur.

- Antagonism of sympathomimetic pressor agents, such as ephedrine, pseudoephedrine, and tyramine.

DRUG INTERFERENCE WITH LABORATORY TESTING

Mirtazapine has not been found to interfere with any known laboratory tests.

MANAGEMENT OF OVERDOSE

Overdose experience with mirtazapine is limited. Reported effects have included tachycardia, disorientation, drowsiness and impaired memory. Overdoses of 10–30 times the maximum recommended mirtazapine dose produced no serious adverse effects in six patients. Overdoses of 30 and 50 times the normal daily dose produced no complications in two patients.

- Institute usual supportive care.
- Serum levels are generally not clinically useful in guiding patient management.

- Monitor for evidence of serotonin syndrome.
- There is no specific antidote to mirtazapine.

SEROTONIN NOREPINEPHRINE REUPTAKE INHIBITING ANTIDEPRESSANTS

This class of antidepressants exerts action through a combination of serotonin and norepinephrine reuptake inhibition. These agents may offer advantages over the more selective antidepressants in the treatment of depression, and they have a different side effect profile. This class of antidepressants includes venlafaxine and duloxetine.

Venlafaxine

PHARMACOLOGY

Venlafaxine is a serotonin and norepinephrine reuptake inhibitor (SNRI).

PHARMACODYNAMICS

Venlafaxine is a bicyclic antidepressant that has been referred to as an atypical or "second-generation" antidepressant. In order of decreasing potency, it selectively inhibits uptake of serotonin, norepinephrine, and dopamine. It does not inhibit monoamine oxidase, and does not show the degree of anticholinergic, sedative, or cardiovascular effects other commonly used antidepressants exhibit. No affinity for central muscarinic-cholinergic, dopaminergic, histaminic, opioid, benzodiazepine, or alpha-1-adrenergic receptors has been demonstrated for venlafaxine or its major active metabolite, O-desmethylvenlafaxine. Venlafaxine is a racemic mixture; whereas the pharmacological profile of the levo(-) isomer is similar to that of the racemate, the dextro(+) isomer is primarily a serotonin uptake inhibitor.

PHARMACOKINETICS

Absorption
- About 92% of an oral dose of venlafaxine is absorbed.
- Absorption is not affected by administration with food.
- Administration of venlafaxine with food may decrease gastric adverse side effects.

Distribution
- Venlafaxine and O-desmethylvenlafaxine, the major active metabolite, are approximately 30% protein bound.
- Due to extensive first-pass metabolism, only 12.6% of an oral dose of venlafaxine is available in the systemic circulation.
- Time to peak concentration for the regular release tablet is 1–2 hours in adults; for the extended-release preparation, 5.5 hours.

ANTIDEPRESSANTS

Metabolism and excretion
- Venlafaxine is metabolized via the cytochrome P-450 isoenzyme 2D6.
- Undergoes extensive first-pass metabolism to three major metabolites, only one of which, O-desmethylvenlafaxine, is active.
- Venlafaxine and O-desmethylvenlafaxine are equipotent in their antidepressant activity.
- Approximately 1–10% is excreted in the urine as unchanged drug; about 30% is excreted in the urine as the active metabolite.
- Another 6–19% is excreted in the urine as the two inactive metabolites.
- The elimination half-life for the parent compound is dose dependent and averages 5 hours in adults.
- The elimination half-life for O-desmethylvenlafaxine is 11 hours.
- Neither venlafaxine nor its metabolites are dialyzable.
- Venlafaxine and O-desmethylvenlafaxine are excreted in breast milk.
  ○ Concentrations are respectively 2.5 and 2.7 times higher in milk than in maternal plasma in breastfeeding women.
  ○ Although no adverse effects were observed in breastfed infants of mothers treated with venlafaxine, caution is recommended in the use of venlafaxine in breastfeeding women.

INDICATIONS

Venlafaxine is indicated in the treatment of adult depression, GAD, and social anxiety disorder. There are presently no approved indications for venlafaxine in pediatric psychopharmacology.

Possible indications
- Depression in pediatric age group.
- Anxiety disorders in pediatric age group.
- OCD in children and adults.
- Premenstrual dysphoric disorder in adolescents and adults.
- Neuropathic pain syndromes.

DOSING AND DURATION OF TREATMENT

Available drug preparations
- Tablets 25 mg, 37.5 mg, 50 mg, 75 mg, and 100 mg
- Extended-release capsules 37.5 mg, 75 mg, and 150 mg

Before initiating treatment
- Obtain a routine pediatric examination, including height, weight, blood pressure, and heart rate.
  ○ Venlafaxine may elevate blood pressure.

General dosing suggestions
Little published data on the use of venlafaxine in the pediatric age group is available to date. Thus the following dosing suggestions are largely extrapolated from the adult literature.

- Effective dose range of venlafaxine for depression is 75–225 mg/day.
- Initiate venlafaxine treatment at 75 mg/day and titrate upward by 75 mg into the therapeutic dose range, depending on individual patient tolerability and effectiveness.
  - Venlafaxine immediate-release tablets are given in two or three divided daily doses.
- Initiate the extended-release preparation at 75 mg once in the morning or evening. Titrate upward by 75 mg into the therapeutic dose range, depending on individual patient tolerability and effectiveness.

Medical Monitoring
- Periodic blood pressure and pulse monitoring while on drug is recommended.
  - Venlafaxine has been associated with increased blood pressure in adults.

Discontinuing venlafaxine treatment
When discontinuing venlafaxine after more than 1 week of therapy, it is recommended that the dose be tapered. Patients who have received venlafaxine for 6 weeks or more should have their dose tapered gradually over at least a 2-week period.

DRUG CONTRAINDICATIONS

Absolute contraindications
- Hypersensitivity to the agent
- Concurrent use of MAOI drugs. Do not use venlafaxine within 2 weeks of discontinuing an MAOI. Do not use an MAOI for at least 7 days after stopping venlafaxine.

Relative contraindications
- History of seizures
- History of mania/hypomania
- Sustained increases in blood pressure associated with venlafaxine
- Patients with recent myocardial infarction or unstable heart disease
- Renal impairment or cirrhosis of the liver (reduction in dose may be necessary)

DRUG SIDE EFFECTS

Venlafaxine is generally well tolerated.
- Common venlafaxine side effects
  - Abnormal ejaculation, anorgasmia, impotence
  - Anorexia, constipation, weight loss
  - Diarrhea, dyspepsia
  - Anxiety, dizziness, insomnia, nervousness, somnolence, tremor
  - Asthenia
  - Dry mouth, nausea, vomiting
  - Sweating, rash, blurred vision, mydriasis
- Uncommon but potentially serious venlafaxine side effects
  - Abnormal bleeding

   ○ Activation of mania/hypomania
   ○ Hepatitis
   ○ Hypertension
   ○ Hyponatremia
   ○ Seizures

DRUG–DRUG INTERACTIONS

Venlafaxine is a weak inhibitor of the CYP2D6 system and has few drug–drug interactions.

DRUG INTERFERENCE WITH LABORATORY TESTING

Venlafaxine has not been found to interfere with any known laboratory tests.

MANAGEMENT OF OVERDOSE

Somnolence is the most commonly observed overdose effect with venlafaxine. Other observed effects include seizures, tachycardia, hypotension, hypertension, diaphoresis, hyponatremia, and ventricular dysrhythmias (rarely). Of 14 pediatric cases of venlafaxine ingestion with doses ranging from 18.75 to 75 mg (2.1–5.5 mg/kg), only one patient developed minor effects (lethargy). Children ingesting 5.5 mg/kg or less are unlikely to develop significant clinical toxicity. Seizures have developed in adults after ingestion of 1.4 grams or more.

• Institute usual supportive care.
• Serum levels are generally not clinically useful in guiding patient management.
• Monitor for evidence of serotonin syndrome.
• There is no specific antidote to venlafaxine.

Duloxetine

Duloxetine is a recently released SNRI that affects reuptake of both serotonin and norepinephrine and lacks affinity for muscarinic and histaminergic receptors. Little pediatric experience to date has accrued with this agent. It is effective in the treatment of adult depression and for the management of peripheral pain of diabetic neuropathy.

PHARMACOLOGY

Pharmacodynamics
Duloxetine is a potent inhibitor of neuronal serotonin and norepinephrine reuptake and a less potent inhibitor of dopamine reuptake. It appears to have little affinity for dopaminergic, adrenergic, cholinergic, histaminergic, opioid, glutamate, and GABA receptors. Duloxetine does not inhibit monoamine oxidase. The antidepressant action and pain inhibitory actions of duloxetine are believed to be related to its potentiation of serotonergic and noradrenergic activity in the CNS.

PHARMACOKINETICS

Absorption
• Well absorbed after oral dosing.
• Maximum plasma concentration occurs 6 hours after oral administration.
• The presence of food and evening dosing (as contrasted with morning dosing) delay the time to maximal plasma concentration from 6 hours to 10 hours.

Distribution
• Highly (>90%) bound to proteins in human plasma, predominately binding to albumin and alpha-1-acid glycoprotein.

Metabolism and elimination
• Undergoes extensive metabolism involving both the CYP2D6 and CYP1A2 enzyme systems. Metabolites found in plasma include:
  ○ 4-hydroxy duloxetine glucuronide
  ○ 5-hydroxy duloxetine sulfate
  ○ 6-hydroxy duloxetine sulfate
• About 70% of oral dose appears as metabolites in urine; about 20% is excreted in feces.
• The elimination half-life in adults is between 11 and 16 hours.

INDICATIONS

Duloxetine is indicated in the treatment of adult depression and adult diabetic peripheral neuropathic pain. Duloxetine is not FDA approved at present for any pediatric psychopharmacological indication in children < 18 years old.

There are no randomized, controlled clinical trials of duloxetine in the pediatric age group at present.

DOSING AND DURATION OF TREATMENT

Available drug preparations
• Capsules 20 mg, 30 mg, and 60 mg

Before initiating treatment
• Obtain a routine pediatric examination, including height, weight, blood pressure, and heart rate.

General dosing suggestions
Duloxetine has not yet been studied in the pediatric age group. Thus these dosing suggestions are extrapolated from the adult literature.

• Effective dose range for adult depression is 40–60 mg/day.
  ○ No evidence that doses greater than 60 mg/day confer any additional benefits.
  ○ Generally given once daily or in two divided daily doses.
• The effective dose range for adult diabetic peripheral neuropathic pain is 60 mg given once daily.

ANTIDEPRESSANTS

• Initiate duloxetine at a low dose of 20 mg once daily and titrate upward by 20 mg until the therapeutic dose range is achieved, depending on individual patient tolerability and effectiveness of the drug.

Discontinuing duloxetine treatment

Withdrawal symptoms associated with abrupt duloxetine discontinuation have been reported. It is recommended that the dose of duloxetine be withdrawn gradually by 10–25% every 2–4 days until drug discontinuation.

DRUG CONTRAINDICATIONS

• Hypersensitivity to duloxetine
• Concomitant use in patients taking MAOIs. Do not use duloxetine within 14 days of discontinuing treatment with an MAOI. At least 5 days should be allowed after stopping duloxetine before initiating treatment with an MAOI.
• Narrow-angle glaucoma.
  ○ Duloxetine is associated with an increased risk of mydriasis; its use should be avoided in patients with uncontrolled narrow-angle glaucoma.

DRUG SIDE EFFECTS

• Common duloxetine side effects
  ○ Nausea, dry mouth, constipation, decreased appetite
  ○ Fatigue, somnolence
  ○ Increased sweating
  ○ Blurred vision
  ○ Insomnia
  ○ Sexual: decreased libido, abnormal orgasm, and erectile dysfunction in males

DRUG–DRUG INTERACTIONS

• Inhibitors of CYP1A2 and 2D6 will increase the plasma concentration of duloxetine; these agents include fluvoxamine, fluoxetine, and paroxetine.
• Duloxetine will increase the plasma concentrations of TCAs, phenothiazines, and type 1C antiarrhythmic agents.
  ○ Duloxetine and thioridazine should not be coadministered because of the potential for elevated thioridazine plasma levels and increased risk for prolonged cardiac QTc interval and arrhythmias.

DRUG INTERFERENCE WITH DIAGNOSTIC LABORATORY TESTS

Duloxetine has not been found to interfere with any known laboratory tests.

MANAGEMENT OF OVERDOSE

To date there is limited experience with duloxetine poisoning in adults and none in the pediatric age group. No cases of fatal duloxetine overdose have been reported.

- Institute usual supportive care.
- Serum levels are generally not clinically useful in guiding patient management.
- Monitor for evidence of serotonin syndrome.
- There is no specific antidote to duloxetine.

TRICYCLIC ANTIDEPRESSANTS

With the advent of SSRIs the use of tricyclic antidepressants (TCAs) in pediatric psychopharmacology has diminished. There exists ongoing clinical concern about the toxicity of TCAs, especially cardiac side effects in youngsters. Presently, there are eight reports of sudden death in children receiving desipramine (N = 6) or imipramine (N = 2) at therapeutic doses, generally in combination with other psychiatric agents (Green, 2001). These children were being treated for a variety of disorders, including anxiety, ADHD, conduct problems, and depression. Although not proven, cardiac arrhythmias are suspected in their deaths (Gundersen & Geller, 2003; Varley & McClellan, 1997). There also is concern about the potential lethality of TCAs if taken in overdose by depressed children and adolescents. As a result, clinical use of TCAs for depression in the pediatric age group has declined.

Despite these concerns, TCAs continue to be prescribed for children and adolescents for a variety of conditions. These include obsessive–compulsive disorder (OCD), major depressive disorder (MDD), attention-deficit/hyperactivity disorder (ADHD), anxiety disorders, and enuresis. The FDA has approved TCAs in the pediatric age group only for the treatment of OCD (clomipramine) and enuresis (imipramine). This section discusses imipramine, desipramine amitriptyline, nortriptyline, and clomipramine. After a discussion of each agent, a general discussion occurs concerning medical monitoring of TCAs, contraindications, side effects, drug–drug interactions, and management of TCA overdose.

Imipramine

PHARMACOLOGY

Imipramine is a tertiary amine tricyclic antidepressant.

Pharmacodynamics
Imipramine, like other tricyclic antidepressants, blocks the reuptake of norepinephrine and serotonin, preventing their degradation and increasing their availability. This results in a decreased turnover of these amines. Effects on the D1 dopamine receptor may also be important in the mediation of the drug's antidepressant activity. However, the relation of this effect to antidepressant activity has not been demonstrated. Evidence suggests that tertiary amines such as imipramine block the reuptake of serotonin more than the reuptake of norepinephrine.

Imipramine is beneficial in the treatment of enuresis. Its effects appear to be unrelated to changes in sleep architecture, the anticholinergic or antiadrenergic properties of imipramine, or effects on thyroid-releasing-hormone-induced urinary urgency. In patients with nocturnal polyuria, imipramine has a vaso-pressin-independent antidiuretic effect attributed primarily to increased tubular reabsorption of urea, and to a lesser extent, to decreased sodium and potassium excretion.

PHARMACOKINETICS

Absorption
• Imipramine is 94–96% absorbed after an oral dose.
• The bioavailability from tablet and from syrup formulations appears to be equivalent.
• Absorption is not affected by food.

Distribution
• 90% protein bound.
• At steady state, tissue concentrations are greatest in the lung followed by the brain, the adipose tissue, and plasma.
  ○ The pulmonary repository gives imipramine an exceedingly large volume of distribution and acts as a reservoir that increases the drug's time to elimination.

Metabolism and excretion
• First-pass metabolism occurs with extensive metabolism to conjugated and nonconjugated metabolites.
  ○ The N-demethylation of imipramine is under pharmacogenic control of CYP2C19.
  ○ The N-desmethyl metabolite of imipramine is desipramine and is pharmaco-logically active.
  ○ The desipramine-to-imipramine ratio in plasma exists in a wide range between 0.3 to 15.0
  ○ Other imipramine metabolites include
    ▪ 2-hydroxy imipramine (pharmacologically active)
    ▪ 2-hydroxydesipramine (active)
    ▪ The serum concentration of the hydroxy metabolites may have some rela-tionship to imipramine's toxicity.
• The amount of imipramine or desipramine in breast milk is small; no reports of adverse events with nursing infants.
• The elimination half-life of imipramine in children ranges from 6 to 15 hours.
• Imipramine is not dialyzable.

INDICATIONS

Imipramine is labeled for the treatment of adult depression and enuresis in children.

Possible indications
• Panic disorder in adults and children
• Urinary incontinence

- Anxiety disorders in the pediatric age group, such as separation anxiety and school refusal
- Depression in the pediatric age group
- ADHD in the pediatric age group and in adults

Controlled studies of imipramine for depression in children and adolescents appear in Table 5.2. Controlled studies for other indications, such as ADHD or anxiety, are discussed in their respective chapters.

DOSING AND DURATION OF TREATMENT

Available drug preparations
- Solution for injection: 12.5 mg/1 mL
- Tablets 10 mg, 25 mg, 50 mg, and 75 mg
- Capsules for once-daily dosing: 75 mg, 100 mg, 125 mg, and 150 mg

Before initiating treatment
Imipramine is associated with many potential adverse cardiovascular effects. A medical work-up is required before drug initiation.

- Screen patients for a medical history and a family medical history of cardiovascular disease, including syncope, prolonged QTc syndromes, and history of cardiac arrhythmias. Patients with a significant cardiovascular history, or whose families have a history of early cardiovascular disease, may not be candidates for a trial of imipramine.
- Obtain a routine pediatric examination, including height, weight, blood pressure, and heart rate.
- A nonclinically significant baseline EKG is required before imipramine can be prescribed.
  - Do not administer in patients with a QTc > 500.
  - Caution is advised in patients with a QTc > 450.

GENERAL DOSING SUGGESTIONS

ADHD
- The dose range for ADHD is between 1.5 mg/kg/day and 5 mg/kg/day.
- There is no relationship between imipramine (plus desipramine) plasma levels and response in ADHD.
- Imipramine is generally given on a tid dosing schedule to young children and a bid dosing schedule to early adolescents.
  - In adults imipramine can be prescribed once daily.

DEPRESSION
- In children the initial starting dose is 1.5 mg/kg/day given in 1–4 divided doses, with dose increases of 1 mg/kg every 3–4 days.
- The daily dose should not exceed 5 mg/kg/day, and children receiving doses of 3.5 mg/kg/day or more should be closely monitored.
- Adolescents should initially receive 30–40 mg/day.

- Doses exceeding 100 mg/day are generally not necessary.
- Imipramine plus desipramine trough serum levels between 125 and 250 ng/ml may correlate with improvement in pediatric and adult depression (Preskorn et al., 1989).

ENURESIS
- Children age 6 and over should initially receive 25 mg orally, 1 hour before bedtime.
- If satisfactory response does not occur within 1 week, the dose may be increased by 25 mg/day.
  - The dose range in enuresis is 2.5 mg/kg/day.
- Children under 12 may receive a maximum daily dose of 50 mg.
- Children over 12 may receive a maximum dose between 75 and 100 mg.
- Imipramine plus desipramine serum levels of around 80 ng/ml have been reported therapeutic in enuresis (DeGatta et al., 1984).

Discontinuing imipramine treatment
Imipramine is known to have a discontinuation syndrome upon abrupt medication withdrawal. A gradual taper by 10–25% of the full dose every 3–4 days is recommended

Desipramine

Desipramine is a secondary amine and active metabolite of imipramine; it is used as an antidepressant.

PHARMACOLOGY

Desipramine is a tricyclic antidepressant.

PHARMACODYNAMICS

Desipramine, like other tricyclic antidepressants, blocks the reuptake of norepinephrine and 5-hydroxy-tryptamine, preventing their degradation and increasing their availability. Evidence suggests that secondary amines such as desipramine block the reuptake of norepinephrine more than the reuptake of serotonin.

PHARMACOKINETICS

Absorption
- Rapidly absorbed from the gastrointestinal tract.

Distribution
- Highly distributed and concentrates in lung, brain, and serum.

Metabolism and excretion
- Metabolized in the liver, and approximately 70% is excreted in the urine.
- Extensive first-pass hepatic metabolism occurs.
- There is one active metabolite, 2-hydroxydesipramine.
- The average elimination half-life in adults is 17 hours.
  - "Slow" metabolizers may have a half-life of up to 77 hours.

- Up to a 36-fold difference in desipramine plasma level may be noted among individuals taking the same oral dose.
- Concentrations of desipramine found in maternal breast milk are approximately equal to those in serum.
  - Withdrawal symptoms have been reported in newborns exposed to desipramine in utero.
  - Neonatal withdrawal symptoms have been reported to include colic, cyanosis, rapid breathing, and irritability.

INDICATIONS

Desipramine is indicated in the treatment of adult depression. Safety and efficacy in the pediatric age group have not been established.

Possible indications
- ADHD in children, adolescents, and adults.
- Enuresis in children.

Table 5.2 lists controlled studies of desipramine in pediatric depression. Controlled studies for other indications, such as ADHD, appear in the respective chapter.

DOSING AND DURATION OF TREATMENT

Available drug preparations
- Tablets 10 mg, 25 mg, 50 mg, 75 mg, 100 mg, and 150 mg

Before initiating treatment
- Screen patients for a medical history and a family medical history of cardiovascular disease, including syncope, prolonged QTc syndromes, and history of cardiac arrhythmias. Patients with a significant cardiovascular history, or whose families have a history of early cardiovascular disease, may not be candidates for a trial.
- Obtain a routine pediatric examination, including height, weight, blood pressure, and heart rate.
- A nonclinically significant baseline EKG is required before desipramine can be prescribed.
  - Do not administer in patients with a QTc > 500.
  - Caution is advised in patients with a QTc > 450.

GENERAL DOSING SUGGESTIONS

ADHD
Although desipramine is not labeled by the FDA for the treatment of ADHD, it has been studied and found to be effective in this condition.

- The dose range in ADHD is between 2–5 mg/kg/day.
- Serum desipramine levels do not correlate with clinical response in ADHD.

ANTIDEPRESSANTS

- Desipramine is generally given on a tid dosing schedule to children and a bid dosing schedule to adolescents with ADHD.
- Initiate dosing at 25 mg/day and titrate by 25–50 mg weekly, according to clinical response.
  - A dose of 150 mg/day should not be exceeded.

DEPRESSION
- For children 6- to 12 years old: the dose range is between 1–3 mg/kg/day given in three divided daily doses.
  - The maximum desipramine dose is 5 mg/kg/day.
- For adolescents: the dose range is 25–150 mg given in two divided daily doses.
  - The therapeutic plasma range in depression is 100–300 ng/ml.

ENURESIS
- Desipramine 50–75 mg/day has been found effective in the short-term treatment of enuresis in children.

Discontinuing desipramine treatment
Desipramine is known to have a discontinuation syndrome upon abrupt medication withdrawal. A gradual taper by 10–25% of the full dose every 3–4 days is recommended.

Amitriptyline

PHARMACOLOGY

Amitriptyline is a tertiary amine tricyclic antidepressant.

PHARMACODYNAMICS

Amitriptyline blocks the reuptake of norepinephrine and serotonin in the CNS. Evidence suggests that tertiary amines such as amitriptyline block the reuptake of serotonin more than the reuptake of norepinephrine.

PHARMACOKINETICS

Absorption
- Readily absorbed after oral dosing.
- Absorption is not affected by food.

Distribution
- 90% protein bound.
- At steady state, tissue concentrations are greatest in the lung, followed by the brain, the adipose tissue, and plasma.
  - The pulmonary repository gives amitriptyline an exceedingly large volume of distribution and acts as a reservoir that increases time to elimination.

Metabolism and excretion
- First-pass metabolism occurs with extensive metabolism to conjugated and nonconjugated metabolites.

○ The N-demethylation of amitriptyline is under pharmacogenic control of CYP2C19.
○ The N-desmethyl metabolite of amitriptyline is nortriptyline and is pharmacologically active.
• The serum half-life of amitriptyline in adults is around 24 hours.

INDICATIONS

Amitriptyline is labeled for the treatment of depression in children $\geq$ 12 years old and in adults.

Possible indications
• Migraine headache in adults and children.
• Polyneuropathic pain in adults.

Controlled studies of amitriptyline for depression in children and adolescents appear in Table 5.2.

DOSING AND DURATION OF TREATMENT

Available drug preparations
• Tablets 10 mg, 25 mg, 50 mg, 75 mg, 100 mg, and 150 mg
• Injectable: 10 mg/1 mL

Before initiating treatment
• Screen patients for a medical history and a family medical history of cardiovascular disease, including syncope, prolonged QTc syndromes, and history of cardiac arrhythmias. Patients with a significant cardiovascular history, or whose families have a history of early cardiovascular disease, may not be candidates for a trial.
• Obtain a routine pediatric examination, including height, weight, blood pressure, and heart rate.
• A nonclinically significant baseline EKG is required before amitriptyline can be prescribed.
○ Do not administer in patients with a QTc > 500.
○ Caution is advised in patients with a QTc > 450.

GENERAL DOSING SUGGESTIONS

Depression
• For the treatment of depression in children, the initial starting dose is 25 mg/day. The dose may be titrated upward by 25 mg every 3–5 days, as tolerated. The usual dose range is 50–100 mg/day.
○ Smaller children may begin amitriptyline at 10 mg/day.
• Generally given in three divided doses to young children and two divided doses to adolescents.

Discontinuing amitriptyline treatment

Amitriptyline is known to have a discontinuation syndrome upon abrupt medication withdrawal. A gradual taper by 10–25% of the full dose every 3–4 days is recommended.

Nortriptyline

PHARMACOLOGY

Nortriptyline is a secondary amine tricyclic antidepressant.

PHARMACODYNAMICS

Nortriptyline, like other tricyclic antidepressants, blocks the reuptake of norepinephrine and 5-hydroxy-tryptamine, preventing their degradation and increasing their availability. This results in a decreased turnover of these amines, but the relation of this effect to antidepressant activity has not been demonstrated. Secondary amines such as nortriptyline appear to block the reuptake of norepinephrine more than the reuptake of serotonin.

PHARMACOKINETICS

Absorption
• 60% absorbed after an oral dose.

Distribution
• Very highly protein bound, 86–95%.

Metabolism and excretion
• Undergoes extensive first-pass metabolism.
• Has three active metabolites:
  ○ 10-hydroxynortriptyline has similar therapeutic effects but only half the potency and is less anticholinergic and less cardiotoxic than the parent compound.
  ○ E-10-hydroxynortriptyline has equal potency to nortriptyline.
  ○ Z-10-hydroxynortriptyline has equal potency to nortriptyline.
• Breastfed infants do not have measurable serum levels of nortriptyline, nor do they display any adverse reactions.

INDICATIONS

Nortriptyline is approved by the FDA for the treatment of depression in adults.

Possible indications
• Postherpetic neuralgia in adults
• ADHD in children, adolescents, and adults
• Nocturnal enuresis

Recent controlled studies of nortriptyline in pediatric depression appear in Table 5.2.

DOSING AND DURATION OF TREATMENT

Available drug preparations
• Capsules 10 mg, 25 mg, 50 mg, and 75 mg
• Oral solution 10 mg/5ml

Before initiating treatment
• Screen patients for a medical history and a family medical history of cardiovascular disease, including syncope, prolonged QTc syndromes, and history
  of cardiac arrhythmias. Patients with a significant cardiovascular history, or
  whose families have a history of early cardiovascular disease, may not be candidates for a trial of nortriptyline.
• Obtain a routine pediatric examination, including height, weight, blood pressure, and heart rate.
• A nonclinically significant baseline EKG is required before nortriptyline can
  be prescribed.
  ◦ Do not administer in patients with a QTc > 500.
  ◦ Caution is advised in patients with a QTc > 450.

General dosing suggestions
Although nortriptyline is not recommended for use in children, several authors
have provided dosing guidelines for pediatric patients (Geller et al., 1985). The
recommended dose in adolescent patients is 30–50 mg/day in divided doses.
The total daily dose may be given once daily. Plasma concentrations in the
range of 50–150 ng/mL are considered therapeutic for depression in adolescents and adults.

  Single-dose pharmacokinetics of nortriptyline can be used to predict steady-
state plasma levels and to suggest doses for depressed pediatric patients
(Geller et al., 1985). Patients 5 to 9 years old ($n = 11$) received a single oral
dose of 25 mg; patients 10 to 16 years old received a single dose of 50 mg. Nortriptyline levels were measured 24 hours after dosing. Based on these results,
the following pediatric dose guidelines are suggested:

Predicted doses from 24-hour nortriptyline plasma levels after a
single dose of 25 mg administered to 5- to 9-year-olds

24-hour plasma level (ng/mL)	Suggested total daily dose (mg)*
6–10	50–75
11–14	35–40
15–20	25–30
21–25	20

Predicted doses from 24-hour nortriptyline plasma levels after a single dose of 50 mg administered to 10- to 16-year-olds

24-hour plasma level (ng/mL)	Suggested total daily dose* (mg)
10–14	75–100
15–19	50–75
20–24	40–50
25–29	35
30–34	30
35–40	25
Over 40	20

*Note: The total daily dose should be divided and given twice daily.

NOCTURNAL ENURESIS
Suggested doses for the treatment of nocturnal enuresis in children are as follows:

Age (yrs)	Weight (kg)	Daily Dose (mg)
6–7	20–25	10
8–11	25–35	10–20
Over 11	35–54	25–35

The dose should be administered one-half hour before bedtime. Treatment should not generally continue for more than 3 months.

Discontinuing nortriptyline treatment
Nortriptyline is known to have a discontinuation syndrome upon abrupt medication withdrawal. A gradual taper off nortriptyline by 10–25% of the full dose every 3–4 days is recommended.

Clomipramine

Clomipramine is a tricyclic antidepressant that has demonstrated efficacy in the treatment of OCD.

PHARMACOLOGY

Clomipramine, like other tricyclic antidepressants, blocks the reuptake of norepinephrine and 5-hydroxy-tryptamine, preventing their degradation and increasing their availability. Clomipramine is a potent inhibitor of the reuptake of serotonin as compared to the reuptake of norepinephrine. However, the primary metabolite, desmethylclomipramine, primarily inhibits the reuptake of norepinephrine.

PHARMACODYNAMICS

The drug is classified as a tertiary amine tricyclic antidepressant with very potent inhibition of serotonin uptake. The therapeutic effects of clomipramine in OCD are mediated via serotonergic mechanisms.

PHARMACOKINETICS

Absorption
• Absorption is highly variable and can range from 20% to 78%.
• Food does not affect absorption.
• Grapefruit juice has been shown to inhibit CYP3A4, causing an increase in the concentrations of drugs that require CYP3A4 for metabolism. This inhibition can result in an increased risk of clomipramine toxicity.

Distribution
• Highly protein bound.

Metabolism and excretion
• Several different cytochrome P-450 pathways metabolize clomipramine, including CYP1A2, 3A4, and 2D6.
• Undergoes extensive first pass metabolism.
• Has two metabolites, 8-OH clomipramine and 8-OH desmethylclomipramine.
  ○ Desmethylclomipramine is an active metabolite.
  ○ OCD responders have a trend toward lower plasma clomipramine to desmethylclomipramine ratios.
• The elimination half-life of clomipramine is 19–37 hours (mean, 32 hours).
• Its half-life may be lengthened at higher doses (200–250 mg/day).

INDICATIONS

Clomipramine is labeled by the FDA for the treatment of OCD in children 10 years and older, and in adults.

Possible indications
• Depression in adolescents and adults
• Anxiety disorders in adolescents and adults
• ADHD in children, adolescents, and adults

Recent studies of clomipramine for the treatment of OCD are discussed in the chapter on OCD.

DOSING AND DURATION OF TREATMENT

Available drug preparations
• Capsules 25 mg, 50 mg, and 75 mg

ANTIDEPRESSANTS

Before initiating treatment
- Screen patients for a medical history and a family medical history of cardiovascular disease, including syncope, prolonged QTc syndromes, and history of cardiac arrhythmias. Patients with a significant cardiovascular history, or whose families have a history of early cardiovascular disease, may not be candidates.
- Obtain a routine pediatric examination, including height, weight, blood pressure, and heart rate.
- A nonclinically significant baseline EKG is required before clomipramine can be prescribed.
  - Do not administer in patients with a QTc > 500.
  - Caution is advised in patients with a QTc > 450.

General Dosing Suggestions
- Clomipramine is sedating; give the larger portion of the daily dose at bedtime.
- In older adolescents and adults, a single dose at bedtime may be sufficient.

OCD (10 yrs. and older)
- Initiate clomipramine at a dose of 25 mg at bedtime. Titrate the dose upward every 5–7 days to a daily maximum of 100 mg or 3 mg/kg/day, whichever is less, over the first 2 weeks. Subsequently, the dose may be increased gradually to a maximum of 200 mg/day or 3 mg/kg/day, whichever is less.
- Serum levels have not been established in OCD. However, some evidence suggests that levels of 100–250 ng/mL (clomipramine) plus 230 to 550 ng/mL (desmethylclomipramine) may be effective in OCD.

TCA medical monitoring
Tricyclic antidepressants are associated with increased risk for cardiovascular side effects. As mentioned previously, there are reports of eight children who died abruptly while receiving desipramine and imipramine at therapeutic (nontoxic) doses. These cases are all complicated by other factors, such as the concomitant medicines that these children were receiving. However, most pediatric psychopharmacologists believe that cardiac arrhythmias, possibly caused or exacerbated by TCA use, was a cause in their deaths (Green, 2001). As such, the clinical use of TCAs requires careful monitoring of cardiovascular functioning. A discussion of the EKG and normal blood pressure parameters appears in the Appendix 3. The following table presents parameters suggested as guidelines for cardiovascular monitoring in children and adolescents receiving TCAs. Children prescribed TCAs, whose vital signs and EKG parameters exceed these thresholds, should have their dose reduced or drug discontinued, with careful medical follow-up to assess safety.

TCA CONTRAINDICATIONS

The following are contraindications to the use of TCAs.

Absolute contraindications
- Concomitant use of MAOIs

Table 5.6 Guidelines for Cardiovascular Parameters in Children and Adolescents Treated With Tricyclic Antidepressants

Cardiovascular Parameter	Children	Adolescents
Heart rate	≤ 130 beats per minute	≤ 120 beats per minute
Systolic blood pressure	≤ 120 mmHg	≤ 140 mmHg
Diastolic blood pressure	≤ 80 mmHg	≤ 90 mmHg
EKG PR interval	< 200 msec	< 200 msec
EKG QRS interval	≤ 120 msec	≤ 120 msec
EKG QTc interval	≤ 460 msec	≤ 460 msec

- Hypersensitivity to TCAs
- Use in patients during acute recovery after a myocardial infarction

Relative contraindications
- Cardiovascular disease, including prolonged QTc syndromes, recurrent syncope, or arrhythmias
- History of urinary retention
- Hyperthyroidism
- History of mania/hypomania
- Increased intraocular pressure
- Narrow-angle glaucoma
- Renal or hepatic function impairment
- Seizure disorder
- Sulfite hypersensitivity (injectable forms only)

TCA SIDE EFFECTS

TCAs are known to have many side effects. The following table presents TCA side effects.

Table 5.7 Tricyclic Antidepressant Side Effects

Common
- Cardiac: tachycardia, postural hypotension, palpitations
- Gastrointestinal: constipation, nausea, dry mouth, vomiting
- CNS: fatigue, somnolence, dizziness, headache
- Ocular: blurred vision
- Genitourinary: urinary retention

Uncommon but potentially serious
- Cardiac: arrhythmias, syncope, QTc prolongation, QRS prolongation, sudden death
- Seizures
- Hematological: neutropenia, agranulocytosis, thrombocytopenia
- Gastrointestinal: jaundice

TCA Drug–Drug Interactions

TCAs have many potential drug-drug interactions. Some of these interactions are presented in the following table.

ANTIDEPRESSANTS

Table 5.8 Tricyclic Antidepressant Drug–Drug Interactions TCAs interact with:

Drug	Interaction
Alcohol	↑ Sedation and hypotension
Bupropion	↑ Risk of lowering the seizure threshold
Carbamazepine	↓ TCA plasma levels
Cimetidine	↑ TCA toxicity
Clonidine	↓ Hypotensive effects of clonidine
MAOIs	↑ Risk of hypertensive crisis
Neuroleptics	↑ TCA toxicity
Oral contraceptives	↑ TCA toxicity
Phenothiazines	↑ TCA toxicity
Quinidine	Bradycardia, palpitations
SSRIs	↑ TCA toxicity

DRUG INTERFERENCE WITH LABORATORY TESTING

TCAs have not been found to interfere with any known laboratory tests.

TCA OVERDOSE

TCAs can be fatal in overdose. In the United States TCAs accounted for over 13,000 poisonings in 2000, and they were the second largest category of drugs causing death by overdose (Shader, 2003, p. 32). Because of its noradrenergic potency, desipramine may be associated with greater risk of fatal outcome in poisoning than other TCAs. However, all TCAs carry this concern. Common signs of TCA overdose include CNS depression, seizures, hypotension, and cardiac dysrhythmias (potentially fatal). Cardiac dysrhythmias most commonly result from sodium channel blockade with widening of the QRS complex seen on EKG. Dysrhythmias are rate dependent and are more likely to occur with tachycardia. Therefore, patients with tachycardia after TCA overdose should not be considered medically stable. QTc interval prolongation because of potassium depletion may also occur with TCA overdose. Anticholinergic delirium may develop. Toxicity generally develops within 6 hours of overdose. In contrast to overdose with nontricyclic antidepressants, serum levels are very useful clinically in guiding patient management in TCA overdose. This is because EKG abnormalities and the potential for cardiovascular arrhythmias correlate with TCA serum levels. Management of TCA overdose includes the following.

• TCA overdoses are assumed to be life threatening.
• Range of toxicity:
  ○ Moderate to serious: 10–20 mg/kg; 15 mg/kg may be fatal in children.
• Monitor vital signs following overdose.
• Hypotension and bradycardia have been reported.
• Monitor fluid and electrolyte status in symptomatic patients.
• Cardiac monitoring is necessary and required.
• Monitor for seizures and changes in mental status changes.

- Administer activated charcoal and gastric lavage.
  ○ Use of Ipecac is contraindicated.
- Other: rhabdomyolysis, renal failure, ARDS, and/or acidosis may complicate severe TCA overdose.

Treatment includes consideration of the following:

- Seizure: Consider the use of IV benzodiazepines or barbiturates.
- The airway must be protected.
- Drug interactions: Avoid the use of flumazenil, procainamide, physostigmine, quinidine, and disopyramide.
  ○ These agents may increase EKG QRS widening, QTc interval prolongation, and/or cardiac conduction disturbances.
- Monitor the patient with serial ECGs, continuous cardiac monitoring, arterial blood gas measurement, and serial mental status examinations.

MONOAMINE OXIDASE INHIBITORS

Monoamine oxidase inhibitors (MAOIs) are primarily used to treat adults with depression that is unresponsive to antidepressant drugs of other classes. There is almost no clinical use of MAOIs in child psychiatry at present because of concerns about the potential toxicity of this class of drugs if strict dietary guidelines are not followed.

There are two forms of monoamine oxidase (MAO), which have different substrate specificity. Type A MAO deaminates norepinephrine, serotonin, and normetanephrine; type B MAO deactivates dopamine and phenylethylamine. MAOIs irreversibly poison the MAO enzyme, preventing MAO deactivation of monoamines. When MAO is deactivated, the patient must follow a tyramine-free diet. Failure to adhere to the diet can result in severe and life-threatening hypertension. The diet must be followed for up to 2 weeks after MAOI discontinuation in order to allow the synthesis of new MAO enzyme in the body. MAOIs have many drug–drug interactions, including severe ones with TCAs. A 2-week washout period after discontinuing a MAOI and before initiating treatment with a TCA is crucial. It is also contraindicated to add a TCA to an ongoing MAOI treatment, because a hypertensive crisis may result. Emergent treatment with chlorpromazine 25 mg may temporarily treat tyramine dietary-induced hypertension while medical treatment is sought.

MAOI drugs presently approved by the FDA include phenelzine (Nardil®), which is approved for use in adolescents at least 16 years old, and tranylcypromine (Parnate®), which has been approved for use in depression only for adults. Phenelzine and tranylcypromine both inhibit MAO-A and MAO-B (mixed function inhibitors). L-deprenyl (Eldepryl®) and selegiline (at low dose) are MAOIs that are specific for MAO-B. At higher doses selegiline becomes nonspecific in its MAO substrate. Clorgyline is an MAOI that is specific for MAO-A.

Use of MAOIs is presently not recommended in pediatric psychopharmacolgy and is not further discussed here.

FUTURE ANTIDEPRESSANTS IN PEDIATRIC PSYCHOPHARMACOLOGY?

There are several antidepressants that are presently unavailable for clinical use in the United States that are of potential future interest in pediatric psychopharmacology. These agents include reversible inhibitors of MAO-A (RIMAs) and selective norepinephrine reuptake inhibitors. These agents have been used in Europe for several years, largely for depression in adults. At present none of these agents is indicated for use in pediatric psychopharmacology but may become more important in the future.

Meclobemide

Meclobemide is the prototypical RIMA and has been effective for adult depression in international controlled trials (Walkup et al., 2003). As a reversible inhibitor of MAO-A, it does not require the tyramine-free dietary restrictions that clinical uses of irreversible MAOIs require. Currently, moclobemide is not available in the United States.

Reboxetine

Reboxetine represents a novel class of antidepressant; the selective noradrenergic reuptake inhibitors (NRIs). Reboxetine has been available in Europe since 1997 for the treatment of adult depression. It achieves its antidepressant effects through selective inhibition of norepinephrine reuptake. This agent shows little or no affinity for muscarinic, histaminergic, alpha-1-adrenergic, serotonin, or dopaminergic receptors. Reboxetine is well absorbed after oral dosing and reaches peak plasma levels within 2.5 hours. The half-life ranges between 12 and 16 hours in adults. Reboxetine is metabolized via the CYP3A4 system and is a weak competitive inhibitor of the CYP2D6 and CYP3A4 systems. As such, reboxetine demonstrates little drug–drug interactions. There are no data at present supporting the use of reboxetine in children and adolescents. However, given its noradrenergic profile, it may have potential uses in ADHD, depression, and anxiety (Walkup et al., 2003). Currently, reboxetine is unavailable in the United States.

CLINICAL USE OF ANTIDEPRESSANTS IN CHILDREN AND ADOLESCENTS

Duration of Treatment

Depression and anxiety disorders have a high rate of relapse across an individual's lifespan. For an episode of depression or anxiety it is now recommended that if a patient responds to antidepressant treatment, medication should be continued for an additional 9–12 months to prevent relapse of the index episode. Premature discontinuation of antidepressant therapy is associated with high rates of relapse in mood disorders (AACAP, 1998; Emslie et al., 2004).

Early-onset depression or anxiety disorders in the pediatric years may be associated with a worse prognosis and more discrete illness episodes across the patient's lifespan than mood disorders that first appear in the adult years. As such, robust treatment for pediatric mood disorders is recommended. After a successful course of antidepressant treatment, patients should be periodically reassessed to determine the need for continued treatment.

Medical Monitoring for Increased Suicidality

In October 2004 the FDA issued a black box warning for all antidepressants used in the pediatric age range. There are concerns that antidepressant use can exacerbate suicidal thinking and behaviors in certain vulnerable children and adolescents who are treated with these agents. The FDA warning emphasizes the need for careful clinical monitoring of young patients receiving antidepressants. The prescribing clinician should assess for worsening of depression or suicidality, especially at the initiation of therapy or when the dose is increased or decreased. Patients who experience symptoms of anxiety, agitation, disinhibition, panic attacks, insomnia, irritability, hostility, impulsivity, akathisia, hypomania, or mania may be at an increased risk for worsening depression or suicidality. If these symptoms are observed, therapy should be reevaluated. It may be necessary to discontinue medications when symptoms are severe, sudden in onset, or were not part of the patient's initial symptoms. The FDA recommends that after antidepressant initiation the patient should be evaluated at weekly intervals for the first 4 weeks, then monitored every other week for the second 4 weeks, and then assessed every 3 months while on the drug, as necessary.

Lack of Response to Initial Antidepressant Treatment

When starting antidepressant therapy, a low initial dose will minimize adverse effects; the dose should then be increased until an adequate response is achieved. Gradual introduction of treatment is of particular importance in the very young, as they may be more susceptible to adverse effects (AACAP, 1998). There is generally a delay of about 2 weeks before any therapeutic benefit is observed, and at least 6–8 weeks before maximum improvement in depressive symptoms occurs. The delay in onset of antidepressant effect may relate to a combination of pharmacokinetic and neurochemical factors. The onset of action is similar with all currently available antidepressants; none has been shown definitively to work faster than any other. Patients should not be considered nonresponders to the chosen antidepressant medication until they have been maintained at an adequate dose for at least 12 weeks. Patients with a partial response at 12 weeks should continue for a further 2 weeks before being considered nonresponders. Treatment failure is often due to subtherapeutic dosing strategies. Where lack of compliance is thought to be responsible for subtherapeutic doses, therapeutic serum drug monitoring (where available) may be helpful.

In those who show little or no response to an adequate trial of the first-choice antidepressant, two strategies exist: either switching to another antidepressant or adding another drug (augmentation) (AACAP, 1998; Birmaher &

Brent, 2003). An SSRI should be the initial treatment for pediatric depression. If no response occurs with adequate dosing after an adequate duration, recommendations are to switch to a second SSRI. Monotherapy with an antidepressant of a different chemical class, such as bupropion, mirtazapine, or venlafaxine, is then suggested.

Antidepressant augmentation strategies may be considered next (Birmaher & Brent, 2003). Medications that have been used in augmentation strategies include lithium and thyroid hormone. Another method is to combine different classes of antidepressants. Although this has been used successfully in the treatment of drug-resistant depression, it may result in enhanced adverse reactions or interactions and is therefore considered controversial and should only be used under expert consultation.

6. Mood Stabilizers

The mood stabilizers include lithium, anticonvulsants, and atypical antipsychotic medications. This chapter discusses mood stabilizers in pediatric psychopharmacology primarily for the treatment of early-onset bipolar disorders. The chapter on conduct disorder and aggression discusses mood stabilizers in the treatment of explosive aggression. Atypical antipsychotics are only briefly mentioned in this chapter. A more complete discussion of these agents is found in the chapter on antipsychotics. Among the mood stabilizing drugs used in psychiatry, this chapter discusses lithium, divalproex, carbamazepine, and lamotrigine. Newer anticonvulsants such as oxcarbazepine, gabapentin, and topiramate are only briefly discussed. There are very few studies of the treatment of children and adolescents with early-onset bipolar disorder. The strongest evidence of antimanic action in this age group is for lithium, divalproex, and recently for olanzapine and adjunctive risperidone. Evidence on new antiepileptics and other novel treatments is very limited or nonexistent in pediatric psychopharmacology.

No single definition of mood stabilizer is agreed upon, and, in fact, the Food and Drug Administration (FDA) does not recognize the term. Ideally, a mood stabilizer should do the following:

• Treat both the depressive and manic phases of acute bipolar illness.
• Prevent recurrence of both depressive and manic phases without worsening other phases of the illness.

No one compound accomplishes all of this, and it is for this reason that the average adult and child patient with bipolar illness receives multiple medications.

Bipolar disorder is very difficult to recognize and diagnose in youth because it often does not present with the same symptom criteria established for adults. Children are more likely to have a chronic course, with mixed symptoms of depression and mania simultaneously overlapping, and often cycling daily from silly, giddy, and amusing highs to depressed lows with suicidal ideation and behaviors.

Table 6.1 Recent Studies of Mood Stabilizers in Pediatric Bipolar Disorder

Study	Medication	Methodology	Age	Duration (weeks)	Dose/Average Serum Level	Outcome
Delbello et al., 2002	Divalproex + quetiapine add-on	RCT	Adolescents	6	DVP = 102 μg/L; quetiapine = 50–450 mg	DVP + quetiapine > DVP + placebo
Findling et al., 2003	Lithium + DVP	Open	Children and adolescents	20	DVP = 79.8 μg/L; Li = 0.9 mEq/L	Combination safe and effective
Geller et al., 1998	Lithium	RCT	Adolescents	6	0.9 mEq/L	Effective
Kafantaris et al., 2004	Lithium	RCT discontinuation trial	Adolescents	2	0.99 mEq/L	Li not effective
Kowatch et al., 2000	Lithium, DVP, carbamazepine	Open with random assignment	Children and adolescents	6	Li = 0.8–1.2 mEq/L; DVP = 85–110 μg/L; CBZ = 7–10 μg/L	ES[a] Li = 1.06; DVP = 1.63; CBZ = 1.0

RCT = randomized controlled trial; DVP = divalproex; Li = lithium; CBZ = carbamazepine.
[a]ES: effect size

Table 6.2 Mood Stabilizers for Bipolar Children and Adolescents

Generic Name	U.S.Trade Name	How Supplied (mg)	Starting Dose (outpatients)	Target Dose	Serum Level	Therapeutic Cautions
Carbamazepine Carbamazepine XR	Tegretol Tegretol XR	100, 200 100, 200, 400	7 mg/kg/day 2–3 daily doses	Based on response and serum levels	8.9–11 mg/L	Monitor for CYP drug interactions
Lithium Lithium Lithium	Lithobid Eskalith Cibalith-S	300 (and 150 generic) 300 or 450 CR Lithium 5cc = 300 mg	25 mg/kg/day 2–3 daily doses	30 mg/kg/day 2–3 daily doses	0.8–1.2 mEq/L	Monitor for hypothyroidism; avoid during pregnancy
Oxcarbazepine	Trileptal	150, 300, 600	150 mg bid	20–29 kg (900 mg/day) 30–39 kg (1,200 mg/day) > 39 kg (1,800 mg/day)	N/A	Monitor for hyponatremia
Valproic acid Divalproex sodium	Depakene Depakote DR Depakote ER	250 syrup 125, 250, 500 250, 500	15 mg/kg/day 2–3 daily doses	20 mg/kg/day 2–3 daily dose	50–120 mg/L	Monitor liver functions and for pancreatitis; avoid during pregnancy

MOOD STABILIZERS

Symptoms of bipolar disorder in the pediatric population can resemble, or co-occur with, those of other common childhood-onset mental disorders, such as ADHD and major depression. In addition, symptoms of bipolar disorder may be initially mistaken for normal emotions and behaviors of children and adolescents. But unlike normal mood changes, bipolar disorder significantly impairs functioning in school, with peers, and at home with family. As a result of recent advances, children can now be diagnosed with bipolar disorder before puberty. However, no medications are as yet approved by the FDA for mania in the pediatric age group.

Once the diagnosis of bipolar disorder (BPD) is made, the treatment of children and adolescents is based mainly on experience with adults, since there is very limited data on the efficacy and safety of mood stabilizing medications in youth (McClellan & Werry, 1997). The essential treatment for this disorder in adults involves the use of appropriate doses of mood stabilizers, most typically lithium and/or valproate, which are often very effective for controlling mania and preventing recurrences of manic and depressive episodes. Anticonvulsants with the best evidence for mood stabilization are divalproex, through its enhancement of GABA, and lamotrigine, through its blockade of glutamate release. Other anticonvulsants appear to have efficacy in BPD, particularly carbamazepine (CBZ), which is mechanistically similar to lamotrigine and valproate (VPA). However, several anticonvulsants do not appear to have much of a role in BPD, particularly gabapentin and topiramate. It is noteworthy that these two agents act via a mechanism of action that is different from divalproex, carbamazepine, or lamotrigine. The difference in mechanisms may help explain the different therapeutic profile of each medicine in treating bipolar illness.

Research on the effectiveness of these and other medications in children and adolescents with bipolar disorder is sparse, yet ongoing. Like most medications used in pediatric psychopharmacology, use of these agents outpaces their evidence base for effectiveness and safety in children and adolescents. The use of these agents remains largely "off label" and is not approved by the FDA in pediatric psychopharmacology.

LITHIUM

Lithium is a monovalent cation with antimanic, antipsychotic, and antidepressant activity. It has been used safely in adults with bipolar disorder in the United States for over 30 years and remains widely used to treat this illness. As maintenance treatment lithium is the only drug shown to reduce risk of suicide in patients with mood disorders (Bowden et al., 2002).

Pharmacology

PHARMACODYNAMICS

Lithium is an element of the alkali metal group. Preclinical studies have shown that lithium alters sodium transport in nerve and muscle cells and causes a shift toward intraneuronal metabolism of catecholamines, but the specific biochemical mechanism of lithium action in mania is unknown.

PHARMACOKINETICS

Absorption
- Absorption of lithium is rapid, with peak serum concentrations occurring within 0.5–2 hours.
- No significant difference in bioavailability exists following oral administration of lithium carbonate capsules or lithium citrate liquid.
- Liquid lithium achieves higher peak serum levels and has a faster time-to-peak plasma concentration than do lithium tablets.
- Standard lithium carbonate and the slow-release form provide equivalent steady-state serum lithium levels.
- Completely absorbed when given after food, but when given on an empty stomach, lithium can cause diarrhea.
- May result in decreased absorption.
- Lithium should be administered after meals.

Distribution
- Lithium is distributed widely in both intra- and extracellular fluids and is not protein bound.
- In young patients with normal renal function the volume of distribution is about 20% greater than for adults.
- In patients with renal insufficiency the volume of distribution is about 20% less than for adults.

Metabolism and excretion
- Elimination half-life is about 24 hours and is prolonged in patients with compromised renal function.
- 90–98% of a dose is excreted unchanged in the urine.

Effects on pregnancy and breastfeeding
- Lithium is excreted in breast milk.
- In pregnant women receiving lithium, neonatal lithium doses range between 0% and 30% of the maternal dose on a per kilogram basis.
- Adverse effects have been reported in breastfeeding infants in association with maternal use of lithium (Tunnessen & Hertz, 1972).
- Poor neonatal muscle tone, cyanosis, heart murmur, T-wave changes on electrocardiography, lethargy, and hypothermia.
- According to the American Academy of Pediatrics, lithium should be given to nursing mothers with caution.
- If use is unavoidable, monitor the infant for side effects such as restlessness, weakness, and hydration status.
- Bottle feeding is a safe alternative.

Indications

Lithium carbonate is indicated in the treatment of manic episodes of manic–depressive illness in adults. Lithium maintenance therapy prevents or diminishes the intensity of subsequent episodes in those manic–depressive adult patients with a history of mania.

MOOD STABILIZERS

Lithium is FDA approved for the treatment of manic episodes of bipolar disorder in patients at least 12 years of age.

Possible indications
- Cluster headache (adults)
- Conduct disorder with impulsive, explosive aggression (children, adolescents, adults)

Dosing and Duration of Treatment

- $0.5–1.5$ g/m^2 in divided doses for the acute phase
- The maintenance dose should be adjusted to maintain lithium serum concentrations of 0.5 to 1.2 mmol/L.
- Doses in children should not exceed adult doses.

Available lithium preparations
There are multiple available lithium preparations. The following table presents some of these formulations.

Table 6.3 Available Preparations of Lithium

Generic	Brand Name	Strength (mg)
Lithium carbonate	Eskatlith®	300
Lithium carbonate	Lithium carbonate	300
Lithium carbonate	Lithonate®	300
Lithium carbonate	Lithotabs®	300
Slow-Release Formulations		
Lithium carbonate slow-release	Eskalith CR®	450
Lithium carbonate slow-release	Lithobid®	300
Syrup Formulation		
Lithium citrate syrup	Cibalith®	8 mEq/5 ml = one 300 mg tablet

Before initiating treatment
Before initiating treatment with lithium, baseline laboratory tests assessing renal, thyroid, hematological, and chemistry status must be completed. Pregnancy status in women of child-bearing age must be assessed.

- Renal function tests, including serum creatinine and blood urea nitrogen
- Urinalysis with specific gravity
- Complete blood count with differential
- Thyroid function tests
- Electrocardiogram
- Pregnancy testing
- Electrolytes
- Serum chemistries, including calcium and phosphorus levels

General dosing suggestions
- Initiating treatment is determined by age and weight (see following table).

Table 6.4 Lithium Dosing and Administration in Children and Adolescents

Child Weight	Initial Lithium Dose on a tid schedule (mg)
Children < 12 years:	
> 25 kg	150/150/300
25–40 kg	300/300/600
50–60 kg	600/300/600

1. Obtain trough lithium levels every other day during titration phase.
2. Stop when two consecutive lithium levels are between 0.6 and 1.2 mEq/L.
3. Then adjust dose gradually, according to clinical efficacy and side effects.

Children > 12 years:
1. Begin at 150 mg/day.
2. Increase dose by 150–300 mg every 5–7 days.
3. Doses of 900–1200 mg/day usually yield a lithium level between 0.6 and 1.2 mEq/L.

General Guidelines:
1. Give lithium in three to four daily divided doses.
2. Check lithium level five days after initial dose, and then every 5 days during dose adjustment.
3. Obtain a trough lithium level drawn 10–12 hours after last dose and before the next dose.
4. Target lithium level is 0.6–1.2 mEq/L.
5. Do not exceed level of 1.4 mEq/L (low therapeutic index [i.e., toxic dose to effective dose ~3]).
6. Monitor closely for side effects/toxicity during lithium titration phase.

Adapted from Weller EB, Weller RA, and Fristad MA. Lithium dosage guide for prepubertal children. *J Am Acad Child Adolesc Psychiatry* 25:92–95, 1986.

- Lithium is a drug with a low toxicity/therapeutic index and careful serum monitoring is mandatory.
- It is important to assess the familey's ability to keep appointments for therapeutic serum lithium monitoring.
- Serum levels must guide therapy.
- Serum levels, not oral dose, are correlated with both benefit and toxicity in patients prescribed lithium.
- Standards for interpreting lithium levels are based on measurements taken 10–12 hours after an oral dose (usually immediately before the first A.M. dose; a trough blood level).
- Maintain a constant lithium dose for 5 days to achieve steady-state serum concentrations before obtaining a lithium serum level.
- Obtain levels until two consecutive levels are in the therapeutic range.
- The therapeutic range is a serum lithium level between 0.6 and 1.2 mEq/L.
- Do not exceed a serum level of 1.4 mEq/L.
- Adjust the lithium dose based on serum level, side effects, and clinical response.
- Immediate-release tablets are usually given 3 or 4 times daily, whereas controlled release tablets are usually given twice daily.
- To switch a patient from immediate-release lithium to controlled-release tablets, the same total daily dose should be administered.
- If the morning and evening doses are unequal, then the larger dose should be given in the evening.
- If the current lithium immediate-release dose is not a multiple of 450, then administer the lower closest dose.

MOOD STABILIZERS

• If closer titration is needed, then immediate-release capsules may be added to controlled-release lithium preparations.
• Lithium tolerance is greater during the acute manic phase, probably due to increased glomerular filtration during manic episodes, and decreases when manic symptoms subside. Therefore, adjust the lithium dose based on levels obtained in various phases of the illness. Patients who cycle into depression from mania may suddenly become lithium toxic, as their renal function decreases during the depressed phase of the illness.
• Use in patients less than 12 years old is not recommended due to a lack of information regarding safety and effectiveness.

Medical monitoring
At approximately 3-month intervals for the first year and 6-month intervals thereafter, monitor the following laboratory tests:

• Renal function tests, including serum creatinine or creatinine clearance, BUN, and urine osmolality or urine-specific gravity or 24-hour urine volume
• Complete blood count with differential
• Thyroid function tests
• Electrocardiogram
• Electrolytes
• Serum calcium and phosphorus levels

Table 6.5 Lithium Laboratory Investigations

Test	Before Starting Lithium	Every 6 Months	Every 12 Months
ECG	Yes		Yes
Electrolytes	Yes	——	——
CBC, differential[a]	Yes	——	——
BUN, creatinine[b]	Yes	Yes	——
Urinalysis	Yes	——	——
Fasting blood sugar[c]	Yes	——	——
T3 T4 TSH TBG[d]	Yes	Yes	Yes
Calcium,[e] PO4	Yes	——	Yes
Pregnancy test	Yes	Optional	Optional
Physical exam and general medical History	Yes	Yes	Yes

[a] Obtain new baseline WBC with expected leucocytosis 4–6 weeks after lithium begins; neutrophils most increased.
[b] Check renal function every 2–3 months during first 6 months of treatment.
[c] Helps establish baseline to determine later if lithium is significantly altering glucose tolerance; hypoglycemia greater risk from lithium.
[d] Many women who develop hypothyroidism do so within first 2 years; 6-month monitoring recommended. Men and women euthyroid after 2 years can be monitored yearly.
[e] Obtain serum calcium again 2–6 weeks after lithium begins. Further assays should be done if clinical symptoms of hypercalcemia are seen: neuromuscular signs, ataxia, apathy, dysphoria, depression. Levels approaching 11 mg/dl should be followed closely.

Discontinuing lithium treatment
• Although abrupt withdrawal of lithium has not been found to be associated with withdrawal effects, rapid cessation has been associated with increased

instability of bipolar symptoms and increased suicidal ideation in bipolar adults, compared with more gradual tapering of lithium (Baldessarini et al., 1996).

Contraindications

• Patients with severe cardiovascular or renal disease
• Evidence of severe physical debilitation or dehydration
• Sodium depletion
• Brain damage
• Conditions requiring low sodium intake

Absolute contraindications
• Severe debilitation, dehydration, or sodium depletion
• Significant cardiovascular disease
• Significant renal impairment

Relative contraindications
• Breastfeeding an infant
• Debilitated or elderly patients
• Discontinue lithium at least 1 week before initiating electroconvulsive therapy (ECT) and withhold lithium for several days after completing ECT.
• Pregnancy
• Protracted diarrhea, sweating, or concomitant infection with elevated core body temperature may decrease tolerance to lithium.
• Significant cardiac disease, organic brain damage, restricted dietary salt intake, or diuretic requirement
• Sodium depletion may increase the possibility of lithium intoxication.

Side Effects

Lithium is a drug with a low toxicity threshold. At serum levels only slightly higher than therapeutic levels, signs of lithium toxicity may appear. The relationship between serum lithium level, clinical side effects, and toxicity is presented in the following table.

Drug–Drug Interactions

Lithium has been used extensively for many years and is know to interact with numerous medications.

Management of Overdose

• Determine serum lithium concentration and severity of intoxication:
  ○ Mild to moderate: 1.5–2.5 mEq/L
  ○ Severe: 2.5–3 mEq/L
  ○ Fatal: Levels greater than 3–4 mEq/L may be fatal, especially in patients on chronic lithium therapy.

MOOD STABILIZERS

Table 6.6 Lithium Carbonate Serum Level, Clinical Side Effects, and Toxicity

Therapeutic Lithium Levels (0.6–1.2 mEq/L)	Mild to Moderate Toxicity (1.4–2.0 mEq/L)	Moderate to Severe Toxicity (2.0–2.5 mEq/L)	Severe Toxicity ≥ 2.5 mEq/L
Central Nervous System	Central Nervous System	Central Nervous System	Central Nervous System
Hand tremor	Dizziness	Coma	Seizures
Memory impairment	Drowsiness	Choreoathetoid movements	
Concentration difficulties	Dysarthria	Clonic limb movements	Renal
	Agitation	Convulsions	Oliguria
Endocrine	Coarsening hand tremor	Delerium	
	Lethargy	EEG changes	
Hypothyroidism	Muscle weakness	Fainting	Renal failure
	Vertigo	Hyperreflexia	Death
Gastrointestional		Leg tremors	
		Muscle fasciculations	
Diarrhea	Gastrointestional	Nystagmus	
Edema	Abdominal pain	Vision blurred	
Nausea	Diarrhea		
Weight gain	Dry mouth		
	Nausea	Gastrointestional	
Renal	Vomiting	Anorexia	
		Nausea	
Polydipsia		Vomiting	
Polyuria			
Nocturnal enuresis		Cardiovascular	
		Cardiac arrhythmia	
Dermatological		Sinus node dysfunction	
Acne		Pulse irregularities	

Adapted from Maxmen JS and Ward NG. *Psychotropic Drugs Fast Facts* (3rd ed.) New York: Norton, 2002, p. 255.

- Intoxication effects include the following:
  ○ Patients with mild intoxication may develop nausea, vomiting, tremors, hyperreflexia, agitation, and ataxia.
  ○ Moderate intoxication includes CNS depression, muscle rigidity, and hypertonia.
  ○ Patients with severe toxicity may develop seizures, myoclonus, hypotension, and coma.

Table 6.7 Lithium Drug–Drug Interactions
Lithium interacts with:

Drug	Interaction
Angiotensin-converting enzyme inhibitors	↑ Serum lithium level
Acetazolamide	↓ Serum lithium level
Alcohol	↑ Serum lithium level
Antithyroid medications	Lithium increases thyroid suppression
Bronchodilators	↓ Serum lithium level
Calcium channel blockers	↑ Risk for lithium-induced neurotoxicity
Corticosteroids	↓ Serum lithium level
Diuretics (osmotic)	↓ Serum lithium level
Diuretics (potassium sparing)	Safest to use with lithium
Diuretics (thiazide)	↑ Risk for lithium-induced neurotoxicity
Nonsteroidal anti-inflammatory drugs	↑ Risk for lithium-induced neurotoxicity
Tricyclic antidepressants	↑ Serum lithium level
Valproic acid	↑ Serum lithium level

- Lavage if within 1 hour of presumed fatal overdose.
- Lithium is not adsorbed to activated charcoal.
- Syrup of ipecac may be useful in the hospital setting in alert and conscious children with large recent lithium ingestions, whose nasogastric tube is too small to retrieve whole pills and large fragments.
- Administer IV normal saline to maintain adequate urine output and to enhance renal clearance of lithium.
- Hemodialysis is indicated for moderate to severe intoxications. Hemodialysis is highly effective because of lithium's lack of protein binding and its small volume of distribution in the body. Indications for hemodialysis include the following:
  ○ Severe neurotoxicity
  ○ Moderate neurotoxicity and serum lithium levels that do not decline by at least 20% in 6 hours
  ○ Renal failure
  ○ Serum lithium level $\geq$ 4 mEq/L, even in the asymptomatic patient
- Dysrhythmia may occur and treatment should follow standard guidelines for the specific arrhythmia encountered.
- Little correlation exists between serum lithium levels and severity of intoxication in acute lithium overdoses.

Drug Interference with Diagnostic Laboratory Testing

Table 6.8 Lithium Effects on Laboratory Tests

Laboratory Test	Results
Blood Serum Tests	
^{131}I uptake	↑
T_3	↓
T_4	↓
Leukocytes	↑
Eosinophils	↑
Platelets	↑
Lymphocytes	↓
Na^+, K^+	↑ or ↓
Ca^{++}, Mg^{++}	↑ or ↓
Serum phosphate	↓
Parathyroid hormone	↑
Glucose tolerance	↑ or ↓
Creatinine	↑
Urine Tests	
Glycosuria	↑
Albuminuria	↑
VMA	↑
Renal concentrating ability	↓
Electrolytes	↑ or ↓
EKG	
Benign, reversible T-wave changes	Flattening, isoelectricity, inversion
Rate	Bradycardia
Conduction abnormalities	Sinus node dysfunction

Adapted from Maxmen JS and Ward NG. *Psychotropic Drugs Fast Facts* (3rd ed.). New York: Norton, 2002, p. 252.

MOOD STABILIZERS

DIVALPROEX SODIUM

Divalproex was the first drug, other than lithium, reported to be efficacious for the treatment of bipolar disorder (Bowden, 2004). Since then, the effectiveness of divalproex—alone, in combination with other agents, and as maintenance therapy—has been investigated in a number of studies. As a monotherapy, clinical studies revealed that divalproex was superior to lithium with regard to being effective in a broader patient population: patients with depressive symptoms concurrent with their mania, patients who previously responded poorly to lithium, patients with more lifetime episodes, and those with specific symptoms of elation/grandiosity and reduced need for sleep. In addition, divalproex had superior efficacy to carbamazepine and equivalent efficacy to the antipsychotic agent olanzapine in manic patients with psychotic manic features, and patients showed much better tolerability to divalproex than carbamazepine, antipsychotics, and, in particular, lithium (Denicoff et al., 1997). Recently, combination therapy (mood stabilizers plus antipsychotic agents) has shown some advantages compared with monotherapy.

Manic symptoms in adolescents have been observed to improve to a greater extent when divalproex was coadministered with an antipsychotic rather than with either agent used alone (DelBello et al., 2002). Although only a few maintenance studies have been conducted to date, randomized studies have indicated consistent trends toward greater efficacy of divalproex than lithium, and significant superiority over placebo on most, although not all, measures (Bowden, 2004). In general, divalproex appears to provide a generally well-tolerated treatment that is efficacious for a broad spectrum of manic states and appears to improve outcomes during maintenance treatment. The use of this anticonvulsant is increasing in pediatric psychopharmacology for conduct disorder, early onset bipolar disorder, and externalizing behavior disorders (Rana et al., 2005).

Pharmacology

PHARMACODYNAMICS

Although the mechanism of action is presently unknown, it is postulated that divalproex effects are mediated through the function of brain gamma-aminobutyric acid (GABA), specifically by increasing brain concentrations of this inhibitory transmitter by inhibiting GABA-aminotransferase and succinic semialdehyde dehydrogenase, enzymes involved in the synthesis and degradation of GABA. Selective increases of GABA with divalproex treatment have been reported to occur in synaptosomes, primarily in areas of high GABA activity. Alternately, it has been postulated that divalproex may selectively enhance postsynaptic GABA responses. Another hypothesis contends that the drug's efficacy is a result of its direct effect on neuronal membranes and its reduction of excitatory transmission by aspartate. There is some evidence that divalproex may inhibit the reuptake of GABA into the glia and nerve endings. There may also be concordance with lithium's mechanism of action via the attenuation of protein kinase C and signal transduction activity (Product Information, Depakote 2002).

PHARMACOKINETICS

Absorption
• Divalproex rapidly absorbed after oral administration.
• A slight delay in absorption occurs when the drug is administered with meals, but this does not affect the total absorption.

Distribution
• Divalproex is rapidly distributed throughout the body.
• Peak serum levels occur approximately 1–4 hours after a single oral dose.
• The serum half-life of valproic acid is typically in the range of 6–16 hours.
• Half-lives in the lower part of the above range are usually found in patients taking other antiepileptic drugs.
• Valproic acid is strongly bound (90%) to human plasma proteins.

Metabolism and excretion
• Divalproex is primarily metabolized in the liver.
• 70–80% of the parent drug is eliminated principally in the urine, with minor amounts eliminated in the feces.
• Increases in dose may result in decreases in the extent of protein binding and variable changes in valproic acid clearance and elimination.
• Breast milk levels range from 1% to 10% of the maternal serum level.
• A 3-month-old developed thrombocytopenic purpura and anemia attributed to valproic acid transferred via breast milk.
• Clearance decreases with increasing age.
• Clearance is increased by coadministration of carbamazepine.

Indications

• Divalproex is indicated for the treatment of
• Manic symptoms in bipolar disorder in adults
• Seizures in the pediatric and adult age range.

Dosing and Duration of Treatment

Available divalproex sodium preparations
• Capsule: 250 mg and 500 mg
• Capsule: gelatin enteric-coated 250 mg and 500 mg
• Intravenous liquid: 100 mg/ml
• Sprinkles: 125 mg caplets
• Solution for injection: divalproex sodium injection, equivalent to 100 mg of valproic acid per mL, is a clear, colorless solution in 5 mL single-dose vials.
• Syrup 50 mg/ml: alcohol-free, gluten-free, lactose-free, sulfite-free, and tartrazine-free.
• Bottles of 450 mL
• Tablets: 125 mg, 250 mg, and 500 mg
• Tablets: enteric coated 125 mg, 250 mg, and 500 mg
• Tablets: extended release 250 mg and 500 mg

MOOD STABILIZERS

Before initiating treatment
Before initiating divalproex treatment, baseline laboratories must be obtained

• CBC, differential, and platelet counts
• Liver function tests
• Determine concentrations of concomitant antiepileptic drugs (if any).
• Serum amylase levels

Table 6.9 Dosing of Divalproex Sodium by Child Weight (based on 15 mg/kg/day)

Weight (kg)	Total daily dose (mg)	Number of 250 mg capsules or teaspoonsful of syrup given daily		
		Dose 1	Dose 2	Dose 3
10–24.9	250	0	0	1
25–39.9	500	1	0	1
40–59.9	750	1	1	1
60–74.9	1000	1	1	2
75–89.9	1250	2	1	2

General dosing suggestions
Divalproex is generally administered orally in pediatric psychopharmacology. Dosing is based on weight in the pediatric population.

• The therapeutic serum range in adult acute mania is between 50–125 mcg/mL. The serum range for pediatric bipolar illness has yet to be determined. Adult serum levels are used to guide divalproex therapy for bipolar illness in children and adolescents.
  ○ A good correlation has not been established between daily dose, serum levels, and therapeutic effect in bipolar illness.
• The recommended initial dose in children is 15 mg/kg/day.
• Increasing the dose at 1-week intervals by 5 to 10 mg/kg/day is recommended until symptoms are controlled or side effects preclude further increases.
• The maximum recommended dose is 60 mg/kg/day.
• When the total daily dose exceeds 250 mg, it should be given in a divided daily regimen.
  ○ A 500 mg enteric-coated capsule may be substituted for two 250 mg capsules.
• Patients who experience gastrointestinal irritation may benefit from administration of valproic acid with food or by a progressive dosage increase from an initial low level.
• The capsules should be swallowed without chewing to avoid local irritation of the mouth and throat.

Medical monitoring
• Divalproex therapy has occasionally been associated with the development of acute pancreatitis. Abdominal pain, nausea, vomiting, and/or anorexia can be

symptoms of pancreatitis that require prompt medical evaluation; if pancreatitis is diagnosed, valproate should be discontinued.

• The probability of thrombocytopenia increases significantly at a total trough divalproex plasma concentration above 110 mcg/mL in females and above 135 mcg/mL in males.

• Serious or fatal hepatotoxicity may be preceded by nonspecific symptoms such as malaise, weakness, lethargy, facial edema, anorexia, and vomiting. In patients with epilepsy, a loss of seizure control may also occur. Hepatic failure occurs most frequently within the first 6 months of treatment. Children under 2 years of age are at increased risk.

• Clinical evidence of hemorrhage, bruising, or a disorder of hemostasis/coagulation is an indication for reduction of dosage or withdrawal of therapy pending hematological investigation.

• Hyperammonemia with or without lethargy or coma has been reported and may be present in the absence of abnormal liver function tests; if elevation occurs, divalproex should be discontinued.

• Because divalproex may interact with other antiepileptic drugs, periodic serum level determinations of concurrently administered antiepileptics are recommended, especially during the early part of therapy.

• There is an association between divalproex use and polycystic ovary syndrome and hyperandrogenism in epileptic women. This association appears most pronounced in women who begin divalproex treatment before 20 years of age than in women who initiated divalproex use at 20 years or older (Rasgon, 2004).

• A complete blood count (CBC), differential, and platelet count should be undertaken at periodic intervals and prior to planned surgeries.

• Liver function tests should be performed at frequent intervals, especially during the first 6 months of therapy, although no cases of hepatotoxicity have been reported in medically well children over age 2 years receiving divalproex monotherapy.
  ○ Clinical monitoring for signs of hepatotoxicity is more important than routine assessment of LFTs, which has little predictive value.

• Carnitine deficiency may occasionally arise during long-term use of valproate; although it is unclear whether carnitine supplementation is of value in children receiving valproate, some neurologists consider it justified in selected cases.

Discontinuing treatment
• In general, withdrawal should be gradual to minimize risk.
• Unless safety concerns require a more rapid withdrawal, the dose of valproate should be tapered over a period of at least 2 weeks.

Contraindications

Absolute contraindications
• Hepatic disease or significant hepatic dysfunction
• Hypersensitivity to valproate, valproic acid, or divalproex sodium

MOOD STABILIZERS

• Patients with known urea cycle disorders
• Pregnancy
• Polycystic ovary disease in females of child bearing age.

Relative contraindications
• Children under the age of 2 years
• Concomitant use of other agents that affect platelet function
• Concomitant use of CNS depressants
• Hepatic dysfunction
• Pancreatitis

Side Effects

Divalproex can cause side effects such as nausea, trouble sleeping, and dizziness. More serious side effects are rare but can occur and include liver function problems, pancreatitis, and a severe allergic reaction. The range of common and uncommon divalproex side effects is listed below:

Table 6.10 Divalproex Sodium Side Effects

Common
  • Alopecia
  • Gastrointestional
    ○ Abdominal pain
    ○ Anorexia
    ○ Dyspepsia
    ○ Constipation
    ○ Diarrhea
    ○ Nausea
    ○ Vomiting
    ○ Changes in weight
  • Neurological
    ○ Ataxia
    ○ Tremor
    ○ Amnesia
    ○ Emotional lability
    ○ Headache
    ○ Sedation
    ○ Dizziness
  • Ophthalmological
    ○ Diplopia
    ○ Ambylopia
    ○ Blurred vision
    ○ Nystagmus
  • Rash

Uncommon and serious
  • Neonatal congential malformations in infants born to women receiving valproate during pregnancy
  • Hepatic failure
  • Pancreatitis
  • Polycystic ovaries in females of child bearing age
  • Thrombocytopenia

Drug–Drug Interactions

Divalproex has many drug–drug interactions. In combination with other antiepileptics it may produce severe hepatic dysfunction, especially when given to children less than 2 years old. In combination with lithium divalproex may increase the risk for neurotoxicity. Divalproex may potentate the CNS depressant action of alcohol. The concomitant use of valproic acid and clonazepam may produce absence status. Caution is recommended when valproic acid is administered with drugs that affect coagulation, e.g., aspirin and warfarin.

Table 6.11 Divalproex Drug–Drug Interactions
Divalproex interacts with:

Drug	Interaction
Lithium	↑ Risk of neurotoxicity
Phenothiazines	↑ Valproic acid serum levels
Phenytoin	↑ Risk of neurotoxicity
Primidone	↑ Risk of neurotoxicity
Salicylates	↑ Valproic acid serum levels
Tricyclic antidepressants	↑ TCA serum levels
Warfarin	↑ Unbound warfarin

Adapted from Maxmen JS and Ward NG. Psychotropic Drugs Fast Facts (3rd ed.). New York: Norton, pp. 298–303, 2002.

Management of Overdose

• Naloxone has been reported to reverse the CNS depressant effects of divalproex overdose.
• Because naloxone can theoretically reverse the antiepileptic effects of divalproex, it should be used with caution.
• Because divalproex is absorbed very rapidly, gastric lavage may be of limited value.
• Apply general supportive measures, with particular attention to the prevention of hypovolemia and the maintenance of adequate urinary output.

Drug Interference with Laboratory Testing

• Divalproex is partially eliminated in the urine as a ketone-containing metabolite that may lead to a false interpretation of the urine ketone test.
• There have been reports of altered thyroid function tests associated with divalproex therapy; the clinical significance is unknown.
• Divalproex therapy has been associated with false urinary glucose test values.

CARBAMAZEPINE

Carbamazepine has been given as an alternative to lithium in adult patients with bipolar disorder. Its use in pediatric bipolar disorder is less clear (McClellan & Werry, 1997). Carbamazepine may conceivably have a role in patients with nonclassical bipolar features such as rapid cycling or mixed manic–depressive states. Carbamazepine has been used in combination with lithium, particularly in patients unresponsive to either drug alone.

MOOD STABILIZERS

Table 6.12 Mood Stabilizer Effects on Laboratory Tests

Generic Name	Blood/Serum Test	Result	Urine Test	Result
Carbamazepine	Calcium	↑		
	BUN	↑	Albuminuria	↑
	Thyroid function	↓	Glycosuria	↑
	*LFT	↑		
	WBC, platelets	↓		
	RBC	↓		
	Sodium	↓		
Clonazepam	*LFT	↑		
Valproic acid	*LFT	↑	Ketone tests	False +
	WBC, platelets	↓		
	Thyroid function	↓		
	Ammonia	↑		

Adapted from Maxmen JS and Ward NG. *Psychotropic Drugs Fast Facts* (3rd ed.). New York: Norton, p. 304, 2002.
* LFT tests are AST/SGPT, alkaline phosphatase, LDH, and billirubin. Increases in transaminases (SGOT, SGPT, and LDH) are usually benign; increases in billirubin and other tests suggest hepatotoxicity.

Pharmacology

PHARMACODYNAMICS

Carbamazepine is structurally similar to the tricyclic antidepressant imipramine. It is an anticonvulsant and specific analgesic for trigeminal neuralgia. It appears to act by reducing polysynaptic responses and blocking posttetanic potentiation. Carbamazepine is chemically unrelated to other anticonvulsants or other drugs used to control the pain of trigeminal neuralgia. The exact mechanism of action remains unknown. Like divalproex and lamotrigine, carbamazepine blocks voltage-gated sodium channels. Other anticonvulsants that are less effective in the treatment of bipolar disorder, such as topiramate and gabapentin, do not share this mechanism.

PHARMACOKINETICS

Absorption
• The carbamazepine tablet is 70–79% absorbed.
• Carbamazepine liquid suspension is 96% absorbed.
• Peak serum concentrations for the oral suspension occur in 3–4 hours.
• Peak serum concentrations for the tablet preparation occur in 11–12 hours.
• More frequent administration of lower doses of the suspension may be indicated to avoid toxicity, compared to the tablet formulation.
• Food increases the absorption of carbamazepine.

Distribution
• Highly protein bound and lipid soluble.

Metabolism and excretion
• The half-life of carbamazepine ranges between 25 and 65 hours for a single dose.
• 98% metabolized by the liver.

- Induces its own metabolism (autoinduction) during prolonged treatment. Autoinduction is generally complete within 3 to 5 weeks with a fixed dosing regimen. Carbamazepine serum levels may decline during the period of autoinduction on a constant daily dose.
  - ◦ With increasing carbamazepine doses in children, a dose-dependent autoinduction process is seen.
- Carbamazepine metabolism occurs via cytochrome P-450 3A4.
- Carbamazepine breast milk concentrations are reported to be approximately 24–69% of that found in maternal plasma.
- Breastfed newborns have developed serum carbamazepine levels between 15% and 65% of maternal serum levels. Caution is advised in nursing mothers receiving carbamazepine.
- Higher levels of carbamazepine metabolites are seen in patients receiving concomitant divalproex or lamotrigine therapy.
- The metabolite carbamazepine-10,11-epoxide is partly responsible for carbamazepine intoxication. The epoxide metabolite is toxic and its presence must be assessed if carbamazepine toxicity is suspected.

Indications

Carbamazepine is FDA approved for

- Adult and pediatric seizures
- Adult trigeminal and glossopharyngeal neuralgia

There currently exists no approved indication for carbamazepine in adult or pediatric psychiatric disorders.

Possible indications
- Adult bipolar disorder
- Pediatric bipolar disorder
- Disorders of impulsivity and explosive aggression
- Adult psychotic disorders.

Carbamazepine has not been as well studied in pediatric psychopharmacology as it has been in pediatric seizure disorders and adult psychopharmacology. To date there are no randomized, placebo-controlled clinical trials of carbamazepine in the treatment pediatric bipolarity. The use of this medication in the pediatric population has significantly out-paced the scientific literature supporting its use in pediatric psychopharmacology.

Dosing and Duration of Treatment

Available carbamazepine preparations
- Tablets: 100 mg and 200 mg chewable
  - ◦ Should be taken with food.
- Extended-release tablets: 100 mg, 200 mg, and 400 mg

MOOD STABILIZERS

- Capsule: 300 mg extended release
  - May be taken with or without food.
  - The contents of capsules may be sprinkled over food (such as a teaspoonful of applesauce or other similar food products); the capsule or its contents should not be crushed or chewed.
- Suspension: 100 mg/5 mL oral suspension
  - Should be taken with food.
  - Should be administered on a 3–4 times/day schedule.
  - Should not be administered simultaneously with other liquid medicinal agents or diluents.
- When adding carbamazepine to existing anticonvulsant therapy, the drug should be added gradually while other anticonvulsants are maintained or gradually decreased.
- The exception is phenytoin, which may have to be increased.
- When converting patients from immediate-release carbamazepine to extended-release capsules, the same total daily mg dose of carbamazepine should be administered.

Before initiating treatment
Before initiating carbamazepine treatment, baseline laboratory tests should be obtained.

- Complete blood count, differential, and platelets: Carbamazepine is often associated with benign neutropenia; very rare and sometimes fatal cases of agranulocytosis and aplastic anemia have occurred.
- Hepatic function tests (alanine aminotransferase, aspartate aminotransferase, alkaline phosphatase)
- Serum electrolytes
- Blood urea nitrogen (BUN) and creatinine

General dosing suggestions
- The dosage of carbamazepine should be adjusted to meet the needs of the individual patient, based upon clinical efficacy and monitoring of blood levels.
- Loss of efficacy has been reported when carbamazepine tablets are exposed to humid conditions.
- Carbamazepine should not be administered simultaneously with other liquid medications or diluents. The suspension will produce higher peak levels than the same dose given as a tablet; therefore, patients should be started on lower doses of the suspension and increased slowly.
- Carbamazepine therapeutic serum levels for seizure disorders range between 4 and 12 µg/mL. It is suggested that these plasma levels also be used to treat psychiatric disorders with carbamazepine.

For children under the age of 6 years:

- The initial recommended dosage is 10–20 mg/kg/day administered in divided doses two or three times a day (chewable or conventional tablets) or four times a day (suspension).

- The dose may then be increased in weekly intervals to obtain the desired clinical response.
- Maintenance doses may be given either 3 or 4 times a day for both tablets and the suspension.
- The maximum recommended dose is 35 mg/kg/day.

For children ages 6 to 12 years

- The initial recommended carbamazepine dose is 100 mg twice a day (tablets or sustained-release tablets) or 50 mg (one-half teaspoonful) four times a day (suspension).
- Adding 100 mg per day in weekly intervals, using a twice-daily regimen for sustained-release tablets or a three or four times a day regimen for conventional tablets or suspension, is continued until the desired clinical response is obtained.
- The usual maintenance dosage is 400–800 mg a day; the maximum daily dosage is generally 1000 mg/day or less for 6- to 12-year-old children.

For children over 12 years of age

- The initial recommended carbamazepine dose is 200 mg twice a day (tablets or sustained-release tablets) or 100 mg (one teaspoon four times a day [suspension].
- Adding 200 mg per day in weekly intervals, using a twice-daily regimen for sustained-release tablets or a three or four times a day regimen for conventional tablets or suspension, is continued until the desired clinical response is obtained.
- The usual effective maintenance doses range between 800 and 1000 mg/day in children 12–15 years and up to 1200 mg in patients over 15 years old.
- The recommended maximum dose of carbamazepine suspension is 1000 mg/day in children 6–15 years of age, 1200 mg/day in children over 15 years.

Medical monitoring
- Therapeutic drug monitoring of serum carbamazepine levels is mandatory with use of this agent.
  - Levels drawn during the first few weeks of therapy or when the dose is changing should be cautiously interpreted, due to autoinduction of liver enzymes.
  - Routine monitoring of the 10,11 epoxide metabolite may also be required during carbamazepine therapy, as serum carbamazepine levels alone may not be adequate to detect toxicity in some patients. Total carbamazepine metabolite serum levels above 9 μg/mL are associated with greater side effects than lower levels.
- A complete blood count, differential, and platelet count should be obtained 2 weeks after initiating carbamazepine and again 4 weeks later.
- Periodic hematological monitoring should occur every 6 months on this agent.

MOOD STABILIZERS

- Serum electrolytes should be obtained after 4 weeks on drug and then monitored every 6 months thereafter.
- Liver function tests should be obtained after 4 weeks on drug and then monitored every 6 months thereafter.
- Periodic complete urinalysis and BUN determinations are recommended for patients treated with this agent because of observed renal dysfunction.

If significant bone marrow depression develops, the manufacturer recommends the following:

- Immediately discontinue carbamazepine.
- Perform daily CBC, differential, platelet, and reticulocyte counts.
- Complete a bone marrow aspiration and trephine biopsy and repeat as necessary to monitor recovery.
- Other specific studies that might help include:
  - White cell and platelet antibodies
  - Fe^{59}-ferrokinetic studies
  - Peripheral blood cell typing
  - Cytogenetic studies on marrow and peripheral blood
  - Bone marrow culture studies for colony-forming units
  - Hemoglobin electrophoresis for A_2 and F hemoglobin
  - Serum folic acid and B_{12} levels.

Discontinuing therapy
Abrupt discontinuation of carbamazepine may result in symptoms of withdrawal, such as anxiety, muscle twitching, tremors, weakness, nausea, and vomiting. A slow tapering of the drug is recommended. One common recommendation is to decrease the total carbamazepine dose by 10% each day, although more gradual reductions have also been used.

Contraindications

Absolute contraindications
- Hypersensitivity to carbamazepine or tricyclic antidepressants
- History of bone marrow depression
- Concomitant use of MAOIs.
- Pregnancy; increased risk of major congenital abnormalities during the first trimester of pregnancy.

Relative Contraindications

- Liver dysfunction
- Kidney dysfunction
- Hypersensitive reaction to other drugs, including other anticonvulsants such as phenytoin or phenobarbital
- Increased intraocular pressure
- History of adverse hematological reaction to any drug
- History of cardiac disease

- Patients with underlying mental illness may experience activation of latent psychosis or agitation
- Cross-sensitivity between carbamazepine and oxcarbazepine occurs in 25–30% of patients.
- Can also occur with phenytoin.

Side Effects

Side effects of carbamazepine can include dry mouth and throat, constipation, problems urinating, dizziness or drowsiness, nausea, vomiting, or loss of appetite. Rare but serious side effects include the risk of hematological problems and liver inflammation. Rash may occur with carbamazepine use and should prompt drug discontinuation. A listing of common as well as serious side effects follows:

Table 6.13 Table Carbamazepine Side Effects

Common
- Blurred or double vision or nystagmus
- Clumsiness or unsteadines, confusion, dizziness, drowsiness, lightheadedness
- Hypertension, hypotension
- Nausea, vomiting
- Pruritic and erythematous rashes, urticaria, photosensitivity reactions

Serious
- Acute renal failure, renal toxicity, hyponatremia, dilutional or water intoxication (SIADH)
- Aplastic anemia, agranulocytosis, pancytopenia, bone marrow depression, thrombocytopenia
- Leukopenia, leukocytosis, eosinophilia, acute intermittent porphyria
- Arrhythmias, atrioventricular (AV) heart block, congestive heart failure, syncope
- Hepatitis
- Hypocalcemia
- Toxic epidermal necrolysis, Stevens–Johnson syndrome, aggravation of disseminated lupus erythematosus

Drug–Drug Interactions

Carbamazepine has been used extensively for many years and is known to interact with numerous other medications. Some of these interactions are listed in the following table.

Table 6.14 Carbamazepine Drug–Drug Interactions
Carbamazepine interacts with:

Drug	Interaction
Anticoagulants	↓ Serum warfarin levels
Fluoxetine	↑ CBZ serum levels
Glucocorticoids	↓ Serum levels of glucocorticoids
Lithium	↑ Risk of neurotoxicity
Macrolide antibiotics	↑ CBZ serum levels
Oral contraceptives	↓ Serum levels of contraceptives, leading to breakthrough bleeding or pregnancy in females of child-bearing age
Theophylline	↓ Levels of theophylline and increased asthma symptoms
Tricycic antidepressants	↓ Antidepressant serum levels, increased risk of cardiac arrhythmias
Valproate	↑ CBZ serum levels, ↓ serum levels of valproate

CBZ = Carbamazepine.

MOOD STABILIZERS

Management Of Overdose

The lowest known oral lethal pediatric dose in a 3-year-old girl is 1.6 grams. Mild intoxication may cause drowsiness, ataxia, slurred speech, nystagmus, dystonic reactions, hallucinations, and vomiting. Coma, seizures, respiratory depression, dysrhythmias, decreased myocardial contractility, pulmonary edema, and hypotension may occur with severe intoxication. Acute renal failure has occurred following a massive overdose.

The first signs and symptoms appear 1–3 hours following ingestion of the extended-release form of carbamazepine. Neuromuscular disturbances are most prominent. Cardiovascular disorders are usually milder, with severe cardiac complications occurring only when very high doses (> 60 g) have been ingested.

General measures
- Ipecac-induced emesis is not recommended because of the potential for CNS depression and seizures.
- Activated charcoal may enhance elimination, but has not been shown to affect outcome.
- Gastric lavage may be helpful if it can be performed within 1 hour after ingestion.
- Monitor for hypotension, dysrhythmias, respiratory depression, and need for endotracheal intubation.
- Evaluate for hypoglycemia, electrolyte disturbances, hypoxia, and rhabdomyolysis.
- Isotonic IV fluid is indicated in case of hypotension.
- If hypotension persists, administer dopamine.
  - In children begin infusion at 0.1 mcg/kg/min and titrate to desired response.
- IV benzodiazepines are indicated in case of seizures.
  - In children begin diazepam 0.2–0.5 mg/kg, repeat every 5 min, as needed, or lorazepam 0.05–0.1 mg/kg.
- Consider phenobarbital if seizures recur after diazepam 30 mg (adults) or 10 mg (children >5 years).
- In case of rhabdomyolysis administer sufficient normal saline to maintain urine output of 2–3 mL/kg/hr. Monitor input and output, serum electrolytes, creatinine kinases, and renal function. Diuretics may be necessary to maintain urine output.
- Urinary alkalinization is not routinely recommended.

Drug Interference with Laboratory Testing

(See Table 6.11, Mood Stabilizer Effects on Laboratory Tests).
  Carbamazepine may:

- Cause a false increase in perphenazine serum levels.
- Increase free thyroid T4 and T3 fractions.

LAMOTRIGINE

Although lamotrigine is the best-studied new anticonvulsant in adults with bipolar disorder, its efficacy in adult acute mania is not well established. Lamotrigine has efficacy in acute bipolar depression, in the long-term maintenance treatment of bipolar depression, and is FDA indicated for the treatment of bipolar depression. Lamotrigine has generated interest in pediatric psychopharmacology. However, there presently are no controlled trials supporting its use for any disorder in this population. This section relies largely on the extant adult psychiatry literature for lamotrigene.

Table 6.14 Studies on Lamotrigine (Adult)

Study	Methodology	Results
Bowden Calabrese et al., 2003	Double-blinded study of Manic or Hypomanic patients with bipolar I disorder: lamotrigine $n = 59$ lithium $n = 46$ placebo $n = 70$	Lamotrigine 200–400 mg daily and lithium titrated to serum levels of 0.8–1.1 mEq/L were both statistically superior to placebo
Calabrese, Bowden et al., 2003	Double-blinded study of Depressed patients with bipolar I disorder: lamotrigine $n = 221$, lithium $n = 121$ or placebo $n = 121$	Both lamotrigine 200–400 mg daily and lithium titrated to serum levels of 0.8–1.1 mEq/L were statistically superior to placebo
Frye et al., 2000	Randomized, double-blinded cross-over study: bipolar I, $n = 11$ bipolar II, $n = 14$ unipolar, $n = 6$ (Of the bipolar, 23 were rapid-cycling)	Lamotrigine 275 mg/day superior to gabapentin 4000 mg/day lamotrigine superior placebo percentages of those who had responded by 6 weeks: 52% for lamotrigine 26% for gabapentin 23% placebo
Martin et al., 1999	Randomized healthy young adults, $n = 17$	Topiramate 5.7 mg/kg, lamotrigine 7.1 mg/kg, or gabapentin 35 mg/kg Improvement on topiramate. Gabapentin and lamotrigine had only minimal effects

Pharmacology

Lamotrigine is a drug of the phenyltriazine class, which is chemically unrelated to existing antiepileptic drugs.

PHARMACODYNAMICS

• Lamotrigine is thought to act on voltage-sensitive sodium channels.
• Lamotrigine may also inhibit the release of excitatory amino acid neurotransmitters.

PHARMACOKINETICS

• The time to peak concentration, elimination half-life, and volume of distribution are independent of dose.

Absorption
• Rapidly and completely absorbed following oral administration.
• Peak plasma concentrations are achieved in 1–5 hours.

MOOD STABILIZERS

• When administered with food, the rate of absorption is slightly reduced, but the extent of absorption remains unchanged.

Distribution
• Approximately 55% bound to human plasma proteins.
• This binding is unaffected by therapeutic concentrations of phenytoin, phenobarbital, or valproic acid.
• Lamotrigine does not displace other antiepileptic drugs (carbamazepine, phenytoin, phenobarbital) from protein binding sites.

Metabolism and excretion
• Elimination half-life of lamotrigene in adults is approximately 33 hours.
• Predominantly metabolized in the liver by glucuronic acid conjugation.
• Has no active metabolites.
• Approximately 70% of drug is recovered metabolized in the urine.
• Lamotrigine is excreted in human breast milk.
   ○ Because of the potential for adverse reactions from lamotrigine in nursing infants, breastfeeding is not recommended while taking this medication.

Indications

Lamotrigine is FDA approved in the treatment of the following disorders.

• In adult bipolar disorder, lamotrigine is indicated as maintenance therapy to delay the time to occurrence of mood episodes.
• In adult and pediatric Lennox–Gastaut syndrome associated seizures
• In adult and pediatric partial seizure disorders

There are presently no FDA approved indications for lamotrigine in pediatric psychopharmacology.

Possible Indications
• Pediatric bipolar disorder
• Disorders of impulse dyscontrol and emotional lability

Dosing and Duration of Treatment

• Safety and efficacy in pediatric patients with bipolar disorder under the age of 18 have not been established.
• Safety and efficacy in pediatric patients with epilepsy under the age of 16 have not been established, except for those with partial seizures and Lennox–Gastaut syndrome.

Available lamotrigine preparations
• Chewable tablets: 5 mg and 25 mg
   ○ Chewable dispersible tablets may be swallowed whole, chewed, or dispersed in water or diluted fruit juice; if the tablets are chewed, drink a small amount of water or diluted fruit juice to aid in swallowing.

○ Only whole tablets of the chewable dispersible tablets should be used; doses should be rounded down to the nearest whole tablet.
○ To disperse lamotrigine chewable dispersible tablets, add the tablets to a small amount of liquid (1 teaspoon, or enough to cover the medication); approximately 1 minute later, when the tablets are completely dispersed, swirl the solution and consume the entire quantity immediately.
• Tablets: 25 mg, 50 mg, 100 mg, 150 mg, and 200 mg

Before initiating treatment
The following laboratory tests are recommended at baseline before initiating lamotrigine therapy.

• CBC, differential, and platelet count
• Liver function tests
• Determine concentrations of concomitant antiepileptic drugs.

General dosing suggestions
Because initial high lamotrigine doses and rapid dose escalation have been associated with Stevens–Johnson syndrome and toxic epidermal necrolysis, it is highly desirable to initiate lamotrigine therapy at a low dose and titrate the dose cautiously. Because divalproex may inhibit the metabolism of lamotrigine and increase risk of toxicity, extra caution is advised when both drugs are administered concurrently.

• Lamotrigine is initiated at 12.5 mg once a day.
• Lamotrigine should be increased no more than 12.5 mg every week in the pediatric population.
  ○ Faster titration schedules have been associated with increased risk of rash.
• Usual maintenance dose of lamotrigine in patients not taking enzyme-inducing drugs such as carbamazepine is 200 mg/day (see "Lamotrigine Drug–Drug Interactions," Table 6.15.
• Lamotrigine dose titration when added to an existing divalproex regimen:
  ○ 12.5 mg/day every other day for 2 weeks
  ○ Then 12.5 mg/day for 2 weeks
  ○ Then 25 mg/day for 1 week
  ○ Then 50 mg/day for 1 week
  ○ Then 100 mg/day
  ○ The usual maintenance dose of lamotrigine in patients taking divalproex is 100 mg/day.
• When discontinuing valproic acid, the dose of lamotrigine should be doubled over a 2-week period in equal weekly increments.
• Lamotrigine dose titration, when added to enzyme-inducing antiepileptic drug regimens such as carbamazepine:
  ○ 25 mg/day orally for 2 weeks
  ○ Then 50 mg/day for 2 weeks in divided doses
  ○ Then 100 mg/day for 1 week in divided doses
  ○ Then 200 mg/day for 1 week in divided doses

MOOD STABILIZERS

- ○ Then 300 mg/day for 1 week in divided doses
- ○ Then may increase up to the usual maintenance dose of 400 mg/day in divided doses.
- When discontinuing an enzyme-inducing drug such as carbamazepine, the dose of lamotrigine should remain the same for the first week and then should be decreased by half over a 2-week period in equal weekly decrements.
- Liver disease: With moderate liver dysfunction, the initial, escalation, and maintenance doses should be reduced by approximately 50%; with severe impairment the initial, escalation, and maintenance doses should be reduced by approximately 75%.
- Renal impairment: May need to decrease maintenance dosage in patients with severe renal impairment.

Medical monitoring
- A therapeutic plasma concentration range has not been established for lamotrigine.
- Obtain a CBC, differential, and platelet count 2 weeks after initiating lamotrigine, 4 weeks later, and then every 6 months thereafter while receiving maintenance therapy.
- Obtain liver function tests 2 weeks after initiating lamotrigine, 4 weeks later, and then every 6 months thereafter while receiving maintenance therapy.
- Determine concentrations of concomitant antiepileptic drugs.

Discontinuing treatment
In general, withdrawal of an antiepileptic drug should be gradual to minimize risk. Unless safety concerns require a more rapid withdrawal, the dose of lamotrigine should be tapered over a period of at least 2 weeks.

Contraindications

Absolute contraindications
- Hypersensitivity to lamotrigine

Relative contraindications
- Renal, hepatic, or cardiac functional impairment
- Risk of suicide attempt (overdose)

Stevens–Johnson syndrome
Administration of lamotrigine or concomitant administration of valproic acid with lamotrigine may increase the risk of Stevens–Johnson syndrome (SJS), toxic epidermal necrolysis (TEN), or other potentially life-threatening rashes. Pediatric patients receiving lamotrigine appear to have a higher incidence of rash, SJS, and TEN than adult patients.

- SJS is an extreme allergic reaction to a drug, to certain bacterial or viral infections, or to food. SJS usually presents with painful, blistery lesions the skin and the mucous membranes of the mouth, throat, genital region, and eyes.

Lesions may erupt over 2–3 weeks. Because the skin has extensive blistering and ulceration, it resembles a severe burn. SJS may cause serious ocular problems, such as conjunctivitis, iritis, corneal blisters and erosions, and corneal ulcerations. In some cases, the ocular complications from SJS can be disabling and lead to severe or complete vision loss.

• TEN is a more serious form of SJS, leading to severe blistering of the skin and mucous membranes encompassing more than 10% of the total body surface area.

• SJS and TEN are potentially fatal and death occurs in up to 15% of untreated cases.

• The overall mortality rate is between 1% and 3%.

There exists no specific treatment for SJS and TEN once they occur. Treatment may require hospitalization and is largely supportive, including immediate discontinuation of the offending agent, meticulous skin care, analgesia, correction of fluid and electrolyte imbalances, and treatment of any secondary infection. High dose corticosteroids may shorten the duration of SJS and TEN. Full recovery may take 4–6 weeks.

The following table presents medications potentially associated with SJS and TEN.

Table 6.15 Medications Potentially Associated with Stevens–Johnson Syndrome and/or Toxic Epidermal Necrolysis

Antibiotics	Sulfa
	Penicillins
	Gentamycin
	Ciprofloxacin
	Tetracycline
Antiepileptic	Carbamazepine
	Lamotrigine
	Phenobarbital
	Phenytoin sodium
Nonsteroidal anti-inflammatory	Ibuprofen
	Oxyphenbutazone
	Naproxen
	Indomethacin
Diuretics	Furosemide

Side Effects

Withdrawals due to adverse events occur in approximately 10% of newly diagnosed patients treated with lamotrigine monotherapy.

• *Common side effects*
  ○ Minor skin rash
  ○ Headache
  ○ Nausea
  ○ Vomiting
  ○ Ataxia, poor coordination
  ○ Blurred vision, diplopia
  ○ Dizziness, drowsiness

MOOD STABILIZERS

- *Serious side effects*
  - ◦ Amnesia
  - ◦ Anemia, eosinophilia, leukopenia, thrombocytopenia
  - ◦ Angioedema
  - ◦ Erythema multiforme
  - ◦ Hepatic failure (rare), hepatic necrosis (rare)
  - ◦ Seizures
  - ◦ Stevens–Johnson syndrome, toxic epidermal necrolysis

It is important to inform parents and patients to notify the child's doctor immediately if any rash occurs.

Drug–Drug Interactions

Lamotrigine is associated with many potential drug–drug interactions. The following table lists some of these interactions.

Table 6.15 Lamotigine Drug–Drug Interactions
Lamotrigine interacts with:

Drug	Interaction
Carbamazepine	↓ Lamotrigine serum levels
Lithium	No significant interactions
Methsuximide	↓ Lamotrigine serum levels
Oral contraceptives	↑ ↓ Lamotrigine serum levels
Oxcarbazepine	↓ Lamotrigine serum levels
Phenobarbital	↓ Half-life of lamotrigine
Phenytoin	↓ Half-life of lamotrigine
Primidone	↓ Lamotrigine serum levels
Rifampin	↓ Half-life of lamotrigine
Ritonavir	↓ Lamotrigine serum levels
Sertraline	↑ Lamotrigine serum levels and ↑ risk for toxicity

Management of Overdose

The highest known overdose of lamotrigine occurred in a 33-year-old female who ingested between 4000 and 5000 mg lamotrigine. The patient presented to the emergency room comatose and remained comatose for 8 to 12 hours, experienced near-complete recovery over the next 24 hours, and completely recovered by 72 hours.

- There is no specific antidote for lamotrigine.
- General supportive care is indicated, including frequent monitoring of vital signs and close observation of the patient.
- Observe for rash.
- If indicated, emesis should be induced or gastric lavage should be performed.
- It is uncertain whether hemodialysis is an effective means of removing lamotrigine from the blood.

Drug Interference with Laboratory Testing

Lamotrigine has not been associated with any assay interferences in clinical laboratory tests.

MEDICAL MANAGEMENT OF PEDIATRIC PATIENTS RECEIVING MOOD STABILIZERS

The following table summarizes the recommended laboratory monitoring of the child or adolescent prescribed mood stabilizers.

Table 6.16 Mood Stabilizer General Recommendations For Laboratory Monitoring

Laboratory	Lithium	Divalproex	Carbamazepine	Lamotrigine
CBC + differential	1, 2, 4	1, 2, 4	1, 2, 4	1, 2, 4
Platelet count	1, 2, 4	1, 2, 4	1, 2, 4	1, 2, 4
TSH[a]	1, 4	1, 4	1, 4	
LFT[b]	———	1, 4	1, 2, 4	1, 2, 4
LBCr[c]	1, 2, 4	1, 2, 4	1, 4	———
Chemistry screen	1, 4	———	———	———
Urinalysis[d]	1, 2, 4	———	———	———
Pregnancy test	1, 4	1, 4	1, 4	1, 4
Serum drug level	1, 2, 3, 4	1, 2, 3, 4	1, 2, 3, 4	———

[a] Thyroid stimulating hormone
[b] Liver function tests
[c] Electrolytes, blood urea nitrogen, creatinine
[d] Urinalysis + specific gravity
1 = at baseline; 2 = at 2–4 weeks after drug initiation; 3 = with dose titration; 4 = every 6–12 months while at a therapeutic dose

Mood stabilizers are associated with many potential side effects. Management strategies to manage common mood stabilizer side effects are discussed below.
- Weight gain
  - Provide education about diet and exercise.
  - Provide referral to a nutritionist.
  - Topiramate titrated to point of appetite suppression (100–150 mg).
  - Zonisamide titrated to point of appetite suppression (100–200 mg).
  - Sibutramine 10 mg po qd.
- Sedation
  - Dose medication at bedtime.
  - Divide the daily dose.
- GI upset
  - Dose medication with food.
  - Use sustained- or extended-release preparations of medication.
  - Use concomitant histamine blockers (e.g., ranitidine, nizatidine).
- Physiological tremor
  - Check blood levels of medication (may indicate supratherapeutic levels).
  - Divide dose or change to sustained- or extended-release preparation.
  - Initiate a trial of propranolol titrated to 20–30 mg po bid or tid.

NEWER ANTICONVULSANTS WITH POTENTIAL UTILITY AS MOOD-STABILIZING AGENTS

None of the newer anticonvulsant agents discussed below has been shown effective in large placebo controlled trials for acute mania in either the adult or pediatric age group. Although the clinical profiles of these newer anticonvulsants do not appear to overlap markedly with lithium, divalproex, carbamazepine, or lamotrigine (except, perhaps, for oxcarbazepine), they may offer important new future options for relieving a variety of specific target symptoms in patients with bipolar disorder. More controlled trials are needed to assess the effectiveness of novel antiepileptic medications in bipolar disorder. At present, none of these agents is indicated in the treatment of any pediatric psychiatric disorder.

Gabapentin

Open reports suggest usefulness of gabapentin as an adjunct in adult bipolar disorder. No studies are presently available in pediatric psychopharmacology.

- Gabapentin was found useful in the treatment of 22 adults with mania, hypomania, or schizoaffective disorder in an open-label, safety and flexible-dose study. The average gabapentin dose was 1440 mg/day (Cabras et al., 1999).
- In a retrospective study, gabapentin add-on therapy was somewhat effective in a subset of patients with heterogeneous mood disorders (unipolar major depressive disorder [$n = 10$], bipolar disorder type I [$n = 13$], bipolar disorder type II [$n = 19$], or bipolar disorder NOS [$n = 8$]). Response rates were approximately 15–20% (Ghaemi et al., 1998).

Oxcarbazepine

Oxcarbazepine is chemically and clinically similar to carbamazepine. It requires no blood-level monitoring, making it more tolerable for patients. Its side effect profile is considerably more benign than carbamazepine. The available data for oxcarbazepine use in adult bipolar disorder is limited. No studies are presently available to guide use in pediatric psychopharmacology.

- An open-label study of 18 adult patients with bipolar disorder taking lithium for at least 1 month (levels 0.53–0.87 mEq/L) were prescribed adjunctive oxcarbazepine to a maximum dose of 2400 mg/day. This study found that adjunctive oxcarbazepine might be a useful add-on medication in the treatment of bipolar disorder not satisfactorily controlled by lithium (Benedetti et al., 2004).
- A retrospective chart review reported the results of 56 adult inpatients with bipolar disorder, depression, or psychosis treated with adjunctive oxcarbazepine. The average oxcarbazepine dose was 831 mg/day. The authors concluded that oxcarbazepine might be useful as an adjunct mood stabilizer in patients with a variety of bipolar, depression, and/or psychotic disorders (Centorrino et al., 2003).

Tiagabine

Tiagabine does not appear to be useful in acute mania and is not currently recommended for treatment of any phase of bipolar disorder.

Topiramate

Topiramate is reported to be effective in acute mania and rapid-cycling bipolar disorder in several open studies of adults. No topiramate studies are presently available in pediatric psychopharmacology.

M
O
O
D

S
T
A
B
I
L
I
Z
E
R
S

7. Antipsychotics

Antipsychotics are classified into two large groups: the first-generation antipsychotics (typical antipsychotics, conventional antipsychotics, or neuroleptics) and the second-generation antipsychotics (atypical antipsychotics). Antipsychotic medications are not disease-specific; they provide clinical benefit for a range of syndromes in children, adolescents, and adults. In adults, antipsychotics help in the treatment of the psychotic symptoms of schizophrenia and in both the manic and depressive phases of bipolar illness. In children and adolescents, they are prescribed for severe tic disorders, explosive aggression and conduct problems in youngsters with autism and developmental delay, for conduct disorder, psychosis, psychotic depression, and for early-onset bipolar disorder.

The prototypical first-generation antipsychotics (FGAs) are chlorpromazine and haloperidol. The group also includes fluphenazine, perphenazine, and molindone, to name but a few. The prototypical second-generation antipsychotic (SGA) is clozapine, and the group includes olanzapine, risperidone, ziprasidone, quetiapine and, most recently, aripiprazole.

Phenothiazines, such as the dye methylene blue, were synthesized in Europe beginning in the late 19th century. In the 1930s a phenothiazine, promethazine, was found to have antihistaminic and sedative properties but was not found to be very effective in the treatment of severe psychiatric disorders. In 1950 Charpentier synthesized chlorpromazine in France while searching for phenothiazine derivatives with anesthesia-potentiating actions. The recognition by Delay and Deniker in 1952 that this antihistamine, when prescribed to psychiatric patients, quieted psychosis ushered in the era of modern psychopharmacology. In 1957 Janssen discovered the antipsychotic properties of haloperidol. These agents have been widely prescribed since their introduction in the 1950s. The efficacy of the FGAs (neuroleptics) was found to be associated with dopamine D2 receptor occupancy. Succeeding compounds with increasing potency of D2 receptor occupancy were developed. Presently there are more than three dozen FGAs formulated worldwide. Their utility is hampered by an adverse events profile that includes tardive dyskinesia (TD), akathisia, extrapyramidal symptoms (EPS), and cognitive blunting. The FGAs are more effective at treating the positive symptoms of schizophrenia, such as auditory and visual hallucinations, than they are for the treatment of negative symptoms, such as anergia, abulia, amotivation, and blunted affect.

In the early1960s, while attempting to develop a novel tricyclic antidepressant, clozapine was synthesized. Thus began the era of the atypical or SGAs. These compounds are atypical in that they have a low affinity for dopamine D2 receptors and a high affinity for serotonin 5HT2A receptors. In general, their adverse event profile is more benign than the FGAs and includes weight gain, hyperglycemia, an increased risk for Type II diabetes mellitus, and hyperprolactinemia, though there is much intercompound variation. In contrast to the FGAs, their use is associated with significantly lower risk of developing TD and EPS.

FGAs have been studied in pediatric psychopharmacology since the 1960s. Now, because of their serious adverse side effect profile, they are more rarely used and less frequently studied in child psychiatry. With the exception of risperidone, almost all of the methodologically controlled research on SGAs has focused on adults. SGAs have been less well studied in pediatric psychopharmacology. However, controlled data are accumulating on the use of SGAs in children and adolescents, especially in those with developmental delay, autism, psychotic conditions, and conduct disorder. This chapter focuses on the use of SGAs in pediatric psychopharmacology, with briefer coverage of the FGAs.

SECOND-GENERATION ANTIPSYCHOTICS

The SGAs currently in clinical use in pediatric psychopharmacology are shown in the following table.

Table 7.1 Second-Generation Atypical (SGA) Antipsychotic Medications

Generic Name	Brand Name	Drug Class	Daily Dose Range (mg)[a]	Chlorpromazine Dose Equivalents (mg)[b]	Potency
Aripiprazole	Abilify	Dihydrocarbostyril	1–30	7.5	Medium
Clozapine	Clozaril	Dibenzodiazepine	25–900	100	Low
Olanzapine	Zyprexa	Thienobenzodiazepine	2.5–20	5	Medium
Quetiapine	Seroquel	Dibenzothiazepine	25–800	100	Low
Risperidone	Risperdal	Benzisoxazole	0.25–6	2	High
Ziprasidone	Geodon	Benzisothiazolyl	20–160	20	Medium

[a]Data for adult dose ranges
[b]Per 100 mg of chlorpromazine

Pharmacology

Heterocyclic dibenzepines are substituted benzamides and contain a seven-member central ring. These compounds include loxapine, molindone (an FGA),

and the SGAs clozapine, olanzapine, and risperidone. Quetiapine is a diben-
zothiazepine, ziprasidone belongs to the benzisothiazolyl class, and aripiprazole belongs to the dihydrocarbostyril class.

PHARMACODYNAMICS

The SGAs are defined as atypical because they possess a relatively low affinity
for D2 receptors compared with the FGAs, and a high affinity for serotonin
receptors, especially 5HT2A receptors. This results in a clinical profile characterized by a substantially reduced incidence of extrapyramidal side effects and
risk for tardive dyskinesia. They are also active alpha-1-adrenergic antagonists,
which may result in hypotension as a side effect. Many SGAs, such as clozapine, have effects at acetylcholine receptors as well.

PHARMACOKINETICS

Absorption
SGAs are readily absorbed from the GI tract. Higher bioavailability is achieved
through intramuscular administration. As a class, they are highly lipophilic,
protein bound, and accumulate in the brain, lung, breast milk, and other tissues. In addition to oral administration, several SGAs are available in other formulations.

• Risperidone, olanzapine, and clozapine are available in an orally disintegrat-
  ing tablet that is absorbed when placed under the tongue.
• Ziprasidone is available as an intramuscular formulation.
• Risperidone is available as a long-acting depot intramuscular formulation.

After oral administration detectable serum levels are achieved within 2–4
hours. After intramuscular injection serum levels are detectable within 15–30
minutes.

Distribution
Antipsychotics are highly lipid soluble, quickly cross the blood–brain barrier,
and may accumulate in obese individuals. They are highly protein bound to
plasma proteins and have relatively large volumes of distribution. These
lipophilic compounds can have concentrations in brain tissue 10 times that of
serum.

Metabolism and excretion
Antipsychotics are all metabolized in the liver via the hepatic cytochrome P450
(CYP) enzymes through one or both of the following pathways:

• Phase I: oxidation and dealkylation, and/or
• Phase II: conjugation to glucuronides, sulfates, and acetylated compounds.

Generally, it is oxidation by the genetically determined hepatic microenzymes
that renders these lipophilic compounds water soluble and excretable in urine.

Most of the oxidized metabolites are inactive, with the exception of clozapine metabolites. Elimination of SGAs from plasma is more rapid than from highly lipophilic tissues such as brain and lung. Cigarette smoking decreases bioavailability of the SGAs through induction of CYP450 enzymes. Pharmacokinetic data on the time to maximum drug concentration and serum half-life are reported in the following table. Please note that this information is from adult studies because the pediatric pharmacokinetics for these agents have not yet been well characterized.

Table 7.2 Pharmacokinetics of Second-Generation Antipsychotics

Compound	Dose (mg.)	Tmax (hours) Avg (range)	T½ (hours) Avg (range)
Aripirazole	15	3–5	75
Clozapine	200	2.5 (1–6)	8 (4–12)
Olanzapine	15	6 (NR)	30 (21–54)
Quetiapine	NR	1.5	6
Risperidone	1	1	20
Ziprasidone	20	6–8	7

Pharmacokinetic data for adults; no available data for children.
NR = not reported.

THERAPEUTIC DRUG MONITORING AND SGAS

In adults there exists some evidence that therapeutic drug monitoring (TDM) may improve efficacy and safety in patients treated with the SGAs. Positron emission tomography (PET) enables measurement of antipsychotic drug occupancy of dopamine D2 receptors and reveals that CNS receptor occupancy correlates better with plasma concentrations than with dose of the antipsychotic. TDM should be considered for the following.

• When patients develop side effects at below therapeutic doses.
• When patients do not respond to prescribed medication in the clinically standard dose range.
• If there is a question of medication compliance on the part of the patient.

In adults with psychotic disorders, optimal plasma levels and their relationship to therapeutic effects have been described for the following SGAs.

• Clozapine (350–600 ng/mL)
• Risperidone (20–60 ng/mL)
• Olanzapine (20–80 ng/mL)

For ziprasidone and aripiprazole, data in adults on therapeutic drug concentrations are presently not available.

In children only one small study of TDM is available for clozapine. In six children with schizophrenia, clinical improvement was seen in five of six subjects at a clozapine serum level of 289 ng/ml and a norclozapine serum level (an active metabolite) of 410 ng/ml (Frazier et al., 2003).

Indications

The SGAs are not currently FDA approved for manufacturer's advertising for any psychiatric condition in child and adolescent psychopharmacology. In adults these agents have indications for the treatment of schizophrenia and bipolar disorder.

Possible indications
• Explosive aggression in conduct disorder
• Disruptive behaviors and agitation in youngsters with developmental delay (mental retardation, autism, or pervasive developmental disorders)
• Tic disorders and Tourette's syndrome
• Adolescent-onset bipolar disorders
• Childhood and adolescent onset schizophrenia
• Early-onset psychotic depression
• Psychotic symptoms in organic mental disorders
• Disruptive behaviors and agitation in youngsters with traumatic brain injury

STUDIES IN PEDIATRIC POPULATIONS

Controlled studies of SGAs in pediatric psychopharmacology are presented in the following table.

Other studies of SGAs in pediatric psychopharmacology have also been completed and include the following.

• In an open trial of 11 adolescents (ages 12–17 years) with childhood-onset schizophrenia refractory to other antipsychotic agents, clozapine was given at an initial dose of 12.5–25 mg/day and increased every 4 days by one or two times the starting dose to a maximal possible dose of 900 mg/day. The mean dose at week 6 of the trial was 370 mg/day. Clozapine appeared effective, with more than half the subjects improving, and well tolerated. Careful monitoring for hematological side effects was completed during the clinical trial (Frazier et al., 1994).
• Remschmidt et al. (1994) reported a retrospective study of 36 adolescent inpatients diagnosed with schizophrenia who were treated with clozapine following treatment failures on at least two other antipsychotic drugs. Patients were between 14 and 22 years old. Clozapine doses ranged from 50 mg to 800 mg/day. Symptom improvement was seen in 75% of the patients. Three patients showed no improvement. Six patients developed side effects that required clozapine discontinuation, including leukopenia, hypertension, tachycardia, and EKG abnormalities.
• Risperidone was beneficial in children and adolescents with pervasive developmental disorder. Starting doses of 0.25 mg were given twice daily and increased in 0.25 mg/day increments every 5 to 7 days (Fisman & Steele, 1996). Optimal doses ranged from 0.75 to 6 mg daily in these children.

Table 7.3 Controlled Studies of Second-Generation Atypical Antipsychotics in Pediatric Psychopharmacology

Study (year)	Drug	Disorder	Number of Subjects	Age Range (yrs)	Dose (mg/day)	Duration	Outcome
Aman et al. (2002)	Risperidone	MR + disruptive behaviors	118	5–12	0.02–0.06 mg/kg/day	6 weeks	Improvement in conduct problems, aggression, and hyperactivity
Buitelaar et al. (2001)	Risperidone	MR + disruptive behaviors	38	Adolescents	1.5–4 mg/day	6 weeks	Improvement in disruptive behaviors
Delbello et al. (2002)	Quetiapine + divalproex	Adolescent bipolar disorder	30	12–18	Divalproex 20 mg/kg + quetiapine up to 450 mg/day	6 weeks	Addition of quetiapine to divalproex significantly improved bipolar symptoms
Findling et al. (2000)	Risperidone	Conduct disorder	20	6–14	0.7–1.5	10 weeks	Improvement in conduct symptoms
Kumra et al. (1996)	Clozapine vs. haloperidol	Early-onset schizophrenia	21	Avg age = 14	Clozapine avg dose = 176 mg/day; haloperidol avg dose = 16 mg/day	6 weeks	Clozapine superior to haloperidol
McCracken et al. (2002)	Risperidone	Autism + disruptive behaviors	101	5–17	0.5–3.5	8 weeks	Improvement in aggression, tantrums, irritability, and SIB
Sallee et al. (2000)	Ziprasidone	Tic disorder	28	7–17	40	8 weeks	Ziprasidone appears effective
Scahill et al. (2003)	Risperidone	Tic disorder	34	6–62	Avg dose = 2.5	8 weeks	Risperidone effective
Van Bellinghen & de Troch (2001)	Risperidone	MR + disruptive behaviors	13	6–14	Mean dose = 1.2 mg/day	4 weeks	Improvement in disruptive behaviors

MR = mental retardation; SIB = self-injurious behavior

- A small study of olanzapine pharmacokinetics in children and adolescents with schizophrenia has been completed (Grothe et al., 2000). Eight inpatients (ages 10–18 years) with treatment-resistant childhood-onset schizophrenia received olanzapine (2.5–20 mg/day) over 8 weeks. Blood samples collected during dose titration and at a steady state provided pharmacokinetic data. The final evaluation at week 8 included extensive sampling for 36 hours after a 20 mg dose. Results showed that olanzapine concentrations in these eight pediatric patients were of the same magnitude as those for nonsmoking adult patients with schizophrenia, but may be as much as twice the typical olanzapine concentration in adult patients with schizophrenia who smoke. Olanzapine pharmacokinetic evaluation revealed an apparent mean oral clearance of 9.6 +/− 2.4 L/hr and a mean elimination half-life of 37.2 +/− 5.1 hours in these young patients.
- Quetiapine therapy was effective in the reduction of motor and phonic tics in pediatric patients with Tourette's disorder (Mukaddes & Abali, 2003). In a prospective open-label study (n = 12) patients 8–16 years of age (11 boys, 1 girl) with Tourette's disorder received 8 weeks of quetiapine therapy at an initial dose of 25 mg daily, titrated to maximum doses of 75 mg/day (under 12 years) or 100 mg/day (12 years and older). The mean dose of quetiapine was 72.9 mg/day with a range of 50–100 mg/day. The mean total tic score of the Yale Global Tic Severity Scale was significantly reduced from baseline to 4 weeks (61.17 vs. 30.67, respectively; p < 0.01) and from baseline to 8 weeks (61.17 vs. 24.17, respectively; p < 0.001). All 12 patients demonstrated a 30%–100% improvement in tic severity (mean change, 61.91; 95% CI = 50. 03–73.79 for week 8). Mild, transient sedation was reported in three patients; however, extrapyramidal adverse effects and statistically significant weight gain were not observed (Mukaddes & Abali, 2003).
- An open-label quetiapine trial was completed in psychotic adolescents. Quetiapine was initiated at a dose of 25 mg twice daily and reached 400 mg twice daily by day 20. Quetiapine significantly improved both positive and negative symptoms of schizophrenia, and the medication appeared well tolerated (McConville et al, 2000). In an extension of this trial, all 10 patients continued open-label treatment with quetiapine (initial 800 mg/day titrated over 2 weeks to optimal dose; mean dose 600 mg/day) for up to 88 weeks. Significant improvements in mean scores from baseline to endpoint were seen at all time points through week 64 for the Brief Psychiatric Rating Scale (BPRS) and Clinical Global Improvement (CGI) Severity of Illness scale (p < 0.05). Improvements in mean scores on the Scale for Assessment of Negative Symptoms (SANS) were significant through week 52 (p < 0.05). Quetiapine was well tolerated and adverse events were mild to moderate, with somnolence (60%), headache (50%), and pharyngitis (40%) being reported most frequently. Extrapyramidal symptoms were not observed during the trial; however, 30% of patients reported increases in mean weight and body mass index as a "mild" adverse event (McConville et al, 2003).
- Kumra et al. (1998) studied olanzapine in eight treatment-refractory pediatric patients who had developed schizophrenia by age 12 years. At last two different FGA (neuroleptic) trials had not previously been successful in each of the

subjects. For the eight patients treatment benefits accrued on olanzapine over and above those found on FGAs over an 8-week open trial.
- An open-label study of aripiprazole was completed in 23 children, ages 6–17 years old, with conduct disorder (Findling Blumer et al., 2003). Aripiprazole dosing was initiated at 1 mg/day for children and 5 mg/day for adolescents. Treatment was associated with improvements in the symptoms of conduct disorder. The most common side effects were dyspepsia, vomiting, somnolence, and lightheadedness.

Choosing A Second-Generation Antipsychotic

Atypical antipsychotics are not currently FDA approved for any pediatric neuropsychiatric disorder. Nevertheless, these agents are commonly used for a variety of psychotic disorders, tic disorders, bipolar disorders, and conduct disorders in referred children and adolescents. Risperidone is the best studied agent in the pediatric age range to date.

Before initiating treatment with SGAs
- Complete a baseline physical examination and medical history. An examination within the 6–12 months previous to the start of medication is generally sufficient in the medically healthy child and adolescent.
- Obtain a careful history of any metabolic disorders and/or diabetes in the patient and family. SGAs are associated with weight gain in children and adolescents, which could exacerbate risk for metabolic disorders.
  ○ If a positive family history for diabetes is found, obtain a fasting blood glucose, cholesterol, and lipid panel prior to initiating treatment with an SGA.
- Obtain a baseline weight and body mass index.
- Complete a baseline Abnormal Involuntary Movement Disorders (AIMS) examination. Although these agents are associated with a low risk of abnormal involuntary movement disorders, they can occur. A baseline examination is necessary to compare against, should the child develop abnormal involuntary movements while on the drug.

Monitoring during SGA treatment
- Follow weight monthly.
- Calculate a body mass index every 4–6 months while on the drug.
- Complete a follow-up AIMS examination for abnormal involuntary movement disorders every 6–12 months while on the drug.

RISPERIDONE

Risperidone (Risperdal®) was approved by the FDA for marketing in the United States in 1993. It has a high affinity for blocking dopamine D2 receptors and serotonin 5HT2A receptors. These actions are thought responsible for its antipsychotic action. It also antagonizes alpha-1 and alpha-2 adrenergic and H1 (histamine) receptors, causing the side effects of hypotension and sedation, respectively.

Available risperidone formulations
- Tablets: 0.25 mg, 0.5 mg, 1 mg, 2 mg, 3 mg, and 4 mg
- Oral solution: 1 mg/ml
- Orally disintegrating tablets: Bioequivalent to oral risperidone tablets and available in 0.5 mg, 1 mg, and 2 mg strengths.
- Risperidone IM:
  - Available as a long-acting depot injection.
  - Safety and efficacy of risperidone IM in the pediatric age range have not been established.
  - Recommended dosing 25 mg intramuscularly every 2 weeks for adults with schizophrenia.
  - For adult patients not responding to 25 mg IM, the dose may be increased to 37.5 or 50 mg at intervals of at least 4 weeks.
  - Maximum dose for adults should not exceed 50 mg given every 2 weeks.

General risperidone dosing suggestions
- The safety and effectiveness of risperidone in children and adolescents ≤ 15 years old have not been established conclusively. However, risperidone has been studied in controlled clinical trials in children and adolescents.
- For children and adolescents less than 15 years of age, initiate risperidone at the lowest possible dose and titrate upward every 3–7 days within a dose range of 0.25–6.0 mg/day.
  - Above a daily dose of 6 mg/day extrapyramidal side effects may appear.
  - Risperidone doses above 6 mg/day have not been demonstrated to have any increased clinical efficacy compared to lower doses in children and adolescents.
- For prepubertal children give risperidone in two to three divided daily doses.
- For adolescents ≥ 16 years of age, initiate risperidone at 0.5–1.0 mg/day and titrate upward every 3–7 days within a dose range of 0.25–6.0 mg/day.
  - In postpubertal adolescents, give risperidone in two divided daily doses or one dose at bedtime.
- Starting at a lower dose and titrating the dose more slowly are associated with less risk for side effects than initiating treatment at higher doses and titrating the dose rapidly upward.

OLANZAPINE

Olanzapine (Zyprexa®) was approved by the FDA for marketing in the United States in 1997. In addition to antagonizing dopamine D2 and serotonin 5HT2 receptors, olanzapine blocks acetylcholine and adrenergic alpha-1 receptors. Olanzapine's actions at dopamine and serotonin receptors are thought responsible for its antipsychotic action. Its action at acetylcholine receptors cause anticholinergic side effects and its action at adrenergic receptors increases the incidence of hypotension.

Available olanzapine formulations
- Tablets: 2.5 mg, 5 mg, 7.5 mg, 10 mg, and 15 mg
- Orally disintegrating tablets: 5 mg, 10 mg, 15 mg, and 20 mg

General dosing suggestions
- The safety and efficacy of olanzapine have not been established for children and adolescents ≤ 17 years old.
- For adolescents, a single initial dose of 5–10 mg given at bedtime is recommended. Further titration within a dose range of 5–20 mg/day should occur at weekly intervals to allow steady-state serum concentrations to develop.
- Olanzapine doses > 10 mg/day have not been shown to increase efficacy, and the safety and tolerability of doses > 20 mg/day have not yet been demonstrated.
- Starting at a lower dose and titrating the dose more slowly are associated with less risk for side effects than initiating treatment at higher doses and titrating the dose rapidly upward.

QUETIAPINE FUMURATE

Quetiapine fumarate (Seroquel®) was FDA approved for marketing in the United States in 1997. This agent antagonizes dopamine D1, D2, 5HT1A, 5HT2, and 5HT3 receptors, which is thought responsible for its antipsychotic action. It also blocks adrenergic alpha-1 and alpha-2 receptors and H1 histamine receptors, which are thought to mediate the side effects of hypotension and sedation, respectively. Quetiapine has no appreciable anticholinergic effects.

Available quetiapine formulations
- Tablets: 25 mg, 100 mg, and 200 mg

General dosing suggestions
- The safety and efficacy of quetiapine have not been established for children and adolescents ≤ 17 years old.
- For adolescents ≥ 18 years old with psychotic disorders, initiate quetiapine at a dose of 25 mg bid. Increase every 3–7 days depending on effectiveness and tolerability to a dose range from 200 to 800 mg, given in two divided daily doses.
  ○ Some symptoms of aggression, anxiety, and sleep disturbance may respond to lower doses.
- Starting at a low dose and titrating the dose more slowly are associated with less risk for side effects than initiating treatment at higher doses and titrating the dose rapidly upward.

ZIPRASIDONE

Ziprasidone (Geodone®) was FDA approved for marketing in the United States in 2001. Ziprasidone demonstrates high affinity for dopamine D2 and D3 receptors and for serotonin 5HT2 receptors. The antagonism of these receptors is thought responsible for ziprasidone's antipsychotic action. It blocks adrenergic alpha-1 receptors, which may result in increased risk for hypotension, and has moderate affinity for H1 histamine receptors, which may cause sedation. Ziprasidone has received very little research attention in pediatric psychopharmacology; little is currently known about its use in children and adolescents.

Almost all available data have accrued from studies of adults with psychotic disorders.

Available ziprasidone formulations
• Capsules: 20 mg, 40 mg, 60 mg, and 80 mg
• Ziprasidone IM injection: 20 mg per mL.
  ○ 1.2 mL of sterile water must be added to each single-dose IM vial and the vial shaken vigorously until all drug is dissolved.
• The safety and effectiveness of the IM formulation have not been tested in the pediatric age group.

Ziprasidone precaution
• *Precaution:* In adult schizophrenia ziprasidone trials, a dose-dependent lengthening of the EKG QTc interval was found. Lengthening of the QTc was also found in a small prospective study of children and adolescents given ziprasidone (Blair et al., 2005). Patients with a history of prolonged QT syndromes should not be given ziprasidone. Prolonged QT syndromes are clinically identified by a family history of unexplained and recurrent syncope and early sudden cardiac death, with or without a family history of congenital deafness.
• Due to concerns of additive effects on prolongation of the QT interval, ziprasidone should not be given with medications that prolong QTc, such as moxifloxacin, chlorpromazine, pentamidine, pimozide, droperidol, quinidine, mefloquine, thioridazine, or mesoridazine.
• The pediatric psychopharmacologist may wish to consider a baseline and on-drug EKG when using ziprasidone (Blair et al., 2005).

General dosing suggestions
• The safety and efficacy of ziprasidone have not been established for children and adolescents ≤ 17 years old.
• For adolescents ≥ 18 years old with psychotic disorders, initiate ziprasidone at 20 mg bid and titrated upward by 20–40 mg every 3–7 days.
  ○ For psychotic disorders the effective dose range of ziprasidone is 40–160 mg/day, given in two divided daily doses.
• Starting at a low dose and titrating the dose more slowly are associated with less risk for side effects than initiating treatment at higher doses and titrating the dose rapidly upward.

ARIPIPRAZOLE

Aripiprazole (Abilify®) was FDA approved for marketing in the United States in 2002. It is a novel antipsychotic with partial agonist/antagonist properties and may possess a unique mechanism of action. The efficacy of the drug in adult schizophrenia appears related to partial agonist activity at D2 and 5HT1A receptors. Antagonist activity at 5HT2A receptors has also been speculated. In vitro data have indicated D2 agonist activity of aripiprazole at presynaptic autoreceptors, with antagonist activity at postsynaptic D2 receptors. The dual effects of aripiprazole are unlike those of conventional antipsychotic drugs and other atypical agents. Aripiprazole also exhibits relatively high affinity for dopamine D3 receptors. Preclinical and clinical data suggest that these actions minimize extrapyramidal and endocrine (e.g., prolactin increase) side effects. Aripiprazole is only just beginning to be studied in pediatric psychopharmacology; most data are from adults. Data from open-label trials of conduct disorder (Findling, Blumer et al., 2003) and a controlled trial of tic disorders (Sallee et al., 2000) in children and adolescents suggest that the dose range for children might be lower than that for adults with schizophrenia.

Available aripiprazole formulations
• Tablets: 5 mg, 10 mg, 15 mg, 20 mg, and 30 mg

General dosing suggestions
• The safety and efficacy of aripiprazole have not been established for children and adolescents ≤ 17 years old.
• Based on the two aripiprazole pediatric trials currently available (Findling, Blumer et al., 2003; Sallee et al., 2000):
  ○ Initiate aripiprazole at a dose of 1 mg in children < 25 kg in weight; 2 mg in children 25–50 kg in weight; 5 mg in children 50–75 kg in weight; 10 mg in youngsters ≥ 70 kg in weight.
  ○ Titrate every 3–7 days to an optimum dose within a range of 1–30 mg/day.
  ○ Steady state aripiprazole serum concentrations are attained within 14 days of a dose change (Findling, Blumer et al., 2003).

CLOZAPINE

Clozapine (Clozaril®) was approved by the FDA for marketing in the United States in 1989. Unlike FGAs (neuroleptics), clozapine blocks both dopamine D1 and D2 receptors and appears to preferentially block dopamine receptors in CNS limbic regions more than in striatal regions. This action may account for a very low prevalence of movement disorders reported with clozapine use. Clozapine has effectiveness in treating both the negative and positive symptoms of schizophrenia and may have a beneficial effect on tardive dyskinesia in patients with a preexisting antipsychotic-induced abnormal involuntary movement disorder. Clozapine has efficacy in adult schizophrenia even for patients whose symptoms did not improve on other antipsychotics.

However, a serious adverse event profile limits the use of clozapine in clinical populations. Because of the increased risk for serious and life-threatening hematological side effects and seizures, the use of clozapine is appropriate only for severely impaired patients with bipolar disorders or schizophrenia who have not clinically responded to trials of at least two other antipsychotic medications or who cannot tolerate the side effects of other agents, resulting in subtherapeutic and ineffective doses.

Contraindications to clozapine
• Hypersensitivity to the agent
• Myeloproliferative disorders

- Uncontrolled epilepsy
- A history of clozapine-induced agranulocytosis or severe granulocytopenia
- Clozapine should not be administered together with agents known to cause agranulocytosis or to suppress bone marrow functioning (i.e., carbamazepine).
- Myocarditis: Clozapine is associated with an increased risk of fatal myocarditis. Patients with myocarditis should not be prescribed clozapine.

Available clozapine formulations
- Tablets: 25 mg and 100 mg

Before initiating clozapine treatment
- Patients must have a severe psychotic disorder that has not responded adequately to at least 2 previous antipsychotic medication trials.
- A thorough physical examination and medical history must be completed prior to initiating a trial of clozapine.
  ○ Patients with a history of seizures must be on an anticonvulsant that does not suppress their bone marrow and results in good seizure control before the initiation of clozapine.
  ○ Patients with a history of bone marrow disease are not candidates for a clinical trial of clozapine.
  ○ Patients with a history of myocarditis are not candidates for a clinical trial of clozapine.
- Because of the known propensity of clozapine to induce seizures, the clinician might consider a baseline and on-drug EEG. Clozapine dose appears to be an important predictor of seizures, with greater risk at higher clozapine doses.
- Baseline pulse and blood pressure: Clozapine can induce hypotension in patients.
- Baseline weight: Clozapine can cause weight gain in patients. Increased body mass index is associated with increased risk for metabolic disorders and Type II diabetes.
  ○ For patients with a history of diabetes or familial metabolic disorders, obtain a baseline fasting glucose and lipid profile.
- *The patient must be enrolled in a clozapine monitoring protocol.* This is mandatory for all patients. Clinicians can obtain details about enrolling the patient at the patient's local pharmacy or through the drug manufacturer.
- Mandatory hematological monitoring:
  ○ Because agranulocytosis is reported to occur in association with administration of clozapine in between 1% and 2% of patients, hematological monitoring is mandatory.
  ○ Baseline complete blood count with differential must be obtained. To prescribe clozapine:
    ▪ The baseline white blood count (WBC) must be $\geq 3,500/mm^3$.
    ▪ The baseline absolute neutrophil count (ANC) must be $\geq 1,500/mm^3$.

Table 7.4 Clozapine Hematology Monitoring for the First Six Months of Therapy*

WBC (mm³)	ANC (mm³)	Action
Baseline: ≥ 3500	Baseline: ≥ 1500	Initiate clozapine and weekly hematological monitoring.
> 3000	> 1500	Continue clozapine and weekly hematological monitoring.
Cumulative drop in count ≥ 3000 and total count between 3000–3500	> 1500	Initiate twice weekly hematological monitoring
2000–3000	> 1500	Discontinue clozapine; initiate daily blood monitoring; observe patient for signs and symptoms of flu-like illness
≤ 2000	≤ 1000	Obtain hematology consult; consider bone marrow aspiration to ascertain granulopoietic status.
—	≤ 500	Agranulocytosis—medical emergency

*If no abnormal hematological events occur with weekly monitoring for the first 6 months of clozapine, then monitoring may occur on an every-other-week basis. Adapted from *2003 Physician's Desk Reference*. Montvale, NJ: Thompson PDR.

Medical monitoring during clozapine treatment
- The following table presents decision rules for clozapine treatment based on weekly hematological monitoring.
- Follow weight monthly.
- Follow pulse and blood pressure with clozapine dose changes.
- Complete the AIMS examination for involuntary abnormal movement disorders every 6–12 months.

General dosing suggestions
- Clozapine is not recommended for use in children ≤ 15 years old.
- For adolescents ≥ 16 years old, initiate clozapine at a dose of 12.5 mg once or twice daily.
  - The dose can be increased by 25 mg to 50 mg as tolerated, to reach a target dose of 300 to 450 mg/day for treatment-resistant psychotic disorders.
  - Subsequent dose increases of a maximum of 100 mg can be made once or twice weekly.
  - The total daily clozapine dose should not exceed 900 mg/day.

Important clozapine adverse effects
- *Agranulocytosis:* Defined as an absolute neutrophil count ≤ 500/mm³. Agranulocytosis is a medical emergency; clozapine should be immediately discontinued. Medical care and hematology consult should be sought immediately. The highest incidence of agranulocytosis occurs within the first 4–10 weeks after initiating clozapine. In the United States, since 1997, 585 cases of agranulocytosis, with 19 fatalities, out of a total clozapine-treated patient population of 150,409, have been described (*Physician's Desk Reference*, 2003).
- *Seizures:* Administration of clozapine is associated with an increased incidence of seizures that is dose dependent (Green, 2001).
  - At doses < 300 mg/day: 1%–2% develop seizures.
  - At doses from 300 to 599 mg/day: 3%–4% develop seizures.
  - At doses from 600 mg to 900 mg/day: 5% develop seizures.

• *Myocarditis:* In adults receiving clozapine, an increased association with myocarditis has been reported. Postmarketing U.S. surveillance data of clozapine-treated patients revealed: 30 reports of myocarditis with 17 fatalities in 205,493 patients. The risk of myocarditis in clozapine-treated patients appears to be 17–322 times greater than the general population (Physician's Desk Reference, 2003). The possibility of myocarditis should be considered in clozapine-treated patients who present with unexplained fatigue, dyspnea, tachypnea, fever, chest pain, and/or EKG abnormalities.

Common Side Effects

Second-generation atypical antipsychotics are frequently used in child and adolescent psychopharmacology. However, they are associated with a wide range of side effects. The following table presents some of the general side effects associated with these agents.

Table 7.5 Side Effects of Atypical Antipsychotics

Cardiovascular	Hematological
• Dizziness	• Agranulocytosis
• Tachycardia	• Leukopenia
• EKG QTc lengthening	• Neutropenia
• ↓ Blood pressure	Neurological
Endocrine	• Extrapyramidal side effects
• ↑ Prolactin	• Seizures
• Menstrual irregularities	• Sedation
• Gynecomastia	Sexual
• ↑ Type II diabetes mellitus	• Anorgasmia
Gastrointestinal	• ↓ Libido
• Constipation	• Ejaculatory dysfunction
• Steatohepatitis	Urological
• ↑ Appetite	• Urinary retention
• Weight gain	

• *Cardiovascular effects:* Atypical antipsychotic medications have several potential cardiovascular side effects. Many of these agents exert strong effects on alpha adrenergic receptors and may cause hypotension. Anticholinergic effects can cause a tachycardia. Some atypicals such as ziprasidone may cause prolonged QTc intervals, which can lead to a fatal dysrhythmia. The risk for ziprasidone on prolonging the QT interval appears less than for the FGAs pimozide, droperidol, and thioridazine, which are all associated with particularly high risk of dose-related QTc changes.

• *Endocrine effects:* Treatment with these agents may lead to increases in plasma prolactin due to dopamine D2 receptor blockade in the neurohypophysis. Consequences of prolactin elevation include amenorrehea, galactorrhea, menstrual irregularities, breast enlargement, gynocomastia, and sexual dysfunction. Clozapine has little to no prolactin elevation (Montgomery et al., 2004).

  ○ Prolactin-sparing antipsychotics include clozapine, olanzapine, quetiapine, ziprasidone, and aripiprazole.

  ○ Prolactin-elevating antipsychotics include FGA such as haloperidol and SGA such as risperidone.

- *Gastrointestional effects:* Increases in serum liver function tests (elevated transaminases) have been reported with the clinical use of these agents.
- *Anticholinergic effects:* May cause constipation.
- It appears that histamine H1 and serotonin 5HT2C receptor blockade is associated with the marked weight gain that may be seen with use of these agents. When compared to adults, SGA-induced weight gain may be more problematic for children and adolescents. Among the newer antipsychotics, long-term treatment with clozapine and olanzapine carries the highest risk of weight gain. Quetiapine and risperidone carry a moderate risk of weight gain, and ziprasidone and aripiprazole have a low risk of weight gain (Misra et al., 2004).
- Marked weight gain increases risks for insulin resistance and development of Type II diabetes. This may be especially true for children who have a family history that is positive for diabetes. The relative risk of glucose intolerance and Type II diabetes has been reported to be highest with clozapine and olanzapine, moderate with quetiapine and risperidone, and lowest with ziprasidone (Misra et al., 2004).
- *Hematological effects:* Decreases in the white blood cell count or other blood dyscrasias may occur with all SGAs, although not as frequently or as seriously as for clozapine. When they occur, these hematological changes usually emerge during the first 2 months of drug therapy.
- *Neurological effects:*
  ○ Sedation: Besides weight gain, the most common side effect in youngsters prescribed SGAs is sedation. Histamine receptor blockade appears to mediate this side effect. Sedation may impair children's and adolescent's daily life and cause them to appear drugged.
  ○ Seizures: With the exception of clozapine (see above), seizure induction with SGAs appears uncommon. Unless there is a prior history of an abnormal EEG, epilepsy, or other neurological disorder, SGAs (except clozapine) are generally not associated with a high risk of seizures.
  ○ Extrapyramidal side effects (EPS): Include acute parkinsonian symptoms, acute dystonic reactions, and akathisia. Compared to adults, younger patients appear more susceptible to developing antipsychotic-induced EPS. Other serious neurological side effects include tardive dyskinesia and neuroleptic malignant syndrome. It appears that SGAs are less likely to cause these side effects compared to FGAs. However, they have all been reported with use of risperidone, olanzapine, quetiapine, ziprasidone, and aripiprazole. Tardive dyskinesia has not yet been reported with use of clozapine.
- *Sexual effects:* Ejaculatory difficulties, impotence, anorgasmia, and reduced libido have been reported to occur occasionally with clinical use of SGAs.
- *Urological effects:* Urinary hesitancy has been reported in both adults and children with use of SGAs.

Drug–Drug Interactions

SGAs have the potential for several drug–drug interactions. These are listed in the following table.

Table 7.6 Atypical Antipsychotic Drug–Drug Interactions

Atypical Antipsychotic	Drug	Interaction
Clozapine	Fluvoxamine	↑ Serum concentration of clozapine
Clozapine	Pheytoin, carbamazepine, barbiturates	↓ Serum concentration of clozapine
Olanzapine	Smoking cigarettes	↓ Serum concentration of olanzapine
Quetiapine	Ketoconazole	↑ Serum concentration of quetiapine
Quetiapine	Phenytoin, carbamazepine, barbiturates, rifampin, glucocorticoids	↓ Serum concentration of quetiapine

Management of Overdose

Symptoms of toxicity

Overdose information with SGAs remains limited, especially in the pediatric age group. Most information is from adult atypical antipsychotic overdose reports. In general, symptoms may include CNS depression, somnolence, slurred speech, ataxia, and dizziness. Acute extrapyramidal symptoms, including cogwheel rigidity, tremors, trismus, and severe dystonia have been reported with SGA overdose. Tachycardia and EKG changes may occur, including QTc prolongation, QRS widening, and premature ventricular contractions. With ziprasidone overdose EKG QTc prolongation must be especially considered. Hepatic toxicity may occur with elevated liver transaminases. Clozapine overdose may result in bone marrow suppression and blood dyscrasias.

General supportive measures

Appropriate supportive measures should be instituted. There is no specific antidote to SGAs. The possibility of multiple drug involvement should be considered. Following a toxic ingestion:

• Serum levels of SGAs are not readily available at most facilities and are not useful for guiding therapy after overdose.
• Monitor respiratory function and vital signs.
• Monitor blood pressure.
• Obtain an EKG and institute continuous cardiac monitoring because of the potential for tachydysrhythmias.
• Monitor liver function tests.
• Monitor for CNS depression, seizures, and extrapyramidal reactions.
• Emesis is not recommended due to the potential for CNS depression and seizures.
• Monitor pulse oximetry and/or arterial blood gases in patients with respiratory depression.

FIRST-GENERATION ANTIPSYCHOTICS

Although the FGAs continue to be used in pediatric psychopharmacology, their use has decreased with the availability of the newer SGAs. FGAs have many side effects, such as increased risk for EPS, tardive dyskinesia, and anticholinergic effects that make them difficult to use. Some FGAs, such as thioridazine and pimozide, cause QTc prolongation on the EKG and increase risk for fatal arrhythmias such as torsades de pointes. The following table provides an overview of the FGAs.

This section briefly reviews several FGAs that continue to be widely used in children and adolescents: chlorpromazine, thioridazine, haloperidol, pimozide, prolixin, and molindone.

Chlorpromazine

Chlorpromazine (Thorazine®) is the prototype FGA and is used in children and adolescents for the treatment of psychotic disorders and for severe behavioral problems such as explosive aggression. This agent may also have some usefulness in treating severe hyperactivity, impulsivity, and agitation found commonly in youngsters with severe ADHD, although it is not as effective as stimulant medications for this purpose. Chlorpromazine may also be used as an antiemetic in the treatment of postoperative nausea and vomiting or following radiation or cytotoxic drugs.

FDA-approved indications for chlorpromazine
in pediatric psychopharmacology
• Children ≥ 6 months of age with severe behavioral problems and/or psychotic conditions.

Possible indications
• Severe ADHD
• Severe agitation and/or explosive aggression in children and adolescents with developmental delay and/or autism spectrum conditions.

Contraindications to chlorpromazine use
• Chlorpromazine may lower the CNS threshold for seizures; *this agent should not be given to seizure-prone individuals.*
• Hypersensitivity to the agent.

Available formulations
• Tablets: 10 mg, 25 mg, 50 mg, 100 mg, and 200 mg
• Syrup: 10 mg/5 ml
• Rectal suppositories: 25 mg and 100 mg
• Concentrate: 30 mg/1 mL and 100 mg/1 mL
• IM injection: 25 mg/1 mL

General dosing suggestions
• *Oral:* 25 mg/kg every 4–6 hours as needed. Initiate treatment at a dose of 10–25 mg for children and 25–50 mg for adolescents. Titrate upward by 25–50 mg twice weekly until a dose range between 50 and 600 mg is reached. For severe psychotic or aggressive symptoms, doses ≥ 200 mg/day may be needed. For

Table 7.7 First-Generation Antipsychotics

Generic/Brand Name (Manufacturer)	Dose Range (mg)	Potency	Therapeutically Equivalent Oral Dose (mg)	Side Effects			Approved Age for Use
				Sedation	Autonomic[a]	Extrapyramidal Reaction[b]	
Chlorpromazine Thorazine (SmithKline Beecham)	10–1000	Low	100	+++	+++	++	Over 6 months
Thioridazine[c] Mellaril (Sandoz)	10–800	Low	100	+++	+++	+	2 years
Mesoridazine Serentil (Boehringer Ingelheim)	10–400	Low	50	+++	++	+	12 years
Loxapine[c] Loxitane (Lederle)	5–100	Medium	15	++	+ – ++	++ – +++	16 years
Molindone Moban (TEVA)	5–225	Medium	10	++	+	+	12 years
Perphenazine[c] Trilafon (Schering)	2–64	Medium	10	++	+	++ – +++	12 years
Trifluoperazine[c] Stelazine (SmithKline Beecham)	1–40	High	5	++	+	+++	6 years
Thiothixene[c] Navane (Roerig)	1–60	High	5	+	+	+++	12 years
Fluphenazine[c] Permitil, Prolixin (Schering, Apothecon)	0.25–10	High	2	+	+	+++	16 years
Haloperidol[c] Haldol (McNeil)	0.25–15	High	2	+	+	+++	3 years
Pimozide[d] Orap (TEVA)	0.5–10	High	10	+	+	+++	Over 12 years

Adapted from Green WH. *Child and Adolescent Psychopharmacology (3rd ed.)*, Philadelphia: Lippincott, Williams & Wilkins, p. 105, 2001; and Findling RL, McNamara NK, Gracious BL. Antipsychotic agents traditional and atypical. In: Martin A, Scahill L, Charney DS, Leckman JF (Eds.), *Pediatric Psychopharmacology Principles and Practice*. New York: Oxford University Press, p. 329, 2003.

[a]Alpha-antiadrenergic and anticholinergic effects.

[b]Excluding tardive dyskinesia, which appears to be produced to the same degree and frequency by all agents.

[c]Available generically.

[d]Only indicated for Tourette's disorder that has not responded to other standard treatments; not approved for use in psychoses.

young children with rapid metabolic rates, give chlorpromazine in three or four divided daily doses. For adolescents, give in one or two daily oral doses.

- *Rectal suppositories:* 1 mg/kg every 6–8 hours as needed.
- *Intramuscular injections for children ≤ 12 years old:* 0.5 mg/kg every 6–8 hours as needed. Chlorpromazine is a hypotensive agent. When giving IM injections, the clinician should follow the blood pressure.
  ○ For children ≤ 5 years old the maximum IM dose is 40 mg/day.
  ○ For children 5–12 years old the maximum IM dose is 75 mg/day.
- *Intramuscular injections for adolescent's ≥ 13 years old:* 25 mg every 6–8 hours as needed. Chlorpromazine is a hypotensive agent. When giving IM injections, the clinician should follow the blood pressure.
  ○ For adolescents ≥ 13 years old the maximum IM dose is 125 mg/day.

Thioridazine Hydrochloride

Thioridazine (Mellaril®) has undergone extensive revisions to its labeling since 2000. A boxed warning indicating that thioridazine has been shown to prolong the QTc interval in a dose-related manner is now included in the labeling for this agent. Medications with this potential, such as thioridazine, have been associated with fatal cardiac arrythmias such as torsades de pointes. Consequently, the use of thioridazine for the treatment of childhood severe behavioral problems, explosive aggression, ADHD and conduct problems, mood lability, and poor frustration tolerance is no longer approved by the FDA. At the present time, thioridazine is only indicated for the treatment of schizophrenia in patients who have failed to respond adequately to adequate clinical medication trials of at least two previous antipsychotics because of lack of efficacy and/or intolerable side effects.

FDA approved indications for thioridazine in pediatric psychopharmacology
- Children ≥ 2 years old who meet diagnostic criteria for schizophrenia and who fail to show an acceptable clinical response to adequate courses of treatment with at least two other antipsychotic medications.

Contraindications to thioridazine use
- Genetically related reduced levels of cytochrome P4502D6 activity. This occurs in about 7–10% of the Caucasian population, and results in diminished metabolism of thioridazine and increased risk for QTc lengthening and fatal cardiac arrythmias.
- Concomitant fluvoxamine, propranolol, fluoxetine, paroxetine, and/or pindolol use: These agents inhibit the metabolism of thioridazine.
- Patients with congenital long QT syndrome.
- On baseline EKG, a QTc interval > 450 msec.
- A history of cardiac arrhythmia.

Available formulations
- Tablets: 10 mg, 15 mg, 25 mg, 50 mg, 100 mg, 150 mg, and 200 mg
- Concentrate: 30 mg/1 mL
- Suspension: 25 mg/5 mL, 100 mg/5 mL

General Dosing Suggestions:
- *Children 2 to 12 years old:* The usual dose range of thioridazine is from 0.5 mg/kg/day to 3 mg/kg/day. Initiate thioridazine at a dose between 10 and 25 mg and titrate upward twice weekly by 10 mg to 25 mg depending on tolerability and effect. For prepubertal children, thioridazine should be given in three or four divided daily doses.
- *Adolescents ≥ 13 years old:* Initiate thioridazine at a dose between 25 and 50 mg and titrate upward twice weekly by 25–50 mg depending on tolerability and effect. A maximum thioridazine dose of 800 mg/day is recommended to minimize the risk of pigmentary retinopathy that is reported to develop at higher thioridazine doses.

Haloperidol

Haloperidol (Haldol®) comes in a variety of formulations and continues to be used in pediatric psychopharmacology, frequently for emergent pharmacotherapy in the treatment of aggression or acute behavioral agitation in the context of a psychiatric disorder. Haloperidol is a high-potency FGA and has a side effect profile characterized by low rates of anticholinergic symptoms and high rates of EPS and long-term risk for tardive dyskinesia. This agent is labeled for use in the treatment of psychotic disorders and Tourette's syndrome in children older than 3 years of age. Only after the failure of treatment with psychosocial interventions and nonantipsychotic medications has haloperidol been approved for treating children with severe behavioral disorders, such as explosive hyperexcitability, impulsive aggression, severe conduct problems, mood lability, poor frustration tolerance, and difficulty with sustained attention.

FDA approved indications for haloperidol in pediatric psychopharmacology
- Psychotic disorders and Tourette's syndrome in children ≥ 3 years old
- Explosive aggression in children ≥ 3 years old, only after psychosocial interventions and nonantipsychotic medications have failed to achieve a satisfactory clinical response.

Contraindications to haloperidol use
- hypersensitivity

Available formulations
- Tablets: 0.5 mg, 1 mg, 2 mg, 5 mg, 10 mg, and 20 mg
- Concentrate: 2 mg/1 mL
- IM injection: 5.0 mg/1 mL
- Haloperidol decanoate, a long-acting depot IM preparation: Haldol Decanoate 50 and Haldol Decanoate 100 contain 50 mg and 100 mg of haloperidol, respectively. The safety and efficacy of haloperidol decanoate have not been established in the pediatric age group. The decanoate formulation is used primarily for treating adults diagnosed with chronic schizophrenia.

General dosing suggestions
- For children 3–12 years old and weighing between 15 and 40 kg: Initiate haloperidol at a dose of 0. 5 mg daily and titrate upward by 0.5 mg increments at weekly intervals. Haloperidol should be given in two or three daily divided doses in younger children.
  - Therapeutic dose range for nonpsychotic behavioral disorders and Tourette's syndrome in children: 0.05–0.075 mg/kg/day.
  - Therapeutic dose range for psychotic disorders in children: 0.05–0.15 mg/kg/day.
- For adolescent's ≥ 13 years old or bigger children weighing ≥ 40 kg: Initiate haloperidol at a dose between 0.5 and 5 mg/day depending on symptom severity. Haloperidol should be given in one or two divided daily doses in older adolescents.

Pimozide

Pimozide (Orap®) is an FGA that is labeled for the treatment of motor and vocal tic suppression in patients with Tourette's syndrome who have failed to respond to other standard treatments, such as haloperidol. This agent is not intended as a treatment of first choice, because pimozide increases the risk for EKG QTc prolongation. Sudden, unexpected deaths have occurred in patients taking doses of pimozide greater than 10 mg/day. Pimozide should not be used for behavioral disturbances, aggression, or psychotic disorders in children and adolescents.

FDA approved indications for pimozide in pediatric psychopharmacology
- Severe Tourette's syndrome in children ≥ 2 years old who have not responded adequately to a trial of a standard medication, such as haloperidol.

Contraindications to pimozide use
- In the treatment of mild motor and vocal tics, because its risk–benefit ratio is unfavorable in all but severe tic symptoms.
- Use of other drugs that may exacerbate tics, such as stimulants or bupropion.
- In patients with a history of congenital long QT syndrome, unexplained and recurrent syncope, and/or a history of cardiac arrhythmias.
- Use of other medications that also prolong the QTc interval, such as thioridazine or ziprasidone.
- Use of other medications that inhibit pimozide's metabolism (thus increasing pimozide plasma concentrations and increasing risk for QTc prolongation). These include macrolide antibiotics, azole antifungal agents, protease inhibitors, nefazodone, and zileuton.
- Pimozide may lower the CNS threshold for seizures and should not be given to patients with uncontrolled seizure disorders.

Available formulations
- Tablets: 1 mg and 2 mg

General dosing suggestions
- For children and adolescents 2–17 years old: Pimozide should be initiated at low doses and titrated upward slowly. Initiate treatment with a dose of 0.05 mg/kg/day at bedtime and increase every 3–5 days by 0.5 mg to a maximum of 0.2 mg/kg/day, not to exceed 10 mg/day. Unexplained deaths and seizures have been reported when the pimozide dose exceeds 10 mg/day.

Mandatory medical monitoring
- A baseline and on-drug EKG are mandatory for cardiac monitoring during pimozide treatment.

Fluphenazine Hydrochloride

Fluphenazine (Prolixin®) is a high-potency FGA with little anticholinergic effects but increased risk for EPS and long-term tardive dyskinesia. Because it is available in a variety of formulations, it is sometimes used to treat acute aggression and behavioral dyscontrol in children and adolescents with psychiatric disorders. However, it is labeled by the FDA only for the treatment of psychotic disorders in adolescents.

FDA approved indications for fluphenazine in pediatric psychopharmacology
- Psychotic disorders in children ≥ 12 years old.

Contraindications to fluphenazine use
- hypersensitivity

Available formulations
- Tablets: 1 mg, 2.5 mg, 5 mg, and 10 mg
- Elixir: 0.5 mg/1 mL (or 2.5 mg/5 mL)
- Concentrate: 5 mg/1 mL
- Injectable preparation: 2.5 mg/1 mL
- Decanoate preparations for parenteral administration: Fluphenazine enanthate 25 mg/1 mL and fluphenazine decanoate 25 mg/1 mL.
  ○ The safety and efficacy of these preparations have not been established in the pediatric age group.
  ○ The decanoate formulation is used primarily for treating adults diagnosed with chronic schizophrenia.

General dosing suggestions
- Adolescents ≥ 12 years old: Initiate fluphenazine at a dose of 1–2.5 mg at bedtime and titrate twice weekly to a daily dose between 2.5 and 10 mg. The dose should be divided and administered in two or three divided doses.

Molindone Hydrochloride

Molindone (Moban®) is a medium-potency FGA that is one of the few antipsychotics to exert no effects on the EKG QTc interval. It is also one of the few antipsychotics that is weight neutral. In some patients, molindone even promotes weight loss. It is approved for the treatment of psychotic disorder.

FDA approved indications for fluphenazine in pediatric psychopharmacology
• Psychotic disorders in children ≥ 12 years old.

Contraindications to flupenazine use
• hypersensitivity

Available formulations
• Tablets: 5 mg, 10 mg, 25 mg, 50 mg, and 100 mg
• Concentrate: 20 mg/1 mL

General dosing suggestions:
• Adolescents ≥ 12 years old: The usual starting dose of molindone for the treatment of early-onset psychotic disorders is between 50 and 75 mg per day. The dose may be titrated every 3–5 days by 25–50 mg, up to a maximum of 225 mg/day. The dose should be split and given in two or three daily divided doses.

Trifluoperazine Hydrochloride

Trifluoperazine (Stelazine®) is a high-potency FGA with little anticholinergic effects but increased risk for EPS and long-term tardive dyskinesia. It is recommended for the treatment of psychotic disorders in children and adolescents.

FDA approved indications for trifluoperazine in pediatric psychopharmacology
• Psychotic disorders in children ≥ 6 years old.

Contraindications to trifluoperazine use
• hypersensitivity

Available formulations
• Tablets: 1 mg, 2 mg, 5 mg, and 10 mg
• Concentrate: 10 mg/1 mL
• IM injection: 2 mg/1 mL
  ○ There is currently little experience in the use of IM trifluoperazine in the pediatric age group.

General dosing suggestions
• *Children 6–12 years old:* A starting dose of 1 mg once or twice daily is recommended. The dose may be titrated upward by 1 mg to 2 mg twice weekly depending on patient tolerability and effectiveness. Generally, trifluoperazine doses ≥ 15 mg/day are required for therapeutic benefits to occur in psychotic disorders.
• *Adolescents ≥ 13 years old:* Initiate trifluoperazine at a dose between 1 and 5 mg once or twice daily. The dose may be titrated upward by 2–5 mg once or

twice weekly. For adolescents, doses of 15–20 mg daily are generally optimal. Occasionally, the dose may have to be increased to a maximum recommended daily dose of 40 mg in adolescents.

Side Effects

FGAs have many side effects in children and adolescents. Adverse effects of greatest concern include the impact of sedation on cognition and the effects of extrapyramidal symptoms (EPS). Of particular concern is the development of tardive dyskinesia in youngsters prescribed FGAs over a long period of time during development. Usually, high-potency FGAs cause less anticholinergic effects, fewer autonomic nervous system effects, and less sedation than the low-potency FGAs. However, high-potency agents may increase risk for EPS and tardive dyskinesia compared to low potency FGAs. The following table lists FGA treatment-emergent side effects.

Table 7.8 Possible Side Effects of First-Generation Antipsychotics

Allergic: urticaria, photosensitivity, angioneurotic edema
Autonomic nervous system: orthostatic hypotension, sexual dysfunction
Anticholinergic: decreased secretions (dry mouth, dry eyes, nasal congestion), blurred vision, mydriasis, exacerbation of narrow-angle glaucoma, constipation, urinary retention
Cardiovascular: tachycardia, prolonged QTc interval (especially thioridazine and pimozide), sudden cardiac death
Central nervous system: extrapyramidal effects, dyskinesias, lowering of seizure threshold, sedation, cognitive dulling (probably an anticholinergic effect), neuroleptic malignant syndrome. Suppression of the cough reflex
Endocrine: elevated prolactin levels, gynocomastia, amenorrhea, menstrual irregularities, hyperglycemia, hypoglycemia
Hematological: agranulocytosis, eosinophilia, leukopenia, anemia, thrombocytopenic purpura
Hepatic: elevated transaminases, jaundice
Metabolic: increased appetite, weight gain
Ophtalmologic: blurred vision, pigmentary retinopathy, epithelial keratopathy

Management of Side Effects

General comments
- Side effects may be minimized by introducing FGAs at a low dose and titrating upward slowly (e.g., once or twice weekly).
- Because of the risk for tardive dyskinesia a baseline Abnormal Involuntary Movement Scale (AIMS) must be completed at baseline before introduction of the FGA and repeated every 6 months while on drug.
- There appears to be no added benefit, but an increased risk of inducing side effects, by using FGA doses that exceed the standard dose range. Generally, there exists a therapeutic window for psychotic disorders of approximately 300–1000 mg/day of chlorpromazine equivalents (Green, 2001). Patients receiving more than this window generally do not exhibit added benefit from the higher dose and often develop more side effects.
- Blood pressure monitoring is suggested for children and adolescents receiving low-potency FGAs with autonomic nervous system effects on blood pressure.

ANTIPSYCHOTICS

Monitoring should occur at baseline, on full dose, and during dose increments.

• Anticholinergic side effects and sedation may be minimized by using the lowest effective dose for the patient.

Extrapyramidal side effects, tardive dyskinesia, and neuroleptic malignant syndrome

The management of EPS, TD, and NMS is covered in Chapter 8 on anticholinergics, amantadine, dopamine agonists, and drugs to treat extrapyramidal symptoms and syndromes and is not repeated here.

8. Drugs to Treat Extrapyramidal Symptoms and Syndromes

Neuroleptic- and antipsychotic-induced extrapyramidal side effects (EPS) are diminished by anticholinergic medications, amantadine, antihistamines, benzodiazepines, beta-blockers, and other dopamine agonists. Vitamin E may provide neuroprotective effects in neurons damaged by neuroleptic- and antipsychotic-induced dyskinetic movement disorders. Benzodiazepines and antihistamines are discussed in Chapter 9, on anxiolytics. Beta-blockers are discussed in Chapter 10 on noradrenergic agents. This chapter discusses anticholinergic agents, amantadine, other dopamine agonists, and Vitamin E.

The basal ganglia, including the caudate nucleus, globus pallidus, and putamen, are the main location of the CNS extrapyramidal system that helps modulate motor activity. Dysfunction in the basal ganglia is manifested primarily by the development of involuntary movement disorders (e.g., dystonia, akathisia, Parkinson's symptoms, tremor). The theoretical mechanism for neuroleptic- and antipsychotic-induced EPS is thought to involve the balance between dopamine and acetylcholine availability in the basal ganglia. When neuroleptics and antipsychotics block dopamine receptors, the balance between dopamine and acetylcholine neurotransmission is upset and movement disorders may occur. Up-regulating dopamine systems or down-regulating acetylcholine systems can restore this balance and ameliorate EPS symptoms.

ANTICHOLINERGICS

Anticholinergic agents used in pediatric psychopharmacology include benztropine (Cogentin®, Tremin®), biperiden (Akineton®), procyclidine (Kemadrin®), and trihexyphenidyl (Artane®, Trihexane®, Trihexy-5®). Others in this class include ethopropazine (Parsidol®) and orphenadrine citrate (Norflex®, Dispal®). The former are used more than the last two agents in child and adolescent psychopharmacology and are the focus of discussion here. Before the introduction of levodopa, the anticholinergics were the principal agents used for treating Parkinson's disease. Although they are occasionally used for this purpose, their current main indication is in the treatment of drug-induced EPS.

Pharmacology

The anticholinergics are congeners of atropine. As tertiary amines, they are sufficiently lipophilic to gain access to the central nervous system. Benztropine, the most frequently prescribed anticholinergic agent in psychiatric practice, was synthesized in an effort to combine the beneficial effects of an antihistamine (diphenhydramine) with those of a belladonna alkaloid (atropine).

PHARMACODYNAMICS

- Anticholinergics block the effects of acetylcholine and related agonists at muscarinic acetylcholine receptors.
- Anticholinergics have no effects on nicotinic receptors in automatic ganglia or in neuromuscular junctions.

PHARMACOKINETICS

Absorption
- Anticholinergics are readily absorbed after oral dosing.
- Peak plasma concentrations occur within 1 to 2 hours after oral administration.
- Parental formulations are available for benztropine and biperiden; the onset of action with IM preparations occurs within minutes.
  ○ Onset of action with intramuscular injection does not differ from onset with intravenous administration. Therefore, for these agents IM injection is the preferred route of administration over IV.

Metabolism and excretion
- Anticholinergic agents are metabolized in the liver.
- The half-life in adults of the various anticholinergics ranges between 3 and 24 hours.
  ○ Trihexyphenidyl has a shorter half-life of approximately 3–10 hours in adults.
  ○ Benztropine and biperiden have long half-lives of approximately 12–24 hours.

Table 8.1 Anticholinergic Drug Pharmacokinetics

Drug	Time to Peak Concentration (hrs)	Elimination Half-Life (hrs)	% Oral Bioavailability
Benztropine			
Oral	1–1.5	12–24	Poor
IM	Minutes	12–24	———
Biperiden			
Oral	1–1.5	18–24	29–33
IM	Minutes	18–24	———
Procyclidine	1–2	7–16	75
Trihexyphenidyl	1–1.5	3–4	100

Indications

The established indications for anticholinergic drugs are the same in child and adolescent psychiatry as they are in adult psychiatry. Anticholinergics are generally used to manage neuroleptic- and atypical antipsychotic-induced EPS.

- Emergent treatment of drug-induced acute dystonic reactions.
- Prophylaxis of drug-induced EPS.
  - Drug-induced parkinsonism
  - Drug-induced akathisia

Pertinent Studies

There are few recent studies of anticholinergic medications in child and adolescent psychopharmacology. Most of the pediatric psychopharmacological practice concerning anticholinergic treatment of drug-induced EPS has been extrapolated from adult psychiatry studies or pediatric neurology practice without much actual research completed in child and adolescent psychiatry patients. Pertinent studies are mostly case reports and are described below:

- Casken et al. (2003) describe a 5-year-old girl with idiopathic epilepsy who developed lingual–facial–buccal EPS upon treatment with phenytoin. Phenytoin was discontinued and biperiden introduced. Biperiden successfully treated the EPS.
- Hoon et al. (2001) describe a retrospective chart survey of 22 children with extrapyramidal cerebral palsy and an upper and/or lower extremity involuntary movement disorder. Trihexyphenidyl successfully improved EPS in these children.
- Keepers et al. (1983) describe the successful prophylaxis of neuroleptic-induced EPS with anticholinergic drugs in 215 psychotic inpatients, many of whom were adolescents.
- Teoh et al. (2002) describe a psychotic child with comorbid ADHD who developed EPS on risperidone, methylphenidate, sertraline, tropisetron, and ketorolac. Benztropine successfully ameliorated the EPS.

Choosing an Anticholinergic for EPS

All anticholinergic agents are equally effective in the treatment of medication-induced movement disorders and EPS (e.g., acute dystonia, parkinsonism).

General dosing suggestions
- For treatment-emergent acute dystonic reactions, give anticholinergics, such as benztropine 1–2 mg IM. If not effective, the IM dose may be repeated in 20–30 minutes.
- For prophylaxis of EPS with ongoing neuroleptic or antipsychotic treatment, give an anticholinergic, such as benztropine, orally in two to four daily divided doses.

EXTRAPYRAMIDAL DRUGS

Table 8.2 Anticholinergic Drug Doses

Generic Name	Trade Name	Available Doses (mg) (tablet/capsule color)	Usual Daily Dose	Dose Schedule (in divided doses)
Benztropine	Cogentin®	T: 0.5 (white) T: 1 (white) T: 2 (white) INJ: 1 mg/ml	0.25–4 mg/day 1–2 mg IM	Once daily to tid acute dystonia
Biperiden	Akineton®	T: 2 (white) INJ: 5 mg/ml	0.04 mg/kg/dose 1–2 mg IM	bid to tid acute dystonia
Procyclidine	Kemadrin®	T: 5 (white)	2.5–15 mg/day	bid to tid
Trihexylphenidyl	Artane®	T: 2 (white)	6–15 mg/day	tid to qid
		T: 5 (white) SR: 5 (blue) E: 2 mg/5 ml		

E = Elixer; INJ = Injectable; SR = Sustained release; t = tablet

○ Begin at a low dose of 0.25–0.5 mg bid benztropine and titrate slowly upward.
○ Give anticholinergics in the lowest possible effective daily dose to prevent the occurrence of EPS.

Discontinuing treatment
• The sudden withdrawal of anticholinergic agents such as benztropine or biperiden may cause an anticholinergic withdrawal syndrome.
• The symptoms of an anticholinergic withdrawal syndrome may include:
○ Nervousness
○ Weeping
○ Craving
○ Restlessness
○ Insomnia
○ Vomiting
○ Malaise
○ Headache
○ Blurred vision
○ Hallucinations
○ Motor agitation
• Tapering anticholinergic medication is advised, especially tapering from chronic maintenance therapy at high dose.

Contraindications

• Children under 3 years of age
• Known hypersensitivity to anticholinergic agents
• Tardive dyskinesia
• Untreated narrow-angle glaucoma
• Obstructive gastrointestinal disease

• Predisposition to tachycardia arrhythmias
• Obstructive uropathy

Psychological and physical dependence have been reported with trihexyphenidyl. This anticholinergic agent may be deliberately abused by substance abusers for its stimulating and euphoric effects.

Side Effects

The adverse effects of anticholinergic agents are related to blockade of muscarinic cholinergic receptors in the periphery and in the CNS. Possible side effects are listed in the following table.

Table 8.3 Anticholinergic Drug Side Effects

CNS	URINARY
Psychosis	Urinary retention
Hallucinations	
Confusion	OCULAR
Delirium	Blurred Vision
Tardive dyskinesia	Mydriasis
Memory dyskinesia	Exacerbation of narrow-angle
Hyperthermia and fever	glaucoma
CARDIAC	DERMATOLOGICAL
Cardiac arrhythmias	Oligohydrosis
Tachycardia (most common)	Dry skin
Bradycardia	Dry mucus membranes
	Rash
GASTROINTESTIONAL	
Constipation	
Paralytic ileus	
Esopageal atony	
Nausea	
Vomiting	
Dry mouth	

E X T R A P Y R A M I D A L   D R U G S

Managing anticholinergic side effects
• The atropine-like side effects of anticholinergic agents increase as dose is titrated upward. To minimize side effects use anticholinergic agents in the lowest possible dose.
• Avoid combining anticholinergic agents with drugs known to have anticholinergic properties (e.g., chlorpromazine, thioridazine, chlorpheniramine cough syrup).

Drug–Drug Interactions

Anticholinergic agents should be used cautiously with other medications known to have anticholinergic properties. Drug–drug interactions are described in the following table.

Table 8.4 Anticholinergic Drug–Drug Interactions
Anticholinergic drug interacts with:

Drug	Interaction
Amantadine	↑ Anticholinergic effects, confusion, hallucinations
Antihistamines	↑ Anticholinergic effects
Atenolol	↑ Atenolol plasmal concentration
Belladonna alkaloids	↑ Anticholinergic effects
Betel nut	↓ Anticholinergic effects
Cisapride	↓ Gastric motility
MAOIs	↑ Anticholinergic effects
Phenothiazines	↑ Anticholinergic effects ↓ Phenothiazine serum levels ↓ Phenothiazine effectiveness
Primidone	↑ Sedation
Propranolol	↓ Bradycardia
Tricyclic antidepressants	↑ Anticholinergic effects

Management of Overdose

Symptoms of anticholinergic toxicity include an extremely dry mouth, dry upper respiratory tract, dry skin, elevation of body temperature, confusion, delirium, hallucinations, disturbances of memory, rapid heart rate, blush (due to vasodilation of the cutaneous blood vessels in the blush areas of the body), and decreased sweating. These signs of toxicity can be especially prominent in young children and children less than 3 years old. Anticholinergic toxicity may be fatal in young children; it is rarely fatal in adults.

Management of anticholinergic toxicity
• Supportive measures
• Adequate IV hydration
• Cardiac monitoring.
• Perform gastric lavage or induce emesis in the conscious patient.
• Monitor the airway.
• Apply cold preparations or ice bags to reduce hyperthermia.

PHYSOSTIGMINE

The anticholinergic inhibitor physostigmine salicylate (Antilirium®, Eserine®) may be used to reduce the severity of the CNS effects resulting from anti-cholinergic toxicity. In doses of 0.5 mg–2.0 mg slow IV infusion, physostigmine is effective in counteracting CNS symptoms of confusion, delirium, and coma. Physostigmine is itself potentially toxic and must be administered slowly with careful observation of the patient. Cardiac monitoring and life support measures must be readily available. The duration of action of physostigmine is shorter that the duration of anticholinergic toxicity. Administration of physostigmine usually must be repeated to prevent the recurrence of the symptoms of anti-cholinergic poisoning.

Drug Interference with Laboratory Testing

Increased heart rate on EKG.

AMANTADINE HYDROCHLORIDE

Pharmacology

Amantadine (Symmetrel®, Symadine®) is an antiviral agent that also increases dopaminergic activity in the peripheral and central nervous system. It has pharmacological actions as both an anti-Parkinson and an antiviral drug and was initially marketed as an antiviral agent for the prophylaxis of influenza A. In the 1960s it was discovered to have effects in Parkinson's disease in a patient who received amantadine for protection against the influenza virus. It became standard therapy in the 1970s to provide symptomatic improvement of mild parkinsonian symptoms. In neurology and psychiatry amantadine is used for its dopaminergic properties. These include blockade of dopamine reuptake into presynaptic neurons and facilitation of dopamine release in the CNS.

PHARMACODYNAMICS

- Parkinson's disease and drug-induced EPS: The mechanism of action of amantadine is thought related to increased CNS dopamine release. Amantadine does not possess anticholinergic activity.
- Antiviral: Amantadine inhibits the replication of the influenza A virus. It appears to mainly prevent the release of infectious viral nucleic acid into the host cell by interfering with the function of the transmembrane domain of the viral M2 protein. Amantadine has no activity against influenza B virus.

PHARMACOKINETICS

Absorption
- Amantadine is well absorbed orally.
- The time to peak concentration ranges between 1.5 and 8 hours.
- Bioavailability is 86–94%.
- Follows first-order rate kinetics up to doses of 200 mg/day.
  ○ Doses > 200 mg/day may result in a greater than proportional increase in maximum plasma concentrations (i.e., nonlinear rate kinetics).

Distribution
- Found in cerebrospinal fluid at 75% of the concentration in plasma when given orally.

Metabolism and excretion
- Elimination half-life in adults is 10–14 hours.
- Primarily excreted unchanged in the urine by glomerular filtration and tubular secretion.

EXTRAPYRAMIDAL DRUGS

○ Urinary excretion of amantadine is pH dependent.
• Acidifying the urine will increase the rate of amantadine excretion.
• Excretion is reduced in the elderly and in those with renal insufficiency.

Indications

• The treatment and prophylaxis of signs and symptoms of infection caused by various strains of influenza A virus.
• The treatment of idiopathic Parkinson's disease.
• The treatment of drug-induced extrapyramidal symptoms and reactions.

Pertinent Studies

Amantadine has not been extensively studied in child and adolescent psychopharmacology for the treatment of drug-induced EPS. The majority of clinical trials of amantadine in the pediatric literature concern the treatment of viral influenza. There is also interest in pediatric neurology in using the dopaminergic properties of amantadine to speed the cognitive recovery of traumatic brain-injury patients, in the treatment of children with EPS secondary to brain injury, and in the care of children with early-onset Parkinson's disease. The most novel uses of amantadine in child and adolescent psychopharmacology concern treatment of ADHD symptoms and hyperactivity in autistic children. Amantadine has also been investigated in children who gain weight while receiving atypical antipsychotics or mood stabilizers. Reports include the following:

• King et al. (2001) studied amantadine in 39 autistic children, using doses ranging between 2.5 and 5.0 mg/kg/day. Compared with placebo, trends toward improvement in hyperactive behaviors were noted by clinicians but not by parents. The authors suggest that amantadine might be investigated further in developmentally delayed youngsters with prominent ADHD symptoms.
• Pranzatelli et al. (1994) describe six pediatric cases of acquired parkinsonism in hospitalized children. Anticholinergic agents and/or amantadine improved symptoms in all children.
• Shahar and Andraws (2001) describe the successful treatment with amantadine of organophosphate insecticide poisoning and subsequent parkinsonian and EPS in a 17-year-old female.
• Meythaler et al. (2002) report a controlled pilot study in which amantadine improved cognitive recovery in 35 patients with traumatic brain injury.
• Gracious et al. (2002) report nine children who received amantadine 200–300 mg/day for the stabilization of weight gain caused by atypical antipsychotic or mood stabilizer medications. Decreased weight and body mass index occurred over 14 weeks of amantadine treatment.

Dosing and Duration of Treatment

• Amantadine (Symmetrel®) is available as
○ 100 mg capsule (red)
○ Syrup 50 mg per 5 ml

- Pediatric dosing:
  - Children 1–9 years old: Total daily dose is 4.4–8.8 mg/kg/day.
  - Children 9–12 years old: Total daily dose is 100 mg bid (200 mg/day).
  - Teenagers ≥ 13 years old: Total daily dose ranges from 100 to 300 mg.
- When discontinuing treatment, it is advisable to taper amantadine to avoid rebound exacerbation of symptoms. An amantadine withdrawal syndrome characterized by symptom rebound has been described in patients with Parkinson's disease, upon abrupt amantadine discontinuation.

Contraindications

- Known hypersensitivity to amantadine
- Narrow-angle glaucoma
- Pregnancy
  - Amantadine is embryotoxic and teratogenic in pregnant female rats at approximately 12 times the human dose. Thus, it should not be given to pregnant females, especially in the first trimester of pregnancy.
- History of previous neuroleptic malignant syndrome (NMS).
  - Amantadine is a dopaminergic agent, and cases of NMS apparently caused by it have been reported in the literature.

Side Effects

The side effects of amantadine are listed in the following table.

Table 8.5 Amantadine Side Effects

CNS	GASTROINTESTINAL
Dizziness	Vomiting
Insomnia	Nausea
Depression	Diarrhea
Anxiety	Constipation
Irritability	
Ataxia	OCULAR
Confusion	Visual disturbance
Hallucinations	Corneal opacity
Headache	Corneal edema
Somulence	Light sensitivity
Slurred speech	
Psychosis	URINARY
Seizures	Urinary retention
	Oculogyric reactions
CARDIOVASCULAR	
Congestive heart failure	
Hypertension	
Orthostatic hypotension	

Management of Side Effects

- To minimize the probability of serious side effects, initiate amantadine at a low dose and titrate cautiously using the lowest effective dose.
- Do not discontinue amantadine abruptly.

EXTRAPYRAMIDAL DRUGS

Drug–Drug Interactions

Table 8.6 Amantadine Drug–Drug Interactions
Amantadine interacts with:

Alcohol	↑ Alcohol effect
Anticholinergics	↑ Anticholinergic effect
Antiemetics	↓ Antiemetic effects
Antipsychotics	↓ Antipsychotic efficacy
Cocaine	↑ Stimulation and agitation
Sympathomimetics	↑ Stimulation and agitation

Drug Interference with Laboratory Testing

Decreased leukocyte count on WBC.

BROMOCRIPTINE AND PERGOLIDE

In addition to amantadine, other direct-acting dopamine agonists are occasionally used in pediatric psychopharmacology. These agents include bromocriptine (Parlodel®) and pergolide (Permax®) and are discussed only briefly here. Direct-acting dopamine agonists are used largely in the treatment of adult Parkinson's disease, in hyperprolactinemia secondary to pituitary tumors, and in the treatment of acromegaly. In psychiatry, bromocriptine may be used in the emergent treatment of neuroleptic malignant syndrome. Pergolide is being explored as a treatment for restless leg syndrome and other periodic movement disorders. Pergolide has been designated an orphan drug product for use in the treatment of Tourette's disorder.

Pharmacology

PHARMACODYNAMICS

Bromocriptine and pergolide are ergot derivative dopamine receptor agonists with action at both D1 and D2 receptor sites. Bromocriptine has strong agonist activity at the D2 class of dopamine receptors and is a partial antagonist at D1 receptors. Pergolide has agonistic activity at both D1 and D2 receptors. Pergolide is 10–1,000 times more potent than bromocriptine.

PHARMACOKINETICS

• Both bromocriptine and pergolide are rapidly absorbed, producing peak plasma levels in about 1 hour.

Metabolism and excretion
• Bromocriptine has a half-life of 6–8 hours.
• Pergolide has an extremely short half-life of several minutes, at most; however, its duration of action may last up to 24 hours in adults.

• Both drugs undergo hepatic metabolism and are excreted in urine and feces.

Dosing

• Bromocriptine is available as a 2.5 mg tablet.
• Pergolide is available in 0.05 mg, 0.25 mg, and 1.0 mg tablets.
• For EPS symptoms and Parkinson's disease:
  ○ Bromocriptine oral doses between 2.5 and 7.5 mg/day in two or three divided doses.
  ○ Pergolide doses of 0.05–3.0 mg/day in three divided doses.
• In the treatment of neuroleptic malignant syndrome (NMS), bromocriptine is initiated orally at 5 mg po, and then rapidly titrated to 2.5–10 mg qid until NMS symptoms resolve.

Side Effects

• Dyskinesias and dystonias
• Hypotension
• Dizziness
• Nausea
• Constipation
• Confusion
• Hallucinations

VITAMIN E

Vitamin E, alpha-tocopherol, is a fat-soluble vitamin. Its medical uses include malabsorption disorders, hematological disorders, cardiovascular disease, and retrolental fibroplasias. It is occasionally used in adult psychiatry as a possible neuroprotective agent in patients with neuroleptic-induced EPS and tardive dyskinesia. No reports are presently available to inform pediatric psychopharmacological practice. However, in the clinical setting alpha-tocopherol is occasionally prescribed to children and adolescents with neuroleptic- and atypical antipsychotic-induced dyskinesias.

Neuroleptic and antipsychotic agents are known to produce oxidative stress in patients with acute psychosis. Neuronal dysfunction may result from excess free radical production during catecholamine metabolism. Oxidative stress has been implicated in EPS produced by antipsychotic medications. Vitamin E has antioxidant properties, is a powerful free-radical scavenging agent, and has demonstrated therapeutic efficacy in idiopathic parkinsonism. Although not all studies agree, some support for the effectiveness of vitamin E in neuroleptic- and atypical antipsychotic-induced EPS and dyskinesias has been reported in adult psychiatry. However, vitamin E should not be considered an established treatment for neuroleptic- and atypical antipsychotic-induced EPS and dyskinesias at this time.

EXTRAPYRAMIDAL DRUGS

Pharmacology

In 1936 Evans and coworkers isolated vitamin E from wheat-germ oil. Eight naturally occurring tocopherols with vitamin E activity are now known. The biologically most active form is RRR-alpha-tocopherol, which constitutes about 90% of the tocopherols in animal tissues. Optical isomerism affects vitamin E activity; d forms are more biologically active than l forms. Marketed vitamin E preparations are racemic mixtures of d and l forms.

PHARMACODYNAMICS

• Tocopherols are redox agents and act as antioxidants.
• Vitamin E ameliorates free-radical damage to biological membranes.
  ◦ Vitamin E protects polyunsaturated fatty acids within membrane phospholipids and within circulating lipoproteins.

PHARMACOKINETICS

• Vitamin E is readily absorbed from the gastrointestinal tract; bile availability is essential for absorption.
• Enters the circulation in chylomicrons by way of the lymph.
• Is taken up in chylomicron remnants by the liver and secreted in very low-density lipoproteins.
• Is distributed to all tissues.

Metabolism and excretion
• Vitamin E primarily undergoes hepatic metabolism.
• The half-life after intramuscular injection is approximately 44 hours.

Dosing

• Available as a mega-dose vitamin containing 100 IU of alpha-tocopherol.
• Available as a capsule providing 400 IU of alpha-tocopherol.
• Pediatric doses have ranged between 1 mg/kg/day to 100 mg/day.
• For the treatment of drug-induced dyskinesias in adults, doses are 300–1600 IU per day.

Contraindications

• Intravenous use in infants is contraindicated because of increased hepatic toxicity.

Side Effects

• Nausea
• Diarrhea
• Flatulence
• Abdominal pain
• Fatigue
• Weakness
• Delayed coagulation times in vitamin K dependent patients.

9. Anxiolytics

Benzodiazepines, buspirone, and nonbenzodiazepine sedative hypnotics such as the antihistamines, chloral hydrate, zolpidem (Ambien®), and zaleplon (Sonata®) are used in pediatric psychopharmacology for multiple purposes. These agents provide antianxiety effects in a number of different diagnoses and in acute anxiety-provoking situational settings. Sedative hypnotics are used for sleep induction and preoperative sedation; some are used for situational agitation.

With the exception of the antihistamines and chloral hydrate, almost all of the research on anxiolytics has focused on adults. Although short-term use in children and adolescents is common in specific anxiety-provoking situations, such as preoperative surgical or dental procedures, or for help with acute insomnia, long-term use of these agents is generally not recommended. This chapter discusses the use of benzodiazepines, buspirone, antihistamines, chloral hydrate, zolpidem, and zaleplon in child and adolescent psychopharmacology.

BENZODIAZEPINES

Benzodiazepines (BZDs) have been widely prescribed around the world since their introduction into clinical use in the early 1960s. Chlordiazepoxide (Librium®) was the first BZD to enter the market in 1960, followed by diazepam (Valium®) in 1963. Between 1960 and 1980 BZDs were the most frequently prescribed drug in the United States. Presently, more than 35 BZDs have been formulated and over 10 are available in the United States.

Although the abuse and addiction potential of BZDs continues to be of concern, more recent research has suggested that, compared to other drugs of abuse, such as alcohol, cocaine, heroin, and nicotine, the abuse potential of BZDs has been greatly exaggerated. An exception to this is in addiction-prone populations such as drug addicts and substance abusers who frequently abuse BZDs. These groups use BZDs to augment the euphoric effects of narcotics and to decrease drug-withdrawal symptoms from alcohol dependence or cocaine addiction. However, continued concern about the possible abuse potential of BZDs has limited their use in child and adolescent psychopharmacology. The federal Drug Enforcement Agency (DEA) determines "scheduling" based on potential abuse liability. Benzodiazepines are Schedule IV drugs; some states require triplicate prescription forms.

Pharmacology

Benzodiazepines are so named because their core chemical structure consists of a benzene ring fused with a seven-member 1,4 diazepine ring. Most BZDs include a 5-aryl substituent ring. Although all BZDs have similar pharmacodynamic properties, the pharmacokinetic properties differ because each has different substituents attached to the core ring structure.

Some available BZDs are listed in the following table.

Table 9.1 Benzodiazepines Available in the United States

Brand Name	Generic Name	Manufacturer
LONG-ACTING		
Centrax®	Prazepam	Generic
Dalmane®	Flurazepam	Generic
Klonopin®	Clonazepam	Roche
Librium®	Chlordiazepoxide	Watson
		ICN Pharma
Tranxene®	Clorazepate	Abbott
Valium®	Diazepam	Roche
INTERMEDIATE-ACTING		
ProSom®	Estazolam	Abbott
Xanax®	Alprazolam	Upjohn
SHORT-ACTING		
Ativan®	Lorazepam	Geneva
		Mylan
Halcion®	Triazolam	Pharmacia &
		Upjohn
Restoril®	Temazepam	Mallinckrodt
Serax®	Oxazepam	Wyeth-Ayerst
Versed®	Midazolam	Baxter

PHARMACODYNAMICS

BZDs act throughout the CNS and have a variety of effects. There exists a proposed relationship between site of action and clinical effect.

Site	*Action*
Spinal cord	Muscle relaxation
Brainstem	Anticonvulsant effects
Brainstem reticular formation	Sedation
Cerebellum	Ataxia
Limbic and cortical CNS	Anxiolytic effects

Table 9.2 Drug Effects of Benzodiazepines

CNS
Depress excitability of nerve tissue
Dose-dependent depression of brain function

Neurophysiological
Depress spinal reflexes
Diminish EEG response to brainstem activating stimulation
Increase seizure threshold
Depress neuronal after-discharges in the limbic system
Diminish REM sleep
Suppress stage 4 sleep
Prolong total sleep time
Mild muscle relaxation (high dose only)

Psychomotor
Impair memory
    Impairment of delayed recall
    Anterograde amnesia
Diminish psychomotor speed
Diminish motor coordination

Cardiovascular
Diminish respiratory function

Behavioral
Anxiolysis
Sedation
May increase irritability
May increase arousal (paradoxical disinhibition)

The main site of action of BZDs occurs at the gamma-aminobutyric acid A (GABA$_A$) receptor. GABA is an inhibitory neurotransmitter in the CNS. Heterogeneity occurs among GABA$_A$ receptors when different subunit proteins combine to form slightly different receptors. These subunit proteins are classified into subfamilies given the Greek letters α, β, γ, δ, ϵ, π, θ, and ρ. Complete BZD binding is thought to require the γ subunit. The α subunit mediates pharmacological effects.

The BZD binding site of the GABA$_A$ receptors is further classified into three types depending on their general location in the CNS and their ability to bind different compounds.

• omega$_1$ GABA$_A$ receptors are generally located in the cerebellum and cortical layers.
• omega$_2$ GABA$_A$ receptors are generally located in the cortical layers, hippocampus, striatum, and spinal cord.
• omega$_3$ GABA$_A$ receptors are generally located in the cerebellum.

The main effect of BZDs occurs via positive allosteric modulation. BZDs and GABA bind to separate sites on the GABA$_A$ receptor complex, facilitating the opening of chloride channels. With opening of chloride channels and subsequent ion movement, cellular excitability decreases, resulting in widespread neuronal inhibition in the CNS.

PHARMACOKINETICS

Absorption
- Most BZDs are completely absorbed from the gastrointestinal tract.
  - Clorazepate is the exception; it is a pro-drug that undergoes acid hydrolysis in the stomach and is decarboxylated to form N-desmethyl-diazepam, which is completely absorbed into the bloodstream.
- Most BZDS are not well absorbed from intramuscular injection sites.
  - Lorazepam and midazolam are the exceptions; they can be given IM and are well absorbed.
- Lorazepam can be given sublingually; tablets are well absorbed when placed under the tongue.
- IV administration of BZDs is used only for seizure control and anesthesia.
  - Onset of action is immediate with this route of administration.

Distribution
- BZDs are highly lipid soluble.
  - Quickly cross the blood–brain barrier.
  - May accumulate over time in obese individuals.
- Highly bound to plasma proteins.
- Volume of distribution is high (1–3 L/kg).

Metabolism and excretion
BZDs are all metabolized in the liver via the hepatic cytochrome P450 (CYP) enzymes through one or both of the following pathways:

- Phase I: oxidation and dealkylation, and/or
- Phase II: conjugation to glucuronides, sulfates, and acetylated compounds.

BZDs can be classified based on their metabolic pathways as well as their chemical structures. There are four chemical types:

- *2-keto benzodiazepines* (clorazepate, chlordiazepoxide, diazepam, halazepam, flurazepam)
  - Are pro-drugs; they may be inactive themselves (e.g., clorazepate), but rapidly undergo metabolism to active compounds (i.e., N-desmethyl-diazepam).
  - Have fast onset of action.
  - Are slowly metabolized in the liver.
  - Have a long duration of action.
- *3-hydroxy benzodiazepines* (temazepam, oxazepam)
  - Are active compounds.
  - Are the metabolic products of desmethyldiazepam and do not give rise to further active metabolic products.
  - Are hepatically metabolized rapidly via glucuronidation and then excreted.
  - Have an intermediate duration of action.
- *Triazolo benzodiazepines* (alprazolam, triazolam, estazolam)
  - Are active compounds.

∘ Do not give rise to further active metabolic products.
∘ Are hepatically metabolized first via hydroxylation, then via glucuronidation, and then excreted.
∘ Have an intermediate or a short duration of action.
• *7-nitro benzodiazepines* (clonazepam)
∘ Are active compounds.
∘ Do not give rise to further active metabolic products.
∘ Are hepatically metabolized by nitroreduction and oxidation and then excreted.
∘ Have a long duration of action.

Table 9.3 Pharmacokinetics of Some Oral Benzodiazepines

Generic Name	Speed of Onset (peak plasma level in hours)	Speed of Distribution	Active Metabolites (half-life in hours)	Mean Elimination Half-Life (hours)†
2-KETO BZDS				
Clorazepate	Rapid (1–2)	Rapid	Desmethyldiazepam (30–200)	30–200
Chlordiazepoxide	Intermediate (0.5–4)	Slow	Oxazepam (3–21) Desmethylchlordiazepoxide (18) Demoxepam (14–95) Desmethyldiazepam (30–200) Oxazepam (3–21)	50–100
Diazepam	Rapid (0.5–2)	Rapid	Desmethyldiazepam (30–200) Oxazepam (3–21) 3-Hydroxydiazepam (5–20)	30–100
Prazepam	Slow (2.3–6)	Intermediate	Desmethylediazepam (30–100)	30–200
3-HYDROXY BZDS				
Lorazepam	Slow to Intermediate (1–6)	Intermediate	None	10–20
Oxazepam	Slow to Intermediate (1–4)	Intermediate	None	3–21
TRIAZOLO BZD				
Alprazolam	Intermediate (1–2)	Intermediate	alpha-hydroxy-alprazolam (6–10)	12–15
7-NITRO BZD				
Clonazepam	Intermediate (1–2)	Intermediate	None	18–50

Data for adults; no data available for children and adolescents.
Adapted from Maxmen JS and Ward NG. *Psychotropic Drugs Fast Facts* (3rd ed.). New York: Norton, 2002, pp. 316–317.

IMPORTANT PROPERTIES OF BENZODIAZEPINES

Half-life

It is important to consider a BZD's half-life in assessing potential for adverse events.

- The longer the half-life, the higher the probability it will adversely affect next-day functioning (e.g., sedation, hangover effects).
- The longer the half-life, the more delayed and diminished are its withdrawal symptoms.
- The shorter the half-life, the less the probability of next day hangover effects.
- The shorter the half-life, the greater and more acute are its withdrawal symptoms.

Lipophilic Properties
- High lipophilic BZDs (e.g., diazepam)
  - Enter the CNS rapidly.
  - Have a rapid onset of action.
  - Have a shorter effect.
  - May be associated with a "rush."
- Low lipophilic BZDs (e.g., lorazepam)
  - Enter the CNS more slowly.
  - Have a slow onset of action.
  - Have a more sustained effect.

POTENCY

High-potency BZDs

- Have a relatively high receptor affinity.
- Have greater withdrawal symptoms than low-potency BZDs.

Table 9.4 Sample of Benzodiazepine Drug Potencies

High Potency	Low Potency
Clonazepam	Chlordiazepoxide
Lorazepam	Diazepam
Alprazolam	Clorazepate
Triazolam	Flurazepam
	Oxazepam
	Temazepam

Indications

Benzodiazepines remain very poorly studied in child and adolescent psychiatry. Methodologically controlled studies of their use in pediatric populations are scarce. Most established indications are for adults.

Established indications in children and adolescents
- Seizure disorders
- Pavor nocturnus (sleep terror syndrome)
- Somnambulism (sleepwalking syndrome)
- Muscle relaxation (high dose only)
- Sleep induction (short-term use only: < 2 weeks)
- Preoperative surgical/dental anesthesia

Possible indications in children and adolescents
- Anxiety disorders
  ∘ Panic disorder
  ∘ Separation anxiety disorder
  ∘ Generalized anxiety disorder
- Bipolar disorder in adolescents
- Aggressive dyscontrol
- Tic disorders

To date, the few controlled studies of BZDs completed in children and adolescents for a variety of anxiety disorders have produced decidedly mixed results (see the following table). Case studies and open-label studies support some effectiveness of BZDs for pediatric anxiety disorders but less than the efficacy reported in adult anxiety disorder studies. The only recent novel use of BZDs is their use in tic disorders. Because anxiety may exacerbate the frequency and intensity of motor and vocal tics, anxiety reduction may also reduce tics in children. Little controlled research is presently available about BZD use in pediatric bipolar disorders, panic disorder, generalized anxiety disorder, and emergent episodes of aggressive dyscontrol. The most robust use of BZDs in children and adolescents is for acute surgical and dental preprocedural anxiety reduction, anesthesia, and for short-term use in situational insomnia.

Established indications in adults
- Many more studies of the safety and efficacy of BZDs have been completed in adults.
  ∘ Support the clinical use of BZDs in adults with a variety of anxiety and other disorders.
- The labeled indications for BZDs in adults vary by the type of agent.

The table below presents established indications for some BZDs in adults 18 years and older.

Choosing a Benzodiazepine

Because the efficacy of BZDs has not been established in children and adolescents, neither have precise clinical guidelines been developed for choosing among the various BZDs and for their clinical use. Some general clinical recommendations on choosing a BZD for a child or adolescent patient follow:

- For anticonvulsant efficacy, a BZD with a long half-life is needed to avoid withdrawal effects and break-through seizures.
- For antianxiety efficacy, A BZD with a long half-life is needed to prevent break-through symptoms and provide more continuous antianxiety coverage.
- For the treatment of insomnia, a BZD with a short half-life is needed to minimize sedation and cognitive impairment the following day.
- For the treatment of acute anxiety associated with minor medical or dental procedures, a BZD with a short half-life is needed to minimize carryover medication side effects.

ANXIOLYTICS

Table 9.5 Controlled Studies of Benzodiazepines in Child and Adolescent Psychiatry

Author (year)	Drug	Study Type	Disorder	N (mean/range)	Age Range (Years)	Dose (mg/day or range)	Duration	Side Effects	Outcome
Bernstein et al. (1989)	Alprazolam	RCT	School refusal	8	7–17	1–3	8 weeks	Stomach ache, constipation, dizziness, drowsiness	Some benefit noted
Graae et al. (1994)	Clonazepam	Crossover	Anxiety	15	7–13	0.5–2.0	4 weeks	Sedation, irritability	Some benefit noted; not statistically significant
Lucas & Pasley (1969)	Diazepam	Crossover	Anxiety	12	7–17	5–20	16 weeks	Not reported	
Popoviciu & Corfariu (1983)	Midazolam	P-C	Sleep terrors (pavor nocturnus)	15	6–15	15	2 nights	None reported	Night terrors eliminated
Simeon et al. (1992)	Alprazolam	RCT	Overanxious	17	8–16	0.5–3.5	4 weeks	Mild	Not statistically significant

RCT = randomized, controlled trial; P-C = placebo-controlled

Table 9.6 Approved Indications for Benzodiazepines in Adults

Formulation	Anxiety Disorder	Insomnia	Procedural Sedation	Alcohol Withdrawal	Other
Alprazolam	Yes	No	No	No	Panic disorder
Chlorazepate	Yes	No	No	Yes	
Chlordiazepoxide	Yes	No	No	Yes	
Clonazepam	Yes	No	No	No	Seizures/panic disorder
Diazepam	Yes	No	Yes	Yes	Muscle spasm/seizures
Estazolam	No	Yes	No	No	
Flurazepam	No	Yes	No	No	
Lorazepam	Yes	No	Yes	No	
Midazolam	No	No	Yes	No	
Oxazepam	Yes	No	No	Yes	
Temazepam	No	Yes	No	No	
Triazolam	No	Yes	No	No	

- To minimize acute BZD withdrawal effects upon abrupt dose discontinuation (e.g., patient noncompliance), consider low-potency, long-acting agents such as chlordiazepoxide or diazepam.
- To minimize a euphoric "rush" when BZDs are absorbed into the CNS, consider use of a low lipophilic agent such as lorazepam.

Dosing and Duration of Treatment

Dosing and duration of treatment with BZDs have not been established in child and adolescent psychiatry. Recommendations are generally extrapolated from the adult literature. In the table below, pediatric dosing suggestions for BZDs are calculated from adult doses by assuming a 70 kg average adult weight and converting to milligrams per kilogram and rounding downward. Cited pediatric doses are conservative. In the table below, available doses, minimum age approved for use, general starting dose, general titration schedule, and usual daily dose in milligrams per kilogram are provided for some available long-acting, intermediate-acting, and short-acting BZDs.

Before initiating treatment
- Inquire about the patient's and family's risk for substance abuse.
  ○ Substance abuse is a relative contraindication to BZD treatment.
- No additional pretreatment medical or laboratory work is needed.
- Determine how the effectiveness of BZD therapy is to be measured (e.g., anxiety symptoms, sleep efficacy).
  ○ Determine baseline to be used against an on-drug comparison.

General dosing suggestions
- Initiate BZD treatment with a low dose (e.g., ~20–25% of the usual daily dose).
- Titrate every 5–7 days, assessing effectiveness and side effects.
  ○ Slow titration allows time for BZD accumulation into fat stores and for the production of active metabolites.

Table 9.7 Benzodiazepine Drug Doses

Trade Name	Available Doses (mg) (tablet/capsule color)	Minimum Age Approved for Any Use	Starting Dose (mg/day)	Titration (in mg)	Usual Daily Dose (mg/kg)*	Dose Schedule
			LONG-ACTING			
Centrax®	C: 5 (ivory-white) C: 10 (green-white)	18 years	5	5 weekly	0.2–0.8	Once to twice daily
Dalmane®	C: 15 (orange-ivory) C: 30 (red-ivory)	15 years	15	15 weekly	0.2–0.4	At bedtime
Klonopin®	T: 0.5 (orange) T: 1 (blue) T: 2 (blue)	2 years	0.01–0.03 mg/kg/day	0.25–0.5 mg q ≥ 3 days	0.1–0.2 mg/kg/day	bid–tid
Librium®	W: 0.125/0.25/0.5/1.0/2.0 C: 5 (green-yellow) C: 10 (green-black) C: 25 (green-white) INJ: 100 mg/1 ml	6 years	5	5 weekly	0.2–0.5	bid–qid
Tranxene®	100 mg/2 ml T: 3.75 (blue) T: 7.5 (peach) T: 15 (lavender) SR: 11.25 (blue) SR: 22.5 (tan)	9 years	7.5	7.5 weekly	0.2–0.8	Twice daily
Valium®	T: 2 (white) T: 5 (yellow) T: 10 (blue) INJ: 5 mg/1 ml	6 months	1	1–2.5 weekly	0.1–0.3	bid–qid
			INTERMEDIATE-ACTING			
ProSom®	T: 1 (white) T: 2 (pink)	18 years	0.5	0.5–1 weekly	0.01–0.02	At bedtime

Drug	Formulation	Age	Dose	Dose schedule	mg/kg	Frequency
Xanax®	T: 0.25 (white) T: 0.5 (peach) T: 1 (blue) T: 2 (white) XR: 0.5 (white) XR: 1 (pale yellow) XR: 2 (pale blue) XR: 3 (pale green)	18 years	0.25–0.5	0.25–0.5 q 3–4 days	0.07–0.08	bid–tid
SHORT-ACTING						
Ativan®	T: 0.5 (white) T: 1 (white) T: 2 (white) INJ: 2 mg/1 ml INJ: 4 mg/1 ml	12 years	0.5–1	0.5–1 q 5–7 days	0.03–0.08	bid–qid
Halcion®	T: 0.125 (white) T: 0.25 (blue)	18 years	0.125	0.125 q 3–4 days	0.03–0.08	At bedtime
Restoril®	C: 7.5 (blue-pink) C: 15 (maroon-pink) C: 30 (maroon-blue)	18 years	7.5	7.5 q 3–4 days	0.1–0.4	At bedtime
Serax®	C: 10 (white-pink) C: 15 (white-red) C: 30 (white-maroon) T: 15 (yellow)	6 years	10	10 q 3–4 days	0.15–1.7	tid–qid
Versed®	INJ: 1 mg/1 ml INJ: 5 mg/1 ml	18 years	No approved psychiatric indication—for preoperative anesthesia			

*Doses are for adults, converted to mg/kg by dividing by 70 kg (i.e., the average adult male weight). Doses and indications have generally not been established for children or adolescents.

C = Capsule; INJ = injectable; SR = slow release; T = tablet; W = wafer; XR-extended release

q = every; bid = twice daily; tid = three times daily; qid = four times daily

Sources: Green, 2001; Werry and Aman, 1999; Rosenberg, 2002; Coffey, 1990; Barnett and Riddle, 2003.

• Because a child's drug metabolism is much faster than an adult's, it is generally recommended that multiple daily doses be given to maximize drug effectiveness and minimize the possibility of drug withdrawal effects (e.g., two to four daily doses, depending on the specific BZD).
  ○ This is true even for pediatric use of long-acting BZDs (e.g., twice-daily dosing).

BZD dose equivalencies
Dose equivalencies to some orally administered BZDs are given in the table below.

Table 9.8 Dose Equivalencies for Orally Administered Benzodiazepines

Compound	Dose Equivalency (mg)	Brand Name
Clonazepam	0.25	Klonopin®
Alprazolam	0.5	Xanax®
Triazolam	0.5	Halcion®
Lorazepam	1.0	Ativan®
Diazepam	5.0	Valium®
Clorazepate	7.5	Tranxene®
Chlordiazepoxide	25.0	Librium®
Flurazepam	30.0	Dalmane®
Temazepam	30.0	Restoril®

Adapted from Hyman S and Arana G. *Handbook of Psychiatric Drug Therapy*. Boston: Little, Brown., 1987; Coffey BJ. Anxiolytics for children and adolescents: Traditional and new drugs. J Child Adolesc Psychopharmacol 1(1):57–83, 1990.

Duration of treatment
• Long-term efficacy for BZDs has not been demonstrated for children and adolescents.
• Because problems of drug dependence are highly correlated with length of administration, BZDs should not be used in excess of 4 consecutive months.
• Use for insomnia should be time-limited to less than 2 weeks.
  ○ Tolerance to the sedative effects of BZDs may develop with longer use.

Discontinuing BZD treatment
Patients may develop physiological dependence within the first 2–4 months of chronic (daily) BZD use. These patients are at risk to undergo a true physiological withdrawal syndrome when medication is discontinued.

• Educate patients about the possibility of BZD withdrawal symptoms.
• Gradual BZD taper may minimize withdrawal symptoms, but they still may occur.
• Abrupt BZD discontinuation increases risk for withdrawal symptoms.
• Short-acting, high-potency BZDs (e.g., triazolam, alprazolam, lorazepam) have more risk of withdrawal symptoms upon discontinuation than longer-acting, low-potency agents (e.g., diazepam, chlordiazepoxide).
• Taper BZDs gradually over several weeks to minimize risk of withdrawal symptoms.
• Rebound insomnia may occur when BZDs are tapered.

Contraindications

Absolute contraindications
• Known hypersensitivity to BZDs
• Narrow-angle glaucoma

Relative contraindications
• Patients with alcohol or substance abuse or dependence
• Patients with a history of BZD-induced paradoxical disinhibition

Side Effects

Common, uncommon, and rare BZD side effects are listed in the table.

Table 9.9 Benzodiazepine Side Effects

Common	Uncommon
Sedation	Behavioral disinhibition
Fatigue	Irritability
Decreased cognitive performance	Substance abuse
Decreased psychomotor speed	*Rare*
Diminished coordination	Hallucinations
Diminished REM sleep	Withdrawal seizures
Diminished stage 4 sleep	Blood dyscrasias (leukopenia, thrombocytopenia, agranulocytosis)
	Teratogenicity

Common side effects
• The most common side effect encountered with BZDs is sedation.
  ○ The extent of sedation does not differ among the various BZDs.
• BZDs affect sleep architecture.
  ○ Dream rebound is common upon BZD discontinuation.
• Adverse cognitive changes can occur with BZD use, including memory problems, diminished attentional focus, and reduced cognitive rehearsal of information. These side effects are potentially important in school-age children and adolescents for whom learning new information is crucial and represent a significant risk of BZD prescription to youths.
• Diminished psychomotor performance can occur with BZD use, including reduced motor coordination and increased reaction time. These side effects are also of potential importance for youth in their daily activities and represent a further risk of BZD prescription to this population.

Uncommon side effects
• Behavioral disinhibition, consisting of increased arousal, agitation, temper tantrums, aggression, and irritability, has been described in children taking BZDs.
  ○ Children may be at more risk for BZD-induced behavioral disinhibition than adults.
  ○ CNS neurological impairment may increase risk for BZD-induced behavioral disinhibition.

ANXIOLYTICS

○ An incidence of BZD-induced behavioral disinhibition between 10% and 23% is described in the neurological and anesthesia literatures.
• BZDs are highly abusable in addiction-prone patients.
○ BZD use may be clinically problematic for impulse-ridden or substance-abusing adolescents.
○ BZD use may also be problematic for youth living in a family or neighborhood with known substance abusers.

Rare side effects
• BZD-induced seizures are clinically seen primarily in drug-withdrawal syndromes and occasionally upon abrupt discontinuation of high-dose, high-potency BZDs with short half-lives.
• Hallucinations may occur as a form of CNS disinhibition and sometimes in children who are vulnerable to psychotic disorders.
• Teratogenicity remains a rare theoretical risk of BZD treatment in pregnant females.
○ Early reports of an association with infant cleft palate have not been substantiated by more recent research.
○ Because detailed prospective data from longitudinal studies are not available, however, BZDs must be considered potential teratogens to females of childbearing age.

Management of common benzodiazepine side effects
• *Sedation:* Although there is no specific antidote to the sedative side effects of BZDs, gradual dose elevations, avoidance of high doses, and lowering the dose when necessary may minimize sedative side effects.
• *Cognitive and psychomotor impairment:* Use of low doses, gradual dose titration, a short duration of BZD treatment, and careful monitoring may minimize the impact of BZD-induced cognitive and performance impairment on the child's daily life. Patients and families should be educated about potential cognitive and psychomotor BZD side effects. Caution is advised while driving, using machinery, and during athletic activities.
• *Behavioral disinhibition:* Dose reduction or drug discontinuation is recommended. Sometimes rechallenge with a different agent is useful if medication treatment of the child is therapeutically necessary.
• *Teratogenicity:* Prevention of pregnancy while receiving BZDs is recommended.

Drug–Drug Interactions

Benzodiazepines have a variety of drug–drug interactions that are listed in the following table.

Management of Overdose

The symptoms of acute BZD toxicity include drowsiness, ataxia, mental confusion, slurred speech, tremor, diminished reflexes, and diplopia. Respiratory depression may occasionally occur. BZDs are relatively safe when taken alone in overdose and rarely cause death by themselves. However, when overdose with BZDs is combined with other CNS sedative agents such as alcohol, opiates,

Table 9.10 Benzodiazepine Drug–Drug Interactions

Benzodiazepine	Drug	Interaction
All types	CNS depressants (neuroleptics, antidepressants, opiates, alcohol)	↑ Sedation ↑ Cognitive impairments ↑ Psychomotor impairments ↑ Risk of accidental overdose
All types	Addicting agents	↑ Risk of addiction
Diazepam, chlordiazepoxide	Oral contraceptives	↓ Metabolism of BZD
Alprazolam	Heterocyclic antidepressants	↑ Plasma level of antidepressants
Diazepam, chlordiazepoxide	Phenytoin	↑ Phenytoin plasma levels
All types	Zidovudine (AZT)	↑ Risk of AZT toxicity
All types	Carbamazepine	↓ Carbamazepine plasma levels
Diazepam, chlordiazepoxide	Erythromycin	↓ Metabolism of diazepam and chlordiazepoxide
Diazaepam	Isoniazide	↓ Metabolism of diazepam
All types	Antacids	Delay BZD absorption
Diazepam, lorazepam	Bronchodilators (aminophylline, theophylline)	Antagonize BZD effects
All types	Alcohol	↑ Suicide risk from BZDs

antidepressants, neuroleptics, and/or anticonvulsants, it can be fatal. Because it is frequently unclear if the patient who has overdosed on BZDs has also ingested other drugs, medical evaluation of the patient with known or suspected BZD overdose is always required.

General measures
- Monitor blood pressure and respiratory rate.
- Evaluate laboratory toxicology screen to determine if other drugs and/or alcohol have been ingested.
- Perform gastric lavage.
- Maintain adequate airway.
- Administer IV fluids.

Specific measures
- Flumazenil, a specific benzodiazepine-receptor antagonist, is indicated for the complete or partial reversal of the sedative effects of BZDs. Flumazenil may be used in situations when an overdose with a BZD is known or suspected.
  ○ There exists a risk of seizures in association with flumzenil treatment, especially in long-term BZD users and in overdoses that include cyclic antidepressants.
- Continued monitoring for re-sedation, recurrent respiratory depression, and other residual BZD overdose effects for an appropriate length of time after use of flumzenil is recommended.
- Dialysis is reported of limited value in BZD toxicity.

Drug Interference with Laboratory Testing

Benzodiazepines may
- Increase liver function tests.
- Decrease white blood cell counts.
- Increase slow-wave and low-voltage fast (beta) activity on the EEG.

BUSPIRONE

Buspirone is a novel antianxiety agent that is not chemically classified with other anxiolytics; it is distinct from the BZDs in both structure and function. The drug was marketed as an anxiolytic for adults in 1986 in the United States. Buspirone is not a controlled substance. Although not well studied in pediatric populations, its minimal sedating effects and limited abuse potential make buspirone of potential interest to pediatricians and child psychiatrists.

Pharmacology

Buspirone is an azaspirone and is the only azaspirone presently marketed in the United States. Other azaspirones include gepirone, ipsapione, flesinoxan, and tandospirone (all not available for clinical use in the United States). All azaspirones possess CNS serotonergic effects. All azaspirones increase CNS norepinephrine turnover. Only buspirone has dopaminergic effects.

PHARMACODYNAMICS

- Serotonergic effects of buspirone
  - Acts as an agonist of presynaptic somatodendritic 5HT1A autoreceptors.
  - Has variable antagonistic effects on postsynaptic 5HT1A receptors.
  - Causes down-regulation of 5HT2 receptors.
  - Probably mediate its anxiolytic effects.
  - Clinical anxiolytic effects require 2–4 weeks of chronic buspirone administration.
- Dopaminergic effects of buspirone
  - Has moderate affinity for presynaptic D2 receptors.
  - At high doses, causes a mild elevation in prolactin levels and may cause some extrapyramidal symptoms.
  - Not effective as an antipsychotic agent.
- Noradrenergic effects of buspirone
  - Is metabolized to 1-pyrimidinylpiperaxine (1-PP).
  - Effects of 1-PP include blockade of alpha-2-noradrenergic receptors, an increase in 3-methoxy-4-phenylglycol (MHPG), and an increase in norepinephrine release from the locus ceruleus.
  - Possible efficacy in ADHD.
- BZD–GABA–chloride complex
  - Buspirone does not appear to interact with the BZD-GABA-chloride ionophore complex.
  - Buspirone may have some antagonistic interactions with GABA neurotransmission.
  - Because of its lack of interaction with the BZD-GABA-chloride ionophore complex, buspirone:
    - Does not cause sedation.
    - Is not addicting.
    - Is not an anticonvulsant.
    - Does not cause muscle relaxation.
    - Does not relieve BZD or alcohol withdrawal symptoms.

○ Buspirone does not appear to interact with adenosine, muscarinic choliner-gic, glutamate, glycine, histamine, or opiate CNS systems.

PHARMACOKINETICS

No pharmacokinetic studies of buspirone are presently available for children and adolescents. The following information is based on adult data.

Absorption
• Rapidly absorbed within 1 hour of oral administration.
• Undergoes extensive first-pass metabolism, reducing oral bioavailability.
• Peak plasma levels in adults are reached within 60–90 minutes.
• Food does not change buspirone absorption, but first-pass metabolism is decreased, improving buspirone oral availability.
• Peak plasma level is higher in children, compared to adults.

Distribution
• In the systemic circulation buspirone is greater than 95% protein bound.
• The primary metabolite of buspirone, 1-pyrimidinylpiperaxine (1-PP), is phar-macologically active and has a much greater brain concentration than the par-ent compound.

Metabolism and excretion
• Metabolized primarily by hydroxylation to 6'OH-buspirone and by N-dealky-lation to 1-PP.
• The half-life of buspirone in healthy adult volunteers is 1–11 hours.
• Metabolism is reduced in patients with hepatic cirrhosis and renal disease.
• There is evidence to suggest that buspirone demonstrates nonlinear pharma-cokinetics.
  ○ Dose increases and repeated buspirone dosing may lead to somewhat higher blood levels of unchanged buspirone than would be expected from results of single-dose pharmacokinetic studies.
• Excretion
  ○ 29–63% of dose excreted in urine.
  ○ 18–38% of dose excreted in feces.

Indications

Buspirone has no FDA-approved indications for patients younger than 18 years. Few controlled pediatric studies are presently available. However, because buspirone has little sedating side effects and does not appear abus-able, it is of interest in pediatric psychopharmacolgy.

Possible indications in children and adolescents
The following uses for buspirone are suggested from case reports and open-label pediatric studies. No controlled studies of buspirone in pediatric samples are currently available to support use in these indications.

• Separation anxiety disorder
• Generalized anxiety disorder

- Social phobia
- Chronic aggression and agitation in developmentally delayed children and adolescents
  - Not useful in acute, emergent aggression because buspirone takes 2–4 weeks of use to exert its clinical effects.
- ADHD
  o The primary metabolite of buspirone, 1-PP, exerts noradrenergic effects in the CNS that may be useful in the treatment of ADHD.

Indications in adults
- Generalized anxiety disorder

Recent case reports and open-label studies of buspirone in children and adolescents are found in the following table.

Dosing and Duration of Treatment

Buspirone is without guidelines for clinical use in children and adolescents. Dosage and treatment regimens have not been established for this population. The following information is informed by the adult literature.

Buspirone dosage formulations
- 5 mg (white), scored tablet
- 10 mg (white), scored tablet
- 15 mg (white), scored tablet

Before initiating treatment
- No particular additional workup or laboratory tests are required before starting a child on buspirone.
- If liver disease is suspected, obtain a serum level of alkaline phosphatase (liver isoenzyme, not bone isoenzyme) because decreases in buspirone clearance are directly related to increases in alkaline phosphatase from the liver in patients with hepatic disease.
  - *Note:* Growing children often have elevated nonfractionated alkaline phosphatase from skeletal bone growth. This nonspecific alkaline phosphatase elevation is not a problem for clinical use of buspirone.

General dosing suggestions (tentative and extrapolated from the adult buspirone recommendations)

- Treatment initiation
  - For prepubertal children begin buspirone at 2.5–5 mg twice daily. Titrate upward by 2.5–5 mg every 3–4 days to a maximum daily dose between 20 mg and 40 mg. Give buspirone two or three times daily in divided doses to prepubertal children.
  - For adolescents begin buspirone at 5–10 mg twice daily. Titrate upward by 5–10 mg every 3–4 days to a maximum dose of about 60 mg/day. Give in two or three divided daily doses.

Table 9.11 Case Reports and Open-Label Studies of Buspirone in Child and Adolescent Psychiatry*

Author (year)	Study Type	Disorder	N	Age (Years) (range/mean)	Dose (mg/day) or range)	Duration	Side Effects	Outcome
Buitelaar et al. (1998)	Open	Autistic spectrum and agitation	22	6–17	15–45	6-8 weeks	Abnormal, involuntary movements in one patient	16 patients improved
Hanna et al. (1997)	Case report	GAD	1	4	12.5	22 weeks	None reported	Anxiety improved
Kranzler (1988)	Case report	GAD	1	13	10	8 weeks	Drowsiness	Anxiety improved
Malhotra & Santosh (1998)	Open	ADHD	12	6–12	15–30	6 weeks	Dizziness	ADHD improved
Pfeffer et al. (1997)	Open	Anxiety and aggression	25	8 ± 1.8	50	9 weeks	Agitation, mania, ↑ aggression	Only 3 patients improved
Simeon (1993)	Open	GAD, SAD, phobias	15	6–14	Mean 18.6	4 weeks	Minimal	Anxiety improved
Zwier & Rao (1994)	Case report	Social phobia	1	16	20	2 weeks	Minimal	Anxiety improved

*No controlled studies of buspirone available in children or adolescents.

ANXIOLYTICS

• Therapeutic effects may take 2–4 weeks to appear. It is unusual to observe any effects on anxiety with less than 1 week of buspirone therapy.

Discontinuing treatment
• No significant buspirone withdrawal effects or rebound anxiety is described in the adult literature, even when the drug is abruptly discontinued.
  ◦ Nevertheless, tapering off by approximately 20% every 2–3 days may be prudent and advisable, given the current lack of knowledge about buspirone's CNS effects in young children. Increased caution is also mandated by the drug's present FDA nonlabeled status for use in pediatric populations.

Contraindications

• Contraindicated in patients with known hypersensitivity to the drug.
• Contraindicated in patients receiving MAOIs or who have received MAOIs within the past 14 days.
• Relatively contraindicated in patients with known hepatic or renal disease.

Side Effects

The side effects of buspirone are generally described as mild and as diminishing over time. Buspirone does not impair psychomotor performance; a disinhibition syndrome has not been described. Buspirone causes less sedation than the BZDs, but sedation remains a possible side effect.
Other side effects include
• Dizziness
• Headache
• Nausea
• Nervousness
• Lightheadedness
• Fatigue
• Irritability

Management of common buspirone side effects
• To minimize side effects, start at low doses and increase buspirone gradually.
• For gastrointestinal distress, give buspirone with meals.
• For headache, manage with acetaminophen.
• Dizziness and lightheadedness generally improve with time.

Drug–Drug Interactions

Table 9.12 Buspirone Drug–Drug Interactions
Buspirone interacts with:

Drug	Interaction
Cimetidine	↑ Buspirone plasma levels
MAOIs	↑ Risk for hypertensive crisis
Haloperidol	↑ Haloperidol plasma levels
Trazodone	↑ Risk for hepatic toxicity

Management of Overdose

The most commonly experienced symptoms of toxicity include severe sedation, pinpoint pupils (miosis), and gastrointestinal distress. No deaths have been reported from buspirone overdose. General supportive measures are required. No specific antidote is known to buspirone. The dialyzability of buspirone has not been determined.

Drug Interference with Laboratory Testing

Buspirone may
• Increase hepatic aminotransferases (SGOT, SGPT).
• Decrease platelet count.
• Decrease WBC.

OTHER DRUGS

Other drugs included here are antihistamines, chloral hydrate, and the novel benzodiazipine receptor agonists zaleplon and zolpidem.

Antihistamines

Agents that provide protection against anaphylactic shock by blocking histamine were first described in the 1940s. Since then, antihistamines have achieved widespread use in medicine. They are used to treat allergies, urticaria, atopic dermatitis, pruritis, allergic rhinitis, insomnia, nausea, vomiting, cough, and for preoperative sedation for minor surgical and dental procedures. In neurology and psychiatry they are used to treat neuroleptic-induced extrapyramidal symptoms, symptoms of Parkinson's disease, acute dystonic reactions, anxiety, agitation, and insomnia.

First-generation antihistamines include diphenhydramine (Benedryl®) and hydroxyzine hydrochloride (Atarax®, Vistaril®). These drugs readily cross the blood–brain barrier and cause sedation and have antianxiety properties. Second-generation antihistamines include cetirizine (Zyrtec®), fexofenadine (Allegra®), and loratadine (Clarinex®). These formulations do not cross the blood–brain barrier as readily, and they cause less sedation. Their use is preferred over first-generation agents in the treatment of immunological, allergic, and dermatological diseases. Antihistamines are not scheduled drugs by the DEA.

In child and adolescent psychiatry, first-generation antihistamines are used rather than second-generation agents and are the focus of discussion. Although cyproheptadine (Periactin®) and promethazine (Phenergan®) are also antihistamines, they are not widely used in pediatric psychopharmacology and are not discussed here.

PHARMACOLOGY

Diphenhydramine is an ethanolamine, and hydroxyzine hydrochloride is a piperidine. The structures of antihistamines resemble histamine in that many agents contain a substituted ethylamine moity. The antihistamines differ from

ANXIOLYTICS

histamine by replacing the primary amino group and single aromatic ring with a tertiary amino group, linked by a two- or three-atom chain to two aromatic substituents.

PHARMACODYNAMICS

• The antihistamines act as competitive inhibitors of histamine at H1 receptors.
• Inside the CNS, H1 antagonists have the following effects:
  ◦ Diminished alertness
  ◦ Slowed psychomotor reaction time
  ◦ Sedation
    ▪ Tolerance builds to the sedative effects of antihistamines within 1 week.
  ◦ Decreased motion sickness (thought to be due to anticholinergic effects)
• Outside the CNS, H1 antagonists have the following effects:
  ◦ Smooth muscle contraction
  ◦ Vasoconstriction
  ◦ Increased capillary permeability and the formation of the edema and wheal and flare reaction.
  ◦ First-generation H1 antagonists block muscarinic cholinergic receptors.

PHARMACOKINETICS

There are no current pharmacokinetic data available in children and adolescents. The following discussion is based on antihistamine studies of adults.

Absorption
• Antihistamines are rapidly absorbed when given orally.
• Peak plasma concentrations are generally reached within 2 hours, and sedative effects peak 1–3 hours after dosing.
• Diphenhydramine is available in IM and IV formulations.

Distrib ution
• Widely distributed throughout the body.
• 98–99% protein bound.

Metabolism and excretion
• Have a plasma half-life between 1 and 4 hours.
• Children metabolize antihistamines faster than adults.
  ◦ The half-life in children is only 60% that of young adults.
• The H1 antagonists are metabolized in the liver.
  ◦ Diphenhydramine is mainly metabolized via N-demethylation.
  ◦ Diphenhydramine is able to induce hepatic microsomal enzymes and may increase the rate of its own metabolism.
• Metabolites are excreted unchanged in the urine.

INDICATIONS

First-generation antihistamines have been used for over 30 years in the acute treatment of anxiety, agitation, and insomnia in children and adolescents.

Currently their most appropriate use is for the short-term treatment of insomnia and to treat situational or anticipatory anxiety. Hydroxyzine has gained FDA approval for the short-term treatment of anxiety. Despite widespread clinical use, there are no recent controlled studies of antihistamines in the treatment of anxiety disorders, insomnia, or agitation in pediatric populations. At present antihistamines cannot be recommended as the primary treatment for any chronic child or adolescent psychiatric disorder.

Antihistamines should be used for short-term periods of days to weeks. Longer-term use is not recommended.

- Symptomatic and short-term (< 4 months) relief of anxiety and tension
- Pruritus due to allergic conditions
- Preoperative sedation
- Drug-induced extrapyramidal reactions
- Motion sickness
- Short-term relief of acute situational insomnia

DOSING AND DURATION OF TREATMENT

Before initiating treatment
- No additional medical workup or laboratory tests are needed.

General dosing suggestions
- Diphenhydramine
  ○ Initiate treatment with 25 mg. Titrate upward by 25 mg every 3–4 days for optimal response. Maximum dose is 5 mg/kg/day or 300 mg/day. Give in three or four divided doses each day.
- Hydroxyzine
  ○ Initiate treatment with 10–25 mg. Titrate upward by 10–25 mg every 3-4 days for optimal response. Maximum dose is 50–100 mg/day. Administer in three or four divided doses each day.

Discontinuing treatment

- Medication tapering is recommended because anticholinergic rebound effects have been described with abrupt discontinuation of high-dose antihistamines, especially diphenhydramine.

CONTRAINDICATIONS

- Known hypersensitivity reactions to antihistamines
- Premature and newborn infants
- Antihistamines are contraindicated in a variety of situations depending on their anticholinergic activity:
  ○ Narrow-angle glaucoma
  ○ Urinary outlet obstruction
  ○ Gastrointestional obstruction

ANXIOLYTICS

Table 9.13 Nonbenzodiazepine Sedative/Hypnotic Drug Doses

Generic Name	Trade Name	Available Doses (mg) (tablet/capsule color)	Minimum Age Approved for Any Use	Starting Dose (mg/day)	Titration (in mg)	Usual Daily Dose (mg/kg)	Dose Schedule
Chloral hydrate	Noctec® Aquachloral® Supprettes®	E: 500 mg per 5 ml C: 250 C: 500 S: 324 mg, 500 mg, 648 mg	Infants	250–500	None	25–100 mg/kg Max dose: Infants 1 g/dose Max dose: Children 2 g/dose	Preprocedural only
Diphenhydramine	Benedryl®	T: 25 (generic: various) T: 50 (generic: various) C: 25 (generic: various) C: 50 (generic: various) INJ: 50 mg per 1 ml E: 12.5 mg per 5 ml	Not for neonatal/ premature infants	Children: 10 Adolescents: 25	10 q 3–4 d 25 q 3–4 d	5 mg/kg 5 mg/kg	bid–qid bid–qid
Hydroxyzine	Atarax®	T: 10 (orange) T: 25 (green) T: 50 (yellow) T: 100 (red) E: 10 mg per 5 ml	Not for neonatal/ premature infants	Children: 10 Adolescents: 25	10 q 3–4 d 25 q 3–4 d	50–100 mg/d 50–100 mg/d	bid–qid bid–qid
Hydroxyzine	Vistaril®	C: 25 (green) C: 50 (green and white) C: 100 (green and gray) E: 25 mg per 5 ml	Not for neonatal/ premature infants	25	25 q 3–4 d	50–100	bid–quid
Zaleplon[a]	Sonata®	C: 5 (green/pale green) C: 10 (green/light green)	18 years old	5–10	None	5–10	qhs
Zolpidem tartrate[a]	Ambien®	T: 5 (pink) T: 10 (white)	18 years old	5–10	None	5–10	qhs

[a]No data available in children and adolescents; data from adults.
C = capsule; E = elixer; INJ = injectable; S = suppository; T = tablet

SIDE EFFECTS

Common
- Sedation
- Slowing of psychomotor speed
- Next day "hangover" effects
- Dizziness
- Anticholinergic side effects (especially diphenhydramine)
  ○ Dry mouth
  ○ Constipation
  ○ Urinary retention
  ○ Blurred vision

Uncommon (generally seen with higher doses, especially diphenhydramine)

- Cholinergic rebound and withdrawal symptoms upon abrupt discontinuation from high dose (i.e., > 200 mg diphenhydramine/day)
- Lowered seizure threshold
- Involuntary movement disorders
- Blood dyscrasias
- Hypotension
- Tachycardia

Management of common side effects

- If anticholinergic effects are problematic, switch to a sedative/hypnotic with fewer anticholinergic properties.
- Sedation: Usually tolerance develops to the sedative side effects of antihistamines; if sedation continues to be problematic, reduce dose as necessary.
- Constipation: Consider the use of stool softeners.

MANAGEMENT OF OVERDOSE

The most common symptoms of antihistamine toxicity are sedation and somulence. Children may develop agitation, ataxia, hallucinations, or convulsions. Signs and symptoms of atropine-like effects may be prominent, including facial flushing, fever, dilated pupils, sinus tachycardia, and dry skin and mucus membranes. At high doses the patient may become comatose, which may be followed by cardiorespiratory collapse and death within 2–18 hours.

General supportive measures
- Induce vomiting in the conscious patient.
- Perform gastric lavage.
- Monitor vital signs.
- Administer IV.
- Hypotension may be treated with levarterenol or metaraminol (do not use epinephrine because hydroxyzine may counteract its pressor action).

ANXIOLYTICS

Specific measures
• Hemodialysis is of unclear benefit in antihistamine toxicity.
• Treatment of atropine-like effects is important in severe antihistamine toxicity.
  ○ Consider physostigmine treatment for the presence of anticholinergic-induced supraventicular cardiac arrhythmias (0.5 mg IV slowly over 2–3 minutes, repeated two or three times).

DRUG–DRUG INTERACTIONS

The following table describes drug interactions with antihistamines.

Table 9.14 Antihistamine Drug–Drug Interactions

	Drug	**Interaction**
All antihistamines	Alcohol	↑ Sedation
		↓ Psychomotor speed
		↓ Coordination
All antihistamines	All sedatives (narcotic, recreational, analgesic, psychiatric drugs)	↑ Sedation
		↓ Psychomotor speed
		↓ Coordination
All antihistamines	Anticholinergics (many psychiatric drugs)	↑ Anticholinergic side effects
Hydroxyzine	Epinephrine	↓ Pressor effect

DRUG INTERFERENCE WITH LABORATORY TESTING

Antihistamines do not interfere with laboratory tests.

Chloral Hydrate

Over the years many drugs with diverse structures have been used for their sedative/hypnotic properties. The pharmacological actions of these drugs generally resemble those of barbiturates: a limited therapeutic index, the development of tolerance and physical dependence with chronic use, and the possible development of life-threatening symptoms upon intoxication and overdose. Chloral hydrate is one such drug. As a Schedule IV drug, its clinical use has diminished markedly over the years as safer medications have become available. It is briefly discussed here because it is still used in hospitalized children and adolescents for preprocedural sedation and to achieve immobility for diagnostic procedures such as radiological imaging or EEG.

PHARMACOLOGY

Chloral hydrate is formed by adding one molecule of water to the carbonyl group of chloral.

PHARMACODYNAMICS

• Rapidly metabolized to the active compound trichloroethanol by the liver.
  ○ Significant amounts of chloral hydrate are not found in the blood after its oral administration.

- Trichloroethanol exerts barbiturate-like effects on $GABA_A$ receptors, which probably accounts for chloral hydrate's pharmacodynamic effects.

Metabolism and excretion
- Undergoes reduction by alcohol dehydrogenase in the liver to trichloroethanol.
- Trichloroethanol is conjugated with glucuronic acid and excreted mostly in the urine.
- The half-life of chloral hydrate is approximately 5–10 hours.

INDICATIONS

Because of its toxicity, chloral hydrate is not generally used in ambulatory pediatric psychopharmacology for any indication. Its remaining indication is for preprocedural sedation to cause immobility in children and adolescents undergoing nonpainful diagnostic procedures, generally while in the hospital.

DOSING AND DURATION OF TREATMENT

- Because of its potential toxicity, long-term use of chloral hydrate is not recommended.
- For hospital procedures, chloral hydrate is given orally or rectally at doses between 25 and 100 mg/kg.
  ◦ Doses are not to exceed 1 gram in infants and 2 grams in children.
- A severe withdrawal syndrome may occur with drug discontinuation after chronic use.
- Chronic use of chloral hydrate may cause liver damage and/or renal injury.

SIDE EFFECTS

- Skin and mucus membrane irritation
- Nausea
- Vomiting
- Unpleasant taste
- Lightheadedness
- Malaise
- Nightmares
- Ataxia
- Sudden withdrawal of chloral hydrate after chronic use may cause delirium and seizures.
  ◦ High mortality rate.

Novel Benzodiazepine Receptor Agonists

Hypnotics in this class include zaleplon (Sonata®) and zolpidem (Ambien®). Their chemical structures do not resemble traditional BZDs. However, they interact with ω_1 BZD receptors and appear to potentiate GABAergic neurotransmission. They possess strong sedative effects but only weak anticonvulsant effects. Because they are so strongly sedating, they are used as hypnotics and not as anxiolytics. Zaleplon and zolpidem are both classified as a Schedule IV drug by the DEA.

ANXIOLYTICS

PHARMACOLOGY

- Zaleplon is a nonbenzodiazepine and a member of the pyrazolopyrimidine class of compounds.
- Zolpidem is a nonbenzodiazepine and is classified as an imidazopyridine.

PHARMACODYNAMICS

- Zaleplon and zolpidem bind to the BZD receptor site on $GABA_A$ receptors containing the alpha-1 subunit of the receptor.
- They bind strongly to $omega_1$ BZD receptors but only bind weakly to $omega_2$ and $omega_3$ BZD receptor subtypes. As such, they exhibit strong cortical effects in the CNS but weak effects on the cerebellum (ataxia) and spinal cord (muscle relaxation).

PHARMACOKINETICS

Few pharmacokinetic studies of zaleplon or zolpidem are presently available for children or adolescents. The following information is largely based on adult data.

Absorption
- These agents are rapidly absorbed after oral administration and reach peak plasma levels within 1 hour.
- The bioavailability of zaleplon is approximately 30% because of presystemic metabolism.
- The bioavailability of zolpidem is approximately 70%.
  ○ The oral bioavailability of zolpidem is decreased when administered with food.

Metabolism and excretion
- Zaleplon
  ○ Is metabolized largely by hepatic aldehyde oxidase and to a lesser degree by CYP3A4. Its oxidative metabolites are converted to glucuronides and eliminated in urine. No zaleplon metabolites are metabolically active.
  ○ Its half-life is about 1 hour.
- Zolpidem
  ○ Is metabolized in the liver to inactive metabolites via hydroxylation and oxidation through CYP3A and CYP2D6.
  ○ Its half-life ranges between 1.5 and 3.2 hours; the rate of clearance in children is three times faster than in young adults.

INDICATIONS

Zaleplon and zolpidem are indicated for the short-term (7–10-day) treatment of insomnia in individuals 18 years and older. Presently there are no FDA-approved indications for these drugs in children and adolescents. No controlled research of zaleplon or zolpidem is presently available in youth, and these agents cannot be endorsed for clinical use in the pediatric population at this time.

DOSING AND DURATION OF TREATMENT

- Zaleplon is usually administered in 5, 10, or 20 mg doses for the treatment of prolonged sleep latency in adult patients with transient or chronic insomnia.
  - Zaleplon is not superior to placebo in reducing awakenings during sleep or in increasing total sleep duration.
- Zolpidem is usually administered in doses ranging between 5 mg and 20 mg for the treatment of insomnia.
  - Zolpidem reduces sleep latency (time to fall asleep) and prolongs total sleep time in patients with insomnia, without exhibiting much effect on the sleep architecture of normal subjects.
- There appears to be no rebound insomnia or withdrawal effects upon discontinuation of these agents.
- Rates of next day "hangover" effects are low.
- Tolerance to the sedating effects of these agents does not seem to develop.
- Treatment with these agents for insomnia should not exceed 7–10 days.

CONTRAINDICATIONS

- Known or suspected substance abuse is a relative contraindication to use.
  o Reports have described clinical cases of zolpidem dependence.

SIDE EFFECTS

- Dizziness
- Lightheadedness
- Somnolence
- Headache
- Gastrointestional upset

MANAGEMENT OF OVERDOSE

In reports of overdose from the American and European experience with zaleplon and zolpidem alone, impairment of consciousness has ranged from somnolence to light coma. Only one case each of cardiac and respiratory depression have been reported. In zaleplon overdoses (including that of a 2-year-old child) ranging between 40 mg and 100 mg, no deaths have been reported. In zolpidem overdoses up to 400 mg, all individuals have fully recovered and no deaths have been reported. However, cases involving zaleplon or zolpidem and multiple agents are more complicated and have resulted in death.

- General supportive measures are recommended.
- Gastric lavage should be performed when appropriate.
- Flumazenil, a specific BZD antagonist, is useful in zaleplon and zolpidem overdose toxicity. It competitively antagonizes the binding and allosteric effects of BZDs. Flumazenil is available for IV administration only and has a half-life of about 30-60 minutes. A total of 1 mg of flumazenil given over 2–3 minutes is sufficient to abolish the effects of therapeutic doses of BZDs. Repeat administration of flumazenil may be necessary.

ANXIOLYTICS

• The value of dialysis in zalephon and zolpidem overdose and toxicity is not known.

ZALEPLON AND ZOLPIDEM DRUG-DRUG INTERACTIONS

Table 9.15 Zaleplon and Zolpidem Drug–Drug Interactions

	Drug	Interaction
Zaleplon	Erythromycin	↑ Zaleplon plasma levels
Zaleplon	Rifampin	↓ Zaleplon plasma levels
Zaleplon and zolpidem	Cimetidine	↑ Zaleplon and zolpidem Plasma levels ↓ Alertness
Zolpidem	Imipramine	↑ Anterograde amnesia
Zolpidem	Thioridazine	↓ Alertness
Zaleplon and zolpidem	Alcohol	↓ Alertness, ↓ Psychomotor speed

10. Adrenergic Agents

Medications that alter adrenergic sympathetic nervous transmission have been used in child and adolescent psychopharmacology for a number of years. Clonidine and guanfacine are presynaptic alpha-2-adrenergic receptor agonists that diminish arousal in the locus ceruleus, the CNS hub of the noradrenergic activating system, leading to inhibition of the CNS release of norepinephrine. Beta-adrenergic receptors are ubiquitously distributed in the CNS and in the periphery. These receptors are activated by adrenergic sympathetic nervous transmission and by endocrine catecholamines, such as noradrenaline, in the circulation. Beta-blockers are synthetic adrenergic receptor-blocking agents. Although these agents are generally used in cardiovascular medicine, they are sometimes used for a variety of child and adolescent psychiatric conditions. Like many psychiatric medications used in pediatric psychiatry, their popularity of use outstrips the scientific study of their effectiveness and safety in children and adolescents. Thus, their use in pediatric psychopharmacology remains largely "off-label" and not approved for manufacturer advertising by the FDA. This chapter discusses clonidine, guanfacine, and beta-blockers.

CLONIDINE

Clonidine is a centrally acting alpha-agonist hypotensive agent. Its primary use in medicine is as an antihypertensive. In psychiatry, clonidine is used for a variety of off-label purposes, such as treatment of ADHD, tics and Tourette's disorder, PTSD, opiate withdrawal, alcohol withdrawal, and for severe maladaptive impulsive aggression and conduct problems.

Pharmacology

The alpha-2-adrenergic agonists such as clonidine modulate central noradrenergic activity primarily through their effects on alpha-2-adrenoreceptors. The alpha-2 receptors are broadly distributed throughout the brain and are differentiated into three subtypes: alpha-2A,alpha-2B, and alpha-2C. All three receptor subtypes transduce their signals via the $G_{i/o}$ protein signaling system. The alpha-2A receptor resides in the plasma membrane and is the main alpha-2 subtype found in the brain. The alpha-2A receptor is found in the locus ceruleus, cerebellum, striatum, hypothalamus, thalamus, amygdala, hippocampus, septum, and cerebral cortex. The alpha-2B receptor also resides in the plasma membrane, but its location appears limited to the thalamus. The alpha-2C receptor is expressed intracellularly and has little cell surface localization; it is widely distributed in the striatum, the hippocampus, the cortex, and in the locus ceruleus. Clonidine is a relatively nonspecific alpha-2-adrenergic agonist and binds to all three alpha-2 receptor subtypes. In addition, clonidine binds with moderate to high affinity to other alpha-adrenergic receptors, such as alpha-1-adrenoreceptors. Thus the actions of clonidine are relatively nonspecific.

PHARMACODYNAMICS

The alpha-2A adrenergic receptor functions as an autoreceptor and mediates the potent inhibitory effects of alpha-2 agonists through actions at the locus ceruleus. Somatodendritic alpha-2A-adrenergic autoreceptors diminish the excitability of locus ceruleus adrenergic neurons. Presynaptic alpha-2A-adrenergic autoreceptors mediate the autoinhibition of norepinephrine release from the locus ceruleus. Clonidine nonspecifically stimulates presynaptic alpha- 2A/B/C-adrenergic receptors in the brain stem. This action results in reduced sympathetic outflow from the locus ceruleus and in decreases in peripheral resistance, renal vascular resistance, heart rate, and blood pressure. Reduced sympathetic outflow may be clinically beneficial in psychiatric disorders characterized by adrenergic overarousal, excitability, and impulsive aggression.

PHARMACOKINETICS

Absorption
• Clonidine is completely absorbed after oral administration.
• Peak plasma levels occur within 3–5 hours after oral absorption.

Distribution
• Clonidine is highly lipid soluble.

Metabolism and excretion
• Elimination is 65% by renal excretion and 35% by hepatic metabolism.
  ○ Clonidine has no active metabolites.
• Clonidine has a half-life in adults of approximately 12–16 hours.
• Clonidine has a shorter half-life in children of 8–12 hours.
• The behavioral effects of clonidine in children last 3–6 hours.

Indications

• Clonidine is FDA approved for the treatment of hypertension.
• There currently exist no approved indications for clonidine in psychiatric disorders.

Possible indications

Clonidine is used in pediatric medicine to treat hypertension and in pediatric anesthesia for sedation and analgesia. Clonidine is used in a variety of psychiatric disorders characterized by adrenergic overarousal. Possible indications in child and adolescent psychopharmacology include:

• ADHD
• Tics and Tourette's disorders
• Impulsive aggression and conduct disorders
• PTSD
• Sleep disturbances associated with ADHD, Tourette's disorder, or PTSD

Although the popularity of clonidine use in child psychiatry exceeds the presently available scientific database to support its use, clonidine has been the focus of clinical research over the past two decades. Recent studies in child and adolescent psychiatry are presented in the following table.

Dosing and Duration of Treatment

Available clonidine preparations
• Tablets (Catapress® and generic): scored, white, oval in 0.1 mg, 0.2 mg, and 0.3 mg.
• Catapress-TTS® (transdermal therapeutic system): Skin patch system.
  ◦ TTS®–1: 0.1 mg per day delivery system
  ◦ TTS®–2: 0.2 mg per day delivery system
  ◦ TTS®–3: 0.3 mg per day delivery system
• Injectable clonidine (Duraclon™) for anesthetic use
  ◦ 100 mcg/mL solution.
  ◦ 500 mcg/mL solution.

Before initiating treatment
• Conduct a baseline medical history and physical examination.
  ◦ Include child and family cardiovascular history (e.g., syncope, irregular heart rate, bradycardic arrhythmias, hypertension, hypotension).
  ◦ It is important to emphasize to patient and family the potentially severe consequences that may result from the abrupt discontinuation of clonidine and to emphasize to them the importance of medication compliance with clonidine.
• Baseline pulse and blood pressure
• If medically significant child or family cardiovascular disease history, consider a baseline EKG.

General dosing suggestions
• Oral clonidine
  ◦ Initiate 0.05 mg at bedtime.
  ◦ Increase by 0.05 mg every 4–7 days to a daily maximum of 0.35 mg.
  ◦ Give in divided doses on a tid–qid daily schedule for younger children.
  ◦ Multiple doses reduce risk of daily withdrawal symptoms in between doses.
  ◦ For adolescents give oral clonidine in divided doses on a bid–tid dose schedule.

Table 10.1 Recent Studies of Clonidine in Child and Adolescent Psychiatry

Author (Year)	Study Type	N	Disorder	Age (yrs) (mean/range)	Dose (mg/day or range)	Duration	Side Effects	Outcome
Agarwal et al. (2001)	Crossover	10	Mental retardation + hyperactivity	7.6 ± 0.54	4, 6, 8 mcg/kg/day	12 weeks	Sedation	Hyperactivity improved
Connor et al. (2000)	RT	8	ADHD + aggression	6–16	0.10–0.30	12 weeks	↓ Fine motor speed, sedation	ADHD and aggression improved
Hazell & Stuart (2003)	RCT	38	ADHD + aggression	6–14	0.10–0.20	6 weeks	Sedation, dizziness	Aggression improved when clonidine combined with stimulant
Niederhofer et al. (2003)[a]	RCT	44	ADHD + tics	10.4	0.4–1.2	8 weeks	Sedation	ADHD and tics improved
Gaffney et al. (2002)	RT	21	Tourette's syndrome	7–17	Avg. = 0.18	8 weeks	Sedation	Clonidine = risperdal in ↓ tic severity
Tourette's syndrome Study Group (2002)	RCT	34	ADHD + Tourette's syndrome	7–14	Avg. = 0.25	16 weeks	Sedation	Improved hyperactivity and impulsivity; tic severity ↓.

[a] This study used lofexidine, a medication very similar to clonidine but associated with less hypotension; lofexidine is available in Europe, but not presently in the United States.
RT = randomized trial; RCT = randomized controlled trial

- Clonidine TTS®
  - ○ Use oral preparation to titrate to optimal daily dose.
  - ○ Then switch to same dose TTS® patch.
  - ○ In adults with hypertension, the TTS® patch must be changed every 7 days. However, children metabolize clonidine more rapidly than adults. To prevent clonidine withdrawal, change the TTS® patch every 4–5 days in children and adolescents.

Medical monitoring
- Clonidine is a hypotensive agent. Follow pulse and blood pressure weekly until the dose is stabilized. Then follow pulse and blood pressure every 2 months.
- In children with known cardiovascular disease, consider on-drug EKG and compare to baseline EKG.

Discontinuing clonidine treatment
- Abrupt discontinuation of clonidine can result in hypertension, hallucinations, and agitation.
- Discontinue clonidine gradually, with a 0.05 mg per day decrease every 3–4 days until the drug is discontinued.

Contraindications

Absolute contraindications
- Known hypersensitivity to clonidine

Relative contraindications
- Depression
- Cardiovascular disorders (e.g., syncope)
- Cerebrovascular disorders
- Raynaud's syndrome
- Renal disease
- Liver disease
- Skin disease (TTS® patch only)

Side Effects

Common and uncommon side effects of clonidine appear in the following table.

Sedation
- Very common with clonidine use.
- Can manifest as daytime sleepiness at school.
- Usually most problematic in the first month of clonidine treatment and generally remits progressively thereafter.

Hypotension
- Children frequently experience an approximately 10% reduction in systolic blood pressure when treated with clonidine.

Table 10.2 Side Effects of Clonidine

Common	Uncommon
• Sedation	• Depression
• Hypotension	• Cardiovascular arrhythmia
• Headache	(bradycardia)
• Dizziness	• Retinal degeneration
• Irritability	• Rebound hypertension
• Nausea	• Skin irritation (under the TTS® patch)
	• Raynaud's syndrome
	• Sleep disturbance
	• Vivid dreams/nightmares
	• Sexual dysfunction
	• Dry mouth

• Orthostatic blood pressure changes occur in about 5% of clonidine treated children.

Cardiovascular disease
• Clonidine treatment acutely diminishes cardiac output by 10–20%. During long-term clonidine therapy cardiac output returns to baseline.
• Clonidine decreases peripheral vascular resistance and lowers pulse.
  ○ Although these cardiovascular changes are rarely clinically significant in healthy children and adolescents, the clinician should routinely monitor for signs of exercise-induced cardiovascular intolerance.
  ○ Symptoms of exercise-induced dizziness, lightheadedness, or syncope should prompt clonidine dose reevaluation and possible reduction.

Depression
• Clonidine may cause depression or worsen preexisting depression in vulnerable children and adolescents.
  ○ Clonidine should be used cautiously with depressed youngsters.

Irritability
• May cause a worsening of irritability in some children and adolescents.

Rebound hypertension
• With high dose or chronic clonidine use, abrupt drug discontinuation can result in clinically significant rebound hypertension.
  ○ This appears to be more of a problem with clonidine than with guanfacine.

Raynaud's syndrome
• Characterized by feelings of cold, pain, and blue discoloration of the fingers and toes upon exposure to cold temperatures.
• Clonidine may (rarely) exacerbate this syndrome in patients with preexisting Raynaud's syndrome.

Skin irritation
- May occur under the patch when using the clonidine TTS® system.
  - Frequently changing the site of the patch or using topical hydrocortisone cream may help the affected skin area.

Drug–Drug Interactions

Four cases of sudden cardiac death have been reported to Med Watch in children treated with a clonidine–methylphenidate combination. It should be emphasized that these four cases all had complicated, potentially confounding factors that may have contributed to their deaths. These include previous cardiac disease and concomitant use of other medications. After review, the consensus of expert pediatric psychopharmacologists is that the combination should not be clinically contraindicated, but caution is advised when using clonidine–methylphenidate combination therapy in children with preexisting cardiovascular disease or who are receiving multiple psychiatric medications in combination.

Table 10.3 Some Clonidine[a] Drug–Drug Interactions
Clonidine[a] interacts with:

Acebutolol	Potentiates clonidine action
Alcohol	↑ Sedation
	↓ Blood pressure
Beta-blockers	↑ Rebound hypertension in patients withdrawn from clonidine
Insulin	↑ Hyperglycemia
Levodopa	↑ Parkinson's symptoms
Nitrates	↑ Hypotension
Tricyclic antidepressants	↓ Blood pressure

[a]similar drug-drug interactions for guanfacine

Management of Overdose

With increased popularity of use, clonidine toxicity is increasing in the child and adolescent population. Overdose with clonidine can be a life-threatening emergency. Signs and symptoms of overdose occur within 30 minutes to 2 hours after clonidine ingestion. Children may be more susceptible to clonidine toxicity than adults. As little as 0.1 mg of clonidine has produced toxicity in children.

Symptoms of clonidine overdose include the early development of hypertension followed later by hypotension, bradycardia, respiratory depression, hypothermia, sedation and CNS depression, decreased or absent reflexes, irritability, and miosis. Toxicity may cause reversible cardiac arrhythmias, especially bradycardic arrhythmias. There is no specific antidote to clonidine poisoning.

General measures
- Because clonidine overdose may rapidly cause CNS depression, induction of vomiting with ipecac syrup is not advised.
- Gastric lavage is indicated following recent or large ingestion.

• Administration of activated charcoal may be helpful.
• IV fluids and pressor agents are indicated for hypotension.
• Atropine is indicated for bradycardia.
• Dialysis is not likely to enhance the elimination of clonidine.

Drug Interference with Laboratory Testing

• Increases growth hormone plasma levels
• Increases blood glucose
• Decreases heart rate on EKG

GUANFACINE

Guanfacine is a centrally acting alpha-agonist hypotensive agent. Guanfacine is more specific in its effects on alpha 2 receptors, resulting in less side effects than clonidine. Use of guanfacine is only beginning to be explored in pediatric psychopharmacology, and presently there are few controlled studies to guide clinical practice. In psychiatry, guanfacine is used for the same off-label purposes as clonidine, namely ADHD, tics, Tourette's disorder, PTSD, and maladaptive, impulsive aggression.

Pharmacology

Guanfacine has specific affinity for the alpha 2A receptor, with 100-fold lower affinity for the alpha 2B receptor and 40-fold lower affinity for the alpha 2C receptor. Guanfacine demonstrates little nonspecific binding to other adrenergic receptors (unlike clonidine).

PHARMACODYNAMICS

Guanfacine specifically down regulates alpha 2A receptors in the brain. In addition to decreasing norepinephrine output from the locus ceruleus, guanfacine may have a number of other actions, including effects on non-noradrenergic neurons with subsequent modulation of CNS dopamine and glutamate release. This modulation may partially explain the calming effect of guanfacine (and clonidine).

PHARMACOKINETICS

Absorption
• Guanfacine is more rapidly absorbed into the systemic circulation than clonidine.
• Peak plasma levels occur in 1–4 hours after oral absorption.

Distribution
• Highly lipid soluble

Metabolism and excretion
• Partially metabolized in the liver to glucuronides and sulfate metabolites.
• The kidney excretes 40–75% of guanfacine as unchanged drug.

- Has a longer half-life than clonidine; thus guanfacine may be prescribed to children and adolescents on a bid–tid schedule.
  - In adults, the plasma half-life of guanfacine is approximately 17 hours (range: 10–30 hours).
  - In children, the plasma half-life of guanfacine is approximately 12–14 hours.

Indications

- FDA indicated for the treatment of hypertension.
- Designated an orphan drug for use in the treatment of fragile X syndrome.
- Presently, there are no FDA-approved psychiatric indications for guanfacine.
- Guanfacine use in children under the age of 12 years is not recommended, based on lack of controlled research demonstrating safety and efficacy.

Possible indications
In child and adolescent psychopharmacology, guanfacine is used to adjunctively treat tics in children with Tourette's syndrome, ADHD and tic disorders, and to treat maladaptive aggression in children with ADHD. At present, fewer randomized, controlled studies have been completed with guanfacine than with clonidine in pediatric psychopharmacology. The following table summarizes pertinent research.

Dosing and Duration of Treatment

Available guanfacine preparations
- Tablets (Tenex®, generic): 1 mg (white), 2 mg (blue)

Before initiating treatment
- Follow clonidine guidelines, pages 215–217.

General dosing suggestions
- Initiate at 0.5 mg at bedtime.
- Increase by 0.5 mg every 4–7 days to a daily maximum of 3 mg in divided doses.
- Because guanfacine has a longer half-life than clonidine, it can be given on a tid dose schedule to younger children and a bid dose schedule to adolescents.

Medical monitoring
- Follow clonidine guidelines on pages 215–217.

Discontinuing guanfacine treatment
- Abrupt discontinuation of guanfacine from high dose or chronic use may be associated with a medically significant withdrawal syndrome characterized by rebound hypertension, agitation, and sleep disturbance (similar to clonidine withdrawal).
- Discontinue guanfacine gradually with a 0.5 mg per day decrease every 3–4 days.

ADRENERGIC AGENTS

Table 10.4 Studies of Guanfacine in Child and Adolescent Psychiatry

Author (year)	Study Type	N	Disorder	Age (Years) (mean/range)	Dose (mg/day) or range)	Duration (Weeks)	Side Effects	Outcome
Chappell et al. (1995)	Open	10	ADHD + Tic disorder	8–16	0.75–3.0 mg/day	4–20	Fatigue, headache, dizziness, insomnia	Improvement in tics, no improvement in ADHD
Horrigan & Barnhill (1995)	Open	15	ADHD	7–17	0.5–3.0 mg/day	10	Sedation	Improvement in ADHD
Hunt et al. (1995)	Open	13	ADHD	4–20	0.5–4.0 mg/day	4	Headache, stomachache	Improvement in inattention and hyperactivity
Scahill et al. (2000)	RCT	34	ADHD + Tourette's disorder	7–14	1.5–3.0 mg/day	8	Sedation	Improvement in tics and ADHD

RCT = randomized controlled trial

Contraindications

Absolute contraindications
• Known hypersensitivity to guanfacine.

Relative Contraindications
• Same as clonidine.

Side Effects

Because guanfacine is more specific and selective than clonidine in its actions at the adrenergic receptor, it has fewer side effects than clonidine. The types of side effects are similar to clonidine but less frequent and intense (see Table 10.2).

Drug–Drug Interactions

Guanfacine has been combined with methylphenidate. No cases of sudden cardiac death with this combination have been reported. Guanfacine drug–drug interactions are similar to those reported for clonidine (see Table 10.3).

Management of Overdose

With increased popularity of "off-label" use, cases of acute guanfacine toxicity are rising. The presentation is similar to clonidine poisoning, and management is the same (see pp. 219–220). There is no specific guanfacine antidote.

Drug Interference with Laboratory Testing

• Increases growth hormone plasma levels
• Increases blood glucose
• Decreases heart rate on EKG

BETA-BLOCKERS

Beta-blockers competitively antagonize epinephrine and norepinephrine actions at beta-adrenergic receptors located in the central nervous system and in the periphery. These agents, which include atenolol, metoprolol, nadolol, propranolol, and pindolol, have many labeled indications for use in various cardiovascular disorders. They have no FDA-established indications for use in psychiatric disorders. To date no controlled studies of beta-blockers in children and adolescents with neuropsychiatric disorders have been completed. However, these medications are sometimes prescribed to treat explosive aggression, tremor, antipsychotic-induced akathisia and dyskinesias, specific types of anxiety (e.g., performance anxiety), migraine headache, and neurally mediated syncope in youngsters. In pediatric psychopharmacology propranolol and, to a lesser extent nadolol, are the most investigated agents. Discussion largely focuses on these two beta-blockers.

Pharmacology

Two major subtypes of beta-adrenoreceptors have been identified in the periphery and in the CNS; both types are located on postsynaptic nerve terminals. In the periphery, beta-1 receptors are located in myocardial tissue and mediate cardiac chronotropic and inotropic actions. Beta-1-blockers slow the heart rate and decrease myocardial contractility, thus decreasing cardiac oxygen demand. Beta-2 receptors are located in pulmonary bronchi and in some blood vessels. Beta-2-blockers block beta-2 adrenoreceptor mediated bronchial smooth muscle action, leading to bronchoconstriction. This may be life threatening in patients with asthma or chronic obstructive pulmonary disease. Beta receptors modify the metabolism of carbohydrates and lipids. Catecholamines promote glycogenolysis and mobilize glucose in response to hypoglycemia. Nonselective beta-blockers may adversely affect recovery from hypoglycemia in patients with insulin-dependent diabetes.

In the CNS, beta-1 receptors are the major type of adrenoreceptor. The exception is the cerebellum, where beta-2 adrenoreceptors predominate. Beta-blockers influence the activation of CNS systems that use norepinephrine and epinephrine as neurotransmitters. By down-regulating adrenergic neurotransmission in the CNS, arousal mechanisms that regulate aggressive fight/flight and fear responses may be altered. This is the principal rationale for the use of beta-blocking agents in neuropsychiatry.

PHARMACODYNAMICS

- Beta-blockers are competitive antagonists of beta-adrenoreceptors in the periphery and in the CNS.
- Nonselective beta-blockers block both beta-1 and beta-2 receptors.
  - Propranolol
  - Nadolol
- Selective agents block only beta-1 receptors.
  - Atenolol
  - Metoprolol
- Some beta-blockers have intrinsic sympathomimetic activity and are partial agonists at the beta-adrenoreceptor. This property results in a more intrinsic sympathomimetic tone, which may protect against treatment-emergent bradycardia and hypotension.
  - Pindolol is an example of a beta-blocker with intrinsic sympathomimetic activity.
- Some beta-blockers have quinidine-like membrane-stabilizing activity, especially in high doses, which may protect against ventricular arrhythmias independently of beta-receptor blockade.
  - Propranolol has some membrane-stabilizing activity.

PHARMACOKINETICS

Absorption
- Beta-blockers such as nadolol and propranolol are readily absorbed after oral administration.
- Time to peak plasma concentration is 2–4 hours.

Table 10.5 Beta-Blockers: Pharmacological and Pharmacokinetic Properties

Name	Relative Potency (mg)	Lipophilicity	Site of Action[a]	ISA[b]	MSA[c]	Beta-Receptor Selectivity[d]	Route of Elimination	Half-Life (hrs)
Atenolol	1.0	+	P	−	−	Beta-1	Renal	6–8
Metoprolol	0.5–2.0	+ +	C, P	−	−	Beta-1	Hepatic	3–4
Nadolol	0.5–2.0	+	P	−	−	Beta-1, 2	Renal	20–24
Pindolol	5.0–10.0	+ +	C, P	+	−	Beta-1, 2	Hepatic, renal	3–4
Propranolol	1.0	+ + +	C, P	−	+	Beta-1, 2	Hepatic	3–5

Data in adults; there is little pharmacokinetic data in the pediatric age range.
[a] C = Central nervous system acting; P = Peripheral acting
[b] Intrinsic sympathomimetic activity
[c] Membrane-stabilizing activity
[d] Beta = 1 receptors: heart, brain; Beta-2 receptors: vascular, bronchial, and gastrointestinal

Distribution
• Beta-blockers differ in their lipid solubility.
  ○ Lipophilic beta-blockers readily cross the blood–brain barrier and penetrate the CNS to exert central effects. (e.g., metoprolol, pindolol, propranolol).
  ○ Hydrophilic beta-blockers exert their effects only in the periphery and do not penetrate into the CNS (e.g., atenolol, nadolol).

Metabolism and excretion
• Propranolol and nadolol undergo extensive first-pass hepatic metabolism.
  ○ Only about 20–40% of the original oral dose reaches the systemic circulation.
• Propranolol is extensively metabolized in the liver, with a short half-life of 3–4 hours after first administration and about 6 hours after repeated administration.
  ○ Because of its short half-life, propranolol must be given in two to four doses per day.
• Nadolol does not undergo hepatic metabolism and is excreted unchanged by renal mechanisms; its half-life is long, generally between 20 and 24 hours.
  ○ Nadolol may be given once or twice daily because of its long half-life.

Indications

• Hypertension
• Angina
• Migraine
• Hypertrophic subaortic stenosis

Possible indications
Beta-blockers are not FDA approved for manufacturers' advertising for any condition in child and adolescent psychopharmacology. Possible uses include the following.

• Explosive aggression, rage outbursts, and states of adrenergic hyperarousal
  ○ Especially in organically brain-damaged patients

- Tremor
- Neuroleptic-induced akathisia
- Performance anxiety
- Posttraumatic stress disorder
- Generalized anxiety disorder
- Panic anxiety

Dosing and Duration of Treatment

The next table lists some available beta-blocking agents and their usual doses. Much of the data in this table are extrapolated from adults. Little dosing guidelines are presently available for children and adolescents.

Before initiating treatment
- Document normal cardiovascular functioning.
  - Obtain baseline blood pressure and pulse.
  - Consider a baseline EKG.
- Obtain a medical history.
  - Rule out asthma, obstructive pulmonary disease, diabetes, hyperthyroid disease, syncope, Raynaud's syndrome, and/or abnormal cardiac history.
  - Rule out pregnancy in female patients.
- Obtain a psychiatric history.
  - Beta-blockers may worsen depression in vulnerable patients.

General dosing suggestions
No firm guidelines have been established for the dosing and administration of beta-blockers in child and adolescent psychopharmacology. The following dosing suggestions are obtained from the extant pediatric beta-blocker literature and focus on the two most commonly used beta-blockers: propranolol and nadolol.

- Propranolol
  - The usual starting dose is 10–20 mg administered two times per day. Younger children are generally started on 10 mg/day.
  - The dose is increased, as necessary and tolerated, by 10–20 mg increments every 3–7 days.
  - Because of the short half-life of propranolol, multiple daily doses are required to prevent interdose withdrawal symptoms.
  - The maximum FDA-recommended propranolol dose for children is 16 mg/kg/day.
  - The maximum FDA-recommended propranolol dose for adults is 640 mg four times per day.
- Nadolol
  - The usual starting dose is 20 mg, administered once in the morning.
  - Younger children are generally started on 10 mg in the morning.
  - The dose is increased every 3–7 days by 10–20 mg.
  - The maximum dose ceiling for nadolol is unknown, but studies generally dose between 20 and 240 mg/day.
  - Because of its long half-life, nadolol can be dosed once or twice daily.

Table 10.6 Studies of Beta-Blockers in Child and Adolescent Psychiatry

Author (year)	Drug	Study Type	Disorder	N	Age (yrs)	Dose (mg/day or range)	Duration (Weeks)	Side Effects	Outcome
Buitelaar et al. (1996)	Pindolol	RCT	ADHD	52	6–13	40	4	Marked: hallucinations, paresthesias	Side effects required med. discontinuation
Connor et al. (1997)	Nadolol	Open	Dev. delay	12	9–24	30–220	20	Mild	10 of 12 improved in aggressive behavior
Famularo et al. (1988)	Propranolol	Open	PTSD	11	Avg: 8.5	2.5 mg/kg/day	5	Sedation	Some improvement
Kuperman & Stuart (1987)	Propranolol	Open	Dev. delay, conduct disorder	16	4–24	80–280	12	Sedation, bradycardia	63% improved
Williams et al. (1982)	Propranolol	Open	Brain damage	30	7–35	50–1,600	8–120	Mild	80% improved

RCT = randomized, controlled trial

227

Table 10.7 Beta-Blocker Drug Doses

Generic Name	Trade Name	Available Doses (mg) (tablet/capsule color)	Minimum Age Approved for Any Use (yrs)	Starting Dose (mg/day)*	Titration	Usual Daily Dose (mg/day)	Dose Schedule
Atenolol	Tenormin®	T: 25 (white) T: 50 (white) T: 100 (white) INJ: 5 mg/10 ml	18	25	25 mg every 1–2 weeks	Adults: 50–100 mg/day	Daily
Metoprolol	Toprol-XR®	XR T: 25 (white) XR T: 50 (white) XR T: 100 (white) XR T: 200 (white)	18	12.5–50	25 mg every 3–7 days	Adults: 50–100 mg/day	Daily Daily Daily bid
	Lopressor®	T: 50 (pink) T: 100 (light blue) INJ: 5 mg/5 ml					
Nadolol	Corgard®	T: 20 (blue) T: 40 (blue) T: 80 (blue) T: 120 (blue) T: 160 (blue)	18	20	20 mg every 3–7 days	Adults: 40–240 mg/day	Daily
Pindolol	Visken®	T: 5 (white) T: 10 (white)	18	10	10 mg every 3–7 days	Adults: 20–60 mg/day	bid
Propranolol	Inderal®	T: 10 (orange) T: 20 (blue) T: 40 (green) T: 60 (pink) T: 80 (yellow) LA C: 60 (white/light blue) LA C: 80 (light blue) LA C: 120 (light blue/dark blue) LA C: 160 (dark blue) INJ: 1 mg/ml	18	0.5 mg/kg bid	10–20 mg every 3–7 days	Adults: 2–4 mg/kg/day 120–240 mg/day	bid–qid Daily Daily Daily Daily

*Most dosing for adults; little information available for children and adolescents. T = tablet; INJ = injectable; XR T: extended = release tablet; LA C: long-acting capsule.

228

Medical monitoring
- Beta-blockers are hypotensive agents. Monitor heart rate and blood pressure at each visit.
  - Hold a dose if the pulse ≤ 50 beats per minute in adolescents or ≤ 60 beats per minute in young children.
  - Hold a dose if BP < 90/60.
- Consider an on-drug EKG to compare against a baseline EKG and assess changes in cardiac conduction.

Discontinuing treatment
- Withdraw beta-blockers gradually, especially after chronic or high-dose treatment. Abrupt discontinuation of beta-blockers can lead to a withdrawal syndrome characterized by rebound sympathomimetic side effects such as hypertension, tachycardia, arrhythmias, agitation, and sleep disturbance.
- Generally decrease the beta-blocker by 10–20 mg/day every 3-4 days, making sure vital signs remain stable.

Contraindictions

- Known hypersensitivity to beta-blocker
- Bronchospastic disease (asthma)
- Cardiovascular disease
- Diabetes/hypoglycemia
- Hyperthyroidism
- Raynaud's syndrome
- Depression
- Pregnancy
- Syncope

Side Effects

Beta-blockers have many side effects. Common and uncommon adverse events are listed in the following table. Gradual dose escalation and clinical attention to vital signs and medical monitoring are strategies to reduce the incidence and severity of beta-blocker treatment-emergent adverse events.

Table 10.8 Side Effects of Beta-Blockers

Common	Uncommon
Decreased heart rate	Bronchoconstriction
Sedation	Congestive heart failure
Lethargy	Depression
Impotence	Hallucinations
Vivid dreams	Raynaud's syndrome
	Hypoglycemia
	Hypotension
	Dizziness
	Nausea
	Diarrhea
	Cardiac conduction abnormalities

- Decreased heart rate: Beta-blockers can decrease the pulse to less than 50 beats per minute and block cardiovascular response to the demands of exercise, resulting in dizziness and syncope. It is essential to obtain baseline and on-drug vital signs.
- Raynaud's syndrome: Beta-blockers decrease peripheral circulation. During periods of exposure to cold, the fingers and toes may turn blue, tingle, and become numb and painful.
- Sexual impotence: Sexual side effects, including impotence, may occur commonly with beta-blockers. Adolescents must be warned in advance about such potential side effects.
- Bronchoconstriction: Do not prescribe beta-blockers to patients with asthma or obstructive pulmonary disease.
- Depression: Beta-blockers may induce depression in susceptible individuals. and should be used cautiously in patients with a history of depression.
- Hypoglycemia: Interference with glycolysis is mostly a concern in patients with diabetes. Beta-blockers should be used with caution in diabetics.
- Hyperthyroidism: Beta-blockers should generally be avoided in patients with hyperthyroid disease.

Drug–Drug Interactions

Beta-blockers have several potentially important drug–drug interactions, listed in the following table.

Table 10.9 Beta-Blocker Drug–Drug Interactions
Beta-Blockers interact with:

Anesthetics	↑ Anesthetic agent
Antipsychotics	↑ Antipsychotics
Tricyclic Antidepressants	↑ TCAs
Alpha Adrenergic Agents	↑ Clonidine/guanfacine
Cimetidine	↑ Beta-blockers
Insulin	↓ Insulin
Carbamazepine	↓ Beta-blockers
Estrogens (birth control pills)	↓ Beta-blockers
Nicotine	↓ Beta-blockers
Nonsteroidal anti-inflammatory analgesics	↓ Beta-blockers

Management of Drug Overdose

The clinical signs and symptoms of beta-blocker toxicity include bradycardia, hypotension, bronchospasm, prolongation of cardiac AV conduction time, and sedation. Among patients ingesting large amounts of propranolol, 66% developed seizures. Beta-blockers are generally not dialyzable. In addition to supportive measures, the following should be considered for beta-blocker overdose.

- Bradycardia: Administer atropine 0.25–1.0 mg. If there is no response to vagal nerve blockade, administer isoproterenol cautiously.
- Cardiac failure: Administer digitalization and diuretics.

• Hypotension: Administer vasopressors such as epinephrine.
• Bronchospasm: Administer isoproterenol and aminophylline.

Drug Interference with Laboratory Testing

• Increased liver function tests.
• Decreased rate on EKG.

11. Other Medications

There are several important medications used in pediatric psychopharmacology that have not been reviewed in previous chapters. Atomoxetine is labeled for use in child, adolescent, and adult ADHD. Modafinil is a wake-promoting agent used in narcolepsy that is also sometimes used in ADHD. Children with diurnal and nocturnal enuresis often receive pharmacotherapy with desmopressin (DDAVP) or oxybutynin (Ditropan). Naltrexone is occasionally used in adolescent psychiatry for severe self-injurious behaviors; in child psychiatry naltrexone has been investigated in autistic children. This chapter discusses these important medications.

ATOMOXETINE

Atomoxetine (Strattera™) was originally developed as a noradrenergic antidepressant but failed to achieve this potential. With growing recognition of the importance of noradrenergic mechanisms in attention deficit hyperactivity disorder (ADHD), atomoxetine was tested in clinical trials for childhood, adolescent, and adult ADHD, where it was found effective.

Pharmacology

Two neural systems appear to regulate attention in the CNS. A posterior attentional system mediates disengagement from stimuli, change of attentional focus to new stimuli, and the engagement of attention to new stimuli. This system uses norepinephrine (NE) as the principal neurotransmitter. An anterior attentional system that uses both dopamine (DA) and NE helps the CNS to analyze data and prepare for a response. Increasing both CNS NE and/or DA neurotransmission may theoretically be effective in the treatment of attentional disorders.

Atomoxetine is a potent and specific inhibitor of the presynaptic NE transporter. Its receptor profile shows minimal affinity for cholinergic, histaminic, serotonergic, or alpha-adrenergic receptors. With blockade of the presynaptic NE reuptake pump, CNS noradrenergic neurotransmission is increased with secondary effects on DA systems. These actions are thought to have beneficial effects in ADHD.

PHARMACODYNAMICS

- A significant number of presynaptic NE reuptake transporters in the prefrontal cortex, are indiscriminant in their reuptake of both NE and DA. Blockade of the NE transporter by atomoxetine creates an equivalent increase of both NE and DA in the prefrontal cortex.
- Atomoxetine does not increase DA levels in the nucleus accumbens (the primary CNS DA-mediated reward pathway), which may explain its lack of association with euphoria or reinforcing properties. As a result, atomoxetine appears to have limited drug abuse potential.
- Atomoxetine does not appear to increase DA levels in the striatum (caudate nucleus and putamen), and appears to have a lack of association with motor and vocal tics.

PHARMACOKINETICS

Absorption
- Rapidly absorbed following oral administration.
- Food does not affect the extent of atomoxetine absorption but does reduce the rate of absorption and prolong the time to peak plasma levels by about 3 hours.
- Maximal plasma concentrations are reached in 1–2 hours after oral dosing.

Distribution
- 98% bound to plasma proteins.

Metabolism and excretion
- Extensively metabolized in the liver by the CYP450-2D6 enzyme system.
  - About 7% of the population demonstrates reduced rate kinetics for drugs metabolized by the CYP450-2D6 enzyme system. These patients (poor metabolizers) are at risk for developing high serum levels at low drug doses compared with extensive metabolizers.
- Atomoxetine has low concentrations (about 1%) of 4-hydroxyatomoxetine, an active metabolite.
- Less than 3% of the drug is excreted unchanged in the urine.
- Most of an oral dose of atomoxetine is excreted as 4-hydroxyatomoxetine-O-glucuronide in the urine (80%); the rest is excreted in the feces (17%).
- The elimination half-life is 3–6 hours in extensive metabolizers, 17–22 hours in poor metabolizers.

Indications

- Atomoxetine is currently approved for the treatment of ADHD in children, adolescents, and adults.

Possible indications
- ADHD and Tourette's disorder
- ADHD and depression
- ADHD and anxiety disorders

The available controlled studies demonstrating the safety and tolerability of atomoxetine are presented in the following table.

Dosing and Duration of Treatment

Available atomoxetine preparations
- Capsules (Strattera™): 10 mg (white), 18 mg (gold/white), 25 mg (blue/white), 40 mg (blue/blue), and 60 mg (blue/gold)

Before initiating treatment
- Obtain baseline medical history, vital signs, weight, height, and physical examination data.
- A baseline EKG is not necessary.
- Rule out narrow-angle glaucoma.
- Routine laboratory tests are not required.

Dosing guidelines
Dosing guidelines for atomoxetine are weight based.
 Dosing of children and adolescents up to 70 kg body weight:

- Initiate atomoxetine at 0.5 mg/kg. Increase after a minimum of 3 days to a total dose not to exceed 1.2 mg/kg/day.
- Atomoxetine may be given in a single morning dose or as two evenly divided daily doses in the morning and afternoon/early evening.

Dosing of children and adolescents over 70 kg body weight:

- Initiate atomoxetine at a total daily dose of 40 mg. After a minimum of 3 days titrate to a target total daily dose of approximately 80 mg, given as a single daily dose in the morning or as two evenly divided doses in the morning and afternoon/early evening.
  - If no response is achieved after 2 weeks, the total daily dose may be titrated to 100 mg/day.
- The total daily dose should not exceed 100 mg per day.

Medical monitoring
- Pulse and blood pressure should be checked on full dose.
- Monitor weight.
- Ask about side effects.
- No EKGs are required.

Discontinuing atomoxetine treatment
- Because atomoxetine is a centrally acting agent, it is wise to avoid abrupt drug discontinuation.
- Taper atomoxetine by 20% of the full dose every 2–3 days until the drug is discontinued.

OTHER MEDICATIONS

Table 11.1 Studies of Atomoxetine in Child, Adolescent, and Adult Psychiatry

Author (year)	Study Type	N	Disorder	Age (yrs) (range)	Dose	Duration (weeks)	Side Effects	Outcome
Kratochvil et al. (2002)	Open	184	ADHD	7–15	1–2 mg/kg/day	10	Vomiting, sedation	Atomoxetine effects comparable to MPH
Michelson et al. (2001)	RCT	297	ADHD	8–18	0.5 or 1.2 or 1.8 mg/kg/day	8	Decreased appetite, nausea, dizziness	1.2 mg/kg/day effective and best tolerated
Michelson et al. (2002)	RCT	171	ADHD	6–16	1.0 mg/kg/day	6	Mild	Once daily dosing effective
Michelson et al. (2003)	RCT	536	ADHD	Adults	60–120 mg/day	10	Modest increase in heart rate and blood pressure	Effective
Spencer et al. (1998)	Crossover	22	ADHD	Adults	Avg: 7 mg/day	3	Well tolerated	Effective

RCT = randomized controlled trial; MPH = methylphenidate

Contraindications

• Known hypersensitivity to atomoxetine or other constituents of the product.
• Monoamine oxidase inhibitors: Atomoxetine should not be taken within 2 weeks of receiving an MAOI.
• Narrow-angle glaucoma.

Side Effects

In children and young adolescents
• Dyspepsia
• Nausea
• Vomiting
• Decreased appetite
• Rhinitis
• Headache
• Mild weight loss

In older adolescents and adults
• Constipation
• Dry mouth
• Lethargy
• Decreased appetite
• Insomnia
• Impaired sexual function (erectile disturbance, impotence, abnormal orgasm)
• Urinary hesitancy

Adults appear to have more varied side effects to atomoxetine than children.

Drug–Drug Interactions

Atomoxetine has relatively few drug–drug interactions, shown in the following table.

Table 11.2 Some Atomoxetine Drug–Drug Interactions
Atomoxetine interacts with:

Albuterol	↑ Heart rate and blood pressure
Alcohol	Does not change the intoxicating effects of alcohol
Desipramine	Combination therapy with desipramine does not change the pharmacokinetics of desipramine
Fluoxetine	↑ Serum levels of atomoxetine
Methylphenidate	No ↑ in blood pressure or heart rate with combination therapy
Monoamine oxidase inhibitors	Severe hypertension
Paroxetine	↑ Serum levels of atomoxetine
Quinidine	↑ Serum levels of atomoxetine

• In combination with methylphenidate, no increase in heart rate or blood pressure is noted over increases seen with either agent alone. Atomoxetine alone will increase the systolic and diastolic blood pressure by an average of approximately 1.5 mmHg and increase the heart rate by approximately 5 bpm.

- Fluoxetine and paroxetine inhibit the CYP2D6 enzyme system and can increase serum levels of atomoxetine.
- Quinidine inhibits the CYP2D6 enzyme system and can increase serum levels of atomoxetine.
- Therapy with MAOIs is contraindicated within 2 weeks of receiving atomoxetine.

Management of Overdose

The effects of atomoxetine overdose involving greater than twice the recommended daily dose are unknown. No specific information on the treatment of overdose with atomoxetine is presently available. Therapeutic measures are supportive.

- Gastric emptying and repeated activated charcoal may prevent systemic absorption.
- Monitor carefully.
- Provide supportive care.

Drug Interference with Laboratory Testing

- Does not prolong corrected QT interval on EKG.

MODAFINIL

Modafinil (Provigil®) is a novel wake-promoting agent with properties different from amphetamine or methylphenidate. Modafinil is used to treat excessive daytime sleepiness associated with narcolepsy. The agent does not appear to be a dopamine agonist and exhibits site-specific CNS activity in subcortical brain areas such as the anterior hypothalamus and the central nucleus of the amygdala. These CNS areas are thought to regulate sleep and waking activity. In contrast, amphetamine and methylphenidate activate many CNS areas, including the cortex, basal ganglia, and the nucleus accumbens; these brain areas are not activated by modafinil. Instead, modafinil appears to indirectly activate the frontal cortex via the hypothalamus and/or the tuberomammilary nucleus, thereby promoting wakefulness. Thus modafinil may have more specific actions at precise wake-promoting CNS areas than the stimulants.

Because stimulants such as amphetamine and methylphenidate are also useful in ADHD as well as to promote wakefulness in patients suffering from narcolepsy, modafinil is being investigated as a nonstimulant treatment for child, adolescent, and adult ADHD. Modafinil is listed in Schedule IV of the Controlled Substances Act.

Pharmacology

Orexins are neuropeptides that are produced in the lateral hypothalamus and may be important in the regulation of sleep. Acting on axon terminals, orexin-A and orexin-B can increase the release of the inhibitory neurotransmitter gamma-aminobutyric acid (GABA) and the excitatory neurotransmitter glutamate. Although its mechanism of action remains unknown, modafinil activates orexin-containing neurons, which may explain some of its pharmacological actions on wakefulness. Activation of the frontal cortex via the hypothalamic arousal system may also be beneficial for disorders of attention.

PHARMACODYNAMICS

- The precise mechanism of action by which modafinil promotes cortical arousal and wakefulness is not known.
- Not a direct or indirect dopamine agonist.
- Does not appear to be a direct or indirect alpha-1-adrenergic receptor agonist. However, an intact alpha-1-adrenergic system is required for the actions of modafinil on wakefulness.
- In addition to its wake-promoting effects, modafinil produces psychoactive and euphoric effects.
  ○ Evidenced by self-administration in animal models.

PHARMACOKINETICS

Absorption
- After oral administration, the time to peak plasma concentration is 2–4 hours.
- Time to peak plasma concentration, but not the extent of absorption, may be delayed when modafinil is taken with food.
- Exhibits linear pharmacokinetics, with increases in plasma levels proportional to dose increases.

Distribution
- Total protein binding about 60%, mostly to albumin.
- More affinity for body tissues than for plasma.

Metabolism and excretion
- Primarily eliminated by hepatic metabolism with subsequent renal elimination of metabolites.
- Hydrolytic deamination, S-oxidation, aromatic ring hydroxylation, and glucuronide conjugation are primary metabolic processes responsible for clearance.
- Elimination half-life is 7–15 hours.
- As a racemic product, the half-life of the *l*- isomer is approximately three times longer than the half-life of the *d*- isomer.
- At maintenance doses ≥ 400 mg/day, modafinil may induce its own metabolism by slightly activating enzyme systems CYP1A2, CYP2B6, and CYP2C9.

Indications

- Labeled to improve excessive daytime sleepiness in patients with narcolepsy ≥ 16 years old.

OTHER MEDICATIONS

Possible indications
• ADHD in children, adolescents, and adults

Because wake-promoting agents such as stimulants are also useful in ADHD, modafinil is currently being studied in children, adolescents, and adults with ADHD. Some studies attest to its possible usefulness. However, at the present time modafinil cannot be recommended for routine use in ADHD until more research is completed. Pertinent studies are listed below.

Dosing and Duration of Treatment

Available modafinil preparations
• Tablets (Provigil®): white (oval) in 100 mg and 200 mg (scored) strengths.

Before initiating treatment
• Obtain baseline vital signs, height, weight, and routine physical exam.
• No baseline laboratory or EKG workup is required.
• Assess for history of substance abuse in the family.

General dosing suggestions
• For excessive daytime somnolence in narcolepsy, the dose is 200 mg/day, given as a single morning dose.
  ◦ Doses higher than 200 mg/day did not confer additional benefits.
• The dose in ADHD is not well established.
  ◦ The effective dose range appears to be higher in ADHD than for excessive daytime somnolence in narcolepsy.
  ◦ In ADHD 300–400 mg/day appear to have some benefit over placebo. However, the dose must be individually titrated in the range between 50 and 400 mg/day.
  ◦ For ADHD, modafinil is given in two equally divided doses, A.M. and noon.
  ◦ For ADHD, initiate modafinil at 50 mg bid and titrate every week to a maximum dose of 200 mg bid (A.M. and noon).

Discontinuing modafinil treatment
• In a controlled 9-week trial of adults with narcolepsy, no withdrawal signs were noted upon discontinuation of modafinil.

Contraindications

• Known hypersensitivity to modafinil

Possible contraindications
• May exacerbate depression in vulnerable patients.
• May exacerbate hallucinations and psychosis in vulnerable patients.
• History of hypertension (periodic monitoring is advised).
• Hepatic and/or renal disease (reduce dose).
• Cardiovascular disease (modafinil has been associated with EKG abnormalities in adults; it should be used cautiously in adults with unstable cardiovascular disease).

Table 11.3 Studies of Modafinil

Author (year)	Study Type	N	Disorder	Age (yrs)	Dose	Duration (weeks)	Side Effects	Outcome
Biederman (2003)	RCT	248	ADHD	6–13	Dosing regimens in children < 30 kg: 300 mg A.M.; 200 mg A.M. and 100 mg midday; or 100 mg A.M. and 200 mg midday; dosing in children ≥ 30 kg: 400 mg as split dose	4	Well tolerated; most frequent were insomnia, abdominal pain, anorexia, cough, fever, rhinitis	Significant improvement on school and home versions of ADHD Rating Scale–IV and Conners Rating Scale—Parent version with 300 mg once daily dose (n = 177 completers); significant improvement on school version of ADHD Rating Scale–IV in 200/100 mg group
MacDonald et al. (2002)	Crossover	40	Excessive somnolence in myotonic dystrophy	Adults	200–400 mg/day	2	Headache	Improved somnolence and mood
U.S. Modafinil in Narcolepsy Multicenter Study Group (2000)	RCT	271	Narcolepsy	Adults	200 or 400 mg/day	9	Headache	Effective for excessive sleep in narcolepsy
Rugino & Copley (2001)	Open	11	ADHD	5–15	50–400 mg/day Avg: 195 ± 96 mg	5	Mild	Once daily dosing effective in ADHD
Rugino & Samsock (2003)	RCT	11	ADHD	6–12	200–300 mg/day Avg: 264 ± 50 mg	5	Mild	Modafinil effective compared to placebo in ADHD
Swanson (2003)	Crossover, analog classroom study	48	ADHD	6–13	Dosing regimens in children < 30 kg: 100 200 300 mg; dosing in children ≥ 30 kg: 400 mg as split dose	4	Most frequent were abdominal pain, headache	Significant improvement on the home version of the ADHD Rating Scale–IV in the 300 and 400 mg groups
Taylor & Russo (2000)	Crossover	22	ADHD	Adults	50–400 mg/day Avg: 207 ± 85 mg	2	Mild anxiety, insomnia	Modafinil effective for ADHD

RCT = randomized controlled trial

Side Effects

Modafinil is generally well tolerated. Common side effects are:

• Headache
• Nausea
• Anxiety
• Insomnia
• Depression

Modafinil should be used cautiously in psychiatric patients with a history of mood or anxiety disorders. Modafinil should also be used cautiously in patients with a history of substance use disorders, because this agent appears to have euphoric and reinforcing properties.

Drug–Drug Interactions

Potential modafinil drug–drug interactions are listed in the following table.

Table 11.4 Modafinil Drug–Drug Interactions
Modafinil (Provigil®) interacts with:

Clomipramine	↑ Clomipramine serum levels
Monoamine oxidase inhibitors	Risk of severe hypertension
Carbamazepine	↓ Modafinil serum levels
Ketoconazole	↑ Modafinil serum levels

Management of Overdose

No deaths have been reported in modafinil overdoses of 1000–4500 mg. Symptoms of modafinil toxicity include excitation, agitation, insomnia, and elevated vital signs. Other signs of modafinil overdose include anxiety, irritability, aggressiveness, confusion, tremor, palpitations, nausea, diarrhea, and decreased prothrombin time.

No specific antidote to the toxic effects of modafinil overdose has been identified to date. There are no data to suggest benefits from dialysis, urinary acidification, or alkalinization in facilitating drug elimination from the body.

• Provided supportive care.
• Cardiovascular monitoring is recommended.
• Induced emesis or gastric lavage is recommended if no contraindications exist.

Drug Interference with Laboratory Testing

• Nonclinically significant increase in plasma gamma-glutamyl transferase (GGT).
• Nonclinically significant increase in eosinophil counts.

DESMOPRESSIN ACETATE

Desmopressin (DDAVP) is a synthetic analogue of the pituitary hormone arginine vasopressin, an antidiuretic hormone affecting renal water conservation. DDAVP is used in pediatrics and in child psychiatry for the treatment of nocturnal enuresis and in cranial diabetes insipidus. It has greater antidiuretic activity and a more prolonged duration of action than vasopressin. It also stimulates factor VIII and plasminogen activator activity in the blood, and is used in the management of mild or moderate hemophilia and type I von Willebrand's disease.

Pharmacology

Secretion of vasopressin during the night in normal individuals reduces urine output. It has been suggested that nocturnal enuresis in some children might be due to impaired or delayed nocturnal secretion of vasopressin (AACAP, 2004). Other evidence suggests that maturational delay in specific cortical areas of the CNS might be responsible for nocturnal enuresis. Use of DDAVP in nocturnal enuresis can produce a 30–60% reduction in wet nights, in general, and an approximately 50% overall reduction in nocturnal enuresis while on the medication.

The primary mechanism of action of desmopressin is to increase the permeability of the renal collecting ducts to water, thus diminishing urine output.

PHARMACODYNAMICS

DDAVP results in

• Decreased urine output
• Increased urine osmolality
• A concomitant decrease in plasma osmolality

PHARMACOKINETICS

• The time to an antidiuretic effect
  ○ For intranasally administered DDAVP: 1 hour.
  ○ For orally administered DDAVP: 1–2 hours.
• After multiple doses, the duration of antidiuretic activity is:
  ○ Intranasal: 5–24 hours.
  ○ Oral: 6–12 hours.
• Regardless of the route of DDAVP administration (e.g., oral, subcutaneous, intranasal, intravenous) the plasma terminal half-life is 4–5 hours.

Indications

• Oral DDAVP is indicated for antidiuretic replacement therapy in the management of central diabetes insipidus.
  ○ Not effective in the management of nephrogenic diabetes insipidus.
• Oral DDAVP is indicated for the management of primary nocturnal enuresis.
• DDAVP injection (IV) is indicated for patients with hemophilia A with factor VIII anticoagulant deficiency.

OTHER MEDICATIONS

• DDAVP injection (IV) is indicated for patients with mild to moderate classic von Willebrand's disease (type I).

Dosing and Duration of Treatment

Available DDAVP preparations for nocturnal enuresis
• Tablets: white, in 0.1 mg and 0.2 mg strengths
• Nasal spray: 0.1 ml (10 μg) DDAVP per spray
• Injection: 4 μg/ml (for hematological disorders only).

General dosing suggestions for nocturnal enuresis
• DDAVP tablets: recommended dose range for patients ≥ 6 years old is 0.2 mg at bedtime. The dose may be titrated to 0.6 mg at bedtime depending on tolerability and response.
• DDAVP nasal spray: recommended dose range for patients ≥ 6 years old is 0.2 μg (spray once in each nostril) intranasally at bedtime. The dose may be titrated to 0.4 μg (spray twice in each nostril) if no response. Administer one-half the dose per each nostril.
• DDAVP has been found effective and safe in children with long-term treatment of up to 12 months for primary nocturnal enuresis.

Contraindications

• Individuals with hypersensitivity to desmopressin or to any of the components of DDAVP tablets.
• Use cautiously in patients vulnerable to fluid and electrolyte imbalance, such as those with cystic fibrosis.
  ◦ These patients may develop hyponatremia.
• Use cautiously in patients with hypertension because of the slight pressor effects of intranasal DDAVP.

Side Effects

DDAVP is generally well tolerated; side effects may include:

• Headache
• Nausea
• Flushing (vasodilation)
• Mild abdominal cramps

Drug–Drug Interactions

• DDAVP causes a mild pressor action on blood pressure; in combination with other pressor agents elevated blood pressure may occur.

Management of Overdose

In case of overdose, the dose should be reduced, frequency of administration decreased, or the drug withdrawn according to the severity of the overdose and clinician judgment. There is no known specific antidote for DDAVP. The patient should be medically monitored with supportive care, as necessary.

Drug Interference with Laboratory Testing

None.

OXYBUTYNIN

Oxybutynin (Ditropan®) is an anticholinergic agent that is used as an antispasmodic for the treatment of neurogenic bladder, bladder spasm, overactive bladder, and detrusor muscle instability. Oxybutynin is used to treat overactive bladder with symptoms of urge urinary incontinence, urgency, and frequency.

Pharmacology

PHARMACODYNAMICS

- Exerts a direct antispasmodic effect on smooth muscle and inhibits the muscarinic action of acetylcholine on smooth muscle.
- Relaxes bladder smooth muscle. In patients with conditions characterized by involuntary bladder contractions, oxybutynin increases bladder capacity, diminishes the frequency of uninhibited contractions of the detrusor muscle, and delays the initial desire to void.

PHARMACOKINETICS

Absorption
- Oral absorption is rapid.
- Peak plasma levels occur within 1 hour.
- Antispasmodic activity occurs within 0.5–1 hour, with peak activity occurring within 3–6 hours.
- May be taken with or without food.
- Oral oxybutynin exhibits linear rate kinetics and dose proportional pharmacokinetic properties.

Metabolism and excretion
- Hepatically metabolized to one inactive (phenylcyclohexylglycolic acid) and one active (desethyloxybutynin) metabolite, which are then excreted by renal mechanisms.
- Metabolized primarily by the CYP3A4 enzyme system, found in the liver and gut wall.
- The elimination half-life after oral dosing is 1–2.3 hours.
- The average steady-state plasma concentration for the oxybutynin transdermal system is reached during the second consecutive patch application.

Indications

- The treatment of overactive bladder in adults
- Although used in children, oxybutynin is not labeled by the FDA for use in the pediatric population.

Dosing and Duration of Treatment

Available oxybutynin preparations

- Tablets (Ditropan®): 5 mg
- Extended-release tablets (Ditropan XL®): in 5 mg (yellow), 10 mg (pink), and 15 mg (gray) strengths
- Oxybutynin transdermal delivery system (Oxytrol™): 2.6 and 3.9 mg/day systems

General dosing suggestions
- Children ≥5 years may receive 5 mg of oxybutynin twice a day. Maximum dose is 5 mg three times a day in children.
- The transdermal system is applied twice weekly (every three to four days) in adults with overactive bladder. Little information is available about its use in the pediatric population.

Contraindications

- Hypersensitivity to oxybutynin
- Gastrointestional obstruction
- Megacolon
- Myasthenia gravis
- Paralytic ileus
- Reflux esophagitis
- Ulcerative colitis
- Narrow-angle glaucoma
- Urinary obstruction

Side Effects

Oxybutynin is associated with many anticholinergic side effects, These including:

- Dry mouth
- Constipation
- Headache
- Asthenia
- Somnolence
- Blurred vision
- Sexual dysfunction
- Nausea
- Skin flushing

Drug–Drug Interactions

- Oxybutynin in combination with other anticholinergic medications can exacerbate atropine-like side effects.
- Oxybutynin in combination with cisapride is likely to counteract the gastrointestinal motility normally induced by cisapride.

• Oxybutynin in combination with clomipramine may induce the metabolism of clomipramine.
• Oxybutynin in combination with procainamide may result in additive antivagal effects on cardiac atrioventricular nodal conduction.

Management of Overdose

Overdose with oxybutynin may be associated with anticholinergic effects, including CNS excitation, flushing, fever, dehydration, cardiac arrhythmia, vomiting, and urinary retention. Treatment is symptomatic and supportive. Activated charcoal as well as a cathartic may be administered.

Drug Interference with Laboratory Testing

None.

TOLTERODINE

Although oxybutynin is effective for the symptoms of overactive bladder and urinary incontinence, it is associated with many treatment-emergent side effects, especially dry mouth. Tolterodine (Detrol®) is a muscarinic receptor antagonist that has been shown to be effective for treating the overactive bladder. Tolterodine is more selective than oxybutynin in its effects on bladder smooth muscle, with less reported side effects, including a lower frequency of dry mouth and gastrointestinal side effects. Tolterodine has a longer half-life than oxybutynin, requiring less frequent dosing. This agent is used in adults with overactive bladder. It is not yet approved for use in children, but has been studied and found effective for detrusor hyperreflexia and overactive bladder in the pediatric population.

Pharmacology

PHARMACODYNAMICS

• Tolterodine is a competitive muscarinic receptor antagonist with potent effects on bladder function.
• The main effects of tolterodine are to increase residual urine, reflecting incomplete emptying of the bladder and diminished detrusor muscle pressure.

PHARMACOKINETICS

Absorption
• Rapidly absorbed after oral administration, with peak plasma concentrations occurring within 1–2 hours after dosing.
• Food has no clinically relevant effects.

Metabolism and excretion
• Extensively metabolized by the liver after oral dosing.
• The primary route of metabolism is through the CYP2D6 enzyme system.

OTHER MEDICATIONS

○ About 7% of the population are devoid of CYP2D6 and are classified as poor metabolizers; these individuals will have high serum drug concentrations at therapeutic doses.
- Metabolized to a 5-hydroxymethyl active metabolite.
- In active metabolizers the half-life is 1.9–3 hours.
- In poor metabolizers the half-life is 9.6 hours.

Indications

- The treatment of overactive bladder with symptoms of urge urinary incontinence, urgency, and frequency in adults.
- Not yet labeled for use in the pediatric population, but has been investigated and found safe and effective in children and adolescents with symptoms of overactive bladder.

Dosing and Duration of Treatment

Available tolterodine preparations
- Tablets (Detrol®): white, in 1 mg and 2 mg strengths
- Extended-release capsules (Detrol® LA): 2 mg (blue green) and 4 mg (blue) strengths

General dosing suggestions
The dose of tolterodine for children and adolescents has not yet been established. Suggestions are abstracted from published clinical trials in children.

- Adults: usual daily dose is 1–2 mg given twice daily.
- Children: reported dose range is between 0.5 to 2 mg given twice daily.

Contraindications

- Known hypersensitivity to the agent
- Urinary retention
- Gastric retention
- Narrow-angle glaucoma
- Bladder outlet obstruction
- Gastrointestinal obstruction
- Reduced hepatic function
- Reduced renal function

Side Effects

- Dry mouth
- Constipation
- Headache
- Abdominal pain
- Dry eyes
- Blurred vision

Drug–Drug Interactions

• Fluoxetine (a potent inhibitor of CYP2D6) inhibits the metabolism of tolterodine.
• Macrolide antibiotics (erythromycin, clarithromycin) may inhibit the metabolism of tolterodine, resulting in higher tolterodine plasma levels.
• Azole antifungals (itraconazole, miconazole) may inhibit the metabolism of tolterodine, resulting in higher tolterodine plasma levels.

Management of Overdose

Tolterodine overdose may result in severe central anticholinergic effects.

• EKG monitoring is recommended.
• Medical monitoring and supportive care are recommended.

Drug Interference with Laboratory Testing

None.

NALTREXONE

Naltrexone hydrochloride (generic, Trexane®, ReVia®) is an orally available semisynthetic pure opiate antagonist similar in structure to naloxone. It is a synthetic congener of oxymorphone without any opioid agonist properties and reversibly blocks the subjective effects of intravenous opioids and precipitates withdrawal symptoms in subjects with physical tolerance to opioids. Naltrexone is used primarily as an adjunct to social and psychosocial rehabilitation in recovering adult narcotic addicts. It is also used as an adjunct in the treatment of adult alcohol dependence.

Naltrexone has primarily been investigated in the treatment of children and adolescents with developmental delay, mental retardation, and/or autism and associated behavioral disturbances and communication deficits. Results are generally disappointing, and at the present time naltrexone cannot be recommended as treatment for any child or adolescent psychiatric condition. In adults with developmental delay naltrexone has sometimes been used as a treatment for severe and repetitive self-injurious behavior (SIB). There are two theories that guide naltrexone use in SIB. The pain hypothesis states that in some patients self-injury does not induce pain because excessive basal activity of opioid systems in the CNS has led to an opioid analgesic state. The addiction hypothesis suggests that SIB occurs in developmentally delayed patients because tissue injury releases endogenous opioids that are reinforcing (addicting) to the patient and facilitates repetitive SIB behaviors. In theory, blocking opioids with naltrexone should result in a decrease in repetitive SIB by diminishing endogenous opioid activity in the CNS (Sandman, 1990; Sandman et al., 1993). However, results from controlled trials in adults with severe SIB are decidedly mixed, and opioid blockade is not presently considered a standard treatment for SIB in persons with developmental delay (Buitelaar, 2003).

OTHER MEDICATIONS

Pharmacology

Endogenous opioid ligands were first described in the mid-1970s. Subsequently, a variety of endogenous peptides were identified that have opioid activity, including enkephalins, endorphins, and dynorphins. Endogenous opioids are derived from three distinct precursor molecules, which are the primary products of three separate genes. The precursor proteins are pro-opiomelanocortin (POMC), pro-enkephalin (ProEnk), and pro-dynorphin (ProDyn). These precursor proteins are post-translationally processed by enzymes, resulting in a mixture of endogenous opioids that are tissue-specific and demonstrate a unique anatomical distribution throughout the CNS and the periphery. Three major classes of opioid receptors are known: the μ-receptor, the κ-receptor, and the δ-receptor. All three opioid receptor types exist in the CNS.

PHARMACODYNAMICS

- Naltrexone blocks opioid receptors (antagonism) and possesses undetectable opioid agonistic effects.

PHARMACOKINETICS

Absorption
- Can be given orally.
- Is rapidly absorbed, with approximately 96% of a given dose absorbed from the gastrointestinal tract within 1 hour.
- After oral dosing, bioavailability is 5–40% of a given dose.

Distribution
- 21% bound to plasma proteins.

Metabolism and excretion
- Naltrexone is extensively metabolized in the liver and has a large first-pass effect, in which about 95% of the active dose is converted to active metabolites, including beta-naltrexol.
- Beta-naltrexol is active but weaker narcotic antagonist than naltrexone.
- The elimination half-life of naltrexone appears to be biphasic.
  ○ In the first 24 hours postdosing, the half-life of naltrexone is between 3 to 10 hours.
  ○ A very slow terminal half-life is found after 24 hours, around 96 hours.
- The elimination half-life of beta-naltrexol ranges between 11 and 17 hours.
- The half-life of naltrexone blockade of μ-receptors in the CNS ranges between 72 and 108 hours.
- Excretion is predominantly by renal mechanisms, with a small amount recovered in feces.

Indications

- Currently approved for the treatment of alcoholism and the blockade of the effects of exogenously administered opiates in individuals 18 years of age and older.

- Naltrexone is not currently approved for any indication in child and adolescent psychiatry.

Possible indications
- Naltrexone has been investigated for disruptive behaviors, self-injurious behaviors, and for its effects on communication skills in children and adolescents with mental retardation and autism.
- At this time, the extant literature does not support a clinical indication for the use of naltrexone in child and adolescent psychopharmacology; its use at the present time must be considered experimental.

The following table summarizes pertinent studies of naltrexone in pediatric psychopharmacology.

GENERAL DOSING SUGGESTIONS

Available naltrexone preparations
- Tablets: 50 mg (yellow)

Dosing guidelines
- For both the treatment of autism and for SIB in children and adolescents, dosages of naltrexone have been in the range of 0.5–2.0 mg/kg/day, given as a single A.M. dose.
- Begin naltrexone with 12.5 mg in young children and 25 mg in older children. Increase the dose in 2 days to 25 mg in young children and 50 mg in older children.
- If no treatment effects are noticed in 2 weeks, the dose may be titrated upward to 2.0 mg/kg/day.

Medical monitoring
- Liver function tests should be obtained at baseline and at regular times during treatment.

Contraindications

- Patients who are physically dependent on opioids or in acute opioid withdrawal should not receive naltrexone, because the drug will provoke or worsen an acute withdrawal reaction.
- Patients who are receiving opioid analgesics should not receive naltrexone, because pain will return with opioid blockade and patients may experience opioid withdrawal.
- Patients with hepatitis or liver failure
- History of hypersensitivity to naltrexone

Side Effects

- Sedation
- Decreased appetite
- Vomiting
- Elevated hepatic transaminases

OTHER MEDICATIONS

Table 11.5 Studies of Naltrexone in Child and Adolescent Psychiatry

Author (year)	Study Type	N	Disorder	Age (years) (range)	Dose	Duration (weeks)	Side Effects	Outcome
Campbell et al. (1990)	RCT	18	Autism	3–8	0.5–1.0 mg/kg/day	3	None reported	Significant improvement compared to placebo
Campbell et al. (1993)	RCT	41	Autism	3–8	0.5–1.0 mg/kg/day	3	Minimal	No significant difference in SIB or autistic symptoms
Feldman et al. (1999)	CO	24	Autism	3–8	1.0 mg/kg/day	7	None reported	No significant difference in communication skills
Kolmen et al. (1997)	RCT	24	Autism	3–8	1.0 mg/kg/day	2	Minimal	Small improvement in hyperactivity; no improvement in autism
Willemsen-Swinkels et al. (1996)	CO	23	Autism	3–7	1.0 mg/kg/day	4	Minimal	Small reduction in hyperactivity; no improvement in autism

RCT = randomized controlled trial; CO = cross over design; SIB = self-injurious behavior.

Drug–Drug Interactions

• The concurrent administration of naltrexone and opioid analgesics is contraindicated. Patients must be free of opioids for a minimum of 7–10 days before naltrexone administration to prevent opioid withdrawal.
• Yohimbine and naltrexone administered concurrently increase negative effects, including anxiety and nervousness.

Management of Overdose

There are currently no reports of toxic reactions following ingestion of an overdose of naltrexone.

OTHER MEDICATIONS

12. Herbal and Alternative Medicines

Herbal and alternative medicines are part of a broad group of alternative medical treatments that exist largely outside the institutions where mainstream health care is provided. Alternative medicine comprises a wide range of disparate interventions, including acupuncture, yoga, and various forms of meditation, homoeopathy, reflexology, and herbal remedies. The use of alternative medicine appears to be growing as some traditional physicians increasingly use these treatments in their practices and as some health care insurers begin to include coverage for alternative medicine treatments. The National Institutes of Health (NIH) in the United States now include a National Center for Complementary and Alternative Medicine, which conducts and supports basic and clinical research in this field. This chapter focuses on the use of herbal and alternative medicines in child and adolescent psychiatry, with an emphasis on St. John's wort, melatonin, essential fatty acids, and secretin.

Herbal and alternative medicines are consumed extensively, and their use appears to be increasing. In pediatric practice, between 11% and 55% of parents report giving their children an herbal product in the past 3 months. Few parents will spontaneously discuss their use of alternative medicine products with the physician, unless directly asked. It is important to inquire, because many herbal and alternative remedies have important drug–drug interactions with prescription as well as over-the-counter medications. It is therefore incumbent on health care providers to have knowledge about herbal and alternative medicines, to routinely inquire about their use, and to educate families about the potential risk–benefit ratio and interactions that these products may possess.

REGULATORY ISSUES

Botanical and herbal supplements are regulated in the United States under the Dietary Supplement Health and Education Act of 1994, which classifies these agents as food products and not medicines. Because of this classification, herbal and alternative medicines are not subject to regulation by the FDA, as are other medications. Less rigorous efficacy and safety standards are required of herbal and alternative remedies than are demanded of prescription medications. As a result of the lower regulatory standards, herbal and alternative medicines may lack standardized preparation and are more prone to contamination, substitution, adulteration, incorrect packaging, wrong dosage, and inappropriate labeling and advertising. This state of affairs is causing growing unease among consumers as well as medical professionals. Independent websites that provide consumers with unbiased information about alternative medicine treatments are provided in Appendix 5, Parent Support Resources.

ST. JOHN'S WORT

St. John's wort (*Hypericum perforatum*) is an aromatic perennial flowering bush that is native to Europe and also grows wild in parts of Asia, Africa, Australia, North America, and South America. *Wort* is an old English word meaning plant. Its leaves contain translucent glands. The whole or cut dried flowering tops of *Hypericum perforatum* are gathered during flowering. At least ten agents with potential biological activity have been extracted from the flowers and leaves of the *Hypericum perforatum* bush, including naphthodianthrones, which have reported antidepressant properties. In Germany, St. John's wort is the second most common herbal remedy and is currently used four times more frequently for depression than is the most commonly used prescription antidepressant. In the United States, St. John's wort is the second most commonly purchased herbal product.

Pharmacology

Substances contained in St. John's wort have been found to interact with a number of CNS neurotransmitter systems implicated in depression. St. John's wort is a weak inhibitor of monoamine oxidase. *Hypericum perforatum* inhibits uptake of serotonin, noradrenaline, and dopamine into neurons, potentiating CNS neurotransmission in these neural systems. Extracts of St. John's wort also show affinity for gamma-aminobutyric acid (GABA) receptors.

PHARMACODYNAMICS

• The exact CNS mechanism of action of St. John's wort is presently not known.

PHARMACOKINETICS

• Because the active compounds in *Hypericum perforatum* are not precisely known, little discussion of this agent's pharmacokinetics is possible.
• In adults, the half-life of St. John's wort is estimated to be 6–9 hours.
• In adults, time to peak plasma concentration after oral ingestion is estimated to be about 2–3 hours.
• Some of the constituents of *Hypericum perforatum* appear to be metabolized in the liver.

Indications

- *Hypericum perforatum* is presently not indicated for any medical or psychiatric disease.
- Possible indications and uses of St. John's wort include the treatment of mild to moderate anxiety and depression.
- Possible uses of St. John's wort also include dermatological diseases such as atopic dermatitis.

Hypericum perforatum has been studied the most in adults suffering from mild to moderate depression. Few open studies and no controlled clinical trials are presently available to guide clinical practice in children and adolescents. In adults there exists a growing body of scientific evidence that St. John's wort is effective in mild to moderate depression, compared with placebo. Pooling results from 13 randomized trials in adults with mild depression, a response rate of 55% was found for *Hypericum perforatum*, as compared with a 22% response rate for placebo. In these studies, seven different preparations of St. John's wort, with widely varying daily doses, were assessed (Linde et al., 1996). In a randomized, controlled trial of St. John's wort, extract 600 mg/day, somatoform anxiety improved independently of depression in 160 adult outpatients with somatoform complaints (Volz et al., 2002). However, not all controlled studies of depressed adults are positive. At least two studies conducted in the United States have shown no superiority of *Hypericum perforatum* over placebo. Nevertheless, St. John's wort is presently the best studied herbal remedy and does show promise in the treatment of mild to moderate depression and anxiety in adults.

In an open-label study of St. John's wort in juvenile depression, 33 youths were given *Hypericum perforatum* 450–900 mg per day. Their ages ranged between 6 and 16 years. Twenty-five youths responded with improvement in the primary depression outcome measure. St. John's wort was well tolerated (Findling et al., 2003).

For severe depression and anxiety, and for psychotic depression, *Hypericum perforatum* should be avoided. Prescription antidepressant therapies with known efficacy such as the SSRIs should be used.

Recent investigations suggest an anti-inflammatory and antibacterial effect of hyperforin, which is a major active constituent of *Hypericum perforatum*. In a controlled study, hypericum cream was superior to placebo in the topical treatment of atopic dermatitis (Schempp et al., 2003).

Dosing and Duration of Treatment

There exists a paucity of information about dosing and duration of treatment of St. John's wort in children and adolescents. Most data are extrapolated from the adult literature.

Available preparations of St. John's wort
- Tablets, capsules, drops, and teas.
  - In health food stores or over the Internet.

ALTERNATIVE MEDICINES

- An oil preparation is available for external use only and has no place in the treatment of depression or anxiety.
- Many preparations of St. John's wort contain other ingredients and should be avoided.
- Because production of St. John's wort is not subject to the same rigorous standards as that of prescription medications, the actual amounts of *Hypericum* plant extract used in different preparations may vary considerably. Quality control studies show that the amount of active ingredient (e.g., *Hypericum*) is often very different from the amount advertised on the bottle label. The therapeutic standard for plant extracts is generally considered to be 0.3% *Hypericum*.

General dosing suggestions
- Like other antidepressants, there is a 2–3-week lag in therapeutic onset of action.
- The adult dosage of St. John's wort generally recommended for the treatment of depression is 300 mg of plant extract (0.3% *Hypericum*) orally three times daily.
- There are no data about optimal dose in the pediatric population.
- In children and adolescents, it is suggested that St. John's wort be initiated at 150 mg tid. If no response occurs after 4 weeks, increase the dose to 300 mg tid (Findling et al., 2003).

Duration of treatment
- There are presently no data on duration of antidepressant treatment with St. John's wort. Like other antidepressants, treatment duration of 6–12 months after a positive response is recommended.

Discontinuing St. John's wort
- Although no studies exist to inform treatment, it is recommended that St. John's wort be tapered gradually to avoid any possible withdrawal effects, especially after chronic treatment.

Contraindications

- History of photosensitivity
- Known hypersensitivity to *Hypericum perforatum*
- Pregnancy

Side Effects

Although the extant evidence in adults suggests that St. John's wort is well tolerated (Knuppel & Linde, 2004), this does not mean it is free of treatment-emergent adverse events. Because of the public's perception that herbal remedies are "natural" and thus safe, the side effects of St. John's wort are probably underreported. Common side effects are:

- Gastrointestional symptoms
- Allergic reactions

- Fatigue
- Restlessness
- Headaches
- Hypomanic reactions have been reported.
- Sensitivity reactions to sunlight (photosensitivity) have been reported.
- *Hypericum perforatum* has been shown to have uterotonic actions; use in pregnancy is contraindicated.

Drug–Drug Interactions

Hypericum perforatum can have clinically significant interactions with prescribed medications. St. John's wort is a potent inducer of the cytochrome P4503A4 enzyme system. Clinical use of St. John's wort may result in diminished clinical effectiveness or increased dose requirements for all drugs that are metabolized using the hepatic CYP3A4 system. Because CYP3A4 is involved in the oxidative metabolism of more than half of all drugs, there are potential interactions with a wide variety of medications.

Some potential St. John's wort drug–drug interactions include the following.

- SSRIs, leading to increased serotonergic effects and possible serotonin syndrome.
- Oral contraceptives, leading to enhanced metabolism and contraceptive failure.
- Anticonvulsants, leading to reduced serum levels and break-through seizures.
- Warfarin, leading to reduced serum levels and anticoagulant effects.
- Theophylline, leading to reduced blood levels and reduced anti-asthmatic efficacy.
- HIV protease inhibitors, leading to reduced blood levels and possible loss of HIV suppression.
- Triptans, leading to increased serotonin treatment-emergent adverse effects.

MELATONIN

Melatonin is an endogenous hormone produced by the pineal gland. It is involved in the production of sleep and may play a role in the regulation of circadian rhythms. The hormone may also produce immunostimulatory and cytostatic effects.

Discrete neuroanatomical sites govern the generation of normal sleep and wakefulness. Experimental lesion studies in animals implicate the medullary reticular formation, the thalamus, and the basal forebrain in the generation of sleep. The brainstem reticular formation, the midbrain, the subthalamus, the thalamus, and the basal forebrain have all been suggested to play a role in the generation of wakefulness.

The pineal hormone melatonin is secreted predominantly at night, reflecting the direct regulation of pineal activity by a circadian pacemaker involving the suprachiasmatic nuclei of the hypothalamus and the pineal gland. Melatonin secretion is not dependent on sleep, but also occurs in individuals kept awake at night. Exogenous melatonin is known to increase sleepiness and reduce latency to sleep onset, helping to regulate slow-wave, non-REM sleep.

ALTERNATIVE MEDICINES

Pharmacology

PHARMACODYNAMICS

- Physiological plasma levels of melatonin during daylight hours are very low (<10 pg/ml).
- At night plasma levels increase significantly to an average of around 90 pg/ml between 2 and 4 A.M.
- Melatonin levels remain elevated during sleep and rapidly return to normal daytime values generally around 9 A.M.
- The normal endogenous production rate of melatonin is 28–30 mcg/day.

PHARMACOKINETICS

Absorption
- After oral administration of exogenous *immediate*-release melatonin, the time to peak plasma concentration is 0.5–2 hours.
- After oral administration of exogenous *sustained*-release melatonin, the time to peak plasma concentration is 2–4 hours.
- Oral exogenous melatonin undergoes extensive first-pass hepatic metabolism (up to 60% of an oral dose).
- Plasma levels of orally administered exogenous melatonin appear to be unaffected by the presence or absence of food.

Distribution
- Melatonin is extensively distributed to numerous body tissues, including saliva, seminal fluid, cerebrospinal fluid, ovarian follicular fluid, amniotic fluid, the ovaries, and the pineal gland.

Metabolism and excretion
- Melatonin is metabolized in the liver to 6-hydroxymelatonin and N-acetyl serotonin, which are then excreted in the urine as glucuronide and sulfate conjugates.
- The half-life of melatonin after exogenous oral dosing is 30–50 minutes.

Indications

- Exogenously administered melatonin is not presently indicated for any psychiatric disorder.
- Possible indications in psychiatry include use in sleep disorders such as jet lag, delayed-phase sleep syndrome, and sleep-onset insomnia.
- Melatonin has been designated an orphan drug product for use in the treatment of circadian rhythm sleep disorders in blind patients with no light perception.

In psychiatry, melatonin has been used mostly for the treatment of various forms of sleep disorder. In child and adolescent psychopharmacology, melatonin has been used to treat sleep-onset insomnia in patients with either neurological or psychiatric disorders. The following table summarizes pertinent research on melatonin.

Table 12.1 Studies of Melatonin in Child and Adolescent Psychiatry

Author (year)	Study Type	N	Disorder	Age (years) (range)	Dose (mg/day)	Duration (weeks)	Side Effects	Outcome
Dodge & Wilson (2001)	RCT	20	Developmental disabilities	1–12	5	6	Mild	61% of patients showed improved sleep
Paavonen et al. (2003)	Open	15	Asperger's disorder	6–17	3	2	None reported	Sleep improved in all
Ross et al. (2002)	Open	46	Seizures, blindness, neurological disorders	1–13	2.5–10	Not reported	None reported	73% of patients showed improved sleep
Smits et al. (2001)	RCT	40	Chronic sleep-onset insomnia	6–12	1–5	4	Headache	Significant sleep improvement in those on melatonin
Smits et al. (2003)	RCT	62	Chronic sleep onset insomnia	6–12	5	4	Mild	Significantly sleep improved in those on melatonin

RCT = randomized controlled trial

Dosing and Duration of Treatment

Available melatonin preparations
• Tablets: 1 mg, 1.5 mg, 2 mg.
• Capsule: 3 mg.
• Oral liquid preparation: 1 mg/1 ml.

No systematic dose or duration of treatment has yet been standardized for children and adolescents who receive melatonin. The following suggestions are based on the extant pediatric literature.

General dosing suggestions
• Initiate melatonin at a dose between 0.5 mg and 5 mg at night.
• The effective dose for sleep-onset insomnia appears to be 0.5–10 mg/day.
• The duration of melatonin treatment should be less than 4 weeks. No data are presently available to guide treatment for longer durations.

Contraindications

• Hypersensitivity to any component of the formulation

Precautions
• Liver disease
• History of cerebrovascular disease
• Depression

Side Effects

Melatonin is generally well tolerated. Reported side effects include the following.

• Tachycardia and increased pulse rate
• Sedation
• Depression and dysphoria
• Increased seizures in neurologically impaired children
• Vasodilation and flushing of the skin

Drug–Drug Interactions

• Melatonin will increase sedation in combination with sedating psychotropics.

ESSENTIAL FATTY ACIDS

The CNS contains high concentrations of lipids. Neuronal membranes are composed of phospholipids that are dense in long-chain polyunsaturated fatty acids of the omega-3 and omega-6 type. These fatty acids are essential, meaning that the body cannot manufacture them and they must be obtained through the diet. Essential fatty acids (EFAs), including omega-3 and omega-6 fatty acids, are found in fish oil, flax seed oil, and evening primrose oil dietary supplements. EFAs appear to play a vital role in the regulation of membrane activity in neurons.

Some research suggests that dietary deficiencies in EFAs are associated with behavioral, learning, and attentional impairments in animal models. In humans, EFA deficiency may be associated with a variety of disease states. Some evidence suggests that depressed and bipolar patients may have low levels of omega-3 fatty acids. However, presently there is no definite scientific evidence that EFAs are effective in the treatment of mental disorders. No controlled studies are available to guide clinical practice in pediatric psychopharmacology, and EFA supplementation cannot presently be recommended for the treatment of any psychiatric disorder of childhood.

Typical dosing strategies are similar for children and adolescents. From 3 to 10 grams of refrigerated fish oil or 3 tablespoons of refrigerated flax seed oil per day are divided and given three to four times per day. The EFAs are generally considered safe except when consumed in very large quantities. Side effects may include belching, nausea, and exacerbation of asthma in aspirin-sensitive patients. Because EFAs may inhibit human platelet aggregation and may prolong bleeding time, caution is advised in patients with bleeding disorders.

SECRETIN

Secretin is a 27 amino acid polypeptide that is produced in the intestine and released into the circulation, where it stimulates the release of bicarbonate and water into the duodenum, buffers low pH, and helps pancreatic digestive enzymes to work more efficiently. Human secretin has an amino acid sequence identical to the naturally occurring porcine secretin. Porcine-derived secretin is used intravenously during gastrointestinal endoscopy for specialized tests of pancreatic function.

In rats and pigs secretin receptors have been found in the central nervous system. When injected intracerebrally, secretin decreases locomotor activity in rats. However, there exists uncertainty about the role of secretin in the human brain.

In 1998 a report on a national television show announced the "cure" of an autistic child using secretin. This set off a convulsion of excitement among the parents of autistic children for the off-label use of secretin, and many families pursued this treatment.

Unfortunately, secretin is one of the many treatments that have not withstood the scrutiny of scientific study. A number of well-controlled studies has examined the impact of single and multiple doses of secretin, and investigated human as well as porcine secretin on behavior and social reciprocity in autistic children. These studies have uniformly demonstrated lack of efficacy. Thus, at present, secretin cannot be recommended for the treatment of any childhood psychiatric disorder, including autism.

KAVA

Kava is a beverage prepared from the rhizome of the oceanic kava plant. Kavapyrones appear to have active therapeutic properties and to influence a number of monoamine, amino acid, and neuropeptide transmitters in the CNS.

ALTERNATIVE MEDICINES

Kava has a long history of being used as a ceremonial drink in the Pacific South Sea Islands.

Presently, seven controlled studies of kava compared to placebo in adults for the treatment of anxiety have been completed. Three trials of 198 ambulatory adults assessed 300 mg/day of kava extract (70% kavalactone standardized product) compared with placebo. All trials showed a significant reduction in anxiety with kava extract compared with placebo. An additional four controlled studies have used a variety of kava doses, ranging between 300 mg and 800 mg daily. All studies show a reduction in anxiety compared with placebo. These data suggest that kava extract is helpful in reducing anxiety in adults. No controlled trials of kava extract have presently been completed in anxious children or adolescents.

Adverse effects of kava extract appear to be uncommon, although nausea, sedation, headache, restlessness, and tremor have been reported. There are isolated reports of kava extract-induced hepatotoxicity and acute liver failure. With persistent and excessive use, a reversible scaly skin rash, called "kava dermopathy," may occur.

VALERIAN

Valerian is made from the dried rhizomes and roots of the plant *Valeriana officinalis*. It is an herbal medicine that is often promoted for improving sleep. In adults, the dose for valerian ranges from 2 to 3 grams given three times a day, or at bedtime. No data about dosing in children and adolescents are available.

The available evidence provides little support for the effectiveness of valerian. There are presently nine trials of valerian, all completed in adults. No controlled trials are available in the pediatric population. Interpretation of these trials is quite limited due to methodological difficulties, which include small sample sizes, poor study designs, lack of prespecified inclusion and exclusion criteria for subjects, and unknown composition and dose of valerian preparations used in the various trials. At the present time, valerian cannot be recommended for use in patients.

CONCLUSIONS

Herbal and alternative medicines are used quite commonly in children and adolescents. Parents do not often spontaneously volunteer information about these products unless the clinician directly inquires about their use. Herbal treatments may have clinically significant drug–drug interactions with prescribed medications. In adults, there is a growing scientific database supporting use of St. John's wort in the treatment of mild to moderate anxiety and depression, and for kava extract in the treatment of anxiety. There is evidence to support the use of melatonin for sleep-onset insomnia in children. Little data are presently available to guide clinical practice in children and adolescents for other herbal and alternative medicines.

13. Electroconvulsive Therapy in Adolescents

Electroconvulsive therapy (ECT) in adolescents is an uncommon treatment for severely disabling and treatment-resistant mood disorders. Although it is a controversial intervention, it can be very effective and even life-saving in severe depression, psychotic depression, or mania with risk of imminent harm to self or others, which does not respond to other therapies (e.g., inpatient hospitalization and psychiatric medication; AACAP, 2004). Because it is an invasive procedure, ECT is generally considered a treatment of last resort.

ECT involves a brief passage of current through the brain, via electrodes placed on the scalp. The passage of electrical current through the brain produces a grand mal seizure. For reasons that are as yet not entirely understood, the seizure is effective in relieving the symptoms of severe depression or mania in a majority of patients who undergo the procedure. ECT is never given to preadolescent children, and it is administered to adolescents only infrequently. About 1% of teenagers 13–18 years old admitted to a psychiatric hospital for the treatment of a mental illness receive ECT. Only rarely is the treatment given to persons less than 16 years old.

ECT was first administered to adolescent psychiatric patients in 1942 in France. In 1947 the first American reports on the use of ECT in hospitalized children appeared. Because of concerns about possible harmful effects of ECT in children and adolescents, negative media portrayals of ECT, and the development of psychiatric medications, interest in the practice diminished. With the development of modern brief-pulse ECT machines and modern anesthesia techniques that diminish side effects from the procedure, the use of ECT in adolescents with severe and treatment-refractory mood disorders is again attracting increased attention. In 1990 the American Psychiatric Association published indications for ECT in minors, followed by the Royal College of Psychiatrists in 1995, the Royal Australian and New Zealand College of Psychiatrists in 1999, and the American Academy of Child and Adolescent Psychiatry in 2004.

Although ECT is well researched in adults with psychiatric disorders, published studies of ECT in adolescents are few and involve uncontrolled methodology. The scientific literature generally consists of case reports rather than randomized, controlled studies of the efficacy and safety of ECT in adolescents. Given the ethical concerns about sham-ECT in minors, it is unlikely that controlled trials will ever take place in adolescents. Studies published after 1980 are of better scientific quality than reports published earlier. With these caveats in mind, this chapter discusses ECT use in adolescents.

EVIDENCE OF EFFECTIVENESS

There are currently no controlled trials of ECT in teenagers. Evidence of ECT effectiveness comes from clinical experience and case reports (see the following table).

Table 13.1 ECT Studies in Adolescents

Study (year)	N	Age Range (years)	Diagnoses	Outcome
Cohen et al. (1997)	21	14–19	Depression, bipolar, schizophrenia	100% depression, 75% mania, only partial response in schizophrenia
Ghaziuddin et al. (1996)	11	13–18	Depression, bipolar depression, organic mood disorder	64% response rate
Kutcher and Robertson (1995)	16	16–22	Bipolar depression and mania	Significantly better than those who refused ECT
Moise and Petrides (1996)	13	16–18	Depression, bipolar, mixed diagnoses	76% response rate
Strober et al. (1998)	10	13–17	Depression, bipolar depression	60% response rate
Walter and Rey (1997)	42	14–17	Mixed diagnoses	100% mania, 85% psychotic depression, 51% all diagnosis

Note. All research used retrospective study designs.

Response to ECT in psychiatric patients younger than 19 years was reported by Walter, Rey, and Mitchell (1999). Response rates in adolescents with specific psychiatric disorders after ECT include:

• Depression, 67%
• Psychotic depression, 71%
• Acute mania, 79%
• Bipolar disorder, 71%
• Catatonic states, 72%
• Schizophrenia, 42%

There are no gender differences in response rates. With the exception of schizophrenia, these improvement rates in adolescents are very similar to ECT improvement rates in adults, suggesting that teenagers may respond to ECT in a fashion similar to adults.

INDICATIONS FOR ECT IN ADOLESCENTS

The primary indication for ECT in adolescents is the treatment of severe mood symptoms, depressive or manic, irrespective of their etiology. Mood symptoms occurring in the context of major depression, psychotic depression, schizoaffective disorder, schizophrenia, bipolar disorder, and/or organic brain disorder all may respond to ECT. In mood disorders (e.g., depression, mania) psychotic symptoms may respond as well. However, in psychotic disorders (e.g., schizophrenia) psychotic symptoms do not appear to get better with ECT (AACAP, 2004).

ECT is generally considered a treatment of last resort for severe mental disorders that are resistant to other psychiatric interventions. To be eligible for ECT, the following criteria for severity must be met:

- Severe, persistent, and significantly disabling psychiatric symptoms, including depression, mania with or without psychotic features, schizoaffective disorder, or less often, schizophrenia with a serious mood component.
- Life-threatening symptoms.
  ○ Refusal to eat or drink
  ○ Severe suicidality
  ○ Uncontrollable mania
  ○ Florid psychosis

Before recommending ECT, a clear definition of treatment resistance and the adequacy of previous psychological and pharmacological interventions must be delineated. This analysis requires consideration of the nature, dose, and duration of previous medication interventions as well as the patient's compliance with recommended treatment. Given the safety and effectiveness of modern ECT, and the morbidity, lifetime mortality rates, and seriousness of the psychiatric disorders for which ECT is considered in adolescents, the number of treatments prior to considering ECT should be limited. In other words, the severely psychiatrically ill adolescent who is not getting better with standard treatment should not be allowed to suffer for long periods of time before consideration of ECT.

The scientific literature is beginning to define treatment resistance for severe adolescent depression and bipolar disorder when considering ECT.

For treatment-resistant depression:
- Failure of at least two adequate antidepressant drug trials of at least 8–10 weeks duration each at a therapeutic dose and serum level (if available), without even mild improvement (AACAP, 2004; Ghaziuddin et al., 1996; Walter et al., 1999).

For treatment-resistant bipolar disorder:
- Failure of at least one antipsychotic mood stabilizer/antidepressant combination treatment trial of at least 6 weeks duration, without even mild improvement (AACAP, 2004; Kutcher & Robertson, 1995; Walter et al., 1999).

PREDICTORS OF RESPONSE

- Severe mood symptoms regardless of etiology
- Absence of comorbid personality disorders
- Absence of comorbid substance use disorders

CONTRAINDICATIONS

- Prepubertal children should not receive ECT because of a lack of scientific data in this age group.
- There are no absolute contraindications for ECT. Relative contraindications for ECT in adolescents include:
  - CNS tumors associated with elevated cerebrospinal fluid levels
  - Active chest infection
  - Recent myocardial infarction

ASSESSMENT OF THE ADOLESCENT FOR ECT

For all adolescents for whom ECT is being considered, the following assessment is required.

- A comprehensive psychiatric history and psychiatric diagnosis, according to DSM-IV or ICD-10. ECT is most effective for severe mood symptoms. Definitions of symptom severity are given above.
- A determination of the adequacy of previous psychiatric treatments. ECT is considered a treatment of last resort for severe mood symptoms that are refractory to previous therapies. Current guidelines describing treatment resistance for mood disorders are given above. Documentation of previous pharmacotherapy should include:
  - Each medication prescribed
  - Maximum dose of each medication
  - Duration of treatment for each medication
  - Patient compliance
  - Response of mood symptoms to each medication trial
  - Side effects and treatment emergent adverse effects
- A complete medical history and physical examination should be performed on all adolescents considered for ECT.
  - Although there are no absolute contraindications for modern ECT treatment, in adults the most common causes of peri-ECT mortality are cardiovascular complications.
    - These include cardiac arrythmias, myocardial infarction, congestive heart failure, and cardiac arrest.
  - The goal of medical examination for ECT is to detect any medical condition that may increase the risk for anesthesia or for the ECT procedure itself. Females should have a serum or urine pregnancy test.
- A review of current drug use is mandatory. Most nonessential psychotropic drugs are discontinued prior to ECT. Adverse ECT–drug interactions are given in the following table.

- A baseline assessment of the type and severity of mood symptoms. Prior to ECT adolescents should target mood symptoms using a standardized depression rating scale. During the course of ECT treatment and after ECT therapy, ratings of mood symptoms should be repeated to assess effectiveness.
- A test of memory is required for all adolescents undergoing ECT. Memory assessment must occur before treatment, immediately after the ECT procedure, and at 3–6 months after treatment is finished. Cognitive testing should focus on short-term memory and new knowledge acquisition (AACAP, 2004).
- Consultation with a second child and adolescent psychiatrist who is knowledgeable about ECT and not actively involved in the treatment of the patient is recommended by the extant ECT guidelines. ECT should not proceed unless the treating psychiatrist and consulting psychiatrist are in agreement as to the necessity of the ECT procedure.

Table 13.2 Some ECT–Drug Interactions
ECT may interact with:

Anticonvulsants	↓ Seizure length; ↓ ECT effectiveness
Benzodiazepines	↓ Seizure length ↓ ECT effectiveness
Caffeine	↑ Seizure length
Lithium	↑ Potentiation of anesthetic and muscle relaxant medications; ↑ Risk for organic brain syndrome
Nicotine (high dose only)	↑ Seizure length
SSRIs	↑ Seizure length
Theophylline	↑ Seizure length
Trazodone	↑ Seizure length

DESCRIPTION AND ADMINISTRATION

ECT is administered by the placement of electrodes on the scalp while the patient is under generalized anesthesia and under the effect of a muscle relaxant (modified ECT). For many years, electrodes were traditionally placed on both temples, a procedure called bilateral ECT. Presently, many clinicians apply electrodes to the temporal and parietal regions of the nondominant hemisphere. This is called unilateral ECT, and it results in less cognitive side effects such as memory problems and post-ECT confusion. However, unilateral ECT requires higher doses of electricity to achieve therapeutic effects than does bilateral ECT. ECT is generally administered two to three times a week and 6–12 treatments are usually given in a single course of treatment.

ECT parameters

- *EEG monitoring*: Modern ECT technique mandates the use of EEG monitoring to measure seizure quality and duration. The goal is to achieve a brief bilateral grand mal seizure lasting 20–25 seconds. Seizures lasting 180 seconds or more in adolescents are considered prolonged, and should be terminated by use of intravenous diazepam or additional methohexital.

- *Stimulus dosing*: This term refers to the calculation of a dose of electrical current for each individual patient, as opposed to the older method of using a fixed current dose for all patients.
  - Practitioners should start with electrical doses in the lower range of the ECT machine.
  - Unilateral ECT may require suprathreshold electrical doses 2–2½ times seizure threshold.
  - Bilateral ECT requires lower electrical doses of "just-above" seizure threshold.
    - May have a faster onset of therapeutic effects but is associated with more cognitive side effects.
    - Should be considered when a rapid response is necessary; for example, in those patients who are at emergent risk of harming themselves or others.
  - There is no difference in overall improvement rates according to electrode placement.
- *ECT device*: Old "sine-wave" ECT machines are now obsolete. ECT should be delivered with modern "brief-pulse" machines that are capable of delivering low-dose electrical current.
- *ECT electrical variables*: Select electrical variables to induce a grand mal seizure of 20–25 seconds.
  - Wave frequency 30–70 cycles per second.
  - Pulse width of 0.5–2.0 milliseconds.
  - Total electrical charge 32–576 millicoulombs.
- *Anesthesia*: Modern ECT is delivered with the patient under generalized anesthesia and medically monitored by an anesthesiologist. Commonly used anesthetic induction agents include methohexital, thiopentone, and propofol. Premedication with anticholinergic agents such as atropine may protect against vagal nerve-induced bradycardiac arrhythmias. The patient is given a muscle relaxant to prevent muscle and skeletal injury during the seizure. Suxamethonium is the agent commonly used. Patients are ventilated with 100% oxygen immediately before administering the convulsive stimulus.
- *Site of ECT treatment*: ECT is given in an ECT suite and recovery area with trained psychiatric and anesthetic staff, meeting standards set forth by professional regulatory authorities.
- After the course of ECT is completed, adolescents should be treated prophylactically with an antidepressant or mood stabilizer medication to prevent early relapse of the index mood disorder.

ADVERSE EFFECTS

Modern ECT is generally well tolerated by patients. The side effects of ECT in adolescents are the same as described for adults. Side effects are usually mild and transient.

- The mortality rate associated with ECT in adults is approximately 0.2 per 10,000 treatments. Adolescents are not believed to be at any more risk from ECT than are adults.
  - No deaths from ECT in adolescents have been reported.

- The anesthesia-related mortality rate is approximately 1.1 per 10,000 inductions.
- Late seizures may occur up to 24 hours after the ECT procedure is completed.
  - Neurological consultation should be obtained if late (tardive) seizures occur.
- Common side effects include:
  - Headache
  - General muscle aches
  - Nausea
  - Subjective memory problems
  - Confusion
- Uncommon side effects include:
  - Hemifacial flushing
  - Manic switching
  - Sinus tachycardia

Psychometric studies of cognition
Neuropsychological tests have documented specific cognitive deficits, including attention deficits, delayed verbal retention, and diminished efficiency of long-term memory search up to 5 days after ECT in adolescents. In adults, these cognitive deficits generally resolve over several months. However, few studies of cognitive side effects of ECT in the young have been completed. As such, this issue requires further research and demands that caution be exercised in the use of ECT in teenagers.

The effects of ECT on the developing brain
Evidence from adults who have undergone ECT include assessments of long-term cognitive impairment, magnetic resonance imaging (MRI) studies, patient brain autopsy studies, and measurement of tissue markers of brain injury. None of the evidence to date suggests that ECT is associated with structural brain damage in adults who have undergone the procedure.

The possible effect of ECT on the developing brain in teenagers is an important issue for which little scientific data are presently available to guide ECT practice. It should be noted that the brain continues to develop during the adolescent years. For example, myelination continues throughout adolescence, suggesting that there might be differences in vulnerability to ECT in the young compared with adults. Further research is needed in this area. Because of our lack of knowledge, caution must be given to the prescription of ECT in adolescents.

LEGAL CONSIDERATIONS

Psychiatrists who refer patients for ECT should be familiar with legal aspects of the treatment. In the United States some states have legislated age-related restrictions on the use of ECT.

- In Texas and Colorado, ECT is not permitted in persons < 16 years old.
- In Tennessee, ECT is not permitted in persons < 14 years old.
- In California, ECT is not permitted in persons < 12 years old.

- Most states require independent assessment of juveniles by one or more child and adolescent psychiatrists before ECT may be administered.

INFORMED CONSENT AND ASSENT

Because ECT is an invasive procedure, legal and ethical issues of parent or guardian informed consent and patient assent to the treatment are very important.

- Legal consent for ECT must be obtained from parents/guardians for ECT for all minor adolescents.
- Every effort should be made to obtain the assent of the adolescent who is to undergo the treatment.
- Informed consent and assent should be considered a process, not a single event. Often, the adolescent may initially refuse assent for ECT. As symptoms do not improve or because of side effects of medications, the teenager may change his or her mind later in treatment.
- Some states require a 72-hour waiting period between signing informed consent and initiating ECT. During this period the patient and guardians may change their minds about ECT and withdraw consent. Parents/guardians and adolescents must be informed by staff that their consent for ECT may be withdrawn at any time.

TRANSCRANIAL MAGNETIC STIMULATION

Transcranial magnetic stimulation (TMS) is a novel treatment for psychiatric illness that is receiving research attention in adult psychiatric disorders. Little TMS research is presently available in child and adolescent psychiatry. TMS is briefly mentioned here because it may become an important psychiatric treatment modality in the future.

TMS involves the passage of electrical current through an insulated coil that is in contact with the patient's head. This coil causes a magnetic field to penetrate into the first few millimeters of cortex. TMS is much less invasive than ECT. Unlike ECT, a specific region of the brain is stimulated, and no seizure is induced by the procedure. TMS requires no anesthesia.

Early research results in adults suggest that TMS may be helpful in depression, has few side effects, and is well tolerated by patients. Studies in children and adolescents will be forthcoming but are not presently available. TMS should be considered a research tool and not a clinical treatment modality at present.

Part III
The Disorders and
Their Treatment

14. Attention-Deficit/ Hyperactivity Disorder

Attention-deficit/hyperactivity disorder (ADHD) is one of the most common neuropsychiatric disorders of childhood and adolescence. In child psychiatric populations as much as 50% of clinical referrals may meet criteria for ADHD. In primary care pediatrics practice, 2–10% of children may have ADHD. It is generally a chronic disorder, and symptoms persist in the majority of ADHD youth as they grow into adulthood. Symptoms may change in manifestation as development proceeds from preschool through adult life. For example, in the young ADHD child symptoms of motor hyperactivity may be prominent. In the teenager with ADHD problems with impulsivity and inattention may be the most troubling symptoms. ADHD interferes with many areas of normal development and functioning. If not properly treated, ADHD may predispose a child to psychiatric and social problems in later life.

A
D
H
D

DIAGNOSTIC FEATURES

ADHD is divided into four types.

- ADHD combined type
- ADHD predominantly inattentive type
- ADHD predominantly hyperactive-impulsive type
- For subsyndromal and subthreshold cases there is an ADHD Not Otherwise Specified (NOS) type.

Signs of ADHD may not be observable when the patient is in highly structured or novel settings, engaged in activities that capture his or her interest and curiosity, receiving one-to-one supervision, or in a situation with frequent rewards for prosocial and appropriate behaviors. ADHD symptoms usually worsen in situations that are unstructured, stimulating, or crowded with many other people, loud environments, boring environments, and situations that lack supervision and structure. Thus the clinician evaluating the ADHD child in a

Table 14.1 Diagnostic Criteria for Attention-Deficit/Hyperactivity Disorder

A. Either (a) or (b):
(1) Six (or more) of the following symptoms of inattention have persisted for at least 6 months to a degree that is maladaptive and inconsistent with developmental level:

Inattention
(a) Often fails to give close attention to details or makes careless mistakes in schoolwork, work, or other activities
(b) Often has difficulty sustaining attention in tasks or play activities
(c) Often does not seem to listen when spoken to directly
(d) Often does not follow through on instructions and fails to finish schoolwork, chores, or duties in the workplace (not due to oppositional behavior or failure to understand instructions)
(e) Often has difficulty organizing tasks and activities
(f) Often avoids, dislikes, or is reluctant to engage in tasks that require sustained mental effort (such as schoolwork or homework)
(g) Often loses things necessary for tasks or activities (e.g., toys, school assignments, pencils, books, or tools)
(h) Is often easily distracted by extraneous stimuli
(i) Is often forgetful in daily activities
(2) Six (or more) of the following symptoms of hyperactivity-impulsivity have persisted for at least 6 months to a degree that is maladaptive and inconsistent with developmental level:

Hyperactivity
(a) Often fidgets with hands or feet or squirms in seat
(b) Often leaves seat in classroom or in other situation in which remaining seated is expected
(c) Often runs about or climbs excessively in situations in which it is inappropriate (in adolescents or adults, may be limited to subjective feelings of restlessness)
(d) Often has difficulty playing or engaging in leisure activities quietly
(e) Is often "on the go" or often acts as if "driven by a motor"
(f) Often talks excessively

Impulsivity
(g) Often blurts out answers before questions have been completed
(h) Often has difficulty awaiting turn
(i) Often interrupts or intrudes on others (e.g., butts into conversations or games)
B. Some hyperactive-impulsive or inattentive symptoms that caused impairment were present before age 7 years
C. Some impairment from the symptoms is present in two or more settings (e.g., at school [or work] and at home)
D. There must be clear evidence of clinically significant impairment in social, academic, or occupational functioning
E. The symptoms do not occur exclusively during the course of a Pervasive Developmental Disorder, Schizophrenia, or other Psychotic Disorder and are not better accounted for by another mental disorder (e.g., Mood Disorder, Anxiety Disorder, Dissociative Disorder, or a Personality Disorder)

Code based on type:
314.01-Attention-Deficit/Hyperactivity Disorder, Combined Type: if both Criteria A1 and A2 are met for the past 6 months
314.00-Attention-Deficit/Hyperactivity Disorder, Predominantly Inattentive Type: if Criterion A1 is met but Criterion A2 is not met for the past 6 months
314.01-Attention Deficit/Hyperactivity Disorder, Predominantly Hyperactive-Impulsive Type: if Criterion A2 is met but Criterion A1 is not met for the past 6 months

Coding note: For individuals (especially adolescents and adults) who currently have symptoms that no longer meet full criteria, "In Partial Remission" should be specified.

American Psychiatric Association. *Desk Reference to the Diagnostic Criteria from DSM-V–TR*. Washington, DC: American Psychiatric Association, pp. 65–67, 2000. Reprinted with permission.

novel and structured office setting may not actually observe the child's symptoms during the evaluation.

PREVALENCE

ADHD prevalence rates vary by the population that is sampled, the age of the sample investigated, the diagnostic criteria used (DSM-IV vs. ICD-10), the subtype of ADHD, and the diagnostic instruments that are used (categorical diagnostic interviews vs. rating scales of ADHD symptoms).

- General population prevalence:
  - For school-age children 6–12 years old: 3–12%.
  - For adults: 2–4%.
- Clinically referred populations
  - Child and adolescent psychiatry: 40–60%.
  - Primary care pediatrics practice: 2–10%.
- ADHD subtype prevalence
  - In general population samples
    - Inattentive type most common
    - Combined type next most common
    - Hyperactive-impulsive type least common
  - In psychiatrically referred populations
    - Combined type most common
    - Inattentive type next most common
    - Hyperactive-impulsive type least common

ADHD has been identified in many countries around the world.

ETIOLOGY

ADHD is most often conceptualized as a disorder of catecholaminergic underactivity with dysregulation in dopaminergic and noradrenergic CNS systems. Neuroimaging has revealed ADHD involvement in several CNS regions, including

- Frontal cortex
- Striatum (caudate nucleus, putamen)
- Cerebellum (involved in cognition as well as motor coordination, equilibrium, and balance)

ADHD has a large heritable component; like many medical diseases, ADHD runs in families.

- ADHD heritability rate: 70% (i.e., about 70% of the difference in ADHD symptoms between ADHD subjects and controls can be explained by genetic and not environmental factors).
- About 1 in 5 biological parents of an ADHD child has ADHD him- or herself.
- About 1 in 2 children born to parents with ADHD develops ADHD in childhood.

COURSE OF ILLNESS

ADHD is now conceptualized as a chronic disorder that persists beyond puberty in the majority of individuals who meet diagnostic criteria in childhood. Research has shown that 30–70% of children with ADHD will continue to have symptoms that impair daily functioning as adults. Thus treatment for ADHD should not be stopped at puberty in patients who continue to have disabling ADHD. Adolescents and adults with ADHD can robustly respond to treatment.

The symptoms of ADHD change over the course of child development.

- *Early childhood*: ADHD symptoms are dominated by motor overactivity, fearlessness, low levels of compliance to parental direction, excessive temper tantrums, vigorous and often destructive play, and aggression (biting, hitting).
- *School age*: ADHD symptoms include poorly organized schoolwork, careless errors in school assignments, distractibility, impulsive interrupting, difficulties with "rule-governed" behavior, and aggression.
  - Poor social skills may begin to cause problems for the school-age ADHD child.
  - Poor self-esteem may develop in childhood because of multiple conflicts experienced by the ADHD child in daily life.
- *Adolescence*: ADHD symptoms may include a decrease in frank motor overactivity but continuing "inner restlessness," disorganized school work, inability to complete schoolwork and homework independently, poor peer relationships, and clashes with authority figures.
  - Risky behavior may develop in ADHD teens.
  - Dangerous driving may occur in ADHD teens with driving privileges.
- *Adults*: ADHD symptoms in adults include poor planning and organization skills, distractibility, poor memory, forgetfulness, low academic and occupational performance relative to potential, waiting "to the last minute," social conflicts, increased family and marriage problems, dangerous driving and vehicular accidents, and rule-breaking behaviors. In adults the clinical presentation of ADHD is driven by inattention to performance-based tasks.

Whereas ADHD symptoms in young children are dominated by motor hyperactivity, symptoms in adults are dominated by cognitive symptoms.

Comorbidity in ADHD

Children, adolescents, and adults with ADHD often meet diagnostic criteria for other psychiatric disorders as well. One important key to the successful clinical management of the ADHD patient is the recognition and treatment of comorbid conditions.

- Comorbid disorders in ADHD children
  - Oppositional defiant disorder
  - Conduct disorder
  - Depression
  - Cigarette smoking
  - Anxiety disorders
  - Learning disorders
  - Tic disorders
- Comorbid disorders in ADHD adolescents
  - Substance use disorders
  - Cigarette smoking
  - Conduct disorder

- ○ Depression
- ○ Anxiety disorder
- ○ Bipolar disorder
- Comorbid disorders in ADHD adults
  - ○ Substance use disorders
  - ○ Antisocial personality disorder
  - ○ Depression
  - ○ Anxiety disorders
  - ○ Bipolar disorder

ASSESSMENT

The assessment of ADHD requires a comprehensive psychiatric evaluation with information collected from multiple sources, including the child or adolescent, parents, and teachers. Psychiatric assessment should evaluate the persistence of ADHD symptoms across the child's developing years, age of onset, impairment caused by symptoms, cross-situational presence of symptoms at home, at school, and in the community, and comorbid psychiatric disorders. Educational evaluations should rule out any associated learning disabilities in reading, spelling, writing, or language. Details of the child's classroom placement and any special education services should be obtained. A history of any familial ADHD and comorbid psychiatric disorders should be ascertained. A medical evaluation should be completed (within the previous year). Hearing and/or visual impairments that might cause the child to appear inattentive, and medical conditions that may mimic ADHD (i.e., hyperthyroid, lead poisoning), should be evaluated.

Once a diagnosis of ADHD is clinically established, rating scales may be given to parents and teachers to evaluate the severity of symptoms and comorbid psychopathology. Rating scales used in the assessment of ADHD are presented below.

TREATMENT OPTIONS

The clinical management of ADHD requires a multiple-modality approach that combines psychosocial/psychoeducational and medical interventions. Children with mild ADHD symptoms from intact families may not require medication intervention. However, stimulant medications remain the most effective short-term intervention available for the core symptoms of ADHD.

Psychosocial Interventions

Psychosocial interventions with proven efficacy in ADHD can be classified as those that focus on the family, the school, and the child.

- Family-focused interventions
  - ○ Education about ADHD
  - ○ Support groups (Appendix 5).
    - ■ Children and Adults with ADHD (CHADD).
    - ■ National Attention Deficit Disorders Association (ADDA).

Table 14.2 Rating Scales for Attention-Deficit/Hyperactivity Disorder in Children and Adolescents

Rating Scale	Type of Scale	What Is Assessed?	Age Range (years)	Reliability	Validity	Sensitivity to Change[a]
ACTeRS—Second Edition	Teacher and parent report; adolescent self-report	ADHD and ODD symptoms, prosocial behavior	5–13	++	++	Yes
ADHD Rating Scale—IV	Parent and teacher report; adolescent self-report	ADHD symptom severity	5–18	++	++	Yes
ADHD Symptoms Rating Scale	Teacher and parent report	ADHD symptoms	5–18	++	++	Yes
Attention Deficit Disorder Evaluation Scale—Second Edition	Teacher and parent report	ADHD symptoms	4–18	++	++	Yes
Brown Attention-Deficit Disorders Scales for Children and Adolescents	Teacher and parent report; adolescent self-report	ADHD symptoms, executive cognitive dysfunction	3–18	++	++	??
Conners Rating Scales—Revised	Teacher and parent report	Psychopathology including ADHD symptoms	3–17	++	++	Yes
IOWA Conners Teachers Rating Scale	Teacher report	Inattention and Oppositional behavior	5–11	++	++	Yes
SKAMP	Teacher report	ADHD and ODD classroom impairment	5–11	+	+	Yes
Swanson, Nolan, Pelham—IV (SNAP-IV) Questionnaire	Teacher and parent report	ADHD, ODD, and other internalizing psychopathology	5–11	++	+	Yes
Vanderbilt ADHD Rating Scale	Teacher report and parent report	ADHD, ODD, anxiety/depression	5–11	++	++	??

[a] sensitivity to change means that the rating scale reliably encodes changes in symptoms with treatment.
?? Unclear sensitivity to change.

- ○ Parent management training (PMT)
  - ▪ Generally delivered by a psychologist.
  - ▪ Trains parents to use behavioral techniques to reduce child oppositional behavior and family stress in the home environment.
  - ▪ Uses point/token response–cost behavioral systems.
  - ▪ Teaches parent to effectively communicate with schools about child's ADHD symptoms and behaviors around schoolwork and homework.
- • School-focused interventions
  - ○ Targets ADHD child's
    - ▪ Academic performance
    - ▪ Classroom behavior
    - ▪ Peer relationships
  - ○ Classroom modifications include
    - ▪ Place child in a structured classroom environment.
    - ▪ Place child in front of classroom in close proximity to teacher.
    - ▪ Assure a small class size with high teacher-to-student ratio.
    - ▪ Assure a well-organized daily classroom schedule.
    - ▪ Assure clear rules and consequences in the classroom.
    - ▪ Provide a slowed pace of assignments.
    - ▪ Allow untimed tests.
    - ▪ For the older ADHD child, provide tutoring support for homework.
    - ▪ Use of electronic devices
      - • Such as laptop computers to help the ADHD child organize schoolwork and writing assignments.
      - • Such as PDA devices to help ADHD child remember daily schedules and appointments.
    - ▪ Daily teacher–parent communication about
      - • Classroom behavior
      - • Homework and schoolwork assignments
- • Child-focused interventions
  - ○ Psychosocial therapy to focus on
    - ▪ Impulse control
    - ▪ Anger management
    - ▪ Social skills building
    - ▪ Assessment of any comorbid depression or anxiety
    - ▪ Education about the nature of ADHD
    - ▪ Support for self-esteem
    - ▪ Social conflict resolution skills

A
D
H
D

Medication Interventions

Stimulant medications are the mainstay of treatment and are considered first-line medication interventions in ADHD. Second-line medications include the antidepressants bupropion (Wellbutrin®) and atomoxetine (Strattera®). Other medications used in ADHD are the antihyperatensive agents guanfacine (Tenex®) and clonidine (Catapress®). Modafinil, a wake-promoting agent used in narcolepsy, has been found useful in ADHD. Tricyclic antidepressants such as imipramine and desipramine are helpful in ADHD, but their use is limited because of high rates of side effects and the possibility of cardiovascular toxicity.

The decision to medicate is based on the presence of a diagnosis of ADHD and persistent target symptoms that are sufficiently severe to cause functional impairment at school and usually at home and in social contexts with friends and peers.

- For the ADHD child with mild symptoms, consider behavioral and classroom interventions first. Add medication as a second treatment step if ADHD symptoms continue to cause impairment.
- For the ADHD child with moderate to severe ADHD symptoms, add medication at the initial phase of treatment, together with psychoeducational therapies.
- Weigh the
  - Risks of medication versus the risks of untreated ADHD.
  - Expected benefits of medication relative to other nonmedication treatments for ADHD.
- Before initiating medication therapy, establish a baseline for target symptoms.

STIMULANTS IN ADHD

Indications

Stimulants are used in pediatric psychopharmacology to treat

- ADHD in children ages 6–12 years old
- ADHD in adolescents
- Adult ADHD

Possible indications
Possible indications for stimulants include

- ADHD in preschool children ages 3–6 years old
- Symptoms of ADHD in persons with mild mental retardation (IQ > 55)
- Symptoms of ADHD in persons with autism and autistic spectrum disorders, such as Asperger's disorder (with only mild associated mental retardation or normal cognition)
- Symptoms of ADHD in persons with head injury or traumatic brain injury
- ADHD in children with well-controlled seizure disorders on a stable anticonvulsant regimen
- ADHD and comorbid conduct disorder with impulsive, explosive aggression
- ADHD and mild Tourette's disorder or chronic tic disorder

Recent studies of stimulants in ADHD

Table 14.3 Recent Studies of Stimulants for ADHD

Author (year)	Drug	Study Type	N	Age (yrs) (mean/range)	Dose (mg/day or range)	Duration	Outcome
				CHILDREN 6–12 YEARS OLD			
Biederman et al. (2002)	Adderall XR	RCT	563	6–12	10–30	3 weeks	Effective
Gillberg et al. (1997)	AMP	RCT	62	6–11	5–45	15 months	Long-term treatment effective
Greenhill et al. (2002)	Metadate	RCT	321	6–16	40.7	3 weeks	Effective
MTA (1999)	MPH	RCT	579	7–9.9	30.5	14 months	Medication > behavior therapy
Wolraich et al. (2001)	Concerta	RCT	282	6–12	18–54	4 weeks	Effective
				ADOLESCENTS			
Greenhill et al. (2002)	Concerta	RCT	177	13–18	18–72	2 weeks	Improvement on all measures
Smith et al. (1998)	MPH	Retro	16	12–14	10–30	6 weeks	Stimulants equally effective in ADHD teens and children
				ADULTS			
Paterson et al. (1999)	AMP	RCT	45	19–57	5–35	6 weeks	Effective for ADHD adults
Spencer et al. (1995)	MPH	CO	23	18–60	1.0 mg/kg/day	7 weeks	Higher doses more effective in ADHD adults
Spencer et al. (2001)	Adderall XR	CO	27	19–60	20–60	7 weeks	Effective

RCT = randomized controlled trial; AMP = amphetamine; MPH = methylphenidate; Retro = retrospective study; CO = crossover design

ADHD

Choosing A Stimulant

Stimulants remain the drugs of first choice in the medication treatment of ADHD. About 70% of ADHD children will respond to the first stimulant prescribed. Up to 90% of ADHD children may respond to either the first or second stimulant attempted.

The present standard of care is to initiate treatment for ADHD with either an intermediate-acting stimulant or a long-acting stimulant formulation. Immediate-release preparations may be used to supplement longer-acting stimulants.

- For ADHD patients with symptoms that interfere with functioning only at school or at work, choose an intermediate-acting stimulant.
- For ADHD patients with more severe symptoms that interfere at school/work and also during the after-school/work hours, choose a long-acting stimulant.
- Initiate treatment with either a methylphenidate-based medication or an amphetamine-based medication.
  ○ ADHD response rates do not vary with the type of stimulant compound used.
  ○ ADHD response to stimulants does not vary with the subtype of ADHD; all subtypes respond equally well.
- If the patient does not respond to an adequate trial of the first type of stimulant prescribed (e.g., methylphenidate or amphetamine), switch to the other type of stimulant formulation.
- In the treatment of non-comorbid ADHD, consider second-line and third-line medications (antidepressants, alpha-agonists) only after the patient has failed trials of both a methylphenidate and an amphetamine stimulant formulation.

Stimulant Treatment

Stimulant treatment of ADHD is divided into two phases: initiation and continuation. The therapeutic goals of each treatment phase differ.

Initiation
- The goals of the initiation phase of stimulant treatment are to
  ○ Choose an initial stimulant medication based on results of a comprehensive medical and psychiatric evaluation.
  ○ Establish effectiveness for the symptoms of ADHD.
  ○ Determine safety and tolerability.
  ○ Determine the optimal dose to maximize effectiveness and minimize side effects.
  ○ Time to complete the initiation phase with stimulants for ADHD: about 1 month.
- The goals of the continuation phase of stimulant treatment are to
  ○ Minimize break-through ADHD symptoms.
  ○ Reduce the overall burden of ADHD on the patient's daily life functioning.
  ○ Enhance the patient's daily quality of life.
  ○ If stimulants are effective, continue for the school year. Consider continuation over the summer versus a summer drug holiday when school is over for the year.

- Some ADHD patients require stimulant treatment throughout the entire year.
- Other ADHD patients may discontinue stimulants during the summer months.
- The decision is based on the risks of untreated ADHD on the patient's life versus risks of continuing on stimulant therapy.
  - No algorithm or rule exists to determine if the ADHD patient should have a medication holiday.
  - Decide in consultation with child and parents on a case-by-case basis.

Before treatment:
- Obtain baseline (off-drug) rating scales of ADHD symptoms and severity for the purpose of comparing with on-drug symptoms and treated severity.
- Obtain baseline (off-drug) rating scales of stimulant side effects before drug therapy actually begins.
  - Often parents report that stimulants have side effects when the reported adverse event is really a symptom of ongoing ADHD (e.g., irritability, rebound when stimulant is wearing off, oppositional behavior).
  - If a baseline rating scale of stimulant side effects is obtained before initiating drug treatment, often it will be seen that parent-reported stimulant side effects decrease on drug (i.e., parents are actually reporting symptoms of ADHD, which get better with treatment).
  - Comparing parent-reported on-drug side effects with a pre-drug evaluation facilitates a more accurate picture of true stimulant side effects.
- Educate parents and the child about the expected benefits of drug treatment, possible side effects, and use of the medication.
  - Written materials are helpful for parents and older children.
- Obtain baseline height and weight and plot on a growth curve.
- Determine if child has psychosis, a tic disorder, or other relative contraindications to stimulant therapy.
- It is not necessary to complete blood work, an EKG, or follow pulse and blood pressure in healthy children receiving stimulant mediations.

Titration
- For methylphenidate compounds
  - Initiate treatment at lowest possible dose.
    - For immediate-release methylphenidate, initiate once in A.M. for a day, then twice daily for a day, then three times daily.
    - For intermediate- and long-acting formulations, initiate once daily.
  - Titrate dose weekly.
    - Obtain parent and teacher ADHD rating scales of symptoms and severity once weekly.
    - Obtain parent- or clinician-administered stimulant side effect scales weekly.
  - Titrate through weekly intervals of low-dose, intermediate-dose, and high-dose.
    - Low-dose methylphenidate: ~ 0.3 mg/kg/dose
    - Intermediate-dose methylphenidate: ~ 0.4–0.6 mg/kg/dose
    - High-dose methylphenidate: ~ 0.9–1.2 mg/kg/dose

○ Determine optimal dose based on maximizing effectiveness and minimizing adverse events.

Amphetamine formulations are twice as potent as methylphenidate compounds and are given in one-half the dose.

- For amphetamine compounds, same as above except:
  ○ Low-dose amphetamine: ~ 0.15 mg/kg/dose
  ○ Intermediate-dose amphetamine: ~ 0.2–0.3 mg/kg/dose
  ○ High-dose amphetamine: ~ 0.5–0.6 mg/kg/dose

Response measurement
- Use a reliable and valid ADHD rating scale that is known to be sensitive to drug treatment to measure response.
  ○ Many rating scales are copyrighted and must be purchased from the author(s).
- Compare baseline ADHD severity scores with on-drug ADHD severity scores.
  ○ A true response occurs when the decline in mean (average) on-drug ADHD severity scores is greater than the error of measurement (standard deviation or spread of reported scores across multiple measurements). This can easily be determined with use of a calculator with statistical functions (i.e., mean and standard deviation).
- Obtain completed parent and teacher rating scales weekly as the stimulant titration phase proceeds.
- Determine optimal dose for the patient with ADHD.

Research has documented that ADHD children who respond to stimulants and are in the continuation phase of treatment often have superior outcomes when seen monthly by the physician over the course of the school year than children who are seen less frequently.

Stimulant Nonresponders

If little response is obtained with stimulant treatment, first consider a general reevaluation of the patient, focusing on patient, medication, and family factors.

- Patient factors
  ○ Is the ADHD diagnosis accurate?
  ○ Are there unrecognized comorbid psychiatric diagnoses that influence treatment response?
    ▪ Anxiety
    ▪ Depression
    ▪ Bipolar disorder
    ▪ Conduct disorder
    ▪ Substance use disorders
  ○ Are stimulant side effects interfering with the patient's medication response?
  ○ Is the patient compliant with medication?
- Medication factors
  ○ Is the patient under- or overdosed?

○ Does the medication quickly wear off and ADHD symptoms return (rebound effects)?
○ Are there drug–drug interactions affecting treatment response?
• Family factors
○ Are there increased stressors in the family that contribute to diminished stimulant treatment response in the ADHD patient?
○ Is there a parent with undiagnosed ADHD (or other psychopathology) that is contributing to family stress?
○ Do parents disagree on the necessity of stimulant medication for their child?

Next, prescribe a different stimulant formulation (e.g., an amphetamine formulation in place of a methylphenidate compound). If the patient does not respond or cannot tolerate stimulants, consider bupropion or atomoxetine as second-line treatments for ADHD.

Stimulant Side Effects

Side effect measurement
Use a reliable and valid measure of stimulant adverse events (see Appendix 4).

• Obtain weight and height every 4–6 months in healthy children with ADHD who receive stimulants.
○ Decrements in weight often worry primary care physicians and parents but are expected with stimulant therapy.
  ▪ Weight will rebound when the child stops stimulant therapy.
  ▪ If weight declines across a 25th percentile line on the standardized weight curves for gender and age, consider a stimulant medication holiday.
    • Stimulant medication holidays should last > 2 weeks to achieve weight rebound.
  ▪ There exists no evidence that long-term stimulant therapy will result in permanent weight reduction by adulthood.
○ Small decrements in height have been reported in some (but not all) studies of children receiving long-term stimulant therapy.
  ▪ The effect appears small: 0.8 cm (0.3 inch) per year of stimulant therapy.
  ▪ Other stimulant studies report no effects of medication on ultimate adult height in children receiving long-term stimulant therapy for ADHD.
  ▪ Still other studies suggest that the small height decrements found may represent delayed growth in the ADHD child as a result of ADHD itself and not as a result of stimulant treatment.
• Obtain parent-reported side effect rating scales weekly during the stimulant titration phase.
• Obtain parent-reported side effect rating scales at each office visit during the continuation phase of stimulant treatment.

Management of stimulant-induced side effects
As noted in Chapter 4, commons clinical side effects of stimulants include insomnia, anorexia, nausea, abdominal pain, headache, mood lability, irritability, sadness, moodiness, and weight loss. In the face of a satisfactory clinical response

to stimulants, it is important to attempt to manage side effects clinically, without having to discontinue stimulant medication. Many of these treatment-emergent side effects occur early in the course of stimulant treatment and decline in intensity with time. It is important to distinguish between true stimulant side effects and returning ADHD symptoms late in the day, when stimulant medications are wearing off. The time course of reported side effects may be helpful. Treatment-emergent side effects that develop 1–2 hours poststimulant administration may represent true medication adverse events. Side effects reported as developing late in the day may represent ADHD rebound phenomena, occurring as stimulant efficacy is diminishing. If symptoms represent ADHD rebound, giving a small supplemental dose of stimulant late in the afternoon may help. Suggestions for the management of common stimulant side effects are included below.

GASTROINTESTINAL SYMPTOMS

Administering the medication with meals can help anorexia, nausea, and abdominal pain that may occur. For persistent distress despite administering medication with meals, it may be necessary to change stimulant preparations.

WEIGHT LOSS

Appetite may rebound in the evening when stimulants are wearing off. Offering a high-caloric snack before the child's bedtime may be helpful. Do not force the child to eat. If routine growth monitoring reveals > 25% decrement in weight for age since the start of stimulant medication, switching medication or a medication holiday may be indicated.

INSOMNIA

It is important to determine if sleep difficulties are a true stimulant side effect or are actually a part of the ADHD disorder. It is well known that ADHD children have more sleep difficulties compared with controls, regardless of stimulant treatment. If insomnia represents a true side effect, give stimulant medication earlier in the day or switch to a shorter-acting preparation. Discontinue late afternoon or evening doses of stimulants. Consider supplementing stimulants with clonidine, imipramine, or mirtazapine to help induce sleep in the evening.

DIZZINESS

It is important to assess pulse and blood pressure to help rule out cardiovascular causes of dizziness. Reducing stimulant dose or switching to a long-acting formulation may be helpful.

REBOUND PHENOMENA

Overlapping stimulant doses at least 1 hour before rebound may be useful. Changing to a long-acting formulation may diminish the intensity of rebound symptoms. Consider changing to a longer-acting nonstimulant ADHD medication, such as atomoxetine or bupropion, with or without concurrent stimulant supplementation.

IRRITABILITY AND MOOD LABILITY

Determine if these symptoms are truly stimulant adverse events (i.e., occur 1–2 hours after administration) or represent ADHD rebound symptoms (i.e., occur late in the day when stimulant efficacy is wearing off). A co-occurring mood disorder needs to be assessed if these symptoms are persistent and severe. If symptoms are a stimulant adverse event, consider changing to a different agent (i.e., methylphenidate to amphetamine) or a nonstimulant such as atomoxetine or bupropion.

GROWTH IMPAIRMENT

Consider a medication holiday. Consider switching to a nonstimulant medication.

STIMULANT TOLERANCE

It remains unclear whether behavioral tolerance develops with chronic administration of stimulants. Research indicates that failure to maintain a clinical response at a given dose is more likely to occur at higher stimulant doses and with chronic use (i.e., more than 6 months of continuous use). When parents call to complain about ineffective doses that were formerly effective, physicians should first evaluate whether new stressful family events are occurring. If no stressful precipitating event is found to account for the loss of stimulant efficacy, consider a dose increase or changing the stimulant formulation. If a stimulant effect on ADHD symptoms is truly lost, consider changing to a nonstimulant medication such as bupropion or atomoxetine.

EMERGENCE OF TICS

If a successfully stimulant-treated ADHD child demonstrates onset of a tic disorder, the clinician should first assess the persistence of tics. After a period of time, tics may subside to a baseline frequency and severity. An informed consent discussion should take place with the patient and family to assess whether the benefits of stimulant treatment remain worth the risk of possible tic exacerbation. If tics continue to be problematic, the addition of an alpha-adrenergic agent such as clonidine or guanfacine may be added to ongoing stimulant treatment. Alternatively, the stimulant can be discontinued and treatment with clonidine, guanfacine, desipramine, nortriptyline, or atomoxetine can be initiated. These alternative medications are effective in ADHD and do not exacerbate tic disorders. *Note:* Bupropion may exacerbate tics.

NONSTIMULANTS IN ADHD

About 25–30% of ADHD children will not respond to a stimulant or will have too many side effects to tolerate a stimulant. Antidepressants, alpha-agonists, and other drugs are used if stimulants are poorly tolerated, if only partial treatment response to a stimulant occurs, or in special populations such as children with tic disorders and ADHD.

Recent studies of nonstimulant medications for ADHD

Table 14.4 Recent Studies of Nonstimulant Medications for ADHD

Author (year)	Study Type	N	Age (yrs) (mean/range)	Dose	Duration (weeks)	Outcome
			CHILDREN AND ADOLESCENTS 6–18 YEARS OLD			
			ALPHA-AGONISTS			
Connor et al. (2000)	RCT	8	6–16	Clonidine 0.17 mg/day	12	Effective but not as well tolerated as MPH
Tourette's Syndrome Study Group (2002)	RCT	67	6–12	Clonidine 0.26 mg/day	16	Effective for ADHD and TS
Scahill et al. (2001)	RCT	17	7–14	Guanfacine 3.0 mg/day	8	Safe and effective for ADHD and tics
			ATOMOXETINE			
Michelson et al. (2001)	RCT	297	8–18	1.2–1.8 mg/kg/day	8	Effective
Michelson et al. (2002)	RCT	171	6–16	1.2 mg/kg/day	6	Once-daily administration effective
			BUPROPION			
Barrickman et al. (1995)	CO	15	7–17	3.3 mg/kg/day	2	Effective
Conners et al. (1996)	RCT	72	6–12	3–6 mg/kg/day	5	Effective but effect size < MPH
			MODAFINIL			
Rugino & Copley (2001)	Open	11	5–15	100–400 mg/day	5	May be useful for ADHD
			TRICYCLIC ANTIDEPRESSANTS			
			DESIPRAMINE			
Biederman et al. (1989)	RCT	31	6–17	4.6 mg/kg/day	6	Effective; monitor for cardiovascular side effects (EKG)

Study	Design	N	Age	Dose		Results
NORTRIPTYLINE						
Prince et al. (2000)	Open	32	6–17	1.8 mg/kg/day	6	Effective; monitor for cardiovascular side effects (EKG)
ADULTS **ATOMOXETINE**						
Michelson et al. (2003)	RCT	536	40.2	60–120 mg/day	10	Effective for ADHD adults
Spencer et al. 1998	RCT	22	19–60	76 mg/day avg	3	Effective for ADHD adults
BUPROPION						
Wilens et al. (2001)	RCT	21	20–59	200–400 mg/day	6	Effective for ADHD adults
MODAFINIL						
Taylor and Russo (2000)	CO	22	18–59	207 mg/day avg	2	Suggests modafinil effective for ADHD adults
TRICYCLIC ANTIDEPRESSANTS **DESIPRAMINE**						
Wilens et al. (1996)	RCT	21	19–60	200 mg/day	6	Effective

CO = crossover design; RCT = randomized controlled trial; MPH = methylphenidate

A D H D

Bupropion

The bupropion molecule is similar to amphetamine and is effective in the treatment of childhood, adolescent, and adult ADHD. It may exacerbate tics in ADHD children who are vulnerable to tic disorders, such as those with Tourette's disorder. Bupropion (Wellbutrin®) is effective in adolescent and adult depression. One of its preparations, Zyban®, is FDA-approved for smoking cessation.

- Bupropion is available in
  - Tablets of 75 mg and 100 mg
  - Sustained-release tablets of 100 mg and 150 mg
  - A once-daily extended-release (XL) formulation is currently available to treat depression in adults and is effective in ADHD. The XL preparation is available in 150 mg and 300 mg tablet strengths
- For the child weighing > 25 kilograms
  - Initiate bupropion at 75 mg once daily
  - Titrate by 75 mg weekly on a bid–tid dosing schedule.
- For the smaller child weighing < 25 kg
  - Initiate at 37.5 mg (*Note:* Pills are not scored, so dividing them is difficult).
  - Titrate at 37.5 mg weekly on a bid-tid dosing schedule.
- Effective dose: 75–400 mg per day in two or three divided doses.
- Give bupropion slow-release on a once-daily or bid dosing schedule.
- Give bupropion extended-release on a once-daily schedule.
- No laboratory or EKG monitoring is necessary during bupropion therapy.

Bupropion side effects
- Irritability
- Decreased appetite
- Insomnia
- Worsening of preexisting tics
- Drug-induced seizures, especially at daily doses > 450 mg

Bupropion contraindications
- Allergic reaction to previous bupropion
- Seizure disorder
- Bulimia (bingeing and purging)
- Tourette's and chronic tic disorders

Atomoxetine

Atomoxetine (Strattera®) is a potent and specific norepinephrine reuptake inhibiting antidepressant. It is effective in the treatment of childhood, adolescent, and adult ADHD. It does not appear to have the cardiovascular toxicity of older tricyclic antidepressants. Unlike tricyclic antidepressants, no QTc prolongation on the ECG is noted with atomoxetine.

Atomoxetine does not appear to exacerbate tics. Although generally a second-line agent of choice in the treatment of ADHD, atomoxetine should be considered a first-line medication in the treatment of ADHD for children and adolescents with ADHD and tic disorders.

Atomoxetine was originally called tomoxetine. The name was changed to avoid confusion with tamoxifen, which might lead to errors in dispensing the drug.

- Available in 10 mg, 18 mg, 25 mg, 40 mg, and 60 mg capsules
- Atomoxetine may be given once daily or in two divided doses in the morning and late afternoon or evening.
- For children up to 70 kg
  ○ Initiate atomoxetine at 0.5 mg/kg.
  ○ Titrate after a minimum of three days to a target daily dose of approximately 1.2 mg/kg/day to 1.8 mg/kg/day.
- For children and adolescents weighing more than 70 kg and in adults
  ○ Initiate atomoxetine at a total daily dose of 40 mg.
  ○ Titrate after a minimum of 3 days to a target total daily dose of approximately 80–100 mg/day.
  ○ Do not exceed 100 mg/day total dose.
- Monitor baseline and on-drug pulse and blood pressure.
- Monitor baseline and on-drug height and weight.
- ECG evaluation is not necessary with atomoxetine use.

Clonidine and Guanfacine

Originally used as antihypertensive medications in adults, clonidine (Catapress®) and guanfacine (Tenex®) are considered first-line therapies for children with tic disorders and Tourette's disorder. They are also used in ADHD for impulsive aggression and when tic disorders co-occur with ADHD. Because of the sedative properties of these medications (clonidine > guanfacine), they are also used to initiate sleep in the evening in ADHD children who have initial insomnia.

CLONIDINE

- Available in 0.10, 0.20, and 0.30 mg tablets (scored).
- Clonidine is a short-acting compound, so it must be given up to four times a day.
- Initiate clonidine at 0.05 mg (one-half tablet) at night.
- Titrate by 0.05 mg every four or five days.
- Dose range for tic disorders and ADHD is generally between 0.05 and 0.35 mg/day in three or four divided doses.
- Also available as a transdermal skin patch system (TTS® System) that is worn continuously for up to 7 days in adults and 4 days in children before the patch must be changed.
  ○ Skin irritation is common under the patch.
- Monitor pulse and blood pressure at baseline, during dose titration, and at full dose.
- EKG monitoring is not required.

Clonidine side effects
- Sedation
- Irritability
- Depression

- Rebound agitation and hypertension if a longstanding dose is abruptly discontinued.
  - ○ Taper clonidine by 0.05 mg every 2–3 days to prevent rebound withdrawal and adverse events.
  - ○ Educate parents and the patient about the dangers of abrupt discontinuation.
- Low blood pressure
- Bradycardia

Clonidine contraindications
- Allergic reaction to previous clonidine
- Syncope
- Cardiovascular disorders
- Bradycardiac arrhythmias

GUANFACINE

Guanfacine is approximately one-tenth as potent as clonidine and causes less sedation and irritability. Guanfacine may have more benefits on attention span than clonidine. Clonidine may have more benefits than guanfacine in the treatment of hyperactivity and impulsive aggression.

- Available in 1.0 mg tablets (scored).
- Guanfacine is given in divided doses two or three times daily.
- Initiate therapy at 0.5 mg at night (sedation).
- Titrate by 0.5 mg every 4–5 days.
- Dose range for ADHD and tic disorders is generally between 0.5 and 4.0 mg/day in two or three divided doses.
- No slow-release preparation of guanfacine is presently available, but one is currently under development.
- Monitor pulse and blood pressure at baseline, during dose titration, and at full dose.
- EKG monitoring is not required.

Guanfacine side effects
- Sedation
- Irritability
- Depression
- Rebound agitation and hypertension if a longstanding dose is abruptly discontinued.
  - ○ Taper guanfacine by 0.5 mg every 2–3 days to prevent rebound withdrawal and adverse events.
  - ○ Educate parents and the patient about the dangers of abrupt discontinuation.
- Low blood pressure
- Bradycardia

Guanfacine contraindications
- Allergic reaction to previous guanfacine
- Syncope

• Cardiovascular disorders
• Bradycardiac arrhythmias

Modafinil

Modafinil is a wake-promoting agent that is FDA-approved for use in the sudden sleep attacks of narcolepsy. There is some evidence that modafinil might be useful in the treatment of ADHD in children.

• Available in 100 mg and 200 mg tablets.
  ○ The 200 mg tablet is scored
• Modafinil is given in one daily dose in the A.M., or in two divided daily doses at A.M. and noon (i.e., it is a wake-promoting agent).
• Initiate modafinil at 100 mg in the morning.
• Titrate dose weekly by 50–100 mg.
• Dose range for ADHD is between 100 mg and 400 mg in one or two divided (A.M. and noon) daily doses.
• No laboratory or EKG monitoring is necessary during modafinil therapy.
• Modafinil is a Schedule IV drug.

Modafinil side effects
• Headache
• Nausea
• Depression
• Initial insomnia
• Nighttime awakening
• Stomachache
• Dizziness

Modafinil contraindications
• Allergic reaction to previous modafinil
• Migraine headache

Tricyclic Antidepressants

Tricyclic antidepressants such as imipramine (Tofranil®), desipramine (Norpramin®, Pertofrane®), nortriptyline (Pamelor®, Vivactyl®), amitriptyline (Elavil®), and clomipramine (Anafranil®) are effective in ADHD. However, their use has been largely supplanted by use of the agents discussed above. Tricyclic antidepressants are rarely considered in the treatment of ADHD because of their cardiovascular toxicity, increased risk of death in overdose, and the need to monitor serum levels.

CLINICAL MANAGEMENT OF ADHD WITH COMORBID PSYCHIATRIC DISORDERS

As discussed above, many other psychiatric disorders may co-occur with ADHD.

In children and adolescents with ADHD, higher rates of comorbid oppositional defiant disorder (ODD), conduct disorder (CD), major depressive disorder (MDD), and anxiety disorders are found compared with control youth without ADHD. In adolescents and adults with ADHD higher rates of antisocial personality disorder, substance abuse, bipolar disorder (BPD), MDD, and anxiety disorders are found compared to controls without ADHD. This section reviews treatment for ADHD when the diagnosis is complicated by psychiatric comorbidity.

Oppositional Defiant Disorder/Conduct Disorder

About 50% of ADHD children meet criteria for either ODD or CD. The prevalence of the association between ADHD and ODD/CD varies with the age of the child.

- Children under the age of 12 years who meet criteria for ODD or CD will almost always meet criteria for ADHD.
- In adolescent samples pure CD is more common, and only about 33% of teenage CD patients will also meet criteria for ADHD.

Many studies have compared the response of ADHD + ODD/CD and ADHD alone to stimulant medications.

- When stimulant is compared with placebo in controlled clinical trials, ADHD children with ODD/CD show the same reductions in inattention, impulsivity, and hyperactivity as do non-comorbid ADHD children.
  - Thus childhood antisocial behavior does not seem to attenuate stimulant response for ADHD symptoms.
- In ADHD youngsters with comorbid CD and aggression, stimulants appear to reduce antisocial behaviors in addition to their effects on the core symptoms of ADHD.
  - Although it is not clear if stimulants help impulsive aggression in children without ADHD, they can help decrease the frequency and intensity of aggressive outbursts in children with ADHD.
- The efects of stimulants on adults with ADHD and antisocial personality disorder have not been studied.

Depression

It is not uncommon to encounter children who are demoralized or dysphoric about the consequences of their impulsive ADHD behaviors. Such children appear depressed, but the depression is usually short-lived and generally occurs only after a frustration or a disciplinary event. Thus brief episodes of depressed and/or irritable mood may be common in the ADHD child, occur many times a day, but not necessarily meet the criteria for an MDD. This demoralization will get better as the ADHD is treated.

The syndrome of MDD, identified by a persistently depressed, sad, or irritable mood different from the child's usual personality, lasting for days to weeks, and accompanied by guilt, anhedonia, social withdrawal, and suicidal thoughts, occurs in 15–30% of ADHD children and adolescents.

The clinician treating patients with ADHD must be vigilant for comorbid depressive disorders. True ADHD comorbid with MDD requires treatment of both the ADHD and the depression.

• Stimulants have been safely combined with SSRIs, such as fluoxetine, in children, adolescents, and adults in the treatment of ADHD comorbid with MDD.

Bipolar Disorder

The prevalence of childhood bipolar disorder in children with ADHD is a topic of considerable controversy and debate. This controversy arises out of a lack of consensus as to how to identify the bipolar child. Part of the problem is the high degree of symptom overlap between ADHD and bipolar symptoms (e.g., irritability, mood lability, aggression, hyperactivity/agitation, and sleep disturbance).

In primary care practice the prevalence of childhood bipolar disorder is rare. Among ADHD children a few may have early-onset bipolar disorder. Symptom factors that most differentiate manic children from ADHD children are

• Grandiosity
• Excessively elated mood
• Racing thoughts
• Hypersexuality (in a child with no history of previous or ongoing sexual abuse)
• Decreased need for sleep without feeling tired or fatigued the next day.

Note that excessive, aggressive or explosive behavior does not seem to distinguish between youth with mania and those with ADHD.

If the child is acutely manic as well as having ADHD

• Stabilize manic symptoms and mood cycling first before treatment with a stimulant (Scheffer et al., 2005).
  ◦ Use a mood stabilizer such as lithium, divalproex sodium, carbamazepine, oxcarbazepine (trileptal), or lamotrigene (lamictal).
  ◦ Or use an atypical antipsychotic such as risperidone, olanzapine, quetiapine, ziprasidone, or aripiprizole.
• Once the acute manic symptoms have stabilized, the clinician should reassess the patient for ADHD. If ADHD symptoms continue to be problematic, stimulants may be added to a mood stabilizer regimen to treat continuing ADHD symptoms.

Anxiety Disorders

About 25–30% of children with ADHD meet criteria for an anxiety disorder, compared to 5–15% of comparison youth. Initial studies suggested that the response of ADHD children to stimulant medications was less when comorbid anxiety disorders were present. However, more recent studies have not supported diminished stimulant responses in anxious ADHD youth. In short-term controlled trials, anxious and nonanxious ADHD children have equally robust responses to stimulants (Abikoff et al., 2005).

• In clinical practice the anxious ADHD child should be treated for ADHD first. Because the response to stimulant medication can be assessed quickly and anxious/ADHD children do not generally worsen on stimulant medications, a stimulant trial is the first intervention.

• Should anxiety continue to be a problem, a psychosocial intervention or a trial of an SSRI for anxiety could be implemented in addition to stimulant medication.

Tic Disorders

Controlled studies have demonstrated an association between tic disorders and ADHD that occurs at a rate greater than expected by chance alone.

• In clinical samples of boys with tic disorders, Tourette's disorder co-occurs with ADHD in between 21% and 54% of cases.
• Tic disorders are found at a lesser rate in samples of ADHD children. For example, in the NIMH funded multimodal treatment of ADHD (MTA) study of 579 ADHD children, 10.9% had a comorbid tic disorder.

Methodologically controlled studies have shown that stimulant medications are highly effective for ADHD symptoms, aggression, and social skill deficits in children with Tourette's disorder or chronic tic disorders. However, numerous clinical observations have reported that stimulants exacerbate tic frequency and intensity in ADHD children who have preexisting tic disorders. This has led clinicians to undertreat ADHD in children with tic disorders. There is now a much greater understanding that the consequences of untreated ADHD are more deleterious than the consequences of a mild to moderate tic disorder on the child's social, behavioral, interpersonal, and academic development.

• Controlled studies show that the frequency and severity of tics in ADHD children with preexisting tic disorders treated with stimulants are not different from the frequency and severity of tics in placebo-treated ADHD + tic children.
• Although stimulants may exacerbate a preexisting tic disorder in an individual child, the frequency and intensity of tics generally return to baseline after several months of stimulant treatment.
• In children who develop severe tics with the use of stimulants: Most tics will remit after the stimulant is discontinued.
• There is little evidence that tic disorders are created *de novo* by the introduction of stimulants in children who are not already vulnerable to tic disorders (generally on a heritable basis).

The current standard of care has now evolved to a recommendation to treat moderate to severe ADHD in children with mild to moderate tic disorders.

• Careful informed consent with parents and close monitoring of tic frequency and severity are necessary aspects of treatment.
• Should tics become problematic
  ○ Controlled studies support the use of clonidine, guanfacine, or risperidone in the treatment of comorbid ADHD and tic disorders.

Substance Use Disorders

Despite the documented efficacy of stimulants in the treatment of ADHD, there continues to be public concern that stimulant use in childhood and adolescence increases the risk of substance use disorders. However, the evidence to date on the actual risks of substance use and abuse in stimulant-treated ADHD children is relatively weak. An overwhelming majority of studies finds no evidence that stimulant treatment increases risks for later substance abuse. Indeed, many studies find that stimulant treatment of ADHD actually reduces the risks for later substance abuse.

- In a meta-analysis of six studies including 674 stimulant-treated subjects and 360 unmedicated subjects followed for at least 4 years, the pooled estimate of the odds ratio indicated a 1.9-fold reduction in risk for substance abuse in stimulant-treated ADHD youth (Wilens et al., 2003).
- Risks for substance abuse in ADHD children and adolescents appear to be the result of the untreated disorder and not a result of treatment for the disorder.
- Stimulant treatment of ADHD actually reduces the risk of later substance use disorder.

A separate clinical challenge is the treatment of ADHD in an adolescent or young adult who is already a substance abuser.

- In uncontrolled environments active substance abuse is a relative contraindication to prescribing stimulant medications.
- Antidepressants with known efficacy for the treatment of ADHD and limited abuse potential, such as bupropion or atomoxetine, should be used.
- Treat the substance abuse with
  ○ Random drug testing
  ○ Substance abuse counseling

STIMULANT USE FOR SYMPTOMS OF ADHD IN SPECIAL POPULATIONS

Learning Disabilities

Learning disabilities include expressive and receptive language delays, auditory processing difficulties, and reading disabilities. An overlap between ADHD and learning disabilities is frequently reported in both children and adults.

- A wide range of overlap was reported in some studies.
  ○ Between 10% and 92% of ADHD children also had learning disabilities.
- More recent studies report a smaller overlap of ADHD and learning disabilities
  ○ Between 20% and 25%
  ○ The wide disparity in comorbidity is probably due to different definitions of learning disabilities used in various studies.
- Research supports independence of learning disabilities and ADHD as two separate disorders, although they may frequently co-occur. The two disorders are transmitted independently in families. Neuropsychological testing supports different deficits in ADHD and learning disabilities.
- Learning disabilities typically require specialized psychoeducational interventions.

- Stimulants are not a treatment for specific learning disabilities.
- However, in ADHD children with comorbid learning disabilities, treatment of ADHD symptoms with stimulants can be helpful as part of an overall treatment plan.

Persons with Developmental Delay

ADHD symptoms often occur in children and adolescents with mental retardation or autistic spectrum disorders.

- Stimulants are effective for the symptoms of ADHD in persons with developmental delay.
  - Stimulant effectiveness is greatest when the IQ $\geq$ 55 and the mental age is $\geq$ 4.5 years.
  - Stimulant side effects are greater in persons with developmental delay than in normally developing youths.

Preschool Children

By definition, ADHD has on early age of onset. Preschool children ages 3–6 years old may have serious symptoms of ADHD that require evaluation and treatment.

- Carefully evaluate the preschool child to rule out other causes of ADHD symptoms, such as stressed parents, hearing loss, or normal developmental activity.
- Always attempt parent management behavioral treatment first.
- Only in children who do not get better with behavioral and family treatment should the clinician consider stimulants.
- Preschool ADHD children can respond to stimulant medications.
  - Response rates are lower than for older ADHD children.
  - Side effects are greater for preschool than for older ADHD children.
- Stimulants should not be given to children < 3 years old.

Children with Seizure Disorders

Children with seizure disorders may also meet diagnostic criteria for ADHD.

- Stimulants can be used in ADHD children with seizure disorders if they are on a stable anticonvulsant regimen.
- In children with unstable seizure disorders, stimulants may worsen the seizure disorder.

SUMMARY: AN ALGORITHM FOR THE TREATMENT OF ADHD

Medication algorithms for the treatment of specific disorders may enhance patient outcomes. This is true for the medication treatment of ADHD. A feasibility study showed that a best practices medication algorithm could be developed by expert clinical consensus and implemented in public health settings (Pliszka et al., 2000, 2003). Algorithms for the treatment of ADHD and ADHD comorbid with tic disorders or depression are presented in the following figure.

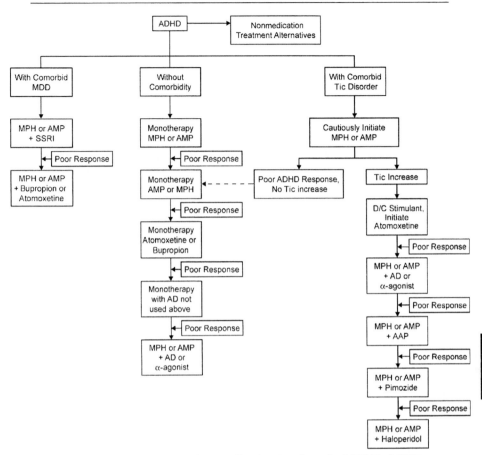

Figure 14.1 An algorithm for the medication treatment of ADHD, ADHD comorbid with major depressive disorder (MDD), and ADHD comorbid with tic disorders.
MPH = methylphenidate; AMP = amphetamine; SSRI = selective serotonin reuptake inhibitor; AD = antidepressant; α = alpha-agonist (clonidine, guanfacine); AAP = atypical antipsychotic. Adapted from: Pliszka et al. and the Texas Consensus. Conference Panel on Medication Treatment of Childhood Attention-Deficit/Hyperactivity disorder. The Texas children's medication algorithm project: Report of the Texas consensus conference panel on medication treatment of childhood attention-deficit/hyperactivity disorder. Part I. *J Am Acad Child Adolesc Psychiatry* 39:908–919, 2000; Green WH. *Child and Adolescent Clinical Psychopharmacology* (3rd. ed.) Philadelphia: Lippincott, Williams & Wilkins, pp. 32–33, 2001; American Academy of Child and Adolescent Psychiatry. Practice parameters for the use of stimulant medications in the treatment of children, adolescents, and adults. *J Am Acad Child Adolesc Psychiatry* 41: 26S–49S, 2002.

15. Tic Disorders and Tourette's Disorder

A tic is a sudden, repetitive motor movement or vocalization that typically mimics some aspect of normal behavior. Tics are brief in duration, generally lasting less than 1 second and have a paroxysmal character usually occurring in bouts. Individual tics can occur singly or multiple tics may occur together. Many tics may be temporarily suppressed. Motor tics vary from simple abrupt movements such as eye blinking, shoulder shrugging, or facial grimacing, to more complicated gestures such as seemingly purposeful behaviors. Vocal tics range between simple sounds such as snorting or throat clearing to complex utterances such as repeating words or even obscene speech (coprolalia). Tics are common in normally developing children and, by themselves, are not necessarily a reason for psychiatric treatment. Simple motor and vocal tics that are mild in nature and do not cause the child impairment usually have a good prognosis without treatment and generally disappear as the child ages into adolescence and young adulthood.

Tic disorders are transient or chronic conditions associated with some impairment in daily functioning, such as impaired self-esteem, difficulties with social acceptance, family conflicts, or school or occupational difficulties that are directly related to the presence of motor and/or vocal tics. Individuals with tic disorders may manifest a variety of other behavioral difficulties, such as disinhibited speech or conduct, motor hyperactivity, attentional deficits, impulsivity, obsessive behaviors, and/or compulsive thoughts.

DIAGNOSTIC FEATURES

The current classification of tic disorders in DSM-IV recognizes chronic motor or vocal tic disorder and transient tic disorder. The diagnostic criteria for these disorders are presented in the following tables.

Table 15.1 Diagnostic Criteria for Chronic Motor or Vocal Tic Disorder

A. Single or multiple motor or vocal tics (i.e., sudden, rapid, recurrent, nonrhythmic, stereotyped motor movements or vocalizations), but not both, have been present at some time during the illness.
B. The tics occur many times a day nearly every day or intermittently throughout a period of more than 1 year, and during this period there was never a tic-free period of more than 3 consecutive months.
C. The disturbance causes marked distress or significant impairment in social, occupational, or other important areas of functioning.
D. The onset is before age 18 years.
E. The disturbance is not due to the direct physiological effects of a substance (e.g., stimulants) or a general medical condition (e.g., Huntington's disease or postviral encephalitis).
F. Criteria have never been met for Tourette's Disorder.

American Psychiatric Association. *Desk Reference to the Diagnostic Criteria from DSM-V–TR.* Washington, DC: American Psychiatric Association, pp. 73–74, 2000. Reprinted with permission.

Table 15.2 Diagnostic Criteria for Transient Tic Disorder

A. Single or multiple motor and/or vocal tics (i.e., sudden, rapid, recurrent, nonrythmic, stereotyped motor movements or vocalizations)
B. The tics occur many times a day, nearly every day for at least 4 weeks, but no longer than 12 consecutive months.
C. The disturbance causes marked distress or significant impairment in social, occupational, or other important areas of functioning.
D. The onset is before age 18 years.
E. The disturbance is not due to the direct physiological effects of a substance (e.g., stimulants) or a general medical condition (e.g., Huntington's disease or postviral encephalitis).
F. Criteria have never been met for Tourette's Disorder or Chronic Motor or Vocal Tic Disorder.

Specify if:
Single Episode or Recurrent

American Psychiatric Association. *Desk Reference to the Diagnostic Criteria from DSM-V–TR.* Washington, DC, American Psychiatric Association, p.74, 2000. Reprinted with permission.

The most severe of the tic disorders is Tourette's disorder (TD) characterized by fluctuating bouts of both motor and vocal tics that wax and wane over time. Named after Gilles de la Tourette who first described the disorder in 1885, TD typically begins early in life and pursues a chronic yet fluctuating course. Tics eventually become persistent and begin to adversely affect the child and family. The range of motor tics can be great, from simple to complex movements and potentially involving almost any voluntary motion. Vocal tics generally begin several years after the onset of motor tics and are usually simple in character (e.g., throat clearing, snorting, coughing, grunting). Complex vocal tics, such as echolalia or coprolalia, occur in only a minority of TD patients, usually after many years of the disorder. The diagnostic criteria for Tourette's disorder are presented below.

In addition to tic symptoms, patients with TD may have other psychological difficulties, including depression and anxiety symptoms. Two comorbid psychiatric disorders appear to be especially prevalent in young people with TD: obsessive–compulsive disorder (OCD) and/or attention-deficit hyperactivity disorder (ADHD). These associated conditions often cause more impairment for the child and family than the tics themselves. As such, the treatment of the patient with TD often involves treatment of these associated disorders. The tics themselves often do not require clinical intervention, especially if they are mild

Table 15.3 Diagnostic Criteria for Tourette's Disorder

A. Both multiple motor and one or more vocal tics have been present at some time during the illness, although not necessarily concurrently. (A tic is a sudden, rapid, recurrent, nonrhythmic, stereotyped motor movement or vocalization.)

B. The tics occur many times a day (usually in bouts) nearly every day or intermittently throughout a period of more than 1 year, and during this period there was never a tic-free period of more than 3 consecutive months.

C. The disturbance causes marked distress or significant impairment in social, occupational, or other important areas of functioning.

D. The onset is before age 18 years.

E. The disturbance is not due to the direct physiological effects of a substance (e.g., stimulants) or a general medical condition (e.g., Huntington's disease or postviral encephalitis).

American Psychiatric Association. *Desk Reference to the Diagnostic Criteria from DSM-V–TR.* Washington, DC, American Psychiatric Association, p. 73, 2000. Reprinted with permission.

and do not cause daily difficulties. One of the clinician's most important tasks is to identify the major sources of distress and impairment in the TD patient and to prioritize the targets for treatment. Sometimes this means tic reduction, often it means interventions directed at associated OCD and/or ADHD.

PREVALENCE

Tics are very common in nonclinically referred community pediatric samples. Most are mild motor or vocal tics that do not warrant clinical intervention. Motor tics are generally more prevalent than vocal tics. Transient tics occur more often than persistent tics in school-age children. Children between the ages of 7 and 11 years appear to have the highest rate of tics.

- The monthly prevalence of any motor or vocal tic over the course of a school year in nonreferred samples of 5- to 15-year-old children ranges between 0.5% and 24%.
  - The monthly prevalence of any motor tic is between 3% and 24%.
  - The monthly prevalence of any vocal tic is much less, around 0.5%.
  - Boys generally have more tics than girls.
- Much less is known about the epidemiology of specific tic disorders. Khalifa and von Knorring (2003) studied the prevalence of tic disorders and TD according to DSM-IV criteria in Swedish school children ages 7–15 years.
  - The overall prevalence rate for any tics was 6.6%.
  - TD occurred in 0.6%.
  - Chronic motor tic disorder occurred in 0.8%.
  - Chronic vocal tic disorder occurred in 0.5%.
  - Transient tic disorder occurred in 4.8%.
  - The prevalence of tic disorder was higher in younger children and males.

COMORBIDITY

Especially in clinically referred children with tic disorders and TD, high rates of comorbidity with other types of psychopathology occur. In a study of the behavioral spectrum of associated psychopathology occurring in a community sample of children and adolescents with tic disorders, the following psychiatric disorders occurred at rates exceeding chance (Kurlan et al., 2002).

- OCD
  - Occurs in about 50% of patients with TD.
- ADHD
  - Occurs in 60–70% of young patients with TD.
  - However, TD occurs in only approximately 7% of ADHD patients.
- Separation anxiety disorder
- Generalized anxiety disorder
- Social phobia
- Simple phobia
- Agoraphobia
- Mania
- Depression
- Oppositional defiant disorder

COURSE OF ILLNESS AND OUTCOME

Tic disorder and TD generally begin early in life. Motor tics begin first, followed by vocal tics several years later. Motor tics have been reported to progress in a rostral–caudal manner, with tics appearing first in muscles of the head and eyes, and then expanding to include the neck, shoulders, arms, and then torso. However, this progression is not totally predictable. Simple tics appear early, followed in some patients by more complex tic behaviors. Tics generally occur in clustered bouts, followed by quiescent periods. Fatigue, anxiety, and stress generally increase tic frequency and severity.

Available epidemiological studies suggest that tic disorders tend to improve in late adolescence and early adulthood. In many cases vocal tics entirely disappear and motor tics become reduced in frequency, number, and intensity. In some individuals tics remit entirely. However when tics do not improve with age, adulthood is the period when the most severe and debilitating forms of tic disorder occur. In addition, comorbid OCD and ADHD may not improve with time and require continuing treatment in patients with TD. Currently, variables that reliably predict the natural course of tic disorders and TD in specific individuals are not known.

ASSESSMENT

Assessment should emphasize a comprehensive evaluation. The clinician should focus on the patient's overall course of development and adaptive functioning and not simply concentrate on the tic disorder. The identification of areas of distress and impairment is important. These areas may relate more to comorbid conditions such as OCD or ADHD than to the tics themselves. Domains to be assessed include:

- Tic location, severity, frequency, complexity, and degree of interference with daily functioning

- Obsessive–compulsive symptoms and behaviors
- ADHD symptoms
- Other comorbid psychiatric disorders
- Adequacy of previous treatments; if pharmacological, adequacy of medication type, dose, duration of treatment, effectiveness, and tolerability
- Family history of neuropsychiatric illness, especially tics, OCD, ADHD, and affective disorders
- Social environment, stresses, and adaptive functioning
- Academic and/or occupational functioning
- Medical and neurological evaluations
  - Evaluate for any relationship between symptoms and sore throats, given the correlation between tics/OCD and beta-hemolytic group A streptococcal infections.

Once a diagnosis of tic disorder or TD is made by clinical evaluation, rating scales can help assess symptom severity and tic typography. Some commonly used rating scales in the assessment of tic disorders are given below.

TREATMENT

Tic disorders can be chronic conditions. By necessity, treatment is long-term and continuity of care is highly desirable. Major components of treatment include psychoeducation of the child and family about the disorder, educational supports for the child, supportive interventions for the family, and treatment with psychiatric medications.

Educational and supportive interventions
- Explaining the nature of tic disorders to the family can have positive effects by reshaping negative expectations concerning the child. Sometimes, family members misconstrue tic behaviors and associated psychopathology as voluntary, intentional, and willfully provocative.
- By educating school personnel about the neurobiological vulnerabilities associated with TD, the child may be seen in a more positive and supportive manner in the classroom.
- Appropriate educational supports should be provided to the child with a tic disorder, as necessary, especially if ADHD is also present.
- Self-help organizations such as the Tourette Syndrome Association can be of assistance to families in providing up-to-date information about the disorder, peer support, and counseling.
- Cognitive–behavioral therapy may help reduce associated anxiety symptoms.

PHARMACOTHERAPY

The mere presence of tics is not necessarily an indication for treatment with psychiatric medications. Many mild cases can be quite adequately managed without the use of medications. Tics exhibit a natural waxing and waning of frequency and severity. This natural course complicates the assessment of

TIC DISORDERS

Table 15.4 Rating Scales for Tic Severity and Tourette's Syndrome in Children and Adolescents

Rating Scale	Type of Scale	What Is Assessed?	Age Range	Reliability	Validity	Sensitivity to Change
Hopkins Motor and Vocal Tic Scale	Parent and clinician-rated	Motor and vocal tic symptoms	Child, adolescent, adult	+ +	+ +	Yes
Tourette's Symptom Severity Scale	Clinician-rated	Tic severity, interference, and impaired functioning	Child, adolescent, adult	+ +	+ +	Yes
Tourette's Syndrome—Clinical Global Impressions	Clinician-rated	Tic-associated impairment in functioning	Child, adolescent, adult	+ +	+ +	Yes
Yale Global Tic Severity Scale	Clinician-rated	Tic number, frequency, intensity, complexity, and interference	Child, adolescent, adult	+ +	+ +	Yes

medication effectiveness in TD. If tics improve with treatment, is it really the treatment or the natural cycle of the disorder? Indeed, the placebo response rate in medication trials for TD is between 6% and 13%.

Indications for pharmacotherapy of tic disorders and TD include
• Symptom severity
• Impairment in daily functioning
• Comorbid psychiatric conditions
• Failure of less invasive treatments to adequately treat tics

Recent medication studies in pediatric tic disorders
and Tourette's disorder
A wide variety of agents is now available to treat tics or tics and comorbid psychopathology. Each medication should be selected on the basis of expected effectiveness and potential side effects. Controlled medication studies in pediatric tic disorders and TD are presented in the following table.

CHOOSING A MEDICATION

Before treatment
• Complete a thorough psychiatric evaluation and document any comorbid psychiatric diagnoses that will be a focus of treatment in addition to the tic disorder.
• Obtain results of a physical exam completed within the 6–12 months prior to initiating therapy.
• Obtain a baseline level of tic symptom severity and associated psychopathology using an established rating scale.
• Obtain baseline ratings of off-drug symptoms to compare against on-drug reported side effects.
• Educate the family about the nature of tics and TD, expected benefits of drug treatment, possible side effects, use of the medication, and expected duration of treatment.
• Determine if the child has any contraindications to medication therapy.

Typical Neuroleptics

Dopamine D2 receptor antagonists remain the most effective tic-suppressing agents in the short-term. Their long-term use is less favorable because of side effects and the possible risk of eventually developing tardive dyskinesia. The most widely used neuroleptics include haloperidol, pimozide, and fluphenazine. Tiapride is a D2 antagonist that is effective for tic suppression but is not available in the United States. The FDA has approved haloperidol and pimozide for labeling in TD.

Haloperidol or pimozide
• Treatment is initiated at low doses (0.25 mg of haloperidol/1 mg of pimozide), given before sleep.

Table 15.5 Controlled Studies of Medications in Children and Adolescents with Tics/Tourette's Disorder

Study (year)	Drug	Study Type	N	Age Range (years)	Dose (mg/day)	Duration	Outcome
Dion et al. (2002)	Risperidone	RCT	24	Adolescents and adults	1–6	8 weeks	Effective
Gaffney et al. (2002)	Risperidone vs. clonidine	RCT	21	7–17	Risperidone 1.5 avg; clonidine 1.75 avg	8 weeks	Risperidone = clonidine; both effective
Gilbert et al. (2000)	Pergolide	RCT	24	7–17	300 μg/day	6 weeks	Effective
Gilbert et al. (2004)	Risperidone vs. pimozide	RCT	19	7–17	Risperidone 1–4; pimozide 1–4	4 weeks	Risperidone > pimozide
Kurlan et al. (1993)	Fluoxetine	RCT	11	Children	20–40	16 weeks	Not effective
Leckman et al. (1991)	Clonidine	RCT	47	7–48	3–5 μg/kg/day	12 weeks	Effective
Sallee et al. (1997)	Haloperidol vs. pimozide	RCT	22	7–16	Haloperidol = 3.5, pimozide = 3.4	6 weeks	Pimozide superior to haloperidol
Sallee et al. (2000)	Ziprasidone	RCT	28	7–17	40	8 weeks	Appears effective
Scahill Leckman et al. (2003)	Risperidone	RCT	34	6–62	2.5 avg	8 weeks	Effective
Scahill et al. (1997)	Fluoxetine	RCT	14	8–33	20	20 weeks	Not effective
Shapiro et al. (1989)	Haloperidol vs. pimozide	RCT	57	8–65	Haloperidol = 10; pimozide = 20	6 weeks	Both haloperidol and pimozide more effective than placebo
Silver Shytle, Sheehan et al. (2001)	Mecamylamine	RCT	29	8–17	2.5–7.5	8 weeks	Not effective
Silver Shytle, Phillip et al. (2001)	Haloperidol and nicotine or placebo	RCT	70	10.4 avg	Nicotine patch 7 mg/24 hrs; haloperidol plasma level = 1.63 ± 2.3	33 days	Improvement with adjunctive nicotine added to haloperidol compared with placebo
Singer et al. (2001)	Baclofen	RCT	10	8–14	60	4 weeks	Effective

RCT = randomized controlled trial

- Doses are titrated every 7–14 days by 0.25 mg–0.5 mg haloperidol or 1 mg pimozide.
- The therapeutic dose range of haloperidol for the treatment of tic disorder or TD is 0.5 mg–6.0 mg/day in divided doses.
- The therapeutic dose range of pimozide for the treatment of tic disorder or TD is 1.0–10.0 mg in divided daily doses.
  - Pimozide is associated with prolonged QTc on EKG. Baseline and on-drug EKG monitoring is recommended. The on-drug QTc should not exceed 30% over baseline. The risk for QTc prolongation increases with increasing pimozide dose.

Fluphenazine
- Fluphenazine is initiated at 1 mg before sleep. The dose is titrated by 1 mg every 7 days until the therapeutic dose range of 2–15 mg/day is achieved. Fluphenazine is given in two or three divided daily doses.
  - Side effects of typical neuroleptics with prolonged use include acute dystonic reactions, akathisia, tardive dyskinesia, weight gain, sedation, depression, and the development of school phobia.
- Duration of treatment of 4–8 weeks is generally sufficient to achieve adequate tic control.
  - Baseline and on-drug monitoring with the Abnormal Involuntary Movement Scale (AIMS) is necessary. The AIMS examination should be completed every 6 months while the patient is on the drug.
  - Akathisia is a subjective, uncomfortable, inner feeling of restlessness that is a treatment-emergent side effect of neuroleptic therapy. Patients may feel an uncontrollable urge to pace. Monitoring for akathisia with the Barnes Akathisia Scale or the Simpson–Angus Scale for extrapyramidal side effects is recommended at each medical monitoring visit for patients receiving neuroleptics.
  - Acute dystonic reactions usually involve a sudden, paroxysmal tightening of the muscles of the jaw and neck after neuroleptic use. Dystonic reactions are emergently treated with anticholinergic agents: diphenhydramine 25–50 mg PO or 25 mg IM or benztropine 0.5-1 mg po or IM. Improvement generally occurs within 15–30 minutes.
  - Monitor weight and body mass index (BMI) especially with long-term neuroleptic therapy.

Atypical Antipsychotics

Atypical antipsychotics combine serotonergic ($5HT_2$) and dopaminergic (D2) antagonism. They have a lower risk of tardive dyskinesia, acute dystonic reactions, and akathisia and are more accepted by patients than neuroleptics. Among this group of agents there is evidence for the tic-suppressing efficacy of risperidone and ziprasidone. Clozapine, which has weak D2-blocking properties but robust $5HT_2$ antagonism, is not effective in suppressing tics, suggesting that D2-blockade is important in tic suppression. At the present time olanzapine, quetiapine, and aripiprazole have not been studied in the treatment of tic disorders in children and adolescents.

- Risperidone is initiated at 0.25 mg (in younger children) to 0.5 mg (in teenagers), given before sleep. The dose is adjusted by 0.25–0.5 mg every 5–7 days while monitoring effectiveness and side effects. The typical dose range is 1–3 mg/day in two to four divided doses.
- Ziprasidone is initiated at 20 mg at night. The dose is adjusted by 20 mg every 5–7 days while monitoring effectiveness and side effects. The clinical dose range is 20–160 mg/day, given in divided doses.
  ○ Ziprasidone is associated with some EKG QTc prolongation. Periodic EKG monitoring while on-drug is recommended.

Side effects
- Atypical antipsychotics are associated with a number of side effects, including weight gain, sedation, akathisia, and increased salivation. Except for weight gain, most treatment-emergent side effects can be managed by dose adjustment.
- Marked weight gain is a problem with most atypical antipsychotics. The rank order of weight gain is clozapine > olanzapine > risperidone > quetiapine > ziprasidone and aripiprazole.
  ○ Weight and BMI must be monitored closely. Prolonged weight gain in adult patients treated with atypical antipsychotics is associated with increased risk for metabolic syndrome, insulin resistance, and Type II diabetes.

Pergolide

Pergolide is a mixed D2-D1 agonist used to alter dopamine activity in the treatment of Parkinson's disease. There is some evidence that pergolide may be helpful in tic suppression. However, until further research supports its use in children and adolescents, pergolide remains a second- or third-line intervention for tic disorders or TD.

- Pergolide is initiated at a dose of 0.05 mg and gradually increased every 3–4 days by 0.1 mg until a therapeutic dose range between 0.15 and 0.30 mg is reached.
- Pergolide is administered in three or four divided daily doses.
- Side effects include dyskinesias, dizziness, hallucinations, dystonias, sedation, and rhinitis.

Alpha-Adrenergic Agonists: Clonidine and Guanfacine

By activating presynaptic noradrenergic autoreceptors in locus ceruleus neurons in the brainstem, alpha-2-agonists such as clonidine and guanfacine reduce CNS noradrenergic neurotransmission. Both clonidine and guanfacine induce tic suppression in children and adolescents.

CLONIDINE

- Clonidine is initiated at 0.05 mg before bed. After 3–4 days the dose is adjusted upward by 0.05 mg, given on a tid–qid dose schedule.

- The effective dose range appears to be between 0.15 and 0.3 mg/day.
- Because clonidine is a hypotensive agent, pulse and blood pressure monitoring is required.
- Side effects include depression, irritability, and mid-sleep awakening.
- Clonidine should not be discontinued abruptly.
  - Withdrawal syndrome has been reported.
- Children and adolescents with a medical history of cardiovascular disease or syncope are not candidates for clonidine.
- Clonidine is available as a tablet or a transdermal patch that is worn on the back and has the advantage of avoiding multiple daily dosing. The patch reportedly has fewer side effects than the oral preparation. However, dermatitis often appears under the patch, requiring application to a different area of the back every day.

GUANFACINE

- Guanfacine is longer acting and less sedating than clonidine, and it appears to have fewer side effects than clonidine.
- Guanfacine is initiated at 0.5 mg in the evening and titrated upward by 0.5 mg on a tid or bid schedule every 3–4 days.
- The therapeutic dose range is between 1.5 mg and 4.0 mg day.
- Vital sign monitoring is recommended because guanfacine is a hypotensive agent.
- Abrupt guanfacine discontinuation is not recommended.
  - A withdrawal reaction has been described.
- Children and adolescents with a medical history of cardiovascular disease or syncope are not candidates for guanfacine.

Other Tic-Suppressing Agents

- Nicotine chewing gum may be an effective tic-suppressing agent alone or in combination with haloperidol.
  - Side effects of nausea and vomiting are common.
- Baclofen is a muscle relaxant with GABA properties. In doses of 20 mg tid it was found effective for tic suppression in a controlled trial.
- Botulinum injections may be effective in reducing tics.
  - Muscle weakness is a side effect.

PHARMACOLOGICAL TREATMENT OF ADHD IN PATIENTS WITH TIC DISORDERS OR TOURETTE'S DISORDER

ADHD occurs more frequently in children and adolescents with TD than would be expected by chance alone. The ADHD symptoms accompanying TD are often a greater source of impairment for children than tic symptoms, per se. Up to 70% of TD patients may have comorbid ADHD. The pharmacological treatment of ADHD in the presence of tics is a common therapeutic challenge.

TIC DISORDERS

Table 15.6 Controlled Studies of Medications in Children and Adolescents with ADHD and Tics/Tourette's Disorder

Study (year)	Drug	Study Type	N	Age Range (years)	Dose (mg/day)	Duration	Outcome
Feigin et al. (1996)	Deprenyl	RCT	24	Mean age 12	10	6 weeks	No significant difference
Gadow et al. (1995)	MPH	RCT	34	6–12	0.2, 0.6, and 1.0 mg/kg/day	2 weeks	No increase in tics; improvement in ADHD
Law & Schachar (1999)	MPH	RCT	91	6–12	1.0 mg/kg/day	1 year	No change in tic frequency between groups; MPH improvement in ADHD
Niederhofer et al. (2003)	Lofexidine	RCT	44	Mean age 10.4	0.4–1.2	8 weeks	Improvements in tics and ADHD
Nolan et al. (1999)	MPH or DEX	RCT-withdrawal	19	6–12	Abrupt placebo substitution for stimulant	Stimulants ≥ 1 year	No change in tics upon placebo substitution
Scahill et al. (2001)	Guanfacine	RCT	34	Mean age 10.4	1.5–3.0	8 weeks	Improvements in tics and ADHD
Singer et al. (1995)	Clonidine or desipramine	RCT	37	7–13	Clonidine 0.05–0.20; desipramine 25–100	6 weeks	Desipramine > clonidine for ADHD and tics
Spencer et al. (2002)	Desipramine	RCT	41	Children and adolescents	3.5 mg/kg/day	6 weeks	Improvements in tics and ADHD
Tourette's Syndrome Study Group (2002)	Clonidine, MPH, or combination	RCT	136	6–12	Avg clonidine dose=0.25; avg MPH dose=26	16 weeks	ADHD improved with clonidine and MPH compared to placebo; no tic differences across the three groups

RCT = randomized controlled trial; MPH = methylphenidate; DEX = dextroamphetamine

314

Stimulants and Tic Disorder

The use of stimulants in children with individual or family histories of tics has been a topic of controversy ever since initial observations suggested that tics are exacerbated with stimulant use. Initial recommendations stated that stimulants were relatively contraindicated in the presence of tics. Given that ADHD is often very impairing and that the most effective treatment for ADHD, stimulants, could not be used, were clinicians left in a dilemma as to how to treat children with tic disorders and ADHD. However, recent methodologically controlled research has begun to challenge the view that stimulants should not be used in children and adolescents with tic disorders.

At least three controlled studies examining tic exacerbation in ADHD+tic disorder children receiving stimulants have reported little or no *average* increase in tic severity scores compared to placebo control. However, individual subjects in these studies did have significant increases in tics severe enough to prompt stimulant discontinuation or the addition of a second medication to control tics. This suggests that although many children with tic disorder and ADHD may benefit from stimulant treatment without tic exacerbation, a subgroup of these children may not tolerate stimulant treatment.

- An informed consent discussion should be held with the family and child about the possibility that tics may be exacerbated by stimulant treatment.
- After an initial stimulant-induced exacerbation, tics often return to a baseline frequency and intensity, despite continuing stimulant treatment.
- Tic disorders and ADHD appear to pursue independent longitudinal courses over development.
  - Tic disorders often remit, despite ongoing stimulant treatment.
  - ADHD appears to pursue a more chronic course over development.
- Methylphenidate preparations in low dose may cause less tic exacerbation than dextroamphetamine preparations in low dose.

Nonstimulant Medication Alternatives for Combined ADHD and Tic Disorder

CLONIDINE AND GUANFACINE

- Alpha-agonists may be useful in diminishing impulsivity, aggression, and hyperactivity symptoms of ADHD, in addition to diminishing tics. These agents are less effective than stimulants in decreasing attention span deficits. The dose range is the same as noted above.

DESIPRAMINE

- Desipramine is a tricyclic antidepressant that appears useful for ADHD and does not appear to exacerbate tics in children with tic disorders and ADHD.
- The dose range is up to 4.6 mg/kg/day given in two or three divided doses.
- Children with a medical history of cardiovascular disease, syncope, or a family history of early-onset cardiovascular disease are not candidates for a TCA trial with agents such as desipramine.

TIC DISORDERS

- Desipramine is associated with prolonged cardiac conduction times on EKG. EKG changes correlate with increasing desipramine serum levels. Baseline and on-drug EKG monitoring are mandated.
  ○ On-drug QTc should not exceed 30% over baseline.
  ○ PR interval should not exceed .20 msec.
  ○ Desipramine has been associated with several reports of sudden death in ADHD children, making clinicians reluctant to use the drug.
- Baseline and on-drug vital sign monitoring are mandated. Desipramine is associated with pulse and blood pressure changes in children.
  ○ Pulse should not exceed 125 bpm.
  ○ BP should not exceed 140/90.
- Serum desipramine plasma monitoring is available and should be used. Slow metabolizers of tricyclic antidepressants occur in 7–10% of the population, resulting in high plasma desipramine levels on low daily doses and increasing the risk for cardiovascular toxicity. Serum levels should be drawn by venipuncture 10–12 hours after the last desipramine dose and before the next one (i.e., a trough level).

ATOMOXETINE

Atomoxetine is a specific noradrenergic reuptake blocker with efficacy in the treatment of ADHD. It is FDA approved for labeling in childhood, adolescent, and adult ADHD. It is not associated with the cardiac side effects of tricyclic antidepressants and does not appear to exacerbate tics in vulnerable children.

- Atomoxetine dosing is weight based; the maximum dose is 1.8 mg/kg/day or 100 mg/day, whichever is less.
- Atomoxetine may be given in a single A.M. dose or on a bid divided dose schedule.
- EKG monitoring is not necessary.
- Vital sign monitoring is recommended.
- For children < 70 kg body weight, atomoxetine is initiated at 0.5 mg/kg and increased after a minimum of 3 days to a target daily dose of 1.2 mg/kg to 1.8 mg/kg.
- For children and teenagers > 70 kg body weight, atomoxetine is initiated at 40 mg and increased after a minimum of 3 days to a target daily dose of 80 mg.
  ○ If no response after 2–4 weeks, the dose may be increased to a maximum of 100 mg/day.

BUPROPION

Bupropion is an aminoketone antidepressant with a norepinephrine and dopamine mechanism of action. It is effective for ADHD in children and adolescents without tic disorders. However, its use in tic disorders is not recommended because it may exacerbate tics. In high doses exceeding 450 mg/day it has been associated with seizures in children.

MODAFINIL

Modafinil is a novel wake-promoting agent that is effective in the sleep attacks of narcolepsy. It is not a stimulant and has a novel mechanism of action. Several open-label and controlled trials report usefulness in pediatric ADHD. Modafinil appears less effective for adult ADHD.

Although not studied in children and adolescents with tic disorders, modafinil has no theoretical reason why it should exacerbate tics; it is not a dopaminergic or noradrenergic agent. With additional research, it may eventually be shown to be a useful second- or third-line agent for children with tic disorders and ADHD.

- Modafinil is initiated at 100 mg/day.
- The dose is increased by 50–100 mg every 3–5 days.
- The therapeutic dose range appears to be between 100 mg and 400 mg/day.
- Modafinil is generally given on a twice daily dose schedule to children and adolescents (A.M. and noon).
- Side effects include depression, headache, dizziness, and stomachache.

Combined Pharmacotherapy

The presence of impairing ADHD and distressing tic disorder is a rational indication for combined pharmacotherapy. Stimulants are often combined with other agents in the treatment of this comorbid condition.

- Stimulants may be combined with either clonidine or guanfacine to treat ADHD and tics.
- Stimulants may be combined with neuroleptics or atypical antipsychotics to treat ADHD and tics.
- Case reports support the usefulness of combined pharmacotherapy with clonidine and clonazepam for comorbid tic disorder and ADHD. Anxiety disorders can exacerbate tic severity; treating comorbid anxiety symptoms and disorders with long-acting benzodiazepines such as clonazepam may decrease tic frequency indirectly, by causing a reduction in anxiety.

PHARMACOLOGICAL TREATMENT OF OCD IN PATIENTS WITH TIC DISORDERS OR TOURETTE'S DISORDER

Up to 50% of children and adolescents with TD may also have comorbid OCD. Often the OCD symptoms are more impairing to the child and family than mild or moderate tics. As such, OCD can become the focus of treatment in such children. In this case, SSRI antidepressants, which are effective for the treatment of OCD, are also effective for the treatment of OCD in the presence of tics. However, SSRIs are not an effective therapy for non-comorbid tic disorders or TD. If comorbid ADHD is also present, the clinician should be aware that SSRIs are not an effective therapy for ADHD.

TIC DISORDERS

Tic-related forms of OCD differ from cases of OCD without a personal or family history of tics. They appear to have a male preponderance, an earlier age of onset, and a predominance of obsessions and compulsions concerning aggression, sex, religion, and symmetry, repeating, and ordering symptoms. Tic-related OCD may be less responsive to monotherapy with SSRIs than non-comorbid OCD.

Combined pharmacotherapy is often indicated to treat moderate to severe symptoms of tics and OCD.

- Risperdal or olanzapine and an SSRI can be combined to target both disorders.
- A neuroleptic and an SSRI can be combined to target both disorders.
- It is advisable to initiate treatment with one agent alone; if clinical response is not adequate to the first agent, titrate the second agent to a stable dose of the first agent.
- The dose ranges of SSRIs are the same as those for OCD alone.
- The dose range of risperdal or olanzapine is the same as for tic disorders.
- The dose range of neuroleptics is the same as for tic disorders.

PEDIATRIC AUTOIMMUNE NEUROPSYCHIATRIC DISORDERS ASSOCIATED WITH STREPTOCOCCAS

Some children may develop new-onset tics or a sudden exacerbation of tic symptoms after group A beta-hemolytic streptococcal infection. Via a process analogous to Sydenham's chorea, infections with group A beta-hemolytic streptococci may trigger autoimmune responses that cause or abruptly worsen some cases of childhood tic disorders (as well as symptoms of OCD).

If pediatric autoimmune neuropsychiatric disorders associated with streptococcas (PANDAS) are suspected, the child should be assessed for evidence of group A beta-hemolytic streptococcal infection.

- A throat culture, antistreptolysin O (ASO), and anti-DNAase B titer should be obtained.
- Interepisode antibody levels are recommended to demonstrate a later rise associated with an intercurrent streptococcal infection and subsequent increase in tic symptoms.

Treatment consists of antibiotic therapy for the streptococcal infection and psychiatric treatment for the tic disorder.

16. Conduct Disorder, Oppositional Defiant Disorder, and Impulsive Aggression

Patients with disorders of excessive, maladaptive, and impulsive aggression are among the most common referrals to child and adolescent psychiatric settings. Up to 60% of patients seen in ambulatory care settings may have problems with conduct disorder, oppositional defiant behavior, and/or aggression that, in part, contributes to the reasons for psychiatric referral. Violent threats and impulsive aggression are very common in child and adolescent psychiatric inpatient settings. Aggressive behavior is a predictor of urgency in emergency mental health services. Disturbances involving maladaptive aggression are extremely costly, involving loss to patients, families, victims, and society, and often portend a poor longitudinal prognosis for the aggressive child or adolescent.

Aggression and antisocial behaviors are heterogeneous in symptom presentation and multifactorial in etiology. A complex interplay between biological and environmental vulnerabilities operating across the levels of the individual, family, and community, over the course of development, is thought to be responsible for the eventual development of maladaptive aggression and antisocial behavior. Maladaptive aggression is associated with many psychiatric disorders, including conduct disorder, oppositional defiant disorder, attention-deficit/hyperactivity disorder, bipolar disorder, depression, Tourette's disorder, substance abuse, personality disorders, psychotic disorders, and some anxiety disorders (i.e., PTSD).

The treatment of disorders of maladaptive aggression requires a multimodal approach involving intervention from multiple interacting systems in the child's life. These include the individual child, parents, family, school, and community. Current treatment emphasizes "wraparound" services involving the child, parents, and family and an array of mental health, juvenile justice, school, and community services, with the overall goal of preventing antisocial recidivism and treating associated mental health issues.

The psychopharmacology of aggression in juveniles suffering from disorders of maladaptive, impulsive, and/or excessive aggression is relatively unexplored. Although medication should never be the first or only treatment

319

intervention for maladaptive aggression in youths, interest in medications for disorders of impulsive, maladaptive aggression is growing. This chapter discusses psychopharmacological interventions for oppositional defiant disorder (ODD) and conduct disorder (CD). Approaches to excessive, maladaptive aggression that occurs independently of a psychiatric diagnosis are also discussed.

OPPOSITIONAL DEFIANT DISORDER

Children and adolescents with oppositional defiant disorder display a recurrent pattern of negativistic, defiant, disobedient, and hostile behavior toward authority figures that is more frequent and intense than is typically observed for individuals of similar age and developmental level. Usually parents are the targets of the child's ODD, but teachers may become involved as well in the child's pervasive hostility. The diagnostic features of ODD are presented below.

Table 16.1 Diagnostic Criteria for Oppositional Defiant Disorder

A. A pattern of negativistic, hostile, and defiant behavior lasting at least 6 months, during which four (or more) of the following are present:
(1) Often loses temper.
(2) Often argues with adults.
(3) Often actively defies or refuses to comply with adults' requests or rules.
(4) Often deliberately annoys people.
(5) Often blames others for his or her mistakes or misbehavior.
(6) Is often touchy or easily annoyed by others.
(7) Is often angry or resentful.
(8) Is often spiteful or vindictive.

Note: Consider a criterion met only if the behavior occurs more frequently than is typically observed in individuals of comparable age and developmental level.

B. The disturbance in behavior causes significant impairment in social, academic, or occupational functioning.
C. The behaviors do not occur exclusively during the course of a Psychotic or Mood Disorder.
D. Criteria are not met for Conduct Disorder and, if the individual is age 18 years or older, criteria are not met for Antisocial Personality Disorder.

American Psychiatric Association. *Diagnostic and Statistical Manual of Mental Disorders 4th Ed. text rev.* Washington, DC: American Psychiatric Association, 2000, pp. 100–102. Reprinted with permission.

Prevalence

The prevalence of ODD varies with the age of the child (younger > older) and the population studied (clinic samples > community samples).

• Prevalence of ODD in nonreferred community samples of children: 2–16%.
• Prevalence of ODD in child and adolescent psychiatric clinics: up to 50%.

Etiology

Research has stressed the importance of social learning and negative reinforcement in the etiology of ODD. "Coercive family process" is a parent–child interpersonal dynamic in which parents and children train each other in oppositional and antisocial behaviors through mutual negative reinforcement. Negative reinforcement is a type of learning in which behavior that leads to avoidance of, or escape from, an aversive situation results in the increased frequency of that behavior in future aversive situations. For example:

- Consider a child with a difficult, irritable temperament who gets irritated, oppositional, and angry when parents ask the child to do something.
- When parents persist in asking the child, the child "ups the ante" and has a temper tantrum.
- To avoid further escalation, the parents "back down" from their request.
- The child learns that getting angry and aggressive "works" to avoid tasks that he or she does not want to do.
- After numerous repetitions of this interplay, the parents become angry and "blow up" at the child.
- To avoid the parents' anger and threats, the child temporarily acquiesces to their request.
- The parents learn that getting angry and aggressive "works" to avoid the child's negative behaviors and increase the child's compliance.
- As this interchange occurs many times a day over the course of the child's development, parents and child "train" each other to believe that getting angry and aggressive works to avoid aversive situations. They negatively reinforce each other to become oppositional and aggressive.
- As the child matures, his or her oppositional, aggressive, and antisocial "coping skills" generalize out of the home to other authority figures in the child's life. An oppositional defiant child has thus been fashioned.

Course of Illness

- ODD behaviors typically emerge 2–3 years before conduct disorder behaviors.
- The onset of ODD is around 6 years old.
- By age 8 it is usually clear that ODD behaviors are in excess of normal oppositional behaviors, and the disorder becomes clarified.
- A clear developmental progression exists between early-onset ODD behaviors and later, more serious, CD, but only for a minority of ODD children.
  ○ About 33% of children with ODD will go on to later CD.
- There is a high rate of other psychopathology that develops in youths with ODD.

CONDUCT DISORDER

Children and adolescents with conduct disorder violate the basic rights of others and/or societal norms. Conduct disorder is highly correlated with aggressive behavior. The diagnostic features of conduct disorder are presented below.

Table 16.2 Diagnostic Criteria for Conduct Disorder

A. A repetitive and persistent pattern of behavior in which the basic rights of others or major age-appropriate societal norms or rules are violated, as manifested by the presence of three (or more) of the following criteria in the past 12 months, with at least one criterion present in the past 6 months.

Aggression to people or animals
(1) Often bullies, threatens, or intimidates others.
(2) Often initiates physical fights.
(3) Has used a weapon that can cause serious physical harm to others (e.g., a bat, brick, broken bottle, knife, or gun).
(4) Has been physically cruel to people.
(5) Has been physically cruel to animals.
(6) Has stolen while confronting a victim (e.g., mugging, purse snatching, extortion, armed robbery).
(7) Has forced someone into sexual activity.

Destruction of property
(8) Has deliberately engaged in fire setting with the intention of causing serious damage.
(9) Has deliberately destroyed others' property (other than by fire setting).

Deceitfulness or theft
(10) Has broken into someone else's house, building, or car.
(11) Often lies to obtain goods or favors or to avoid obligations (i.e., "cons" others).
(12) Has stolen items of nontrivial value without confronting a victim (e.g., shoplifting, but without breaking and entering; forgery).

Serious violations of rules
(13) Often stays out at night despite parental prohibitions, beginning before age 13 years.
(14) Has run away from home overnight at least twice while living in parental or parental surrogate home (or once without returning for a lengthy period).
(15) Is often truant from school, beginning before age 13 years.

B. The disturbance in behavior causes clinically significant impairment in social, academic, or occupational functioning.
C. If the individual is age 18 years or older, criteria are not met for Antisocial Personality Disorder.

Code based on type:
Conduct disorder, childhood-onset type: onset of at least one criterion characteristic of conduct disorder prior to age 10 years.
Conduct disorder, adolescent-onset type: absence of any criteria characteristic of conduct disorder prior to age 10 years.
Conduct disorder, unspecified onset: age at onset is not known.

Specify severity:
Mild: few if any conduct problems in excess of those required to make the diagnosis *and* conduct problems cause only minor harm to others.
Moderate: number of conduct problems and effect on others intermediate between "mild" and "severe."
Severe: many conduct problems in excess of those required to make the diagnosis **or** conduct problems cause considerable harm to others.

American Psychiatric Association. *Diagnostic and Statistical Manual of Mental Disorders 4th Ed. text rev.* Washington, DC: American Psychiatric Association, 2000, pp. 93–100. Reprinted with permission.

Prevalence

Prevalence of CD varies with the population studied (clinically referred or criminal justice vs. community samples), age of children, gender, and community setting (urban > rural communities). Prevalence rates for CD have increased during the past few decades, possibly due to the increase in the adolescent population or improved case-identification.

- Prevalence of juvenile CD in the general population: 1.5–3.4%.
- Prevalence of CD in child and adolescent psychiatry clinics: 30–50%.
- Prevalence of antisocial personality disorder in adults: 2.6%.

Gender effects
At all ages boys are affected with CD more than girls. The gender gap is most pronounced in prepubertal children. As children mature into adolescence the gap between boys and girls with CD narrows.

- Ratio of boys to girls with CD: 3.2:1 to 5:1 in various studies.

Etiology

Conduct disorder is probably the result of a complex interplay between individual biological and social factors and family and community variables. For example, recent research documents a genotype–environment interaction that predicts individual variation in risk for antisocial behaviors and conduct disorder in boys. Adverse childhood experiences such as maternal rejection, repeated loss of a primary caregiver, harsh discipline, and abuse were risk factors for the later development of conduct disorder only in boys who also possessed a genotype characterized by low serum levels of monoamine oxidase A activity (Caspi et al., 2002; Foley et al., 2004). Thus this research elucidates a biosocial mechanism for the development of CD. Risk factors for CD are given below.

Table 16.3 Risk Factors for Conduct Disorder

Individual	Family	Community
*Impulsivity	Harsh parenting	Access to weapons
*Affect dysregulation	Inconsistent discipline	Antisocial peers
*Explosive rage	Lack of monitoring	School failure
*Hyperactivity	*Maternal depression	Overcrowding
*Psychosis	Paternal antisocial behavior	Poverty
*Depression	Parental alcohol abuse	
Substance abuse	Parental drug abuse	
*Irritability	*Parental ADHD	
Low VIQ	Large family size	
Lack of coping skills	Low SES/poverty	
Difficult temperament	Family violence	
Sensation seeking	Abuse	
Low ANS arousal	Neglect	
Male gender	Access to weapons	
Early-onset aggression		
Traumatic stress during development		
Genotype: low levels of MAO-A		

*Possible target for psychopharmacological intervention. VIQ = Verbal Intelligence Quotient; SES = socioeconomic status

Course of Illness

Several longitudinal studies document that for most patients, untreated CD follows a predictably worsening course from childhood through young adulthood, after which it seems to decline in virulence, generally after 30 years of age. The course of CD may be thought of as the steady accumulation of old and new antisocial risk factors as life demands more sophisticated and competent individual skills for successful management as one matures.

• About 40% of youth with CD will go on to develop adult antisocial personality disorder.
• There is a high rate of other psychopathology that develops in youth with CD.

COMORBIDITY IN ODD AND CD

Other psychiatric disorders are found in juveniles with ODD/CD at rates far above chance expectation. The presence of comorbid psychiatric disorders must be evaluated in the clinical assessment of youth with ODD/CD. The clinician must also assess for the presence of family dysfunction, traumatic stress such as abuse, coercive family processes, and parental psychopathology.

Comorbidity in childhood ODD/CD
• ADHD
• Depression
• Early-onset bipolar disorder
• Anxiety disorders, including PTSD
• Reading learning disability
• Other learning disabilities

Comorbidity in adolescent ODD/CD
• ADHD
• Depression
• Bipolar disorders
• Substance use disorders
• Cigarette smoking
• Psychotic disorders
• Anxiety disorders, including PTSD
• Reading learning disability
• Other learning disabilities

PSYCHOPHARMACOLOGICAL TREATMENT OF ODD AND CD

ODD and CD are not considered robustly medication-responsive disorders. The treatment of ODD emphasizes parent management behavioral training and family behavioral therapies focused on interrupting coercive family processes. The treatment of CD emphasizes multimodal psychoeducational wraparound services. Early intervention in childhood appears to be more effective than initial treatment later in adolescence. Therefore, early recognition and treatment of these externalizing behavioral disorders is crucial. Family involvement with the treatment plan is mandatory if treatment is to succeed for the juvenile with

ODD or CD. Evaluation and educational interventions for any associated learning disabilities are important.

Psychopharmacological interventions in ODD/CD often target associated comorbid disorders. Any associated disorder such as ADHD, depression, bipolar disorder, some anxiety disorders, and/or psychotic disorders may be responsive to medication treatment if present in the youth with CD. While ODD/CD may not respond to medications, psychopharmacological treatment of associated psychiatric disorders in the patient with ODD/CD may decrease affiliated antisocial and aggressive symptoms.

IMPULSIVE AGGRESSION

ODD and CD are categorical psychiatric diagnoses. Children and adolescents meeting diagnostic criteria are assigned the diagnosis, or they do not meet diagnostic criteria and are not assigned the diagnosis. Psychiatric diagnoses as categories are either present or absent. Another approach to the problem of aggression in psychiatrically referred juveniles is to consider aggression as a dimensional characteristic of patients that may be continuously present but in varying degrees in many different psychiatric disorders. In the dimensional approach to aggression, psychiatric medications target aggression as a symptom of a disorder, rather than treating the disorder itself. This approach is analogous to the palliative treatment of pain or fever with a medicine, regardless of the underlying medical condition.

When aggression is considered from a dimensional viewpoint, subtypes of aggression may be identified. These are present to varying degrees in patients with a variety of psychiatric disorders. Aggression may become a focus of treatment when it is very maladaptive, intense, frequent, and impairs the individual's life and the lives of those around him or her.

Table 16.4 Characteristics of Maladaptive Aggression

Aggression that is:
Intense
Frequent
Impulsive
Extended in duration
Does not terminate appropriately
Associated with psychiatric illness
Associated with other CNS dysfunction
Explosive
Excessive and disproportionate for the precipitating event(s)
Out of control
Not connected to appropriate social cues in the environment

Categories of aggression are listed below.

Patients may exhibit characteristics of more than one category of aggression. Some of these *categories* of aggression may be targets of medication intervention in psychiatrically referred youths. Different types of aggressive behaviors may occur, especially in the reactive and overt categories. These types are listed in the following table.

Table 16.5 Categories of Aggression and Their Characteristics

Category	Description	Premeditated	ANS Arousal
Overt	Direct confrontation with the environment (hits, kicks, threatens)	Yes or No	↑
Covert	Hidden and furtive (shoplifts, lies, cheats, vandalizes, sets fires)	Yes	↓
Reactive	Defensive response to a perceived threat	No	↑
Proactive	Goal oriented for a purpose; planned (robbing a store)	Yes	↓

Table 16.6 Aggression Type[a]

Type	Description
Verbal	Threats of violence and/or harm to others
Property destruction	Impulsive, explosive destruction of own or others' property or possessions
Self-injurious behavior	Harm to self
Physical assault	Physical attack on another

[a]Most often present in the Overt and/or Reactive categories of aggression.

In general, overt categories of aggression that are impulsive and reactive (defensive) in character and have high autonomic nervous system (ANS) arousal are more responsive to psychopharmacological interventions, regardless of the accompanying diagnosis. Covert aggression and premeditated, proactive (instrumental) forms of aggression are less responsive to medication interventions. These categories of aggression generally require behavioral therapy, community interventions, and/or juvenile justice involvement.

TREATMENT OF EXCESSIVE, MALADAPTIVE AGGRESSION

Psychosocial Treatments

Psychosocial, psychoeducational, and community treatments form the backbone of therapeutic interventions for childhood excessive, maladaptive aggression. These therapies emphasize interpersonal skill building and educational remediation for the aggressive child and should involve parents and families as well as the individual child or adolescent.

Principals of intervention
- Intervention early in a child's life appears to be more effective than interventions given later in life when antisocial behavior patterns are well established and fixed.
  - Early intervention programs that identify at-risk children and families and intervene before the child is 6 years old appear to be very effective

in diminishing risk for later conduct disorder, antisocial behaviors, and aggression.
  ○ Antisocial behaviors become solidified around 10–12 years old.
• Psychosocial interventions must involve the parents as well as the identified child if they are to be effective.
• Interventions administered over longer durations, generally 1–2 years, are more effective than short-term interventions.
• Because many aggressive juveniles have educational deficits (e.g., reading delays), the treatment plan must involve educational assessment and intervention.

Effective psychosocial interventions
Effective psychosocial therapies for aggression and conduct problems emphasize interpersonal skill acquisition. Therapies that primarily encourage the expression of feelings are not effective in externalizing disorders.

• For younger aggressive children 2–6 years old
  ○ Parent management training
• For school-age aggressive children 6–12 years old
  ○ Peer mediation at school
  ○ Anger management training
  ○ Conflict resolution training
  ○ Assertiveness training
  ○ Impulse control training
  ○ Behavioral therapy
• For teenagers
  ○ Cognitive–behavioral therapy

Ineffective psychosocial interventions
• Psychodynamic therapy
• Play therapy
• Group therapy
  ○ Group therapy with antisocial youngsters only encourages the children to learn new antisocial behaviors from one another.
• Psychodynamic-based family therapy

Educational Interventions

Many juveniles with conduct disorder and maladaptive aggression have accompanying learning deficits and disabilities. Common learning deficits in these youngsters include

• Speech disorders
• Expressive language disorders
• Receptive language disorders
• Reading learning disabilities
• Writing learning disabilities

Educational evaluation to assess for the presence of associated learning problems is mandatory in the evaluation of the child or adolescent with conduct disorder and aggression. Educational remediation should be offered, as indicated.

Psychopharmacological Treatments

In general, psychopharmacological treatments for disorders of maladaptive aggression are adjunctive to psychosocial, psychoeducational, and community treatment plans. It is important to assess for an underlying primary psychiatric illness that might predict a response to medication treatment. This approach is outlined below.

CHOOSING MEDICATIONS

- Conduct a thorough psychiatric evaluation.
- Attempt to identify a primary underlying psychiatric illness in which aggression is an associated symptom.
- Treat the primary psychiatric illness.
- Common pediatric psychiatric disorders with excessive, maladaptive aggression as a significant associated symptom include:
  ○ ADHD → consider stimulants, alpha-agonists (guanfacine/clonidine), and/or noradrenergic antidepressants (atomoxetine or bupropion).
  ○ Depression → consider SSRIs.
  ○ Adolescent bipolar disorder → consider atypical antipsychotic agents with or without accompanying lithium and/or mood stabilizers (carbamazepine, valproic acid).
  ○ PTSD → consider SSRIs, clonidine, or atypical antipsychotics.
  ○ Psychotic disorders → consider atypical antipsychotics.
- If a primary underlying psychiatric disorder associated with aggression cannot be identified, begin a target symptom approach to the pharmacological treatment of excessive, maladaptive aggression.
- Use the principles of medication management outlined below.

PRINCIPLES OF MEDICATION USE

When a target symptom approach is used to treat excessive, maladaptive aggression independently of treatment for the primary psychiatric diagnosis, it is important that the clinician adopt a systematic approach. In the absence of a systematic approach the use of adjunctive medication interventions for excessive, maladaptive aggression can easily fail. There exists a real risk that non-methodically conducted medication trials may result in the exposure of aggressive youth to multiple ineffective medications, each with the potential for adverse side effects or drug–drug interactions that may impair their quality of life. A systematic approach is outlined below.

Atypical antipsychotics, lithium, anticonvulsants such as valproic acid and alpha-agonists (clonidine, guanfacine), and, for children with associated ADHD, stimulants have the best research support in the adjunctive medication treatment of symptoms of excessive, maladaptive aggression.

Table 16.7 Principles of Medication Management For Aggressive Children/Adolescents

1. Use medication for aggression based on a medication-responsive psychiatric diagnosis or behavioral–biological rationale—and only after conducting a complete diagnostic assessment.
2. Only use medication for aggression adjunctively within a coordinated multidisciplinary psychoeducational treatment plan.
3. Obtain written informed consent from children's legal guardians and oral assent from children 7 years of age or older for all medication trials.
4. When considering a medication trial for maladaptive aggression, attempt to treat the underlying neuropsychiatric syndrome first.
5. Use the most benign interventions first.
6. Have some quantifiable means of assessing drug safety and efficacy.
    a. Define objective behaviors and quality-of-life measures to be tracked.
    b. Use empirical methods (validated, treatment-sensitive rating scales).
    c. Obtain off-drug baseline data and on-drug treatment data for comparison.
    d. Obtain data at regular intervals during drug treatment.
7. Institute medication trials for aggressive behavior systematically.
    a. Whenever possible, medication should be introduced as a single variable into treatment.
    b. Medication trials should be introduced for preplanned periods of time that have clear beginnings and endings so that drug efficacy can be assessed.
    c. Explore the full dose range of a single medicine using low-, intermediate-, and high-dose conditions before switching to a different medication or adding other medications.
    d. Explore a medication for an adequate length of time (generally, several weeks) before switching to a different drug or adding medicines.
    e. Avoid polypharmacy with multiple drugs all given at subtherapeutic doses.
    f. Follow drug serum levels when available.

Adapted from Connor DF. *Aggression and Antisocial Behavior in Children and Adolescents; Research and Treatment.* New York: Guilford Press, p. 362., 2002.

Atypical antipsychotics
• Reported effectiveness in decreasing hostility, impulsivity, hyperactivity, aggression, and conduct problems in juveniles with conduct disorder, bipolar disorders, psychotic disorders, pervasive developmental disorders, and mental retardation (Pappadopulos et al., 2003; Schur et al., 2003).
• Generally preferred over older, typical neuroleptics in the treatment of juvenile excessive, maladaptive aggression because they have a more benign safety profile.
  ○ Less risk of extrapyramidal side effects.
  ○ Less risk of tardive and withdrawal dyskinesias.
• Block dopamine D2 receptors and serotonin 5HT2A,2C receptors.
  ○ Blockade of 5HT2A receptors may confer some antiaggressive properties to atypical agents.
• Risperidone is presently the most studied atypical agent in the treatment of excessive, maladaptive aggression in children and adolescents.

Lithium
• Reported effectiveness in the treatment of explosive rage attacks in patients meeting clinical criteria for conduct disorder in several controlled studies.
• Overall the research findings are mixed: Three randomized, controlled clinical trials of lithium report some benefits for impulsive, explosive anger attacks in youths with conduct disorder; two controlled studies report no effectiveness for lithium in aggressive youths.
• Serum levels 0.6–1.2 mEq/L in studies for aggression.

Table 16.8 Controlled Studies of Medications for Maladaptive, Excessive Aggression in Children and Adolescents

Author (year)	Diagnosis/Symptoms	Study Type	N	Age (yrs) (mean/range)	Dose	Duration (weeks)	Outcome
ANTICONVULSANTS							
Cueva et al. (1996) (carbamazepine)	CD	RCT	22	9	400–800 mg/d avg serum level = 6.8 µg/ml	6	Equal to placebo
Donovan et al. (2000) (divalproex)	CD/ODD	CO	20	10–18	750–1500 mg/d avg serum level = 82.2 µg/ml	12	↓ CD/ODD symptoms
Steiner et al. (2003) (divalproex)	CD	RCT	58	16	high dose	8	↓ CD symptoms
ANTIDEPRESSANTS TRICYCLICS							
Gordon et al. (1993) (clomipramine)	PDD + anger	CO	24	6–23	avg dose = 152 mg/d	10	↓ Anger attacks but side effects severe
ATYPICAL ANTIPSYCHOTICS							
Findling et al. (2000) (risperidone)	CD	RCT	20	6–14	0.7–1.5 mg/d 0.03 ± 0.004 mg/kg/d	10	↓ CD symptoms
McCracken et al, 2002 (risperidone)	PDD + CD	RCT	49	5–17	0.5–3.5 mg/d avg 1.16 mg/d	8	↓ CD symptoms
Aman et al. (2002) (risperidone)	MR + CD	RCT	55	5–12	0.006–0.092 mg/kg/d	6	↓ CD symptoms
LITHIUM							
Malone et al. (2000)	CD	RCT	40	12.5	900–2100 mg/d avg serum level = 1.07 mEq/L	6	↓ CD symptoms
Klein (1991)	CD	RCT	35	6–15	500–2000 mg/d	5	Equal to placebo
Rifkin et al. (1997)	CD	RCT	33	12–17	500–2000 mg/d	2	Equal to placebo
Campbell et al. (1995)	CD	RCT	50	5–12	avg dose 1248 mg/d avg serum level = 1.12 mEq/L	6	↓ CD symptoms
Campbell et al. (1984)	CD	RCT	61	9	500–2000 mg/d avg serum level = 0.99 mEq/L	6	↓ CD symptoms
STIMULANTS							
Klein et al. (1997) (methylphenidate)	CD + ADHD	RCT	84	12	20–60 mg/d	5	↓ CD + ADHD symptoms
CLONIDINE ADDED TO STIMULANTS							
Hazell & Stuart (2003)	CD/ODD + ADHD	RCT	38	6–14	Clonidine 0.10–0.20 mg/d added to stimulant	6	↓ CD

Diagnosis: CD = conduct disorder; ADHD = attention-deficit/hyperactivity disorder; ODD = oppositional defiant disorder; PDD = pervasive developmental disorder; MR = mental retardation
Study type: RCT = randomized controlled trial; CO = crossover design

- Low therapeutic index to toxic index; careful clinical monitoring is necessary.
- Must be given in three or four divided daily doses to minimize side effects.

Anticonvulsants
- Valproic acid has reported effectiveness in conduct disorder and aggression in two randomized, controlled clinical trials.
  - Serum levels 50–125 μg/ml.
  - Higher doses may be more effective than lower doses for conduct disorder.
- Carbamazepine has not been found effective in one controlled study of conduct disorder.

Alpha-agonists
- Clonidine has been found effective for aggression in conduct disorder in both open-label and controlled trials.
  - Dose range 0.05–0.40 mg given in two to four daily doses.
  - Monitoring of vital signs recommended.
  - EKG monitoring is optional.
- Guanfacine may also have anti-aggressive properties.
  - However, guanfacine has not been investigated in disorders of excessive, maladaptive aggression.

Stimulants
- Aggression often present in children and adolescents with ADHD.
- In juveniles with ADHD, stimulants can decrease associated aggression.
  - A meta-analysis of stimulant effects on aggression in children with ADHD found an effect size of 0.84 for overt aggression-related behaviors and 0.69 for covert aggression-related behaviors (Connor et al., 2002).
- In the absence of ADHD, stimulants are not effective for aggression.

Atomoxetine
- Oppositional defiant behaviors are often present in children and adolescents with ADHD.
- Atomoxetine has been shown to reduce ODD behaviors in ADHD children in doses similar to that of atomoxetine treatment of ADHD.
  - Atomoxetine dose range found effective in ODD: 0.5–1.8 mg/kg/day (Newcorn et al., 2005).

Combined pharmacotherapy
- In ADHD, some evidence suggests that adding alpha-agonists (such as clonidine) or atypical antipsychotics to ongoing stimulant treatment may be helpful to down-regulate excessive, maladaptive aggression.

ALGORITHMS FOR THE MEDICATION TREATMENT
OF AGGRESSION DISORDERS

Treatment algorithms provide one possible way of organizing a systematic clinical approach to medication interventions for children or adolescents with disorders of aggression. Unless the clinician has a systematic approach, there is a real possibility of polypharmacy in which multiple medications are prescribed with no clear understanding of which medication intervention(s) is/are effective. Medication algorithms for aggression are only just beginning to be developed and have not been tested yet in research clinical trials. The following figure describes one such algorithm; it is divided into a *primary treatment approach* and a *target symptom approach*.

Measuring Treatment Response

Because medication interventions for conduct disorder, oppositional defiant disorder, and excessive, impulsive aggression are "off-label" uses, it is important to carefully measure clinical response and side effects to medications. Side effect rating scales for a variety of medications are provided in Appendix 4 at the end of the book.

When treating aggression with medication

- Obtain a baseline rating of aggressive behaviors to be followed.
- Obtain a baseline rating of medication side effects before medication titration begins.
- Follow both the aggression rating scale and the medication side effects scale weekly to monthly to obtain a clinical impression of treatment response and medication side effects.
  ○ Parent completed
  ○ Teacher completed
  ○ Youth completed (for children ≥ 11 years old)
- Consider periodic medication discontinuation (*N* of 1 design) to test medication effectiveness and tolerability.

The table below provides examples of treatment-sensitive, reliable, and valid aggression rating scales.

A CLINICAL APPROACH TO THE AGGRESSIVE CHILD OR ADOLESCENT

It is recommended that the clinician develop a systematic approach to the assessment and treatment of excessive, maladaptive aggression in clinically referred children and adolescents. One such approach is outlined in the following figure.

This approach emphasizes an initial comprehensive evaluation of aggressive behavior and the determination of aggression as adaptive or maladaptive. If aggression is adaptive and, for example, in response to some understandable threat or dispute over a dominance hierarchy or desired resource, psychiatric intervention may not be needed. Other forms of societal, family, or school intervention may be required. If aggression is maladaptive, the clinician must then determine if it is a symptom of a primary underlying psychiatric disorder. If so, then a primary illness approach to treating the underlying disorder will help resolve the associated aggressive behavior. If not, the clinician must adopt

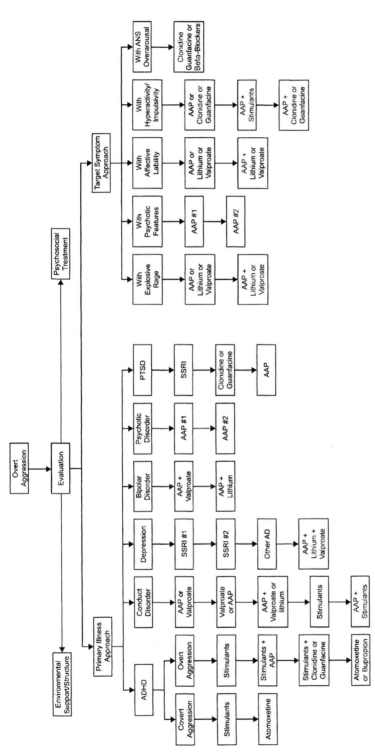

Figure 16.1 A clinical algorithm for the medication treatment of maladaptive aggression in juveniles.
The left side of the algorithm outlines a primary illness approach to the medication treatment of aggression; the right side illustrates a target symptom approach. AAP = atypical antipsychotics; SSRI = selective serotonin reuptake inhibitor; AD = antidepressants; PTSD = posttraumatic stress disorder; ANS = autonomic nervous system. Source: Adapted from Connor DE *Aggression and Antisocial Behavior in Children and Adolescents: Research and Treatment.* New York: Guilford Press, 2002 pp. 389–390. Used with permission. Copyright Guilford Press, 2002.

Table 16.9 Rating Scales for Aggression and Other Related Behaviors in Children and Adolescents

Rating Scale	Type of Scale	What Is Assessed?	Age Range (years)	Reliability	Validity	Sensitivity to Change
Buss Durkee Hostility Inventory for Children	True/false self-report	Hostility	12–17	+	+	??
Children's Aggression Scale—Parent and Teacher Versions	Parent and teacher report versions	Aggression	7–11	++	++	??
Children's Social Behavior Scale and Teacher Form	Peer report	Gender differences in aggression expression	8–12	++	++	Yes
Conners Rating Scale	Parent or teacher report	Hyperactivity and impulsivity	6–17	++	++	Yes
Direct and Indirect Aggression Scale	Peer or self-report	Direct and indirect aggression	8–15	++	++	??
Iowa Conners Teachers Rating Scale	Teacher report	Oppositional and defiant behavior	6–12	++	++	Yes
Overt Aggression Scale	Parent, teacher, or staff report	Four categories of aggression (verbal, property destruction, SIB, assault)	4–17, adults	+	+	Yes
Predatory–Affective Aggression Questionnaire	Parent, teacher, or staff report	Predatory and affective aggression	10–18	+	+	??
Proactive–Reactive Aggression Scale	Parent, teacher report	Proactive and reactive aggression	8–12	++	++	??

SIB = self-injurious behavior; + = fair; + + = good

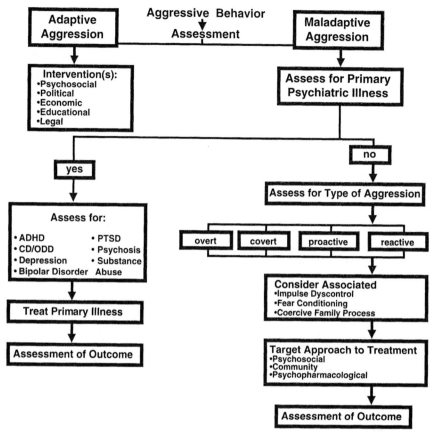

Figure 16.2 A systematic approach to the assessment and treatment of the aggressive child or adolescent.

a target symptom approach to aggression. It is helpful to classify the aggressive behavior along the dimensions of overt versus covert aggression and proactive versus reactive aggression. Overt, impulsive, and reactive (defensive) types of excessive, maladaptive aggression may be more responsive to psychopharmacological agents than other types of aggression. The clinician should carefully assess the patient for the presence of impulse dyscontrol. Impulsive responding can be highly associated with aggression and may be responsive to psychiatric medications. Fear conditioning, as may occur in traumatized children, also is associated with aggressive responding and may respond to medications. If coercive family process is identified, then the treatment plan should emphasize behavioral therapy and not necessarily medication.

17. Mood Disorders

Mood disorders include depression and bipolar illnesses (manic–depressive illness). This chapter discusses both types of disorders in children and adolescents. To begin, definitions of *mood* and *affect* are presented.

- *Mood*: A pervasive and sustained emotion that colors the perception of the world. Common examples of mood include depression, irritability, and anxiety (American Psychiatric Association, 2000, p. 825).
- *Affect*: A pattern of observable behaviors that is the expression of a subjectively experienced feeling state (emotion). Affect refers to fluctuating changes in emotions in contrast to mood, which refers to more sustained and pervasive emotional tone. Common examples of affect include sadness, elation, and anger (American Psychiatric Association, 2000, p. 819).

Mood disorders are a commonly occurring group of serious mental disorders that have a disturbance in mood as the predominant feature. They carry a considerable risk for recurrence across the lifespan and are frequently accompanied by marked psychosocial impairment. They may have an early age of onset in childhood or adolescence and are often intermittent and episodic, yet continuous, into adulthood. In psychiatric nomenclature, mood *episodes* are distinguished from mood disorders and serve as an essential building block in the definition of mood disorders. *Mood episodes* describe the type of mood disturbance, its associated features, duration of disturbance, exclusion criteria, and accompanying impairment. The essential feature of a mood disorder is a clinical course characterized by one or more mood episodes. Mood episodes include major depressive episodes, manic/hypomanic episodes, and mixed depression–manic episodes. The episodes themselves are not specific diagnostic entities but serve as building blocks for each of the specific mood disorder types.

The following figure demonstrates the range of mood subtypes. Individuals may have just one type of illness, such as subsyndromal depression (1), hypomania (2), or both, as is the case in cyclothymic disorder (a subsyndromal type of mild bipolar disorder) (1 + 2).

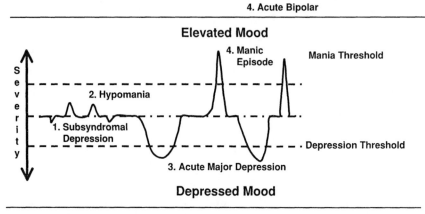

Figure 17.1 The range of mood subtypes.

Bipolar disorder is represented in the figure as a major depressive episode (3) followed by a frank manic episode (4). Rapid cycling bipolar disorder occurs when there are four or more depressive and manic or hypomanic episodes per year. Major depressive disorder occurs when only (3) occurs. Dysthymia occurs when subsyndromal depression (1) exists alone but continuously for more than 2 years. It is not uncommon for pediatric patients to present with subsyndromal depression or dysthymia (1) and progress directly to major depression (3) or incrementally through hypomania (2) to bipolar illness (3 + 4). Pediatric bipolar patients are more likely to cycle rapidly and less likely to respond to medication monotherapy (Wagner, 2004). The following table summarizes mood disorders and their symptoms.

There is no current diagnostic category for patients who have a manic episode (4) alone. They are automatically diagnosed with bipolar illness Type I, despite never having had a major depressive episode (3).

DEPRESSIVE DISORDERS

Major depressive disorder (MDD) is a state of lowered mood, often accompanied by a disturbance of sleep, energy, appetite, concentration, and/or interest. MDD is a syndrome characterized by depressed mood clustered with other symptoms that impair a child's ability to function at home, at school, or in relationship to others. Depressed mood alone does not constitute a depressive disorder. Depression as a mood disorder can include a variety of emotional and physiological symptoms. These are summarized below and are described fully

Table 17.1 Mood Disorders and Symptoms

Disorder/Symptom	Hypomania	Mania	Minor Depression	Dysthymia	Major Depression	Note
Major depressive disorder					X	
Dysthymia					X	Major Depression for more than 1 years duration
Depression NOS						Do not make duration criteria for MDD or do not make full symptom criteria for MDD
Adjustment disorder w/depressed moood			X			Do not make duration criteria for MDD
Bipolar Type I		X			X	Frank mania and major depression
Bipolar Type II	X				X	Hypomania and major depression
Cyclothymia	X		X			Hypomania and subsyndromal depression neither achieves frank Manic or MDD criteria
Bipolar NOS	X	X				Hypomania w/o any evidence of depressive symptoms
Bipolar NOS	X	X			X	Do not make duration criteria for MDD, hypomania or mania; may cycle very rapidly
Mood NOS						Difficulty clarifying dx of depression NOS vs bipolar NOS
Mood disorder general medical condition		X				Mood disorder direct physiological consequence of medical illness
Mood disorder substance abuse						Mood disorder direct physiological consequence of substance abuse

MDD = Major depressive disorder; NOS = not otherwise specified

MOOD DISORDERS

in the DSM-V–TR (American psychiatric Association, 2000). Diagnostic criteria for a depressive episode are presented in the following table.

Table 17.2 Diagnostic Criteria for Major Depressive Episode

A. Five (or more) of the following symptoms have been present during the same 2-week period and represent a change from previous functioning; at least one of the symptoms is either (1) depressed mood or (2) loss of interest or pleasure.

Note: Do not include symptoms that are clearly due to a general medical condition, or mood-incongruent delusions or hallucinations.

(1) Depressed mood most of the day, nearly every day, as indicated by either subjective report (e.g., feels sad or empty) or observation made by others (e.g., appears tearful)

Note: In children and adolescents, can be irritable mood.

(2) Markedly diminished interest or pleasure in all, or almost all, activities most of the day, nearly every day (as indicted by either subjective account or observation made by others)
(3) Significant weight loss when not dieting or weight gain (e.g., a change of more than 5% of body weight in a month), or decrease or increase in appetite nearly every day.

Note: In children, consider failure to make expected weight gains.

(4) Insomnia or hypersomnia nearly every day
(5) Psychomotor agitation or retardation nearly every day (observable by others, not merely subjective feelings of restlessness or being slowed down)
(6) Fatigue or loss of energy nearly every day
(7) Feelings of worthlessness or excessive or inappropriate guilt (which may be delusional) nearly every day (not merely self-reproach or guilt about being sick)
(8) Diminished ability to think or concentrate, or indecisiveness, nearly every day (either by subjective account or as observed by others)
(9) Recurrent thoughts of death (not just fear of dying), recurrent suicidal ideation without a specific plan, or a suicide attempt or a specific plan for committing suicide

B. The symptoms do not meet criteria for a Mixed Episode.
C. The symptoms cause clinically significant distress or impairment in social, occupational, or other important areas of functioning.
D. The symptoms are not due to the direct physiological effects of a substance (e.g., a drug of abuse, a medication) or a general medical condition (e.g., hypothyroidism).
E. The symptoms are not better accounted for by Bereavement, i.e., after the loss of a loved one, the symptoms persist for longer than 2 months or are characterized by marked functional impairment, morbid preoccupation with worthlessness, suicidal ideation, psychotic symptoms, or psychomotor retardation.

American Psychiatric Association. *Desk Reference to the Diagnostic Criteria from DSM-IV to TR*. Washington, DC, American Psychiatric Association, pp. 168–169, 2000. Reprinted with permission.

Mood episodes are described according to their severity (mild, moderate, severe), duration, and frequency as well as their response to either time or treatment (response, remission, partial remission, recovery, relapse, or recurrence).

Diagnostic Features and Subtypes of Mood Disorders

Unlike transient sadness or "the blues," clinical depression causes significant distress and interferes with a child's ability to perform routine daily functions. An episode of MDD is diagnosed when five of nine symptoms are present in the same 2-week period, and where one of the symptoms is either depressed mood or loss of interest or pleasure. Children who are depressed have feelings of sadness, loneliness, irritability, worthlessness, hopelessness, agitation, and guilt that may be accompanied by an array of physical symptoms. The spectrum of

Table 17.3 Major Depressive Disorder Specifiers

- Specifiers for major depressive disorder, full criteria met:
  - Single episode
  - Recurrent
  - Mild
  - Moderate
  - Severe
    - With psychotic features
    - Without psychotic features
- Chronic
  - With catatonic features
  - With melancholic features
  - With atypical features
  - With postpartum onset
- Specifiers for major depressive disorder, full criteria *not* met:
  - In partial remission
  - In full remission
  - Chronic
  - With catatonic features
  - With melancholic features
  - With atypical features
  - With postpartum onset
- Recurrent episodes also earn a *course specifier*:
  - With interepisode recovery
  - Without interepisode recovery
  - Seasonal pattern
- Dysthymia is specified by
  - Early onset (before age 21)
  - Late onset (after age 21)
  - With atypical features

M
O
O
D

D
I
S
O
R
D
E
R
S

depressive illness includes transient sadness and grieving, adjustment disorder, chronic depression such as dysthymia, subsyndromal depression, major depressive disorder, psychotic depression, and bipolar illness. The pattern of depressive symptom presentation can vary widely from patient to patient and suggests that the neurobiology underlying these patterns may differ (Charney & Manji, 2004). Numerous subtypes have been described (unipolar/bipolar, psychotic/nonpsychotic, familial, primary/secondary); therefore, it is plausible to expect different patients to respond to different therapies at different rates.

The clinical picture of pediatric major depressive disorder (MDD) is similar to and extends from studies on adult MDD. There are, however, developmental differences. Prepubertal children with MDD frequently experience somatic and psychomotor disturbances. Symptoms of separation anxiety, phobias, somatic complaints, irritability, and behavioral problems occur more frequently in childhood depression than in adults with depression. Depressed adolescents are more likely to report feelings of hopelessness, anhedonia (disinterest in pleasurable activities), hypersomnia, and weight change than younger depressed children. Psychotic depression, suicidality, suicidal lethality, and impairment of function increase with age (Kaufman et al., 2001). Adolescents also differ from adults in that they exhibit a more fluctuating course characterized by more interpersonal problems, tend not to report pervasive anhedonia, and also make more suicide attempts than depressed adults (Birmaher et al., 1996a; Yorbik et al., 2004).

Emotional symptoms can be expressed verbally or nonverbally and can include: sadness, tearfulness, low self-esteem, obsessive self-critical thoughts, inability to experience pleasure, loss of ambition, loss of interest, indecisiveness, inability to concentrate, irritability, anxiety, anger, pessimism, guilt, helplessness, hopelessness, and suicidal fantasies. Any one or more of the emotional states listed above may be the primary emotional state of a person suffering from depression, not just sadness.

Physiological symptoms can include fatigue, insomnia, increased need for sleep, increase or decrease in appetite, anorexia, digestive problems, constipation, social withdrawal, sexual dysfunction, and hypochondriasis. For children and adolescents, the clinical manifestation of depression varies across developmental stages and diverse ethnic groups, but is generally analogous to adult symptoms.

Heredity, biology, and environment play a contributing role in MDD. Clinical studies have shown a significant correlation between depression and a family history of psychiatric disorders. Various hormonal changes also appear to affect depressive symptoms. In addition, there are strong indications that life events can precipitate depression, and that childhood adversity (e.g., abuse, neglect) is particularly associated with a high risk of both depression and anxiety (Kaufman, 1991).

Prevalence

Major depressive disorder is a common disorder in children and adolescents.

- Population studies of children and adolescents have reported prevalence rates of depression in children between 0.4% and 4.6% and in adolescents, between 0.4% and 8.3%.
- The lifetime prevalence rate of MDD in adolescents has been estimated to range from 15% to 20%, which compares with the lifetime prevalence rate of MDD in adult populations.
- In children, rates of MDD for girls and boys appear to be equal, but this changes in adolescence, where the female-to-male risk is 2:1, the same as it is in adult MDD.

Comorbidity

The majority of children with MDD, 40–90%, suffer from other psychiatric disorders.

- 20–50% also meet criteria for two or more comorbid diagnoses, the most common being anxiety disorders, disruptive behavior disorders and substance use disorders.
- Younger children more commonly manifest separation anxiety disorder and symptoms of oppositional defiant disorder.
- Comorbid substance abuse, conduct disorder, social phobia, obsessive–compulsive disorder, dysthymic syndromes, and general anxiety disorder are more common in adolescents.

• Studies have found high rates of depression and dysthymia in children who have been abused and suffer from PTSD.
• Substance abuse and conduct disturbances tend to appear after the onset of child MDD and may persist after depression remits.

Course of Illness

Depression is often not diagnosed until quite late in an episode, when the burden of the illness has taken a toll on the child and family. The onset of depressive episodes can be either acute or insidious and generally occurs without a clear environmental precipitant. The median duration of a major depressive episode for community pediatric samples is 2–3 months, compared with the duration of depression in clinically referred populations of up to 7–9 months.

• Approximately 90% of major depressive episodes take 1–2 years to remit.
  ○ The remaining 10% become chronic.
• After successful treatment, relapse occurs in 40–60% of depressed patients within 5 years.
  ○ Many factors contribute to, relapse, including the natural history of the illness itself, nonadherence to, or a rapid decrease in, medication or psychotherapy, or exacerbating negative life events.
• The likelihood that a depressed patient will experience recurrence is between 20–60% 1 to 2 years after remission from the index depressive episode, and increases to 70% after 5 years.
  ○ Risk factors for recurrence include earlier age of onset, increased number of previous episodes, severity of the first episode, psychosis, developmental delay, and nonadherence to prescribed treatment.

Longitudinally, baseline depression severity scores on depression rating scales appear to be related to follow-up, with more severe depression predicting increased school problems, substance abuse, tobacco use, sexual activity, and disruptive behavior problems. Actual school performance (e.g., academic grades) seems to be more consistently affected by depression than cognitive and intellectual abilities. In addition, depressed youth appear to be less socially adept than nondepressed peers, although depression does not consistently impair social–cognitive abilities. Indications that depressed youth show mild declines in tested verbal performance over time and that residual problems in social functioning persist after symptomatic recovery suggest that major depression may have significant negative effects on a broad range of important developmental domains in childhood.

Assessment

Identifying patients with depression can be difficult in busy clinical care settings where time is limited, but certain depression screening measures may help diagnose the disorder. Patients who score above the predetermined cutoff levels on screening measures should be interviewed more specifically for a diagnosis of a depressive disorder and its comorbidities. If a clinical diagnosis

MOOD DISORDERS

of depression is found, these patients should be treated. Because individual patients can have variation in depressive symptoms, the use of rating scales can be very helpful in assessing symptom severity and individual response to treatment (Pavuluri & Birmaher, 2004). Commonly used depression rating scales are presented in the following table.

All children for whom there is concern that depressed mood may be present should have a comprehensive clinical psychiatric evaluation. The assessment might include a structured or semistructured psychiatric diagnostic interview to confirm depressed mood and assess for other comorbid psychiatric disorders. Unfortunately, structured and semistructured interviews are very time intensive and more oriented to research environments than busy clinical practices, pediatric or psychiatric. A short screening instrument can very quickly and effectively screen patients for whom there is high suspicion that depressed mood may be present (see preceding table).

- Often with adolescents, very straightforward depression screening questions casually dropped into conversation while performing the physical exam, such as "How have your spirits been lately?" or "How's your mood?" or "Have you been feeling 'blue' a lot lately?" can have very high clinical yield.
- Mother–child and clinician–child agreement increases as a function of the child's age and is consistently attenuated by maternal depression. Depressed mothers may overrate their children's symptomatology as compared with the children's self-reports. Children older than 11 years can reliably report on their depressive feelings.

Once it has been established that a youngster may be experiencing a depressive disorder beyond what one would expect for the child's developmental age, a more careful review of symptoms should be undertaken. A comprehensive clinical assessment must pay attention to a number of specific issues. These include the following:

- Age of onset of the depressive symptoms
- Identification of specific symptoms and their frequency, severity, and associated degree of impairment
- The child or adolescent's insight into the symptoms
- Comorbid anxiety symptoms
- The context and longitudinal course of symptoms
- Developmental history of mood symptoms, including infant temperament and shyness
- School functioning
- Social functioning
- The presence of suicidal thoughts or plans
- The presence of psychotic and/or manic symptoms accompanying depression
- In adolescents, a substance abuse history

Assessment of the family should include:
- The degree to which parents and siblings have become entangled in the child's MDD symptoms

Table 17.4 Screening Measures for Depression in Children, Adolescents, and Adults

Measure	Age Appropriateness (approximate years)	Reading Level (grade)	Spanish Version	Number of Items	Time to Complete (approximate minutes)	Psychometric Properties/Cutoff
CHILDREN AND ADOLESCENTS						
Children's Depression Inventory (CDI)	7–17	1st	Yes	27	10–15	Alpha: 0.81; test–retest: 0.60/above 19
Center for Epidemiological Studies— Depression Scale for Children (CES-DC)	12–18	6th	Yes	20	5–10	Sensitivity: 71% Specificity: 57%/above 14
Center for Epidemiological Studies— Depression Scale (CES-D)	14 and older	6th	No	30	5–10	Sensitivity: 84% Specificity: 75%/above 15
Reynolds Child Depression Scale	8–12	2nd	Yes	30	10–15	Sensitivity: 73% Specificity: 97%/above 73
Reynolds Adolescent Depression Scale	13–18	3rd	No	30	10–15	Alpha: 0.87–0.91; test–retest: 0.80–0.93/refer to manual
Beck Depression Inventory (BDI)	14 and older	6th	Yes	21	5–10	Sensitivity: 84% Specificity: 81%/above 15
ADULTS						
Beck Depression Inventory (BDI)			Yes	21	5–10	Sensitivity: 100% Specificity: 89%/above 15
Beck Depression Inventory—II			Yes	21	5–10	Alpha: 0.92/refer to manual
Beck Depression Inventory-PC (BDI-PC)			Yes	7	Fewer than 5	Sensitivity: 82% Specificity: 92%/above 6
Center for Epidemiological Studies Depression (CES-D)			Yes	20	5–10	Sensitivity: 89% Specificity: 70%/above 15
Edinburgh Postnatal Depression Scale			Yes	10	Fewer than 5	Alpha: 0.87; sensitivity: 85–86%/above 12
Zung Depression Rating Scale			No	20	5–10	Sensitivity: 97% Specificity: 63%/above 49

Information from Beck, 1961; Beck, Steer, & Brown, 1996; Beck, Guth, Steer, & Ball, 1997; Cox, Chapman, Murray, & Jones, 1996; Fendrich, Weissman, & Warner, 1990; Kovacs, 1992; Radloff, 1977; Reynolds, 1986, 1989; Sheikh & Yesavage, 1986; Alexopoulos, Abrams, Young, & Shanoian, 1988; Yesavage, Brink, Rose, Lum, Huang, Adey, et al., 1983; Zung, 1965.

• Biological family history of MDD, BPI, suicide, anxiety disorders, and substance abuse
• Family functioning

The medical workup for a child or adolescent with a mood disorder should include routine pediatric evaluation. Laboratory investigations are at the discretion of the child's primary care physician. Specific medical conditions that may mimic mood disorders should be considered; these are listed in the following table.

Table 17.5 Medically Related Conditions That May Present as Mood Disorder

• Medications (beta-blockers, corticosteroids, benzodiazepines, ranitadine)
• Herbal supplements and remedies
• Drugs of abuse (alcohol, sedatives/hypnotics, cocaine/stimulant withdrawal)
• Over-the-counter medications
• Pregnancy
• Hypothyroidism
• Hyperthyroidism
• B12 deficiency, pellagra (B3 and tryptophan deficiency, high corn diets)
• Cushing's syndrome
• Hypercalcemia
• Hyponatremia
• Diabetes mellitus
• Seizure disorder
• Stroke
• Multiple sclerosis
• Huntington's disease
• Closed head injury
• Viral infections (mononucleosis or influenza)

Once medical conditions have been eliminated as a cause of depression, a psychiatric differential diagnosis needs to be completed. It is important to distinguish depression from other disorders in which depressive symptoms may occur, such as:

• Bipolar I or II.
• Mood disorder due to a general medical condition, in which the mood disorder is due to the direct physiological effects of illness.
• Substance-induced mood disorder, in which the mood disorder is due to the direct physiological effects of a substance, including medication.
• Schizoaffective disorder, which is characterized by 2 weeks of delusions or psychotic symptoms in the absence of prominent mood symptoms.
• Adjustment disorder with depressed mood, which is characterized by depressive symptoms that occur in direct response to an acute stressor.
• Bereavement that occurs in direct response to the loss of a loved one, lasts no more than 2 months, and is not associated with marked functional impairment.
• Nonpathological periods of sadness, which are characterized by short duration, few symptoms, and lack of functional impairment.

Cultural Factors Affecting Assessment

Cultural factors play a significant role in detecting depressive disorders. The tendency to perceive and report distress in psychological or somatic terms is influenced by various social and cultural factors, including the degree of stigma associated with particular symptoms. For example, Hispanic patients may complain of "nerves" (e.g., *ataque de nervios* [American Psychiatric Association, 2000, p. 899]), not depression. Many Chinese-Americans do not consider depressed mood a symptom to report to their physicians and rarely report depressed mood spontaneously. Many are unfamiliar with depression as a treatable psychiatric disorder. Many Chinese-Americans complain of somatic symptoms; only a small few report psychological symptoms such as irritability, rumination, and poor memory. Yet almost all endorse depressed mood when they fill out a survey questionnaire. Most do not know the name of their illness or do not consider it a diagnosable medical illness but attribute their symptoms to preexisting medical problems. Few Chinese-American patients label their illness as a psychiatric condition. Patients generally seek help for their depressive symptoms from general hospitals, lay help, and alternative treaters but rarely from mental health professionals.

Treatment of Depression

Depression may be treated with pharmacotherapy, cognitive–behavioral therapy (CBT), interpersonal therapy (IPT), family therapy, or a combination of these. Medication alone or CBT alone appears to be almost equally effective in the treatment of mild to moderate depression. Treatment rates may increase with the use of both CBT and antidepressant medication concurrently (March et al., 2004). The most current approach to treating adolescent depression emphasizes multimodal intervention programs. It is suggested that the combination of various interventions, such as medication, cognitive–behavioral therapy, and family therapy, may yield the best results for depressed children and adolescents (American Academy of Child and Adolescent Psychiatry Work Group on Quality Issues, 1998; Birmaher et al., 1996a, 1996b).

There is no evidence that psychotherapy alone is effective with severely depressed patients. In general, given the effectiveness of antidepressant medications, most patients with moderate to severe depression will warrant a trial of antidepressant medication in combination with individual and family psychosocial therapies. When psychosis, suicidal ideation, or severe dysfunction is present, medication and perhaps hospitalization are necessary.

Early-onset depression, first occurring in the child or adolescent years, is often episodic with frequent recurrences across the developing years. Effective treatment for depression emphasizes maintenance therapy, either with psychosocial therapies and/or antidepressants, to minimize the severity of episode recurrence. Without maintenance treatment many young patients may experience a recurring course of illness, with serious consequences (Kupfer et al., 1992).

COGNITIVE–BEHAVIORAL THERAPY

CBT is focused on teaching people to recognize fundamental beliefs and expectations that are maladaptive and may influence their behavior and attitudes. Cognitively based techniques are used to change negative views about self, the world, and the future, and behaviorally based techniques are used to modify environmental contingencies and change behavior. The goals are to help the child or adolescent become aware of negative cognitions and the negative impact of these thoughts; and to replace the negative ways of thinking with more positive and constructive thoughts. Techniques such as self-monitoring, self-reinforcement, challenging autonomic thoughts, cognitive restructuring, goal setting, social skills training, and relaxation techniques are used in this approach. Recent meta-analytic reviews have concluded that cognitive–behavioral techniques are effective in the treatment of adolescent depression (Reinecke et al., 1998).

Research evidence indicates that CBT is an effective means of treating adolescent depression and should be used as first-line therapy in mild to moderate depression (March et al., 2004). Mild depression may benefit from psychotherapy alone. Unfortunately, there is no way to predict which individual will benefit from CBT alone. Data suggest that acute, not chronic, mild to moderate MDD symptoms, older age of onset, absence of comorbid psychiatric disorders, and absence of psychosocial stressors are positive predictors of response to CBT alone (Reinecke et al., 1998). Clinical experience suggests that articulateness, intelligence, and insight will also increase the likelihood that CBT will be effective. A 10–20 week course of CBT with follow-up, as needed, provided by a master's- or Ph.D.-level therapist specifically trained in CBT is usually effective. If symptoms have not improved after 2–3 months of CBT, a trial with an SSRI is indicated (American Academy of Child and Adolescent Psychiatry Work Group on Quality Issues, 1998).

INTERPERSONAL THERAPY

This brief therapy approach is a three-phase process that focuses on past and current interpersonal conflict as the basis for depression. The goals of IPT are to decrease depressive symptoms and improve interpersonal relationships. Although originally developed for use with depressed adults, it has been modified for use with adolescents and is referred to in the literature as IPT-A. Preliminary methodologically controlled investigations indicate its effective in treating adolescent depression (Mufson et al., 2004).

FAMILY THERAPY

Family therapy focuses on the role of interactional and reciprocal interpersonal interactions in maintaining depression in the child or adolescent. Individual and family expectations, communication styles, and reward patterns are examined in therapy. This type of therapy is based on the assumption that depressive symptoms represent general dysfunction in the entire family system; and the therapy therefore seeks to improve family communication, alter dysfunctional patterns of interaction, and change maladaptive relationships among family members.

PSYCHODYNAMIC PSYCHOTHERAPY

More than any other intervention approach, psychodynamic therapy attends to developmental issues that are particularly salient during adolescence. This approach assists the adolescent with working on unresolved conflicts. Transference issues, interpretation, and insight are key techniques used. Despite the usefulness of this therapy, there is little methodologically controlled evidence to support its effectiveness.

PSYCHOPHARMACOLOGY IN PEDIATRIC MAJOR DEPRESSIVE DISORDER

Antidepressant use in children and adolescents is currently the subject of controversy. Meta-analytic reviews conducted in the United Kingdom have questioned the risk–benefit profile of antidepressants used in children and adolescents (Whittington et al., 2004). The FDA in the United States reviewed published and unpublished antidepressant studies involving over 4,400 children and adolescents receiving nine different antidepressants for a variety of psychiatric disorders, including depression, obsessive–compulsive disorder, anxiety, and attention-deficit/hyperactivity disorder. The FDA concluded that a small but real risk of increased suicidality existed with the use of antidepressants in pediatric populations, although no deaths by suicide occurred in these medication trials. Antidepressants now carry a black-box warning in the United States discussing the possibility of increased suicidal thinking and dangerous behaviors that can occur in children and adolescents during the early phases of antidepressant treatment. The FDA did not conclude that antidepressants cause suicidality in the young. Rather, they recommended close physician monitoring for suicidality and/or behavioral disinhibition for the first 2 months after the start of antidepressant treatment, when the dose changes, and when discontinuing antidepressant treatment (American Academy of Child and Adolescent Psychiatry, 2004; Yerevanian et al., 2004). In addition, screening of children for possible bipolar disorder prior to antidepressant initiation is now recommended.

Antidepressant medication is warranted when

• Depressive symptoms are severe.
• Symptoms have not been alleviated by psychological and family interventions.
• Psychosis is present.
• Symptoms show no sign of abating.

Available antidepressants and their pediatric dose ranges are given in the following table.

Controlled studies of antidepressants in the child and adolescent populations are presented in the following two tables.

Selective serotonin reuptake inhibitors
SSRIs are currently the antidepressants of choice in pediatric psychopharmacology. Fluoxetine is FDA approved for the treatment of depression in the young (it is also approved for the treatment of obsessive–compulsive disorder in youngsters). Sertraline, paroxetine, and citalopram currently have the support of one controlled study in the treatment of pediatric depression. However, a concern about their use in increasing suicidality in the young exists.

Table 17.6 Available Antidepressant Medications

Drug	Dosage Forms (mg)	Usual Daily Dose (mg/day)	Extreme Dosage (mg/day)	Therapeutic Plasma Levels (ng/mL)
SELECTIVE SEROTONIN REUPTAKE INHIBITORS				
Citalopram (Celexa)	T: 10, 20, 40 LC: 5 mg/5 mL	20–40	10–60	
Fluoxetine (Prozac)	C: 10, 20 LC: 20 mg/5 mL	20	10–80	
Fluvoxamine (Luvox)	T: 25, 50, 100	150–200	50–300	
Escitalopram (Lexapro)	T: 5, 10, 20 LC: 5 mg/5 mL	10–20	5–20	
Paroxetine (Paxil)	T: 10, 20, 30, 40 LC: 10 mg/5 mL CR: 12.5 , 25, 37.5	20	10–50	
Sertraline (Zoloft)	T: 25, 50, 100 LC: 20 mg/1 mL	25–200	50–250	
CYCLIC COMPOUNDS				
Amitriptyline (Elavil and generics)	T: 10, 25, 50, 75, 100, 150 INJ: 10 mg/mL	50–150	50–300	>120[b]
Clomipramine (Anafranil)	C: 25, 50, 75	50–200	50–200	
Desipramine (Norpramin and generics)	T: 10, 25, 50, 75, 100, 150 C: 25, 50	25–150	50–150	>125
Imipramine (Tofranil and generics)	T: 10, 25, 50 C: 75, 100, 125, 150 INJ: 12.5 mg/1 mL	50–200	50–300	>225[a]
Nortriptyline (Pamelor and generics)	C: 10, 25, 50, 75 LC: 0 mg/5 mL	75–100	25–150	50–150
Doxepin (Adapin, Sinequan, and generics)	C: 10, 25, 50, 75, 100, 150 LC: 10 mg/mL	150–200	25–300	100–250
Trimipramine (Surmontil)	C: 25, 50, 100	150–200	50–300	
Protriptyline (Vivactil)	T: 5, 10	15–40	10–60	
Maprotiline (Ludiomil)	T: 25, 50, 75	100–150	50–200	
Amoxapine (Asendin)	T: 25, 50, 100, 150	150–200	50–300	

OTHER COMPOUNDS

Drug	Formulations (mg)		
Bupropion (Wellbutrin)	T: 75, 100 SR: 100, 150, 200 XL: 150, 300	75–225	100–450
Duloxetine (Cymbalta)	C: 20, 30, 60	40–60	40–60
Mirtazapine (Remeron)	T: 15, 30, 45	15–45	7.5–45
Nefazodone	T: 50, 100, 150, 200, 250	200–300	100–600
Trazodone (Desyrel and generics)	T: 50, 100, 150, 300	100–300	100–600
Venlafaxine (Effexor)	T: 25, 37.5, 50, 75, 100 XR: 37.5, 75, 150	75–150	75–225

MONOAMINE OXIDASE INHIBITORS

Drug	Formulations (mg)		
Phenelzine (Nardil)	T: 15	45–60	15–90
Tranylcypromine (Parnate)	T: 10	30–50	10–90

C = capsules; INJ = injectable form; LC = liquid concentrate or solution; SR = slow release; T = tablets; XL, CR, and XR = extended release.
[a]Sum of imipramine plus desipramine.
[b]Sum of amitriptyline plus nortriptyline.

MOOD DISORDERS

351

Table 17.7 TCA Double-Blind Studies in Children with Major Depressive Disorder

Study (year)	N	Diagnostic Assessment	TCA	Dose	Treatment Duration (weeks)	Results
Petti & Law (1982)	6	Clinical	IMI	Up to 5 mg/kg/day	4	IMI ~ placebo
Kashani et al. (1984)	9	DSM-III	AMI	1.5 mg/kg/day	Crossover: each phase 4 weeks	AMI ~ placebo
Preskorn et al. (1986)	30	DICA/DSM-III	IMI	Up to 5 mg/kg/day	6	IMI > placebo
Puig-Antich et al. (1987)	38	K-SADS/RDC	IMI	Up to 5 mg/kg/day	5	IMI ~ placebo
Geller et al. (1989)	50	K-SADS/RDC	NT	"Fixed" plasma level (80 20 ng/ml)	8	NT ~ placebo
Hughes et al. (1990)	31	DICA/DSM-III	IMI	?	6	IMI ~ placebo

TCA = tricyclic antidepressant; DICA = Diagnostic Interview for Children and Adolescents; K-SADS = Schedule for Affective Disorders and Schizophrenia for School-Age Children; RDC = Research Diagnostic Criteria; IMI = imipramine; AMI = amitriptyline; NT = nortriptyline.

Table 17.8 Additional Studies of Antidepressants in Pediatric Psychopharmacology

Study (year)	N/Age in Years/ Duration	Treatment (dose)	Study Design and Measures	% Responders (endpoint analysis): drug vs. PBO
TRICYCLIC ANTIDEPRESSANTS IN ADOLESCENTS				
Kramer & Feiguine (1981)	20/13–17/ 6 weeks	Amitriptyline (200 mg/day) vs. PBO	1–3-week washout; parallel authors' improvement scale	80% vs. 60% (ns)
Geller et al. (1989)	31/12–17/ 8 weeks	Nortriptyline (45–140 mg/day) vs. PBO	2-week PBO washout; parallel CDRS, CGAS	8% vs. 21% (ns)
Kutcher et al. (1994)	42/15–19/ 6 weeks	Desipramine (200 mg/day) vs. PBO	1-week PBO washout; parallel HDRS, BDI, SCL-58	48% vs. 35% (ns)
Kye et al. (1996)	31/12–18/ 6 weeks	Amitriptyline (5 mg/kg/day) vs. PBO	2-week PBO washout, parallel CGI, HDRS, K-SADS-L	90% vs. 90% (ns)
Birmaher et al. (1998)	27/13–17/ 10 weeks	Amitriptyline (average dose: 56 mg/day) vs. PBO	Resistant depression; parallel HDRS, BDI, CGI	77% vs. 79% (ns)
Klein et al. (1998)	45/13–18/ 6 weeks	Desipramine (average dose: 87 mg/day) vs. PBO	2-week PBO washout; parallel CGI, HDRS, K-SADS-L	67% vs. 50% (ns)
SELECTIVE SEROTONIN REUPTAKE INHIBITORS IN CHILDREN AND ADOLESCENTS				
Simeon et al. (1990)	30/13–18/ 7 weeks	Fluoxetine (20–60 mg/day) vs. PBO	1-week PBO washout; parallel HDRS, CGI, SCL-58	66% vs. 66% (ns)
Emslie et al. (1997)	96/8–18/ 8 weeks	Fluoxetine (20 mg/day) vs. PBO	3-week washout; parallel CGI, CDRS	ITT: 56% vs. 33% (p = 0.02) but per protocol 74% vs. 58% (ns)
Milin et al. (1999)	286/13–19/ 12 weeks	Paroxetine (20–40 mg/day) vs. PBO	Parallel K-SADS-L, MADRS	74% vs. 71% (ns)
Keller et al. (2001)	275/13–17/ 8 weeks	Paroxetine (20–40 mg/day) vs. imipramine (200–300 mg/day) vs. PBO	1–2-week washout; parallel CGI, HDRS, K-SADS-L	ITT: 65.6% vs. 52.1% vs. 48.3% (p = 0.02)

(continued)

MOOD DISORDERS

Table 17.8 Additional Studies of Antidepressants in Pediatric Psychopharmacology (Continued)

Study (year)	N/Age in Years/ Duration	Treatment (dose)	Study Design and Measures	% Responders (endpoint analysis): drug vs. PBO
Emslie et al. (2002)	219/8–18/ 8 weeks	Fluoxetine (20 mg/day) vs. PBO	3-week washout; parallel CGI, CDRS	ITT: 65% vs. 53% (ns) but the CDRS-R score was more improved on active drug ($p < 0.01$)
Wagner et al. (2003)	366/6–17/ 10 weeks	Sertraline (50–200 mg/day) vs. PBO	2-week washout; parallel CDRS-R, CGI	ITT: 69% vs. 59% ($p = 0.05$)
Braconnier et al. (2003)	121/12–20/ 8 weeks	Paroxetine (20–40 mg/day) vs. clomipramine (75–150 mg/day)	2-week washout; parallel MADRS, CGI	ITT: 65.1% vs. 48.3% (ns)
Wagner et al. (2004)	174/7–17 8 weeks	Citalopram (20–40 mg/day) vs. PBO	Parallel KSADSL, CDRS	36% vs. 24% ($p < 0.05$)
Emslie et al. (2004)	75/8–18 32 weeks	Fluoxetine (20–60 mg/day) vs. PBO	Randomized relapse prevention, CDRS	Mean time to relapse longer in fluoxetine than PBO group ($p = 0.05$)
March et al. (2004)	439/12–17 12 weeks	Fluoxetine (10–40 mg/day) vs. PBO	Parallel, CDRS	61% vs. 35% ($p = 0.001$)

BDI = Beck Depression Inventory; CDRS = Children's Depression Rating Scale; CGAS = Children's Global Assessment Scale; CGI = Clinical Global Impression—Severity; HDRS = Hamilton Depression Rating Scale; ITT = intent-to-treat analysis; K-SADS-L = Schedule for Affective Disorders and Schizophrenia for Adolescents—Lifetime version, nine-item depression subscale; MADRS = Montgomery–Asberg Depression Rating Scale; PBO = placebo; SCL-58 = 58-item Hopkins Symptom Checklist.
*Results are given according to the protocol primary outcome measure with the exception of the Keller et al. (2001) study, in which the primary outcome measure (HDRS) did not show a significant difference between active drugs and placebo.

There is research suggesting that SSRIs are no more likely to cause suicide in depressed patients compared to other types of antidepressants or placebo (Khan et al., 2003). Additional epidemiological evidence suggests that SSRIs may be beneficial in the young. In the period since 1984, when SSRIs first became available, the rate of completed suicide attempts in the United States has dropped 20%. The national decline in suicide rates appears to be associated with greater use of nontricyclic antidepressants, largely SSRIs (Grunebaum et al., 2004). In Sweden a significant decrease in suicide rates in the adolescent and young adult population temporally coincided with the introduction of the SSRI antidepressants into treatment in that country. This suggests that from an epidemiological perspective, SSRI use may actually decrease suicides in the young (Carlsten et al., 2001). For these reasons and others, SSRIs continue to be valued and prescribed for moderately to severely depressed children and adolescents in the United States.

Available SSRIs consist of six compounds: fluoxetine, sertraline, paroxetine, citalopram, escitalopram, and fluvoxamine. An adequate trial of an SSRI consists of at least 8–12 weeks of medication treatment at maximally tolerated suggested doses. Continued improvement is likely to occur beyond the first 8–12 weeks of treatment. Trials lasting less than 8–12 weeks or at less than maximum tolerated dose may be only partially effective or may fail.

Serotonin norepinephrine reuptake inhibitors

Serotonin norepinephrine reuptake inhibitors (SNRIs) such as venlafaxine and duloxetine have received little attention in pediatric psychopharmacology. Venlafaxine has been studied for ADHD in open-label clinical trials (Motavalli Mukaddes, & Abali, 2004), but no controlled studies have been published to date in pediatric depression. Duloxetine has not yet been studied in pediatric depression.

Tricyclic antidepressants

The tricyclic antidepressants (TCAs) comprise more than 20 compounds. The best studied include imipramine, desipramine, nortriptyline, and amitriptyline. TCAs have FDA approval for the treatment of MDD only in youth at least 12 years of age, despite the fact that MDD is known to occur in children less than 12 years of age. This class of medication has been shown to be effective in several open studies, but there are no double-blind placebo-controlled studies demonstrating benefit over placebo. Although studies generally report success rates of 40–70% for the use of TCAs (Birmaher et al., 1996a), several reviews have concluded that the use of TCAs with adolescents offers no added improvement over placebo treatments. Because of the side effect profile, including possible cardiotoxicity and toxicity in overdose, TCAs should not be considered a first-line choice in the medication treatment of depressive disorders.

Monoamine oxidase inhibitors

Although considered effective for adult depression, monoamine oxidase inhibitors (MAOIs) are not recommended for children and adolescents because of the tyramine-free dietary restrictions imposed by the use of the medication and the difficulties in monitoring food intake in pediatric patients. The use of

MOOD DISORDERS

MAOIs should be reserved for severe depression refractory to any other treatment and when excellent dietary monitoring is assured. Because of the side effect profile, including risks associated with dietary nonadherence and toxicity in overdose, MAOIs should not be considered a first-line choice in the medication treatment of depressive disorders in pediatric psychopharmacology.

Choosing a medication
- SSRIs are the treatment of choice in pediatric MDD.
- Fluoxetine, sertraline, and citalopram all have at least one RCT supporting their safety and efficacy in pediatric MDD.
- Only fluoxetine has been shown to work convincingly (4/4 studies).
- Weaker evidence exists for citalopram (1/3 studies) and sertraline (2 studies when data were aggregated, but neither study alone was sufficiently powered).
- Very weak evidence for paroxetine (only on secondary outcome measures).
  - Paroxetine should be reserved for patients who have failed an adequate trial (maximal dose for at least 8–12 weeks) of the other SSRIs.
- Virtually no evidence exists for the effectiveness of other SSRI/SNRI agents.
- There is no evidence of one SSRI's superiority over another in the treatment of pediatric depressive disorders.

Dose ranges for the commonly used medications to treat depressive disorders in children and adolescents are given in Table 17.5. Based on the above studies it is recommended that fluoxetine be tried first. If the child does not respond, citalopram and sertraline are equally good second agents (the algorithm in Figure 17.2).

Before treatment
- Complete a thorough psychiatric evaluation and document any comorbid psychiatric diagnoses that will be a focus of treatment in addition to MDD.
- Obtain results of a physical exam completed within the 6–12 months prior to initiating therapy.
- Obtain baseline (off medication) rating of depressive symptoms and severity, using an established rating scale.
- Obtain baseline (off medication) rating of symptoms to compare against on-drug reported side effects.
  - Parents may misreport depressive symptoms as side effects of treatment.
- Educate the family about the nature of MDD, expected benefits of drug treatment, possible side effects, use of the medication, and expected duration of treatment.
- Make available written psychoeducational materials about depression and its treatments.
- Determine if the child has any contraindications to antidepressant therapy.

Initiating treatment
Selective serotonin reuptake inhibitors

- Initiate SSRI at the lowest possible dose.
  - Weight-based dosing is not available for SSRIs.

- Titrate dose every 5–7 days until the daily dose is within the therapeutic range.
- Fluoxetine may be given once daily even in young children because if its active metabolites and long half-life.
- If activation, jitteriness, or insomnia occurs as a side effect, reduce the dose and give the majority of the SSRI dose in the morning.
- If sedation is a prominent side effect, give the majority of the SSRI dose in the evening.
- If no response occurs within 2–4 weeks, titrate the SSRI dose into the medium to high dose range for no less than 4 weeks. If no response occurs, switch to a different antidepressant medication.
- High doses of SSRIs other than fluoxetine may require twice daily dosing in young children because of increased metabolism and a shorter half-life compared to adults.

Atypical antidepressants (bupropion, mirtazapine, venlafaxine)
These agents remain poorly studied in pediatric depression and are only briefly mentioned here.

- Bupropion: Generally a treatment for pediatric ADHD, bupropion is occasionally used for adolescent depression. It is generally initiated at a dose of 75 mg/day and titrated upward by 75 mg until a therapeutic dose range between 75 mg and 225 mg/day is achieved. Bupropion is available in immediate-release slow-release, and extended release once daily formulations. The immediate-release compound should be given three times a day to prepubertal children, and twice daily to adolescents. The slow-release formulation should also be given twice a day. Once daily dosing is acceptable with the extended-release bupropion formulation.
- Mirtazapine: Generally not used as a first-line antidepressant treatment. Generally initiated at a dose of 7.5 mg and titrated to a therapeutic dose range between 15 mg and 45 mg given in one or two divided daily doses. As a sedating agent, the majority of the dose should be given at bedtime.
- Venlafaxine: The effective dose range is between 75 mg and 225 mg, generally given in two or three divided daily doses.

Tricyclic antidepressants (imipramine, desipramine, amitriptyline,
and nortriptyline)
- A baseline and on-drug EKG is required for all tricyclic antidepressant use in children and adolescents. EKG parameters for youngsters on tricyclic antidepressants include:
  ○ Heart rate <125 bpm
  ○ QTc <460 msec
  ○ On-drug QTc increase <30% of baseline QTc
  ○ PR interval <0.20 msec
- Baseline and on-drug vital signs are necessary for children and adolescents receiving tricyclic antidepressants.
  ○ Particularly imipramine, which can produce elevated BP and orthostatic hypotension.

M
O
O
D

D
I
S
O
R
D
E
R
S

• Considerable interpatient metabolic variation exists, leading to differing plasma levels on the same dose across different individuals.
  ○ TCA serum levels correlate with toxicity.
• On average, it takes 5–7 days for TCAs to achieve steady state in most children.
• The most common reasons for medication treatment failure are inadequate medication dose and inadequate duration of an antidepressant medication trial.

Imipramine (IMI)
• The only TCA with FDA approval for use in the treatment of MDD in youth 12 years of age and younger.
• Dosing is based on serum levels; the final daily dose ranges between 2–5 mg/kg/day administered in divided daily doses.
• Initiate imipramine at 25 mg to 50 mg for young children or adolescents in the evening.
• Titrate by determining combined imipramine plus desipramine levels on days 7–10.
• Titrate to a trough plasma level of 125–250 ng/ml.
  ○ Use a twice to three times daily dose schedule for prepubertal children.
  ○ Use a twice daily dose schedule for young teenagers.
  ○ Use a once daily dose schedule given in the evening for older teenagers (Tanner Stage 5) and young adults.

Amitriptyline
• Dosing is based on serum levels; the final daily dose ranges between 50 mg and 100 mg or 2–5 mg/kg/day.
• Initiate amitriptyline in the evening at 25 mg to 50 mg. Titrate upward every 5 to 7 days by 25 mg to 50 mg until a therapeutic dose range is achieved.
• Titrate by determining combined amitriptyline plus nortriptyline plasma levels on days 7–10.
• Titrate to a trough plasma level between 125 and 300 ng/ml.
  ○ Use a twice to three times daily dose schedule for prepubertal children.
  ○ Use a twice daily dose schedule for young teenagers.
  ○ Use a once daily dose schedule given in the evening for older teenagers (Tanner Stage 5) and young adults.

Desipramine (DMI)
• Initiate at 10 mg in the evening; the final daily dose ranges between 100 mg and 150 mg per day and 2–3 mg/kg/day administered in divided doses.
  ○ A dose of 150 mg per day should not be exceeded.
• The following clinical parameters are more relevant when titrating desipramine than is an arbitrary maximum amount:
  ○ Serum level (DMI plus 2-OH-DMI) should be kept under 300 ng/ml.
  ○ PR interval on ECG should be less than 200 msec.
  ○ QRS interval on ECG should be less than 120 msec.
  ○ Use a twice to three times daily dose schedule for prepubertal children.

○ Unlike imipramine, there is no significant correlation between DMI plus 2-OH-DMI levels and treatment outcome.
○ Use a once daily dose schedule given in the evening for older teenagers (Tanner Stage 5) and young adults.

Nortriptyline
• Initiate at 10 mg in the evening; the final daily dose ranges between 25 mg and 100 mg per day and 2–3 mg/kg/day administered in divided doses.
○ A dose of 150 mg per day should not be exceeded.
○ In children plasma levels of 60–100 ng/ml are considered therapeutic.
○ In adolescents and adults a plasma level between 50 ng/ml and 150 ng/ml is considered therapeutic.
• Use a twice to three times daily dose schedule for prepubertal children.
• Use once daily for older adolescents (Tanner Stage 5).

Duration of treatment
The treatment of depression is divided into three phases: initiation, continuation, and maintenance. These will vary depending on whether one is treating an initial or recurrent episode of depression.

• Initial antidepressant treatment of the initial depressive episode lasts 6–12 weeks with the goal of achieving symptom remission.
• Continuation antidepressant therapy usually lasts 4–12 months to consolidate remission and prevent relapse of the index depressive episode.
• The goal of maintenance therapy is to prevent recurrence of depressive symptoms.

Most studies of pediatric depressive disorders evaluate acute treatment. There are no controlled clinical trials that evaluate continuation or maintenance, and all recommendations to date have been inferred from adult studies.

The time course to effectiveness varies from medication to medication and from child to child.

• SSRIs may take 2–6 weeks before a treatment effect emerges.
○ A full antidepressant treatment effect may require 8–12 weeks to emerge.
• TCAs may take 2–4 weeks before a treatment effect emerges.
• No medication has immediate effect on depressive symptoms.

A minimum 5-year course of treatment with the same dose and medication used to achieve remission is recommended for adult patients with recurrent MDD (>2 episodes) (Kupfer et al., 1992). Active treatment is an effective means of preventing recurrence beyond 5 years; those adult patients with previous episodes less than 2½ years apart merit continued prophylaxis for at least 5 years. After that time, treatment can cease as long as patients and their families understand not only the high probability of relapse but also the need to restart treatment if symptoms recur. Another strategy is to treat each episode of depression for 6–12 months and then taper therapy. Since recurrence may be

M
O
O
D

D
I
S
O
R
D
E
R
S

infrequent (e.g., once every 8 years), patients should not be treated with pharmacotherapy indefinitely.

Discontinuation of antidepressant therapy

Discontinuation syndromes are related to the sudden discontinuation of compounds with short half-lives. The shorter the half-life of the antidepressant formulation, the greater the likelihood of a discontinuation or withdrawal syndrome. Discontinuation syndromes may mimic recurrence of the disorder or present with the onset of new symptoms. With the exception of fluoxetine, all antidepressants should be gradually discontinued by 10–25% of the full dose every 2–4 days until stopped.

PEDIATRIC DEPRESSION MEDICATION TREATMENT ALGORITHM

An antidepressant treatment algorithm for depressed children and adolescents is presented in the following figure. It is hoped that standardizing medication approaches to the treatment of pediatric depression by the use of algorithms will enhance clinical care and patient outcomes.

Despite FDA concerns about increased suicidality in children and adolescents prescribed SSRI antidepressants, they remain the medication of first choice in the treatment of early-onset depression. Unless there exists a compelling clinical reason not to, fluoxetine should be prescribed as the initial choice, given its indication for pediatric depression by the FDA. If no response to an adequate trial of fluoxetine at an adequate dose occurs in 6–12 weeks, the second step is the prescription of another SSRI. Citalopram, sertraline, and paroxetine all have at least one randomized, controlled trial supporting their effectiveness. If no response occurs to two trials of SSRIs, consideration should be given at step 3 of the treatment algorithm to an antidepressant from another class, such as bupropion, venlafaxine, or mirtazapine.

Antidepressant augmentation strategies have rarely been studied in pediatric psychopharmacology. Results suggest that augmentation strategies are more effective for adult depression than for early-onset depressive disorders. Augmentation strategies include some of the following:

• Combining two different types of antidepressants that have different mechanisms of action; for example, coprescribing an SSRI and bupropion for treatment-resistant depression in an adolescent.
• Lithium augmentation: Adding lithium to the monotherapy of adolescents who remain depressed has been studied in open-label trials and found somewhat effective in depressed adolescents (Strober et al., 1992).

Treatment of depression subtypes

• *Psychotic depression*: Depression complicated by psychotic symptoms occurs when delusions, hallucinations, or illogical and disorganized thinking accompanies severe MDD. True psychotic depression is rare in prepubertal children, but increases in frequency in the adolescent years. It is important for the clinician to recognize psychotic symptoms in a severely depressed teenager, because this type of MDD requires combined pharmacotherapy with

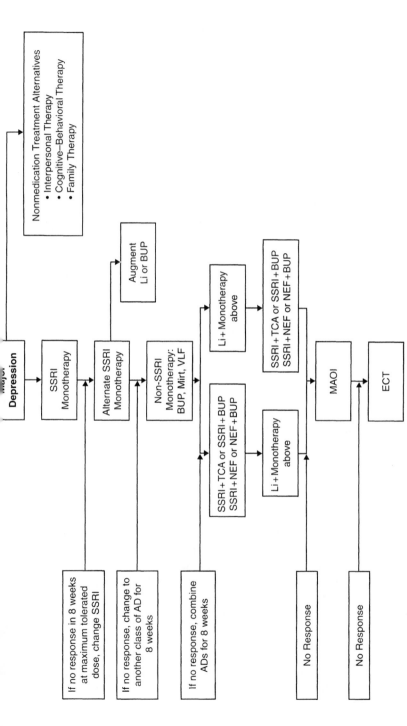

Figure 17.2 Major depression treatment algorithm.

AD = antidepressant; BUP = bupropion; CBT = cognitive–behavioral therapy; ECT = electroconvulsive therapy;
Li = lithium; MAOI = monoamine oxidase inhibitor; Mirt = mirtazapine; NEF = nefazodone; SSRI = selective serotonin reuptake inhibitor; TCA = tricycic antidepressant; VLF = venlafaxine. *Information from Birmaher et al., 2003; Crismon et al., 1999; Hughes et al., 1999.*

MOOD DISORDERS

an antidepressant and an antipsychotic. MDD with psychotic features rarely responds to monotherapy alone (Matthews et al., 2002).

• *Seasonal affective disorder* (SAD): A relatively common cyclical depressive illness characterized by seasonal depressions during winter. It has not been well studied in the pediatric age range. In adults, SAD responds to SSRIs (Moscovitch et al., 2004) or full-spectrum light therapy (Wileman et al., 2001).

• *Adjustment disorder with depressed mood*: Occurring after an environmental stressor, adjustment disorder generally presents with a mild depression and responds to psychotherapy. It is usually time-limited, and medications are rarely required.

BIPOLAR DISORDERS

Description and Diagnostic Features

Bipolar illness (BPI) and bipolar spectrum disorders can occur in children and adolescents and are not as rare as previously thought. Early-onset bipolar disorder in children and adolescents and the discrimination of bipolar disorder from commonly occurring conditions in the pediatric years, such as attention-deficit/hyperactivity disorder (ADHD), is an area of active clinical research (Carlson et al., 2003; Coyle et al., 2003; Leibenluft et al., 2003).

Kraeplin proposed a unitary concept of manic–depressive illness approximately a century ago. Bipolar illness may exist on a spectrum of severity, ranging from problematic mood and affective instability to low-grade sustained mood changes, such as described in the clinical diagnosis of cyclothymia, to hypomania, and finally to frank mania (Kahana et al., 2003). Youth with BPI and its spectrum disorders often exhibit poor academic performance, disturbed interpersonal relationships, legal difficulties, high rates of suicide attempts and completions, high rates of comorbidity with other psychiatric disorders such as ADHD and conduct disorder, and increased rates of substance abuse. Early recognition is the key to effectively treating these often-complicated patients.

Diagnostic criteria for a manic episode, bipolar disorder, hypomanic episode, and cyclothymia are given in the following tables.

The DSM uses a categorical model for making a psychiatric diagnosis. These categorical diagnoses are based on the presence or absence of clusters of signs and symptoms. This method has a high level of reliability but, because it is not based on any etiological factors, diagnostic boundaries in bipolar spectrum illnesses are, to some degree, arbitrary. For example, in DSM-III a manic episode had to last 7 days to meet the duration criteria for bipolar illness. In DSM-III–R the 7-day criterion was dropped in favor of an illness impairment criterion in occupational or social functioning or the requirement of hospitalization because of bipolar disorder. In DSM-IV, the 7-day duration criterion returns with the addition that a shorter duration of illness meets diagnostic threshold criteria for bipolar disorder if symptoms are severe enough to require hospitalization. The division of bipolar disorder into discreet categories may have a great deal of utility in research settings, some utility in adult outpatient psychiatry, less so in adult inpatient psychiatry, and very little utility in pediatric and geriatric psychiatry.

Table 17.9 Diagnostic Criteria for Manic Episode

A. A distinct period of abnormally and persistently elevated, expansive, or irritable mood, lasting at least 1 week (or any duration if hospitalization is necessary).

B. During the period of mood disturbance, three (or more) of the following symptoms have persisted (four if the mood is only irritable) and have been present to a significant degree:
   (1) Inflated self-esteem or grandiosity
   (2) Decreased need for sleep (e.g., feels rested after only 3 hours of sleep)
   (3) More talkative than usual or pressure to keep talking
   (4) Flight of ideas or subjective experience that thoughts are racing
   (5) Distractibility (i.e., attention too easily drawn to unimportant or irrelevant external stimuli)
   (6) Increase in goal-directed activity (either socially, at work or school, or sexually) or psychomotor agitation
   (7) Excessive involvement in pleasurable activities that have a high potential for painful consequences (e.g., engaging in unrestrained buying sprees, sexual indiscretions, or foolish business investments)

C. The symptoms do not meet criteria for a Mixed Episode.

D. The mood disturbance is sufficiently severe to cause marked impairment in occupational functioning or in usual social activities or relationships with others, or to necessitate hospitalization to prevent harm to self or others, or there are psychotic features.

E. The symptoms are not due to the direct physiological effects of a substance (e.g., a drug of abuse, a medication, or other treatment) or a general medical condition (e.g., hyperthyroidism).

Note: Manic-like episodes that are clearly caused by somatic antidepressant treatment (e.g., medication, electroconvulsive therapy, light therapy) should not count toward a diagnosis of Bipolar I Disorder.

American Psychiatric Association. Desk Reference to the Diagnostic Criteria from DSM-IV to TR. Washington, DC, American Psychiatric Association, pp. 169–170, 2000. Reprinted with permission.

Table 17.10 Specifiers of Bipolar I Disorder

Single Manic Episode
• The patient has had just one Manic Episode and no Major Depressive Episodes.
• Schizoaffective disorder doesn't explain the Manic Episode better, and it isn't superimposed on Schizophrenia, Schizophreniform Disorder, Delusional Disorder, or Psychotic Disorder Not Otherwise Specified.

Specify Mixed: If a single episode meets the criteria for Mixed Episode, it would be recorded, for example:
Axis I 296.02 Bipolar I Disorder, Single Manic Episode, Mixed, Moderate
Include any specifiers that apply to this Manic Episode.

Most Recent Episode Manic
• The patient's most recent episode is of mania.
• The patient has had at least one Major Depressive, Manic or Mixed Episode.
• Schizoaffective disorder doesn't explain the above episodes better, and they aren't superimposed on Schizophrenia, Schizophreniform Disorder, Delusional Disorder, or Psychotic Disorder Not Otherwise Specified.

Include any specifiers that apply to this Manic Episode or to the overall course of the disorder.

Most Recent Episode Hypomanic
• The patient's most recent episode is hypomanic.
• The patient has previously had one or more Manic or Mixed Episodes.
• The symptoms cause clinically important distress or impair work, social, or personal functioning.
• Schizoaffective disorder doesn't explain the above episodes better, and they aren't superimposed on Schizophrenia, Schizophreniform Disorder, Delusional Disorder, or Psychotic Disorder Not Otherwise Specified.

Include any specifiers that apply to the overall course of the disorder.

Most Recent Episode Mixed
• The patient's most recent episode is of mixed mania and depression.
• The patient has had at least one Major Depressive, Manic, or Mixed Episode.

(continued)

MOOD DISORDERS

Table 17.10 Specifiers of Bipolar I Disorder (Continued)

• Schizoaffective disorder doesn't explain the above episodes better, and they aren't superimposed on Schizophrenia, Schizophreniform Disorder, Delusional Disorder, or Psychotic Disorder Not Otherwise Specified.

Include any specifiers that apply to this Mixed Episode or to the overall course of the disorder.

Most Recent Episode Depressed
• The patient's most recent episode is Major Depressive.
• The patient has had at least one previous Manic or Mixed Episode.
• Schizoaffective disorder doesn't explain the above episodes better, and they aren't superimposed on Schizophrenia, Schizophreniform Disorder, Delusional Disorder, or Psychotic Disorder Not Otherwise Specified.

Include any specifiers that apply to this Major Depressive Episode or to the overall course of the disorder.

Most Recent Episode Unspecified
• Other than duration, the patient currently or recently meets criteria for Major Depressive, Manic, Mixed, or Hypomanic episode.
• The patient has had at least one previous Manic or Mixed episode.
• These symptoms cause clinically important distress or impair work, social, or personal functioning.
• Schizoaffective disorder doesn't explain the above episodes better, and they aren't superimposed on Schizophrenia, Schizophreniform Disorder, Delusional Disorder, or Psychotic Disorder Not Otherwise Specified.
• The symptoms are not directly caused by a general medical condition or the use of substances, including prescription medications.

Include any specifiers that apply to the overall course of the disorder.

American Psychiatric Association. *Diagnostic and Statistical Manual, of Mental Disorders* (4th ed.). Washington, DC, American Psychiatric Association, pp. 355–358, 1994. Reprinted with permission.

Table 17.11 Diagnostic Criteria for Hypomanic Episode

A. A distinct period of persistently elevated, expansive, or irritable mood, lasting throughout at least 4 days, that is clearly different from the usual nondepressed mood.
B. During the period of mood disturbance, three (or more) of the following symptoms have persisted (four if the mood is only irritable) and have been present to a significant degree:
   (1) Inflated self-esteem or grandiosity
   (2) Decreased need for sleep (e.g., feels rested after only 3 hours of sleep)
   (3) More talkative than usual or pressure to keep talking
   (4) Flight of ideas or subjective experience that thoughts are racing
   (5) Distractibility (i.e., attention too easily drawn to unimportant or irrelevant external stimuli)
   (6) Increase in goal-directed activity (either socially, at work or school, or sexually) or psychomotor agitation
   (7) Excessive involvement in pleasurable activities that have a high potential for painful consequences (e.g., the person engages in unrestrained buying sprees, sexual indiscretions, or foolish business investments)
C. The episode is associated with an unequivocal change in functioning that is uncharacteristic of the person when not symptomatic.
D. The disturbance in mood and the change in functioning are observable by others.
E. The episode is not severe enough to cause marked impairment in social or occupational functioning, or to necessitate hospitalization, and there are no psychotic features.
F. The symptoms are not due to the direct physiological effects of a substance (e.g., a drug of abuse, a medication, or other treatment) or a general medical condition (e.g., hyperthyroidism).

Note: Hypomanic-like episodes that are clearly caused by somatic antidepressant treatment (e.g., medication, electroconvulsive therapy, light therapy) should not count toward a diagnosis of Bipolar II Disorder.

American Psychiatric Association. *Desk Reference to the Diagnostic Criteria from DSM-V–TR*. Washington, DC, American Psychiatric Association, pp. 171–172, 2000. Reprinted with permission.

Table 17.12 Diagnostic Criteria for Cyclothymic Disorder

- For at least 2 years,* the patient has had many periods of hypomanic symptoms and many periods of low mood that don't fulfill criteria for Major Depressive Disorder. The longest the patient has been free of mood swings during this period is 2 months.
- During the first 2 years of this disorder, the patient has not fulfilled criteria for Manic, Mixed, or Major Depressive Episode.
- Schizoaffective disorder doesn't explain the disorder better, and it isn't superimposed on Schizophrenia, Schizophreniform Disorder, Delusional Disorder, or Psychotic Disorder Not Otherwise Specified.
- The symptoms are not directly caused by a general medical condition or the use of substances, including prescription medications.
- These symptoms cause clinically important distress or impair work, social, or personal functioning.

Coding Notes
* In children and adolescents, the time required is only 1 year. After the required 2 years (1 for children), a Manic, Mixed, or Major Depressive Episode may be superimposed on the Cyclothymia. Then, a Bipolar I or II diagnosis may be made concomitant with Cyclothymic Disorder.

American Psychiatric Association. *Diagnostic and Statistical Manual of Mental Disorders,* (4th ed.). Washington, DC, American Psychiatric Association, pp. 365–366, 1994. Reprinted with permission.

Research on bipolar disorder in the pediatric population suggests that the illness may present differently in children and adolescents than in adults (Geller et al., 2002a, 2002b). Prodromal symptoms can appear early—before kindergarten in some children. Early-onset bipolar illness often does not fulfill strict DSM criteria for mania or depression, but has characteristics of rapid cycling and mixed depressive and manic features.

Researchers are beginning to define the characteristics of early-onset pediatric bipolar disorder. Leibenluft and colleagues (2003) give four definitions of bipolarity across three phenotypes in the pediatric population that may prove useful to researchers and clinicians:

- Phenotype 1: Children or adolescents who meet the strict adult DSM-IV criteria for mania or hypomania.
- Phenotype 2A: Those who meet the full symptom criteria but not the duration criteria.
- Phenotype 2B: Those children or adolescents characterized by irritability, not euphoria, and who also meet bipolar duration criteria.
- Phenotype 3: Children and adolescents whose symptoms tend to be more chronic and continuous on a daily basis, rather than episodic.

The fourth category is a rather broad phenotype and is better characterized by mood disorder NOS than bipolar II or bipolar NOS. Symptomatically, Phenotype 2 children present with pervasive irritability, not euphoria or grandiosity. Leibenluft and colleagues (2003) suggest that the early onset of bipolar illness is a complex and heterogeneous disorder representing a severe syndrome characterized by high rates of psychiatric comorbidity, especially ADHD and conduct disorder.

Comorbidity

The identification of BPI and its disorders is often difficult to distinguish from other disorders of childhood. Many youngsters meeting diagnostic criteria for bipolar disorder also meet diagnostic criteria for other comorbid psychiatric disorders—particularly ADHD, MDD, oppositional and conduct disorders, substance use disorders, and aggression. Untangling bipolar illness and ADHD has been a particularly knotty problem in both research and practice.

• *ADHD*: Both ADHD and early-onset bipolar disorders share many clinical symptoms in common. These include impulsivity, irritability and aggression, oppositional behaviors and conduct problems, increased activity, sleep problems, increased rates of adolescent substance abuse, and marked daily impairment. Distinguishing ADHD from early-onset BPI is important because recommended treatments differ. ADHD responds to stimulants and noradrenergic antidepressants. BPI responds to mood stabilizers and atypical antipsychotics. Indeed, stimulants and antidepressants may worsen the clinical symptoms of early-onset bipolar disorder and precipitate mania. Thus distinguishing the two disorders is clinically important.
• Complicating the clinical picture are high rates of comorbidity between the two disorders. Anywhere from 57% to 98% of children with manic symptoms also meet criteria for ADHD. Anywhere from 11% to 23% of children with ADHD also meet diagnostic criteria for BPI (Kim & Miklowitz, 2002). However, research suggests that the two disorders may be clinically distinguished by the presence of five symptoms found in manic children that are not as prevalent in children with ADHD (Geller et al., 2002a, 2002b):
  ○ Grandiosity
  ○ Elation
  ○ Decreased need for sleep without feeling tired or fatigued the nextday
  ○ Racing thoughts
  ○ Hypersexuality in the absence of a history of sexual abuse or neglect
• *Unipolar depression*: Most commonly, adolescents with bipolar disorder present to the clinician with a new-onset depression. About 70% of individuals with an adolescent onset of BPI will have an initial presentation of MDD. About one-third of prepubertal-onset children with depression and about one-fifth of teenage-onset depressives will eventually develop mania. In adolescents, the mean onset of manic symptoms occurs about 4 years after the initial depressive episode, and after two to four depressive episodes have occurred. In such patients it is difficult to distinguish unipolar depression from latent BPI in the absence of any history of mania or the presence of manic symptoms. The distinction is clinically important, however, because standard treatments with antidepressant medications run the risk of precipitating a manic episode in these youths. Characteristics of depression that may help distinguish adolescents presenting with depression who may go on to pursue a bipolar outcome include (DelBello et al., 2003; Strober et al., 1993):
  ○ A biological family history of affective disorders characterized by multiple generations with either unipolar or bipolar illness
  ○ A rapid onset of severe depression
  ○ Psychomotor retardation
  ○ Depression with psychotic features
  ○ Manic activation upon exposure to antidepressant medications

• *Conduct disorder*: Overlapping features of mania and conduct disorder include irritability, hostility, and impulsivity. Inappropriate sexual behaviors and displays of poor judgement, such as stealing parents' credit cards, are also behaviors associated with both BPI and conduct disorder. There exists an elevated risk for conduct disorder among children and adolescents with BPI. Studies have reported a 42–69% rate of CD in youth meeting diagnostic criteria for BPI (Biederman et al., 2003). This research recommends evaluating CD youth for symptoms of BPI, which may be treatable.

• *Substance use disorders*: Research with adolescents meeting criteria for BPI suggests high rates of substance use disorders compared to non-BPI teenagers (Wilens et al., 2004). Findings suggest that BPI, independently of conduct disorder, is a significant risk factor for substance use disorder.

Prevalence

Bipolar disorder affects 0.5–1.5% of individuals in the United States; both males and females are affected equally. Bipolar II is somewhat more common in adult women. A recent community study of adults found that the rate of bipolar I and bipolar II disorders was 3.7%. In adults the bipolar spectrum disorders may be more frequent than the "classic" manic–depressive illness, with lifetime prevalence rates of 3–6.5%. The typical age at onset is late adolescence or early adulthood, placing women at risk for episodes throughout their reproductive years.

Course of Illness

Bipolar disorders are generally episodic, lifelong illnesses with a variable course. The disorder usually begins in early childhood or late adolescence with a peak incidence between 15 and 19 years of age.

• About one-fifth of bipolar adults first experienced symptoms before age 19.
• Around 60% of adults with BPI were younger than 19 years when bipolar symptoms first appeared.
• One-third of patients have symptom onset before age 13.
• Kraepelin found onset of BPI before age 10 in only 0.3% of his adult patients.

Findings from follow-up studies are mixed but trend toward poor evidence for continuity of manic symptoms from the pediatric age range to early adolescence. Follow-up from adolescents who endorse subsyndromal manic symptoms, including hypomania and cyclothymia, report progression to a young adult population with generally high rates of major depression, personality disorder, and anxiety, but not necessarily frank bipolar illness (Hazell et al., 2003).

Geller and her colleagues (2004) recently described the time to recovery from an episode of prepubertal mania. In a 4-year prospective, longitudinal study of 86 children with a mean age of 6.9 years, they found that the time to recovery was 60.2 weeks. In 70 of the children the episode under study was the index episode. Neither gender nor prepubertal status was predictive of mania. The 51 children with mania and psychosis were ill significantly more weeks than the 35 children without baseline psychosis.

Assessment

The assessment of children and adolescents with BPI includes a comprehensive psychiatric evaluation that reviews current and past mood symptoms and comorbid psychiatric disorders. An adequate evaluation obtains information from multiple sources, including the child, parents, and reports on school functioning and interpersonal relationships. Symptoms of BPI must be distinguished from more common childhood mood disorders, conduct disorder, and ADHD and take into account normal developmental excitability. Excitability that is pleasurable, readily suppressible, and does not interfere with daily functioning is not considered symptomatic of BPI or its disorders. These are in contrast to intense mood episodes that are recurrent, bothersome, and interfere with daily functioning. In those suspected of suffering from BPI, an assessment of substance use and suicidal ideation should occur.

Assessment of the child should include:
• Identification of specific symptoms and their frequency, context, and associated degree of impairment
• An assessment of depression and a history of any associated depressive disorders.
  ○ Some patients experience more than one depressive episode prior to their first manic episode.
• The child or adolescent's insight into the symptoms
• Comorbid depression and/or anxiety symptoms
• Comorbid psychotic thinking
• Comorbid suicidality
• Comorbid substance use disorders
• The context, onset, and longitudinal course of symptoms

Assessment of the family should include:
• The degree to which parents and siblings have become entangled in the BPI child's symptoms
• Family dysfunction caused by the BPI symptoms
• Biological family history of BPI and its spectrum disorders, MDD and its spectrum disorders, ADHD, anxiety disorders, and substance abuse disorders

Once a diagnosis of BPI is established, symptom severity can be determined with the use of a reliable and valid parent-report measure, such as the Young Mania Rating Scale (Gracious et al., 2002).

TREATMENT OF PEDIATRIC BIPOLAR ILLNESS

BPI is a spectrum disorder. The nature and severity of symptoms, the degree of comorbid psychopathology, and the impact of the disorder on child and family functioning vary significantly in youngsters with BPI. Mild symptoms such as elevated mood, affective instability, or hypomanic symptoms that are not the source of distress may only warrant monitoring over time without specific treatment interventions.

Psychosocial Therapies

Child- and family-focused cognitive–behavioral therapy is a new and promising psychosocial intervention for pediatric bipolar disorder (Pavuluri et al., 2004). The theoretical framework is based on (1) the specific problems of children and families coping with early-onset bipolar disorder, (2) a biological theory of excessive reactivity in bipolar disorder, and (3) the role of environmental stressors in outcome. Although not sufficient alone for the treatment of BPI, adjunctive individual and family therapy is often useful clinically to help the child and family better understand their child's symptoms and disentangle themselves from the child's behavior at home. Family psychoeducational groups and interventions have been found beneficial for families of children with bipolar disorder (Fristad et al., 2002; Miklowitz et al., 2000).

Psychopharmacology

Psychopharmacology is the principal treatment modality for early-onset bipolar disorders. However, psychopharmacology should never be the sole treatment prescribed, but should occur within the context of a multimodality psychoeducational treatment plan. Specific goals of psychiatric management include

- Establishing and maintaining a therapeutic alliance
- Monitoring the patient's psychiatric status
- Providing education about bipolar disorder
- Enhancing treatment compliance
- Promoting regular patterns of activity and sleep
- Anticipating stressors
- Identifying new mood episodes early in their course
- Assessing any suicidal thoughts or plans, and minimizing functional impairments

Treating bipolar disorder includes treating the acute phase of manic or depressive episodes and preventing recurrence of both manic and depressive episodes. In adults the atypical antipsychotics risperidone, olanzapine, quetiapine, ziprasidone, and aripiprazole have been FDA approved for the treatment of acute mania. Mood stabilizers approved for the treatment of adult bipolar illness include lithium, divalproex, and long-acting carbamazepine. The treatment of bipolar depression remains problematic because antidepressants may precipitate manic episodes in previously stable adults with manic–depressive illness. A combination of olanzapine and fluoxetine has recently been FDA approved for treatment of depression in adult bipolar illness. The mood stabilizer lamotrigine has also been FDA approved for maintenance treatment in bipolar illness and may have effectiveness for depression.

However, research in pediatric psychopharmacolgy for the treatment of early-onset BPI is not sufficiently advanced to inform clinicians specifically about treatment in children and adolescents. Pediatric clinical practice in this area is largely influenced by the adult literature. Pertinent studies of BPI in the pediatric age range are presented in the following table.

MOOD DISORDERS

Table 17.13 FDA-Approved Treatments of Adult *Bipolar Disorder*

Therapy	Acute Mania	Acute Mixed Episode	Bipolar Depression	Bipolar Maintenance
Lithium	X[a]			X
Valproic acid	X[b]			
Lamotrigine			X	X
Olanzapine	X	X		X
Quetiapine	X			
Ziprasidone	X	X		
Risperidone	X	X		
Aripiprazole	X	X		
Olanzapine + fluoxetine			X	

Note: There are no FDA approved indications for medications other than lithium and valproic acid in patients less than 18 years of age.

[a]Lithium monotherapy is approved for both acute mania and bipolar maintenance in patients 12 years of age and older.

[b]Valproate is approved for acute mania in patients 18 years of age and older.

X = FDA approval

These studies suggest that combination therapy, either with an atypical antipsychotic and a mood stabilizer or a combination of two mood stabilizers, is more effective for early-onset BPI than monotherapy. Similar to bipolar adults, children and adolescents with BPI may frequently require combined pharmacotherapy (Kowatch et al., 2003).

Choosing a Medication

Medications for the treatment of pediatric bipolar disorder are presented in Table 17.12.

LITHIUM

Lithium is FDA approved for treatment of the manic episodes of BPI and for maintenance therapy in patients with a history of BPI who are 12 years of age or older. The efficacy of divalproex and olanzapine are measured against lithium. Even though lithium is the best-established treatment for bipolar mania, there is a trend away from its use in favor of other mood stabilizers. This may be due to the range of adverse effects of lithium, the need for adjunctive treatments for psychotic and agitated symptoms, and the clinical difficulty of monitoring levels and physiological parameters that has made the choice of lithium less than desirable. Despite this lack of desirability, lithium remains a remarkably effective treatment, especially in the care of "pure" euphoric mania. The most common difficulty with the use of lithium is underdosing. Lithium serum levels should be maintained at 0.8–1.2 mEq/ml. Many patients tolerate lithium well for long periods, but there is a wide range of potential side effects, the most problematic being life-threatening overdose. Lithium is a drug with a narrow therapeutic index and requires close clinical monitoring.

Before treatment
• Complete a thorough psychiatric evaluation and document any comorbid psychiatric diagnoses that will be a focus of treatment in addition to BPI.

Table 17.14 Medication Studies of Child and Adolescent Bipolar Illness

Study (year)	Drug	Methodology	Sample Size	Age (yrs)	Outcome
Chang et al. (2003)	Divalproex	Open: Children with mood or behavioral symptoms and a parent with BPI	24	6–18	78% responders
DelBello et al. (2002)	Quetiapine + divalproex	RCT	30	12–18	Combination > divalproex monotherapy
Findling Calabrese, et al. (2003)	Divalproex + lithium	Open	90	5–17	Combination effective and safe
Frazier et al. (2001)	Olanzapine	Open	23	5–14	61% responders
Kafantaris et al. (2003)	Lithium	Open	100	12–18	63% responders
Kafantaris et al. (2004)	Lithium	RCT	40	12–18	No difference from placebo
Wagner et al. (2002)	Divalproex	Open	40	7–19	Improvement

RCT = randomized controlled trial

MOOD DISORDERS

371

Table 17.15 Medications Used in the Treatment of Bipolar Disorder in Children and Adolescents

Medication	Usual Daily Starting Dose	Titration Schedule	Target Therapeutic and Maximum Dose	Common Adverse Events	Warnings	Initial Laboratory Tests	Monitoring
Lithium	300–1200 mg	150 mg bid; increase 150 mg q 3 days as indicated	300–900 mg/day; therapeutic levels 0.6 to 1.2 mEq/L qd or bid	Nausea, vomiting, diarrhea, headache, polyuria, polydipsia, tremor, weight gain, fatigue, acne	Neurotoxicity, hypothyroidism, renal function abnormal, NIDDM, proteinuria	CBC w/diff, electrolytes, Ca and PO4, BUN/CR, thyroid function tests	q 2 months Li level 12 hrs post last dose or A.M. before first dose
ANTICONVULSANTS							
Divalproex	15 mg/kg in adolescents; 10 mg/kg in young children	Dose increase: 5–10 mg/kg/day weekly	Plasma level of 50–125 µg/mL	Nausea, vomiting, sedation, weight gain	Hepatic failure, pancreatitis, thrombocytopenia, behavioral deterioration	CBC w/diff blood chemistries, LFTs, platelets, pregnancy test, plasma levels	CBC, platelets, and serum level should be obtained q 3–6 months
Carbamazepine	100–200 mg	100 mg weekly as tolerated	Plasma level 4–12 µg/mL	Nausea, vomiting, dizziness, sedation, rash	Agranulocytosis, aplastic anemia, hepatic toxicity, multiple drug interactions	CBC w/diff, LFTs, platelets, pregnancy test, plasma levels	Plasma levels should be obtained q 3–4 days after dose initiation and upon increasing dose.
Lamotrigine	12.5 mg; double the dose with carbamazepine, halve the dose with divalproex	12.5 mg/day q 2 weeks	200–400 mg/day	Nausea, ataxia, vomiting, constipation; serious adverse	Stevens–Johnson syndrome (prevalence < 1%)	CBC, blood chemistries, LFTs	Parents should be informed to contact the physician if child develops rash
ANTIPSYCHOTICS							
Olanzapine	2.5 mg	2.5–5 mg increments q 5 days	20–40 mg/day	Weight gain, sedation	None	CBC, blood chemistries, LFTs, fasting glucose, lipids, cholesterol	Weight should be monitored throughout treatment
Risperidone	0.5 mg; 0.25 mg for young children	Dose increments: 0.5 mg/day	0.25–6 mg/day	Weight gain, sedation	Hepatotoxicity, hyperprolactinemia, orthostatic BP	CBC, blood chemistries, LFTs	Weight monitoring
Quetiapine	50 mg	Dose increments: 50 mg/day	800 mg/day	Orthostatic hypotension, dizziness, tachycardia, somnolence, weight gain	Development of cataracts	CBC, blood chemistries, LFTs, slit lamp	Examination of the eye lens to detect cataract formation at initiation of quetiapine
Ziprasidone	20 mg	Dose increments: 20–40 mg every 5–7 days	160 mg	EKG QTc prolongation	Cardiac history	EKG, CBC, blood chemistries, LFTs	EKG, weight monitoring
Aripiprazole	1–10 mg	1–5 mg q 5–7 days	1–30 mg	Orthostatic hypotension, dizziness, tachycardia, somnolence	None	CBC, blood chemistries, LFTs	Weight monitoring

Note. All information is based on open studies and case reports.

- Obtain results of a physical examination completed within the 6–12 months prior to initiating therapy.
- Obtain baseline laboratory studies, including renal function tests, serum creatinine, CBC and differential, thyroid function tests (TSH), EKG, pregnancy testing in females of child-bearing age, electrolytes, serum calcium, and serum phosphorus levels.
- Obtain a baseline level of BPI symptom severity using an established rating scale.
- Obtain baseline ratings of drug side effects to compare against on-drug reported side effects.
- Educate the family about the nature of BPI, expected benefits of drug treatment, possible side effects, use of the medication, and expected duration of treatment.
- Determine if the child has any contraindications to lithium therapy, such as pregnancy, cardiac disease, renal disease, and/or thyroid disease.

Initiating treatment
- Initiate lithium at 0.5–1.5 g/m^2 in two divided daily doses for the acute phase of treatment.
- Serum levels must guide therapy.
- Serum levels, not oral dose, are correlated with both lithium benefit and toxicity.
- Obtain levels until two consecutive levels are in the therapeutic range.
- Standards for interpreting lithium levels are based on trough measurements taken 12 hours after an oral dose (usually immediately before the first A.M. dose).
- After initiating a dose change, serum levels should be obtained on the morning of the 5th day before the A.M. dose has been taken.
- Maintain the lithium dose for 5 days to achieve steady state before obtaining next level.
- The therapeutic range is a serum lithium level of 0.6–1.2 mEq/L.
- Do not exceed a serum level of 1.4 mEq/L; *lithium is toxic at high serum levels.*
- The dose may be adjusted based on serum level, side effects, or clinical response.
- Immediate-release tablets are usually given three or four times daily, whereas controlled-release tablets are usually given twice daily.

ANTICONVULSANT MOOD STABILIZERS

Divalproex
Divalproex is approved for the treatment of acute mania in adults, and a few reports have suggested that it may even be more effective in adult cases where dysphoria or a mixed manic–depressed state is present. As with lithium, high serum levels may be necessary in order for some patients to achieve their maximum clinical improvement. Side effects such as weight gain, gastrointestinal distress, and hair loss are common and are more likely to occur at higher doses. Hepatic abnormalities are intermediate in their occurrence, whereas pancreatitis, thrombocytopenia, and polycystic ovary disorder occur rarely.

Before treatment
- CBC, differential, and platelet counts
- Liver function tests
- Concentrations of concomitant antiepileptic drugs
- Serum amylase level

Initiating treatment
- The therapeutic range of divalproex in acute mania is 50–125 mcg/mL.
  ○ Occasionally patients may be controlled with serum levels lower or higher than this range.
- The recommended initial dose is 15 mg/kg/day orally.
- Increase the dose at 1-week intervals by 5–10 mg/kg/day until symptoms are controlled or side effects preclude further dose increases.
- The maximum recommended dose of divalproex in children and adolescents is 60 mg/kg/day.
- Patients who experience gastrointestinal irritation may benefit from administration of divalproex with food or by a slow progressive dosage increase from an initial low level.
- Divalproex sodium capsules should be swallowed without chewing to avoid local irritation of the mouth and throat.
- A good correlation has not been established between daily dose, serum levels, and therapeutic effect.
- When the total daily dose exceeds 250 mg/day, divalproex should be given in a divided daily regimen.

Carbamazepine
Carbamazepine is less widely used in recent years for BPI due to the fact that it is complex to dose, may cause rash, and has multiple side effects. Studies of its efficacy have been conflicting; although clearly effective in some adult patients, at least one early study suggested that short-term benefit was not sustained in the longer term. More recent results have suggested that lithium is more effective in patients with classical bipolar disorder, but that carbamazepine may conceivably have a role in patients with nonclassical features. A long-acting formulation of carbamazepine was recently FDA approved for treatment of adult BPI. Carbamazepine has also been used in combination with lithium, particularly in patients unresponsive to either drug alone; there are suggestions that the combination may be more effective than monotherapy, particularly in patients with a history of rapid cycling.

Carbamazepine has not been as well studied in pediatric psychopharmacology as it has been in pediatric seizure disorders and adult psychopharmacology. To date there are no randomized, placebo-controlled clinical trials of carbamazepine in the treatment of pediatric bipolarity.

Before treatment
- Blood count, differential, and platelets
- Hepatic function tests (AST, alkaline phosphatase)
- Serum sodium and osmolality

- Thyroid function tests (TSH)
- Baseline complete urinalysis, BUN, and creatinine

Initiating treatment
- The dosage of carbamazepine should be adjusted to meet the needs of the individual patient, based upon clinical efficacy and monitoring of blood levels. Therapeutic serum levels of carbamazepine range between 4 and 12 μg/ml.
- For children under the age of 6 years, the initial recommended carbamazepine dosage is 10–20 mg/kg/day administered in divided doses two or three times a day (chewable or conventional tablets) or four times a day (suspension).
- The dose may then be increased in weekly intervals to obtain the desired clinical response; maintenance doses may be given either three or four times a day for both tablets and suspension.
- The maximum recommended dose for children and adolescents is 35 mg/kg/day.
- The usual carbamazepine maintenance dosage is 400–800 mg a day; the maximum daily dose is generally 1000 mg/day or less. For adolescents, the maximum daily dose is 1200 mg/day.
- Carbamazepine should be taken with food to minimize gastrointestional upset upon dosing.

Lamotrigine
Good evidence exists to support the use of lamotrigine as a first- or second-line agent for bipolar depression in adults. Lamotrigine has received FDA approval as a maintenance therapeutic in adult bipolar disorder but not specifically for bipolar depression. Case reports, chart reviews, and open-label studies suggest that lamotrigine may be effective in the treatment of acute mania. However, absence of placebo control groups, small sample sizes, or both hampers almost all current studies of lamotrigine's anti-manic properties. Although lamotrigine appears to have a role in the treatment of bipolar depression, its role in treating acute mania appears less than clear. Concern has emerged about the risk for toxic epidermal necrolysis and Stevens–Johnson syndrome with lamotrigine, especially when co-administered with divalproex or when rapidly titrated. There currently is little available data on lamotrigine for psychiatric disorders in the pediatric age range.

Before treatment
- CBC, differential, and platelet counts
- Liver function tests
- Concentrations of concomitant antiepileptic drugs

Initiating treatment
- Lamotrigine is initiated at 12.5–25 mg once a day.
- Should be increased no more than 12.5 mg to 25 mg every week.
  ○ Faster titration schedules have been associated with increased risk of developing rash.

- ○ When lamotrigine is administered with divalproex, the dose must be cut in half. Valproate may cause hepatic enzyme inhibition and cause elevated lamotrigine plasma levels.
- The usual maintenance dose of lamotrigine is 200–300 mg/day.

Lamotrigine initiation when added to a divalproex regimen:
- 12.5–25 mg/day orally every other day for 2 weeks
- Then 12.5–25 mg/day for 2 weeks
- Then 25–50 mg/day for 1 week
- Then 100 mg/day
- The usual maintenance dose of lamotrigine in patients taking valproic acid is 100 mg/day.
- When discontinuing divalproex, the dose of lamotrigine should be doubled over a 2-week period in equal weekly increments.

Lamotrigine initiation, when added to enzyme-inducing antiepileptic drug regimens such as carbamazepine without valproic acid:

- Initiate lamotrigine at 25–50 mg/day orally for 2 weeks.
- Then 100 mg/day for 2 weeks in divided doses.
- Then 200 mg/day for 1 week in divided doses.
- Then 300 mg/day for 1 week in divided doses.
- Then the dose may be increased up to a maximum maintenance dose of 400 mg/day in divided doses.
- When discontinuing an enzyme-inducing drug such as carbamazepine, the dose of lamotrigine should remain the same for the first week and then should be decreased by half over a 2-week period in equal weekly decrements.

Liver disease: With moderate liver dysfunction, the initial, escalation, and maintenance doses of lamotrigine should be reduced by approximately 50%; with severe impairment by approximately 75%.

Renal impairment: The maintenance dosage of lamotrigine may need to be decreased.

Oxcarbazepine
- Oxcarbazepine is chemically similar to carbamazepine.
- Its use is clinically similar to carbamazepine.
- No blood-level monitoring is required or available, making oxcarbazepine easier to administer than carbamazepine.
- The side effect profile is considerably more benign than that of carbamazepine.
- There is less available data with only three published reports in adult BPD. Two small studies found oxcarbazepine had similar efficacy to lithium and haloperidol in acute mania. None of these reports are randomized, placebo-controlled, and prospective.
- There currently is no methodologically controlled data on oxcarbazepine use in pediatric BPI.

Anticonvulsants used in adult BPI for which no data exist in the pediatric BPI population:

- Gabapentin
- Levetiracetim
- Tiagabine
- Topiramate
- Zonisamide

ANTIPSYCHOTIC MOOD STABILIZERS

Before treatment

Before initiating treatment with any atypical antipsychotic, such as olanzapine, risperidone, quetiapine, ziprasidone, or aripiprazole, the following should be completed:

- Complete a baseline physical examination and medical history.
  - An examination within the 6–12 months previous to the start of medication is generally sufficient in the medically healthy child and adolescent.
- Obtain a careful history in the patient and family of any metabolic disorders and/or diabetes. Atypical antipsychotics are associated with weight gain in children and adolescents, which can exacerbate risk for metabolic disorders.
  - If a positive family history for diabetes is found, obtain a fasting blood glucose, cholesterol, and lipid panel prior to initiating treatment with an atypical antipsychotic.
- Obtain baseline weight and height, and calculate a body mass index.
- Complete a baseline Abnormal Involuntary Movement Disorders (AIMS) examination. Although these agents are associated with a low risk of abnormal involuntary movement disorders, they can occur. A baseline examination is necessary to compare against, should the child develop abnormal involuntary movements while on drug.

Olanzapine

Initiating treatment

- For youth, a single initial daily dose of olanzapine 5–10 mg given at bedtime is recommended. Further titration within a dose range of 5–20 mg/day should occur at weekly intervals to allow steady-state serum concentrations to develop.
- Olanzapine doses > 10 mg/day have not been shown to increase efficacy, and the safety and tolerability of doses > 20 mg/day has not yet been demonstrated.
- Starting at a lower dose and titrating the dose more slowly are associated with less risk for side effects than initiating treatment at higher doses and titrating rapidly upward.

Risperidone

Initiating treatment

- For children and adolescents less than 15 years of age, initiate risperidone at the lowest possible dose, generally 0.25–0.5 mg, in the evening. Titrate the risperidone dose upward every 3–7 days by 0.25–0.5 mg until the therapeutic dose range of 0.25–6.0 mg/day is reached.

○ Above a daily dose of 6 mg/day extrapyramidal side effects may appear.

○ Doses above 6 mg/day have not been demonstrated to have any increased clinical efficacy compared to lower doses in children and adolescents.

• For prepubertal children, give risperidone in two to three divided daily doses.

• For adolescents ≥ 16 years of age, initiate risperidone at 0.5–1.0 mg/day and titrate upward every 3–7 days within a dose range of 0.25–6.0 mg/day.

○ In postpubertal adolescents, give risperidone in two divided daily doses or one dose at bedtime.

• Starting at a lower dose and titrating the dose more slowly are associated with less risk for side effects than initiating treatment at higher doses and titrating the dose rapidly upward.

Quetiapine
Initiating treatment

• For adolescents ≤ 18 years old, initiate quetiapine at a dose of 25 mg bid. Increase every 3–7 days, depending on effectiveness and tolerability, to a dose range of 200–800 mg given in two divided daily doses.

○ Some symptoms of aggression, anxiety, and sleep disturbance may respond to lower doses.

• Starting at a low dose and titrating the dose more slowly are associated with less risk for side effects, especially sedation, than initiating treatment at higher doses and titrating the dose rapidly upward.

Ziprasidone
Before treatment

• *Precaution*: There have been no reports of cardiac adverse events of ziprasidone since it was made available in 2001. However, in the adult schizophrenia ziprasidone trials, a dose-dependent lengthening of the EKG QTc interval was found. Patients with a history of prolonged QT syndromes should not be given ziprasidone. Prolonged QT syndromes are clinically identified by a family history of unexplained and recurrent syncope or early sudden cardiac death, with or without a family history of congenital deafness.

• Due to concerns of additive effects on prolongation of the QT interval, ziprasidone should not be given with medications that prolong QTc, such as moxifloxacin, chlorpromazine pentamidine, pimozide, droperidol, quinidine, mefloquine, thioridazine, or mesoridazine.

• The pediatric psychopharmacologist may wish to consider a baseline and on-drug EKG when using ziprasidone.

Initiating treatment

• For youth, initiate ziprasidone at 20 mg bid and titrate upward by 20–40 mg every 3–7 days. For psychotic disorders the effective dose range of ziprasidone is 40–160 mg/day, given in two divided daily doses.

• Doses as high as 320 mg/day in two divided doses have been reported.

• Starting at a low dose and titrating the dose more slowly are associated with less risk for side effects than initiating treatment at higher doses and titrating the dose rapidly upward.

Aripiprazole

Initiating treatment

Based on the extant aripiprazole pediatric trials currently available:
• In children
  ◦ < 25 kg in weight, initiate at a dose of 1 mg/day.
  ◦ 25–50 kg in weight, initiate at a dose of 2 mg/day.
  ◦ Between 50 and 75 kg in weight, initiate at a dose of 5 mg/day.
  ◦ ≥ 70 kg in weight, initiate at a dose of 10 mg/day.
• Titrate every 3–7 days to an optimum dose within a range of 1–30 mg/day.
• Steady-state aripiprazole serum concentrations are attained within 14 days of a dose change.

Clozapine

Before treatment

• A thorough physical examination and medical history must be completed prior to initiating a trial of clozapine.
  ◦ Patients with a history of seizures must be on an anticonvulsant that does not suppress their bone marrow and results in good seizure control before the initiation of clozapine.
  ◦ Patients with a history of bone marrow disease are not candidates for a clinical trial of clozapine.
  ◦ Patients with a history of myocarditis are not candidates for a clinical trial of clozapine.
• Patients must have severe BPI that has not responded adequately to at least two previous antipsychotic medication trials in order to be eligible for a clozapine trial.
• Because of the known propensity of clozapine to induce seizures, the clinician might consider a baseline and on-drug EEG.
  ◦ Clozapine dose appears to be an important predictor of seizures, with more risk at higher doses.
• Baseline pulse and blood pressure: Clozapine can induce hypotension in patients.
• Baseline weight: Clozapine can cause weight gain in patients.
  ◦ Increased body mass index is associated with increased risk for metabolic disorders and Type II diabetes.
  ◦ For patients with a history of diabetes or familial metabolic disorders, obtain a baseline fasting glucose and lipid profile.
• The patient must be enrolled in a clozapine monitoring protocol. This is mandatory for all patients. Clinicians can obtain details about enrolling patients at the patient's local pharmacy or through the drug manufacturer.
• Mandatory hematological monitoring:
  ◦ Because agranulocytosis is reported to occur in association with administration of clozapine in 1–2% of patients, hematological monitoring is mandatory.

MOOD DISORDERS

○ Baseline (before drug) complete blood count with differential must be obtained. To prescribe clozapine:
  ▪ The baseline white blood count (WBC) must be $\geq 3500/mm^3$.
  ▪ The baseline absolute neutrophil count (ANC) must be $\geq 1500 /mm^3$.

Initiating treatment
- For youth, initiate clozapine at a dose of 12.5 mg once or twice daily.
- The dose can be increased by 25–50 mg/day as tolerated, to reach a target dose of 300–450 mg/day for treatment-resistant disorders.
- Subsequent dose increases of a maximum of 100 mg can be made once or twice weekly.
- The total daily clozapine dose should not exceed 900 mg/day.

Duration of Treatment

- The optimal duration of medication treatment for children and adolescents with BPI is presently unknown.
- Expert consensus suggests 9–18 months of treatment after symptom resolution or stabilization to prevent relapse of the index depressive, manic, or mixed bipolar episode.
- Medications should be discontinued gradually (about 25% every 1–2 months) with careful psychiatric monitoring for any return of BPI.
- BPI is generally a chronic condition; when BPI medication is discontinued, the child should continue to be periodically monitored for the possible return of BPI.
- There exists a high lifetime prevalence of suicide in adults with BPI compared to control samples. Adolescents with BPI are also at risk for suicidality. When BPI medication is tapered and discontinued, the physician should carefully monitor the bipolar patient for any suicidal ideation or plan.

PEDIATRIC BIPOLAR ILLNESS MEDICATION TREATMENT ALGORITHM

Bipolar illness treatment algorithms for children and adolescents are presented in the following figures. It is hoped that standardizing medication approaches to the treatment of pediatric BPI by the use of algorithms will enhance clinical care and patient outcomes (Pavuluri et al., 2004).

Acute Treatment

EUPHORIC OR MIXED/DYSPHORIC MANIA

The first-line pharmacological treatment for classical euphoric or mixed dysphoric (a combination of manic and depressed symptoms) mania is the initiation of either lithium or an atypical antipsychotic. If no response occurs, then lithium or valproate plus an antipsychotic should be prescribed. Short-term adjunctive treatment with a benzodiazepine may also be helpful for insomnia and agitation. For mixed episodes, valproate may be preferred over lithium. Atypical antipsychotics are preferred over typical antipsychotics because of

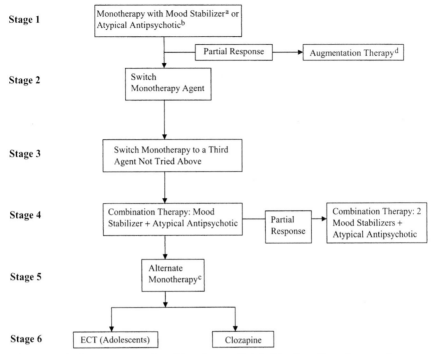

Figure 17.3 A treatment algorithm for pediatric bipolar disorder: acute, manic, without psychosis.
Stages 1–3 are monotherapy with different agents. The duration of each stage of treatment should last 4–6 weeks with a therapeutic serum level where appropriate. Stage 4 and augmentation strategies involve combinations of agents.
[a] Mood stabilizers: lithium, valproate, carbamazepine.
[b] Atypical antipsychotics: risperidone, olanzapine, quetiapine, ziprasidone, aripiprazole.
[c] Alternate monotherapy: lamotrigine, oxcarbazepine.
[d] Augmentation therapy: lithium + valproate or atypical antipsychotic or valproate + atypical antipsychotic or carbamazepine + atypical antipsychotic.
Kowatch RA, Fristad M, Birmaher B, et al. Treatment guidelines for children and adolescents with bipolar disorder. *Journal of the American Academy of Child and Adolescent Psychiatry* 44(3):213–235, 2005.

their more benign side effect profile, with most of the evidence supporting the use of olanzapine, quetiapine, or risperidone in pediatric BPI. Alternatives include carbamazepine or lamotrigine instead of lithium or valproate. Antidepressants should be tapered and discontinued, if possible. Psychosocial therapy should be combined with pharmacotherapy.

When first-line medication treatment at optimal doses fails to control symptoms, recommended treatment options include addition of another first-line

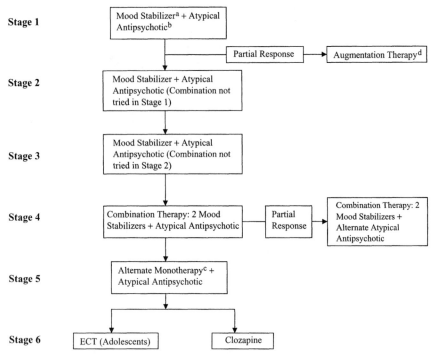

Figure 17.4 A treatment algorithm for pediatric bipolar disorder; acute, manic, with psychosis.
Combination therapy with mood stabilizers and an atypical antipsychotic is emphasized. The duration of each stage of treatment should last 4–6 weeks with a therapeutic serum level where appropriate.
[a] Mood stabilizers: lithium, valproate, carbamazepine.
[b] Atypical antipsychotics: risperidone, olanzapine, quetiapine, ziprasidone, aripiprazole.
[c] Alternate monotherapy: Atypical antipsychotic + either lamotrigine, or oxcarbazepine.
[d] Augmentation therapy: A combination of two mood stabilizers + an atypical antipsychotic
Kowatch RA, Fristad M, Birmaher B, et al. Treatment guidelines for children and adolescents with bipolar disorder. *Journal of the American Academy of Child and Adolescent Psychiatry* 44(3):213–235, 2005.

medication. Alternative treatment options include adding lamotrigine in lieu of an additional first-line medication, adding an antipsychotic if not already done, or changing from one antipsychotic to another. Clozapine may be particularly effective in the treatment of refractory BPI that fails to respond to two or more other atypical antipsychotics. ECT may also be considered for patients with severe or treatment-resistant mania or bipolar depression or if preferred by the patient in consultation with the psychiatrist. In addition, ECT is a potential treatment for patients experiencing mixed episodes or for patients experiencing severe mania during pregnancy. Manic or mixed episodes with psychotic features usually require treatment with an antipsychotic medication.

BIPOLAR DEPRESSIVE EPISODES

The first-line pharmacological treatment for bipolar depression is the initiation of either lithium or lamotrigine. In adult BPI a combination olanzapine–fluoxetine medication has received FDA approval for the treatment of bipolar depression. However, this combination has not been studied in pediatric bipolar patients and presently cannot be recommended for use in children and adolescents. Antidepressant monotherapy is not recommended for depressive episodes associated with bipolar illness. As an alternative, especially for more severely ill patients, simultaneous treatment with lithium and an antidepressant may be helpful. In patients with life-threatening inability to care for themselves, suicidality, and/or psychosis, ECT also represents a reasonable alternative. ECT is also a potential treatment for severe bipolar depression during pregnancy.

When an acute bipolar depressive episode fails to respond to first-line medication treatment at optimal doses, next steps include adding lamotrigine, bupropion, or paroxetine. Alternative next steps include adding other newer antidepressants (e.g., a selective serotonin reuptake inhibitor [SSRI] or venlafaxine) or a monoamine oxidase inhibitor [MAOI]. For patients with severe or treatment-resistant depression or depression with psychotic or catatonic features, ECT should be considered. The likelihood of antidepressant treatment precipitating a switch into a hypomanic episode is probably lower in patients with bipolar II depression than in patients with bipolar I depression. Therefore, the clinician should consider recommending antidepressant treatment earlier in patients with bipolar II disorder who are depressed. Depressive episodes with psychotic features usually require adjunctive treatment with an antipsychotic medication. ECT represents a reasonable alternative.

RAPID CYCLING

"Rapid cycling" refers to the occurrence of four or more mood disturbances within a single year that meet criteria for a major depressive, mixed, manic, or hypomanic episode. These episodes are either clearly separated from one another by a partial or full remission for at least 2 months or a switch to an episode of opposite polarity (e.g., from a major depressive to a manic episode). In patients who experience rapid cycling, identify and treat medical conditions such as hypothyroidism or drug or alcohol use that may contribute to cycling. Certain medications, particularly antidepressants, may also contribute to cycling and should be tapered, if possible. The initial treatment for patients who experience rapid cycling should include lithium or valproate. As an alternative treatment consider lamotrigine. For most patients, multiple medications and combined pharmacotherapy will be required to effectively treat rapid cycling BPI.

MOOD DISORDERS

Maintenance Treatment

Following remission of an acute episode, patients may remain at particularly high risk of relapse for a period of up to 6 months. This phase of treatment is considered the maintenance phase. Maintenance regimens of medication are recommended following a manic episode. Although few studies involving patients with bipolar II disorder have been conducted, maintenance treatment for this form of the illness is also strongly warranted. The medications with the best empirical evidence to support their use in maintenance treatment include lithium and valproate. Possible alternatives include lamotrigine or carbamazepine or oxcarbazepine. If one of these medications is used to achieve remission from the most recent depressive or manic episode, it generally should be continued into the maintenance phase of treatment. Maintenance treatment with ECT may also be considered for patients whose acute episode responded to ECT.

For patients treated with an antipsychotic medication during the acute episode, the need for ongoing antipsychotic treatment should be reassessed upon entering maintenance treatment. Antipsychotics should be discontinued unless they are required for control of persistent psychosis or prophylaxis against recurrence. Although maintenance therapy with atypical antipsychotics may be considered, there is no definitive evidence that their efficacy in maintenance treatment is comparable to lithium or valproate.

For patients who, despite receiving maintenance medication treatment, experience a manic or mixed episode (i.e., a "break-through" episode), the first-line intervention should be to optimize the medication dose. Introducing or resuming an antipsychotic is sometimes necessary. Severely ill or agitated patients may also require short-term adjunctive treatment with a benzodiazepine. For patients who experience a break-through depressive episode while receiving maintenance medication treatment, the first-line intervention should be to optimize the dose of maintenance medication.

During maintenance treatment, patients with bipolar disorder are likely to benefit from concomitant psychosocial interventions that address bipolar illness management (i.e., treatment adherence, lifestyle changes, regular sleep–wake and exercise cycles, early detection of prodromal bipolar symptoms) and interpersonal difficulties. Group psychotherapy may also help patients address such issues as adherence to a treatment plan, adaptation to a chronic illness, regulation of self-esteem, and management of marital and other psychosocial issues. Support groups provide useful information about bipolar disorder and its treatment.

Treatment of Comorbid ADHD

Given high rates of comorbidity between ADHD and pediatric bipolar disorder, there exists concern that treatment of ADHD symptoms with stimulants or noradrenergic antidepressants in bipolar youth might destabilize symptoms of the manic–depressive illness. This issue is further complicated by the fact that many of the symptoms of ADHD are similar to the symptoms of pediatric BPI. Treating ADHD with medication and not recognizing an underlying comorbid BPI may lead to an exacerbation of manic symptoms in such youths.

- Current recommendations for the treatment of ADHD in the context of BPI emphasize the need to treat the bipolar disease first with antipsychotic and/or mood stabilizing medications.
- If ADHD symptoms persist after successful treatment of BPI, then stimulants may safely be added to ongoing bipolar medications without destabilizing comorbid bipolar symptoms (Carlson et al., 2000; Carlson et al., 2004; Scheffer et al., 2005)

18. Psychotic Disorders

Psychosis implies a serious disturbance in an individual's "reality testing." Impaired reality testing is reflected by a number of specific pathological signs and symptoms, including hallucinations, delusions, and disorganized thought processes (Volkmar, 1996). Disorganized thought processes reflect information-processing deficits in psychotic children, adolescents, and adults. Psychotic symptoms occur in a wide variety of neuropsychiatric conditions in children and adolescents and are not pathognomonic for any one disorder. For example, in addition to early-onset schizophrenia, disorganized thought processes and illogical thinking are also found in children suffering from generalized and complex partial epilepsy (Kanner, 2004), in those receiving steroids (Dawson & Carter, 1998) or stimulant medications (Calello & Osterhoudt, 2004) for asthma, in youngsters suffering from bipolar disorder (Pavuluri et al., 2004), as a result of traumatic brain injury (Fujii & Ahmed, 2002), and in traumatized youngsters with PTSD (Janssen et al., 2004).

A thought disorder needs to be distinguished from expressive and receptive language disorders, which are classified as learning disabilities. Hallucinations can be found in youth suffering from illicit substance intoxication, mood disorders such as psychotic depression, sexual and physical abuse, and bereavement following the loss of a loved one (Reimherr & McClellan, 2004). Indeed, in clinical practice, psychotic symptoms occur much more commonly as part of these disorders than in schizophrenic spectrum disorders. Most children who have psychotic symptoms are not schizophrenic. The onset of schizophrenia in childhood is relatively rare (Volkmar, 1996). Types of disorders that may include psychotic symptoms in children and adolescents are given in the following table.

DEVELOPMENTAL CONSIDERATIONS

Developmental issues need to be considered in the assessment of childhood psychotic disorders. Because psychotic symptoms can generally only be assessed by an evaluation of how the child uses language, little is known about

Table 18.1 Child and Adolescent Disorders That May Have Psychotic Symptoms

Psychotic disorders
  • Early-onset schizophrenia
  • Early-onset schizoaffective disorder
Affective disorders
  • Early-onset bipolar disorder
  • Major depression with psychotic features
Anxiety disorders
  • Posttraumatic stress disorder (sexual/physical abuse)
  • Obsessive–compulsive disorder
Pervasive developmental disorders
  • Autism spectrum disorders
  • Pervasive developmental disorders
Adolescent-onset personality disorders
  • Schizoid
  • Schizotypal
  • Borderline
  • Paranoid
Drug-induced toxic psychoses
Neurological conditions
  • Seizure disorders (psychomotor, temporal lobe)
  • Traumatic brain injury
  • Demyelinating diseases
Congenital conditions
  • Velo-cardio-facial syndrome
Bereavement

---

psychotic processes in preschoolers. As a result of cognitive immaturity, preschool children do not yet utilize adult rules of logic and causality. Thus illogical thinking and loose associations of ideas are common in normal preschoolers. After about age 7 years these cognitive styles are not so commonly observed in normally developing children (Isohanni et al., 2004). Hallucinations are rare in children younger than age 8 years. The presence of pervasively disorganized thinking found after age 7 years can clearly be understood as indicating pathology (Caplan et al., 2000).

Psychotic phenomena are relatively uncommon in the elementary school years. Their presence generally indicates severe psychopathology. Hallucinations are much more prevalent in psychotic 6- to 12-year-old children than delusional thinking, probably because of cognitive immaturity. The content of hallucinations in this age group often reflects developmental concerns such as monsters, ghosts, pets, or toys. Delusions are rare in this age group; when they do occur, they are more simply organized and less complex, entrenched, and systematic than in psychotic adults (Volkmar, 1996).

During adolescence the frequency of psychotic illness increases markedly, and symptomatology becomes generally similar to adults. The prevalence of delusional thinking increases markedly after age 17 years in psychotic youth, probably reflecting increased cognitive development. Delusions can become organized, systematized, and elaborate in adolescent psychotic disorders, similarly to adult psychotic disorders. During adolescence hallucinations and disorganized thinking begin to take on an adult psychotic form and appearance (Tolbert, 1996; Volkmar, 1996).

PREVALENCE

Psychosis in children and adolescents is not an uncommon entity. It is estimated that psychosis afflicts approximately 1% of youth in nonreferred community samples and 4–8% of children and adolescents in referred samples. Most of these youngsters do not suffer from schizophrenia but meet diagnostic criteria for a wide variety of other neuropsychiatric disorders. In one large study of the phenomenology of psychosis in psychiatrically referred children and adolescents, 8% reported delusions and/or hallucinations (Biederman et al., 2004). Almost all of the psychotic youngsters also met diagnostic criteria for other disruptive behavioral, mood, or anxiety disorder diagnoses.

COMORBIDITY

Comorbidity is the rule rather than the exception in children who come to the clinician with early-onset psychotic disorders (Biederman et al., 2004; Reimherr & McClellan, 2004). Comorbid conditions may confound accurate diagnosis, affect responses to treatment, and increase the possibility of poorer outcomes in these disorders.

• *Disruptive behavioral disorders*: Premorbid and concurrent ADHD, oppositional defiant disorder, and conduct disorder are noted frequently in children and adolescents with bipolar illness, schizophrenia, and other psychotic disorders. In the sample of Biederman and colleagues (2004), children and adolescents with psychoses were frequently comorbid for externalizing disorders.
  ○ ADHD: 70%
  ○ Conduct disorder: 30%
  ○ Oppositional defiant disorder: 70%
• *Mood disorders*: Youngsters with psychotic symptoms often have accompanying internalizing disorders.
  ○ Major depressive disorder: 40%
  ○ Bipolar disorder: 55%
• *Anxiety disorders*: Youngsters with psychotic symptoms often have accompanying anxiety disorders.
  ○ Multiple anxiety disorders: 65%
  ○ Obsessive–compulsive disorder: 20%
• *Substance abuse*: Up to 60% of adolescents with psychotic disorders my abuse illicit substances.
• *Neurological disease*: Children with epilepsy can develop psychotic signs and symptoms; children who suffer traumatic brain injury may develop psychotic symptoms.

ASSESSMENT

A wide variety of symptoms can be seen in children with psychotic disorders. These may include severe anxiety and unusual fears, odd behaviors, social withdrawal, hallucinations, attacks of disinhibited behaviors, and regression in psychosocial development. Some possible symptoms of psychotic disorders are listed in the following table.

A wide variety of disorders should be considered in the assessment of children and adolescents with psychotic symptoms. These include medical and

---

Table 18.2 Symptoms of Early-Onset Psychotic Disorders

- Strange, vivid, disturbing, and bizarre thoughts
- Language disturbances
- Severe and pervasive anxiety and fears
- Auditory hallucinations
- Tactile hallucinations
- Visual hallucinations
- Diminished interests
- Social withdrawal
- Confused thinking
- Inability to distinguish television/dreams from reality
- Odd behaviors
- Disinhibited behaviors
- Developmental regression
- Problems making and keeping friends

Table 18.3 Patient Assessment in Early-Onset Psychotic Disorders

Developmental and psychiatric history
- Prenatal history
- Early developmental history
- Temperament
- Social history
- Cognitive functioning
- School history

Symptom history
- Assess for psychotic symptoms
- Assess for formal thought disorder
- Symptom onset
- Course of illness

Previous treatment history
- Psychosocial treatments
- Psychopharmacological treatments

Impairment in daily functioning
- School
- Interpersonal
- Family
- Self-care
- Leisure

Medical history
- Pediatric consultation with hearing/vision screens
- Complete physical examination
- Speech evaluation
- Neurological consultation

Laboratory studies
- Complete blood count
- Thyroid function tests
- Metabolic studies
- Liver transaminases
- Chemistry profile
- BUN, creatinine
- Toxicology screen
- Heavy metals screen
- HIV testing (if risk factors present)
- Brain-imaging studies
- Sleep-deprived EEG

neurological disorders as well as psychiatric disorders. Every child with new-onset psychotic symptoms, especially if they occur in the context of an acute mental status change, should have a thorough medical evaluation and neurological screen to rule out the possibility of organic CNS illness. An approach to the clinical assessment of psychotic disorders is provided in the following table.

Once a diagnosis of a psychotic disorder is established by clinical assessment, and once medical and neurological etiologies are ruled out, assessment instruments can be used to determine the extent of psychotic symptoms. These rating scales are not diagnostic assessment instruments such as semistructured and structured psychiatric interviews. Rather, they are useful in quantifying psychotic symptoms in terms of positive symptoms, deficit symptoms, thought disorder, and functional impairment. Some assessment instruments are presented in the following table.

Table 18.4 Assessment Instruments for Assessing Psychotic Symptoms in Children and Adolescents

Instrument	Study (year)	Description	Age Range (years)	Informant
Positive and Negative Syndrome Scale for Children and Adolescents	Fields et al. (1994)	Rates severity of positive and negative symptoms of schizophrenia	6–16	Interview rated parent/child
Children's Psychiatric Rating Scale	Fish (1985)	Rates symptom severity	≤ 15	Interview rated child
Kiddie—Formal Thought Disorder Story Game and Scale	Caplan et al. (1989)	Assesses logical pattern of speech samples	5–13	Child
Thought Disorder Index	Arboleda & Holzman (1985)	Assesses thought disorder from speech samples	5–16	Child

Adapted from Remschmidt H and Hebebrand J. Early-onset schizophrenia. In: Martin A, Scahill L, Charney DS,and Leckman JF (Eds.), *Pediatric Psychopharmacology Principles and Practice.* New York: Oxford University Press, p. 548, 2003.

EARLY-ONSET SCHIZOPHRENIA

Although rare in children and adolescents, the prototypic psychotic disorder is schizophrenia and is briefly discussed here. Schizophrenia is a chronic, severe, neuropsychiatric disorder presenting with significant disruptions in emotional, cognitive, and/or behavioral regulation and with significant impairments in daily life. The disorder is characterized by persistent or recurrent periods of active psychosis, accompanied by progressive deterioration in social, academic, occupational, familial, and self-care functioning. Schizophrenia is generally diagnosed in early adulthood. However, it is often preceded by a very long prodromal period of impairment, characterized by developmental lags in academics and social withdrawal from interpersonal relationships that may insidiously begin in childhood or adolescence.

PSYCHOTIC DISORDERS

Evidence from family, twin, and adoption studies indicates that schizophrenia has a strong hereditable component. As much as 83% of the variance in vulnerability to schizophrenia may be attributable to genetic inheritance. However, complex gene–environment interactions are very important in contributing risk for schizophrenia. For example, only 50% of identical twins whose siblings develop schizophrenia will themselves go on to develop the disorder (Volkmar & Tsatsanis, 2002).

Schizophrenia usually emerges in late adolescence or early adulthood, with 75% of cases emerging between the ages of 17–25 years old. Males tend to become symptomatic 2–3 years earlier than females. The incidence of schizophrenia remains greater for males than for females until mid life (40–50 years old), at which point female rates remain elevated above males for the remainder of life (Torrey, 1995).

Prevalence

- Schizophrenia affects 1% of the general adult population.
- There is very little epidemiological data for adolescent-onset schizophrenia and even less for the preadolescent type. It appears that schizophrenia rarely occurs before puberty (Stayer et al., 2004). Studies suggest that schizophrenia may occur in only 0.01% of nonreferred children living in the community (Tolbert, 1996). The rate of onset increases throughout adolescence and by the end of adolescence has achieved rates of adult prevalence.
- Gender ratio: prepubertal males tend to be affected by schizophrenia 2:1 over prepubertal females. This ratio evens out with increasing age (AACAP, 2001).

Course and Prognosis

Although no longitudinal outcome studies in early-onset schizophrenia have been completed, the consensus is that childhood-onset schizophrenia has a uniformly poor prognosis. There exists an increased risk of suicide or accidental death directly due to behaviors caused by psychotic thinking in at least 5% of those suffering from this disorder (AACAP, 2001).

Assessment

With children and adolescents, the overlap of categorical boundaries between different psychotic conditions and other affective, behavioral, and developmental disorders has led to high rates of misdiagnosing schizophrenia in the young. This appears especially problematic at the time of initial evaluation, before a clear longitudinal course of illness has been established. A cross-sectional diagnosis of schizophrenia at a single point in time is made all the more difficult because the symptoms that comprise the diagnosis are also found in other childhood psychotic disorders, such as bipolar illness, psychotic depression, and substance use disorders. In addition, careful attention must be paid during clinical assessment of early-onset schizophrenia to the possibility of comorbid psychiatric, neurological, and/or medical disorders. The diagnostic criteria for schizophrenia are given in the following table.

Table 18.5 Diagnostic Criteria for Schizophrenia

A. *Characteristic symptoms*: Two (or more) of the following, each present for a significant portion of time during a 1-month period (or less if successfully treated):
(1) Delusions
(2) Hallucinations
(3) Disorganized speech (e.g., frequent derailment or incoherence)
(4) Grossly disorganized or catatonic behavior
(5) Negative symptoms, i.e., affective flattening, alogia, or avolition

Note: Only one Criterion A symptom is required if delusions are bizarre or hallucinations consist of a voice keeping up a running commentary on the person's behavior or thoughts, or two or more voices conversing with each other.

B. *Social/occupational dysfunction*: For a significant portion of the time since the onset of the disturbance, one or more major areas of functioning such as work, interpersonal relations, or self-care are markedly below the level achieved prior to the onset (or when the onset is in childhood or adolescence, failure to achieve expected level of interpersonal, academic, or occupational achievement).
C. *Duration*: Continuous signs of the disturbance persist for at least 6 months. This 6-month period must include at least 1 month of symptoms (or less if successfully treated) that meet Criterion A (i.e., active-phase symptoms) and may include periods of prodromal or residual symptoms. During these prodromal or residual periods, the signs of the disturbance may be manifested by only negative symptoms or two or more symptoms listed in Criterion A present in an attenuated form (e.g., odd beliefs, unusual perceptual experiences).
D. *Schizoactive and Mood Disorder exclusion*: Schizoaffective Disorder and Mood Disorder With Psychotic Features have been ruled out because either (1) no Major Depressive, Manic, or Mixed episodes have occurred concurrently with the active-phase symptoms; or (2) if mood episodes have occurred during active-phase symptoms, their total duration has been brief relative to the duration of the active and residual periods.
E. *Substance/general medical condition exclusion*: The disturbance is not due to the direct physiological effects of a substance (e.g., a drug of abuse, a medication) or a general medical condition.
F. *Relationship to a Pervasive Developmental Disorder*: If there is a history of Autistic Disorder or another Pervasive Developmental Disorder, the additional diagnosis of Schizophrenia is made only if prominent delusions or hallucinations are also present for at least a month (or less if successfully treated).

American Psychiatric Association. *Desk Reference to the Diagnostic Criteria from DSM-V–TR*. Washington, DC, American Psychiatric Association. pp. 153–155, 2000. Reprinted with permission.

TREATMENT OPTIONS

Treatment of the child or adolescent with early-onset psychotic disorders will depend on the nature of the psychiatric disorder present. Treatments for depression and bipolar disorders with psychotic features are presented in Chapter 17. If psychotic symptoms are a result of substance abuse, treatment requires substance abuse rehabilitation as well as psychiatric interventions. This section focuses on the treatment of early-onset schizophrenia.

The treatment of early-onset schizophrenia in children and adolescents is both specific and general. Specific treatments target the characteristic psychotic symptoms of the disorder and often emphasize psychopharmacological interventions. More general treatments address the related psychological, social, educational, and cultural needs of the child and family. Often multiple psychoeducational and psychiatric treatment modalities are needed. In addition to medications, these modalities may include educational interventions at school for the child; family psychoeducation as to the nature, prognosis, and treatment of early-onset schizophrenia; and supportive therapies for the child and family (AACAP, 2001; Volkmar, 1996). The child with early-onset schizophrenia benefits most from a treatment team approach to the illness, which includes the primary care physician, a consulting psychiatrist, an individual and family

Table 18.6 Studies of Atypical Antipsychotics in Children and Adolescents with Early-Onset Schizophrenia

Study (year)	Drug	Diagnosis	Age (mean/range) (yrs)	Treatment Duration (weeks)	Mean Dose (mg/day and range)	Outcome
CONTROLLED STUDY						
Kumra et al. (1996)	Clozapine	Schizophrenia	14.0 ± 2.3	6	176 ± 149	Improvement, clozapine > haloperidol
OPEN STUDIES						
Armenteros et al. (1997)	Risperidone	Schizophrenia	11–18	10	6.6 (4–10)	90% of patients improved
Frazier et al. (1994)	Clozapine	Schizophrenia	12–18	6	370 (125–900)	> 50% of patients improved
Kumra et al. (1998)	Olanzapine	Schizophrenia	6–18	8	12.5–20	25% of patients improved
McConville et al. (2000)	Quetiapine	Psychosis	12–15	3	200 and 800	Improvement
Remschmidt et al. (1994)	Clozapine	Schizophrenia	14–22	22	330 (50–800)	75% of patients improved

therapist, and special education school personnel. Inpatient psychiatric treatment may be needed, particularly when psychotic symptoms become acute, and access to a psychiatric emergency department may occasionally be necessary. An individual practitioner model of care is not suitable for the treatment of children and adolescents with early-onset schizophrenia.

Psychopharmacological Treatments

Medications target the specific positive and negative symptoms of early-onset schizophrenia. Positive symptoms of the disorder include illogical thinking, bizarre thoughts, hallucinations, and delusions. Negative symptoms include social withdrawal, apathy, and lack of motivation. The treatment of early-onset schizophrenia emphasizes the use of atypical antipsychotic medications. Although neuroleptics are effective, their adverse side effect profile, including extrapyramidal side effects (EPS), tardive dyskinesia (TD) with long-term use, and anticholinergic effects with low-potency agents, precludes their consideration as first-line medications for early-onset schizophrenia.

Pertinent studies of antipsychotic medications in early-onset schizophrenia

There are few controlled studies of antipsychotic medications for schizophrenia in pediatric psychopharmacology. Most of the available scientific evidence for antipsychotic effectiveness in children and adolescents comes from clinical experience and open case series. The following table presents some of this evidence.

Despite the lack of controlled clinical trial evidence, second generation antipsychotic medications are felt to play a crucial role in treating the specific symptoms of psychosis in early onset schizophrenia.

CHOOSING AND INITIATING A MEDICATION

Doses of second-generation (SGA) and first-generation (FGA) antipsychotic medications that have been used in pediatric psychopharmacology are given in the following table.

It should be noted that use of these agents to treat early-onset schizophrenia is off-label at this point. However, these agents are frequently prescribed for children and adolescents with psychotic disorders, disruptive behaviors and explosive aggression in the context of autistic disorders and developmental delay, impulsive aggression in conduct disorder, and psychotic symptoms or aggression in organic mental disorders such as epilepsy or traumatic brain injury. In choosing an antipsychotic medication, consider the following:

• No antipsychotic is more effective than any other antipsychotic in the treatment of the positive symptoms of schizophrenia such as delusions and hallucinations, with exception of clozapine. Up to 60% of nonresponders to other FGAs will improve when prescribed clozapine (Remschmidt & Hebebrand, 2003). However, use of clozapine is associated with many potential adverse events, such as seizures and hematological side effects, which require careful clinical

PSYCHOTIC DISORDERS

Table 18.7 Antipsychotic Doses

Generic Names	Chlorpromazine Equivalent Dose (100 mg)	Acute Dose (mg/day)	Range (mg/day)	PRN (mg/po)	PRN (mg/IM)
SECOND-GENERATION ANTIPSYCHOTICS					
Clozapine	75	150–500	75–700	N/A	N/A
Olanzapine	4	5–20	3–30	N/A	N/A
Quetiapine	100	200–800	100–1000	N/A	N/A
Risperidone*	1	2–8	1–16	N/A	N/A
Ziprasidone	15	40–200	20–160	2–25	N/A
Aripiprazole	7.5	1–30	1–30	N/A	N/A
FIRST-GENERATION ANTIPSYCHOTICS					
Chlorpromazine	100	200–1600	25–2000	25–100	25–50
Fluphenazine	2	2.5–20	1–60	0.5–10	1–5
Haloperidol	2	2–40	1–100	0.5–5	2–5
Loxapine	15	60–100	30–250	10–60	12.5–50
Mesoridazine	50	75–300	30–400	10–100	25
Molindone	20	50–100	15–25	5–75	N/A
Perphenazine	10	16–32	4–64	4–8	5–10
Pimozide	0.5	10–12	1–20	N/A	1–3
Thioridazine	100	200–600	40–800	20–200	N/A
Thiothixene	0.5	6–30	6–60	2–20	2–4
Trifluoperazine	5	6–50	2–80	5–10	1–2

*Doses over 6 mg yield less improvement and more side effects than 6 mg or less.

monitoring. As such, clozapine should only be used after failure to respond to two or more previously prescribed antipsychotics.
• SGAs may have more effectiveness against the negative symptoms of schizophrenia (e.g., apathy, amotivation, social withdrawal, emotional blunting) than FGAs.
• Treatment should emphasize SGAs as agents of first choice for early-onset schizophrenia and related conditions, because they have a more benign side effect profile than FGAs. Specifically, SGAs compared to FGAs have a lower risk of TD with long-term use and a lower prevalence of EPS.

Before initiating treatment with antipsychotic medications
• Complete a baseline physical examination and medical history; an examination within the 6–12 months previous to the start of medication is generally sufficient in the medically healthy child and adolescent.
• Obtain a careful history of the patient and family of any metabolic disorders and/or diabetes. SGAs are associated with weight gain in children and adolescents, which could exacerbate risk for metabolic disorders.
   ○ If a positive family history for diabetes is found, obtain a fasting blood glucose, cholesterol, and lipid panel prior to initiating treatment with an SGA.
• Obtain a baseline weight and body mass index.
• Complete a baseline Abnormal Involuntary Movement Scale (AIMS) examination; a baseline examination is necessary to compare against, should the child develop abnormal involuntary movements while on drug.

• If low-potency FGAs such as chlorpromazine are to be used, obtain a baseline pulse and blood pressure; low-potency FGAs have hypotensive effects.

Dose titration
• In adults, the effective dose range of antipsychotics is expressed in chlorpromazine equivalents (see Table 18.7) and ranges between 300 mg and 1000 mg per day of chlorpromazine equivalents. Doses less than this do not appear effective in adult schizophrenia, and doses greater than this appear to increase risk for side effects without conferring any additional therapeutic benefits. Because schizophrenia is so rare in children, the effective dose ranges are not yet known. However, high doses do not appear to result in additional antipsychotic benefits in children, but *do* increase risk for treatment-emergent side effects.
• In children and adolescents a useful rule-of-thumb for antipsychotic dose titration is to initiate medication at a low dose and titrate upwards slowly, monitoring for clinical benefit and/or the emergence of side effects.

MONITORING DURING ANTIPSYCHOTIC TREATMENT

• Follow weight monthly.
• Calculate a body mass index every 4–6 months while on drug.
• Complete a follow-up AIMS examination, searching for abnormal involuntary movement scale every 6–12 months while on drug.
• For low-potency antipsychotics such as chlorpromazine, follow the pulse and blood pressure every 3 months while on a stable dose and after each dose increase.
• EKG monitoring is mandatory with use of thioridazine.
  ○ Consider EKG monitoring with use of ziprasidone.

DISCONTINUING ANTIPSYCHOTIC TREATMENT

Antipsychotic agents should not be stopped abruptly. A variety of withdrawal side effects may occur if patients suddenly discontinue antipsychotics. These may include abnormal involuntary movements, "neuroleptic withdrawal dyskinesias." Generally these movements spontaneously remit, but may cause distress for the patient and family.

• Taper off antipsychotics by 10–25% every 5–7 days when stopping treatment.
• Monitor for the emergence of treatment withdrawal symptoms.

SIDE EFFECTS

A more detailed discussion of side effects is found in Chapter 7; Chapter 8 discusses tardive dyskinesia, neuroleptic malignant syndrome, and EPS adverse events in detail. Some common side effects of antipsychotics and their management are briefly mentioned here.

• *Weight gain*: The atypical antipsychotics commonly cause weight gain in patients, especially clozapine, olanzapine, and risperidone; somewhat for

PSYCHOTIC DISORDERS

quetiapine; and less so for ziprasidone and aripiprazole. FGAs do not appear associated with as much weight gain as SGAs. Molindone is an FGA that is associated with weight *loss* in patients. The management of antipsychotic-induced weight gain is largely clinical; diet and exercise are common strategies. Use of the lowest effective antipsychotic dose is also recommended.

• *Endocrine effects*: Antipsychotics, especially risperidone and FGAs, may cause menstrual irregularities, amenorrhea, gynocomastia, and galactorrhea as a result of increased prolactin levels. Management consists of using the lowest effective dose and switching to prolactin-sparing SGAs such as aripiprazole, olanzapine, quetiapine, or ziprasidone (Haddad & Wieck, 2004).

Psychosocial Treatments

The morbidity of early-onset schizophrenia results not just from the positive and negative symptoms of psychosis, but also from the consequences of the disorder on an individual child's development. Therapeutic interventions must address the needs of the child and family in addition to targeting psychotic symptoms with medications. Thus treatment for the child with an early-onset psychotic disorder is broad-based and designed to address any comorbid psychiatric conditions, such as substance abuse, ongoing stressors, and family factors that may complicate the course of illness (AACAP, 2001).

INDIVIDUAL PSYCHOTHERAPY

• Psychotherapeutic interventions that emphasize skill building, social skills training, and cognitive–behavioral strategies have proved helpful for adults with schizophrenia.
• Traditional psychotherapeutic approaches emphasizing psychodynamic understanding have not proved helpful for people with psychotic disorders.

FAMILY THERAPY

• Family therapy interventions, including problem solving and communication skills training, have decreased relapse rates.
• Family education about the nature of the disorder, manifest symptoms, course, prognosis, and treatment options should always be provided.

EXPRESSED EMOTION

"Expressed Emotion" (EE) refers to family attributes of overprotectiveness of the patient and/or criticism expressed by family members toward the patient. Relapse rates are higher for adults with schizophrenia who live in families characterized by high rates of EE. Reducing family EE may be helpful in preventing relapse in children or adolescents with early-onset schizophrenia.

EDUCATIONAL INTERVENTIONS

Schizophrenia is an information-processing disorder. Thus patients with early-onset schizophrenia have great difficulty in regular school classrooms and often require special educational interventions. They may do best in a classroom characterized by low levels of stimulation, an individualized educational curriculum that recognizes their information-processing strengths and vulnerabilities, and a teaching staff specifically trained to interact with and teach emotionally disturbed youth.

SERVICE CONTINUUM

Youngsters with early-onset schizophrenia often require a variety of services and treatment providers that may include some or all of the following.

• Extensive case management services to access and coordinate the patient's service needs across multiple agencies and providers
• Crisis intervention services
• Family support programs
• Parent advocacy groups
• Access to a psychiatric emergency department and an inpatient child or adolescent psychiatry unit when acute behavioral or symptom deterioration occurs
• In-home services to focus on helping the family reduce EE
• Day treatment or partial hospitalization programs that combine both special education and mental health services
• Vocational and life skills training

PSYCHOTIC DISORDERS

19. Extrapyramidal Syndromes and Central Serotonin Syndrome

Children and adolescents receiving neuroleptic or atypical antipsychotic medications that alter central nervous system (CNS) dopamine signaling and increase D2 receptor blockade may develop extrapyramidal syndromes (EPS). These syndromes include acute dystonic reactions, symptoms of Parkinsonism, akathisia, tardive dyskinesia, and neuroleptic malignant syndrome. Compared with older neuroleptics, the risk of EPS is much less with newer atypical antipsychotics. Clozapine appears to have the least risk of EPS of any atypical antipsychotic agent.

Youngsters receiving multiple psychiatric mediations that affect CNS serotonin neurotransmission may develop central serotonin syndrome. When considering adverse events associated with psychiatric medications, EPS and central serotonin syndrome are important side effects for the practicing clinician to bear in mind.

ACUTE DYSTONIC REACTIONS

Acute dystonic reactions are involuntary muscle spasms and contractions typically involving the muscles of the neck, jaw, mouth, and/or tongue. When the muscles of the eye are involved, an oculogyric crisis may occur in which the eyes roll upward and remain fixed in that position. Rarely in children, acute dystonic reactions may involve muscles of the diaphragm, making coordinated respiration difficult; the smooth muscles of the esophagus, making swallowing difficult; and/or the muscles of the spine, causing opisthotonos. The period of maximum risk for acute dystonic reactions is within hours to 7 days following initiation of neuroleptic or atypical antipsychotic therapy. Occasionally acute dystonic reactions occur when titrating the antipsychotic dose upward from a previously well-tolerated dose.

As far as neuroleptics are concerned, high-potency agents such as haloperidol or pimozide are more likely to precipitate dystonic reactions than low-dose, highly anticholinergic agents such as chlorpromazine. Risk with atypical antipsychotics is less than for typical neuroleptics, but can still occur. Compared

401

with adults, male children and adolescents may be particularly at-risk to develop acute dystonic reactions upon exposure to antipsychotic medications. Untreated acute dystonic reactions may last from a few minutes to several hours, and they may recur in bouts.

Acute dystonic reactions are rapidly treated with anticholinergic drugs and/or antiparkinsonian agents.

- Diphenhydramine 25–50 mg orally.
  ∘ Repeat in 20 minutes if acute dystonic reactions recur.
- Diphenhydramine 25 mg intramuscularly may be used for severe reactions.
- Benztropine 1–2 mg orally; repeat in 20 minutes if acute dystonic reactions recur.
- Benztropine 1 mg intramuscularly may be used for severe reactions.

PARKINSONISM

Symptoms of parkinsonism include tremor, cogwheel rigidity, drooling, a decrease in facial emotional expression, and slowness in initiating voluntary movements (akinesia). Subtle signs of parkinsonism are common when children and adolescents are treated with neuroleptics. Parents may not notice slight signs of akinesia but report that the child seems withdrawn, not emotional, and not spontaneous. The period of maximal risk appears to be within 5–30 days of initiating neuroleptic therapy. The risk of developing parkinsonian symptoms appears to be greater for females, to increase with age, and to increase with duration of neuroleptic therapy. Parkinsonism symptoms can occur with use of atypical antipsychotics, but more rarely than with use of neuroleptics.

Symptoms of parkinsonism respond to antiparkinsonian medications.

- Benztropine 0.5–2 mg given two or three times daily usually provides relief within 1–2 days.

To prevent the development of parkinsonian symptoms, benztropine is often given prophylactically to patients who are receiving neuroleptic medications.

However, the prophylactic use of anticholinergic agents to minimize the risk of acute dystonic reactions or symptoms of parkinsonism from treatment with an antipsychotic drug is somewhat controversial. Anticholinergic agents, by themselves, have side effects that can adversely affect the child. For example, anticholinergic agents cause constipation, dry mouth, may affect memory and cognition, and may exacerbate psychotic symptoms. The clinical decision to use these agents prophylactically must be made on case-by-case basis. Several strategies include the following.

- Beginning with a low dose and titrating the neuroleptic/atypical antipsychotic slowly may obviate the need for additional anticholinergic medication.
  ∘ If acute parkinsonian symptoms occur, they can be treated acutely with anticholinergic agents.

- When anticholinergics are prophylactically prescribed, the goal is to cover the time period of maximum risk for parkinsonian symptoms, generally the first 1–2 months of therapy.
  - Prophylactic benztropine is prescribed at a dose of 0.5–2 mg/day in two or three divided doses.
  - Can usually be discontinued gradually in 4 or 8 weeks to ascertain if it is still necessary for symptomatic relief of parkinsonian symptoms.
    - If acute EPS occur, they can be treated acutely with anticholinergic agents.
- An option for ambulatory child and adolescent patients is to prescribe a small amount of benztropine or diphenhydramine, with an explanation to parents of how it is to be administered should an acute EPS event occur.
  - Take one capsule at the start of a reaction.
  - Take another capsule 20–30 minutes later if there is no improvement.
  - Notify the prescribing physician of the event.
  - Take the child to the emergency room if the reaction is severe.

AKATHISIA

Akathisia is an EPS caused by neuroleptics and, to a lesser extent, atypical antipsychotics. As a medication side effect akathisia needs to be distinguished from increased agitation associated with the primary psychiatric diagnosis being treated. The primary period of risk for the development of akathisia is 5–60 days after beginning neuroleptics. Akathisia results in a subjective sense of intolerable inner restlessness and observable motor overactivity. Symptoms of akathisia include a constant uncomfortable restlessness, a feeling of tension in the lower extremities, an irresistible urge to move one's legs or pace constantly, and/or an inability to sit still. Clinically, signs of akinesia may also occur, such as a blunted affect, emotional withdrawal, and depression. Akathisia is associated with increased suicide attempts in psychotic adults and noncompliance with antipsychotic medication, leading to an increased risk of relapse.

Akathisia is poorly responsive to antiparkinsonian drugs such as benztropine or trihexyphenidyl. Medications that are useful in treating akathisia include:

- Benzodiazepines: clonazepam 0.25–0.5 mg/day
- Beta-blockers: propranolol in divided doses of 20–120 mg/day
- Alpha-agonists: clonidine in divided doses of 0.05–0.3 mg/day
- For treatment-resistant cases, it may be necessary to reduce the antipsychotic dose.

TARDIVE AND OTHER NEUROLEPTIC-RELATED DYSKINESIAS

Dyskinesias are abnormal, writhing, involuntary muscle movements that are caused by long-duration exposure to agents that block D2 receptors, such as neuroleptics and some atypical antipsychotics. Tardive dyskinesia occurs in patients while they are receiving long-term neuroleptic or atypical antipsychotic treatment. In adults, the condition may be irreversible, even with discontinuation of the neuroleptic agent. Withdrawal dyskinesias are more common in children and adolescents. Abnormal involuntary movements appear as the neuroleptic is being discontinued or the dose is being reduced, generally last for days to weeks, and then disappear. To date no cases of irreversible tardive dyskinesia have been described in children or adolescents. Of the atypical antipsychotics, risperidone may be the agent with the highest risk of tardive dyskinesia and other EPS. Clozapine appears to be an atypical antipsychotic with very low risk of EPS.

Typical symptoms of tardive dyskinesia include involuntary choreoathetotic movements of the face, tongue, perioral, buccal, and masticatory musculature and muscles of the neck. More rarely, the torso or extremities may be involved. Even more rarely, the smooth muscles of the diaphragm or esophagus become involved, leading to difficulties in breathing or swallowing. Symptoms of tardive dyskinesia typically begin insidiously after many months to years of neuroleptic or antipsychotic exposure. The risk of developing tardive dyskinesia increases with both total cumulative neuroleptic dose and lifetime duration of treatment. Treatment with older neuroleptics increases risk compared to treatment with newer atypical antipsychotics. In adults, older females appear more at risk than males. Diabetes and a psychiatric diagnosis of affective psychosis may also be risk factors in adults. Concurrent extrapyramidal symptoms and prophylactic anticholinergic use may increase risk in adults. In children and adolescents, mental retardation, neuroleptic treatment (as opposed to treatment with an atypical antipsychotic), an abnormal baseline Abnormal Involuntary Movement Scale (AIMS) score, and total number of risk factors correlate with risk for neuroleptic-related dyskinesias (Connor et al., 2001).

In 1982 Schooler and Kane proposed research diagnostic criteria for tardive dyskinesia.

• Exposure to neuroleptic drugs for a minimum total cumulative lifetime exposure of 3 months.
• The presence of at least "moderate" abnormal involuntary movements on one or more of seven separate body areas (face, lips, jaw, tongue, upper extremities, lower extremities, trunk).
• Absence of other medical, psychiatric, or neurological conditions that might produce abnormal involuntary movements.

These criteria may identify six categories or subtypes of tardive dyskinesia.

• Probable tardive dyskinesia: The patient is either receiving concurrent neuroleptic therapy or is medication free (but with a lifetime history of neuroleptic exposure).
• Masked probable tardive dyskinesia: Within 2 weeks of increasing the dose or resuming neuroleptic therapy, the patient no longer has abnormal involuntary movements.

- Transient tardive dyskinesia: Within 3 months after a patient is diagnosed with probable tardive dyskinesia, and with no increase in the neuroleptic dose, the abnormal involuntary movements disappear.
- Withdrawal tardive dyskinesia: While receiving neuroleptics the patient does not have abnormal involuntary movements; but within 2 weeks following cessation of neuroleptic therapy the patient develops abnormal involuntary movements.
- Persistent tardive dyskinesia: Signs and symptoms of tardive dyskinesia for ≥ 3 months, either while receiving neuroleptics or no longer receiving them but with a lifetime history of exposure.
- Masked persistent tardive dyskinesia: In a patient with ≥ 3 months of abnormal involuntary movements, increasing the neuroleptic dose causes the movements to disappear.

Assessment of Neuroleptic-Induced Dyskinesias

A careful history of drug exposure and examination to determine the typical abnormal involuntary motor movements of dyskinesias are the keys to accurate assessment. It is necessary to carefully consider other neurological or medical causes of dyskinetic movements before assigning a diagnosis of probable tardive dyskinesia.

- A drug history should establish at least a 3-month lifetime history of cumulative neuroleptic or atypical antipsychotic drug exposure.
  - It is important to obtain information on the type of neuroleptic or antipsychotic drug, total months of cumulative exposure, tolerability, side effects, and effectiveness.
- Identify other medications that the patient is receiving.
  - Anticholinergic agents may worsen tardive dyskinesia.
  - Concomitant stimulant therapy in the face of a neuroleptic withdrawal dyskinesia may worsen the abnormal involuntary movements.
  - Rarely, SSRIs may cause a dyskinesia.
  - Dyskinesias have been described with the use of monoamine oxidase inhibitors, lithium, antihistamines, benzodiazepines, and anticonvulsant drugs.
- Examination with a standardized scale such as the Abnormal Involuntary Movements Scale (AIMS) is mandatory (Appendix 4). Ideally, examination should occur at baseline before the start of the antipsychotic drug, and then every 6 months while on drug.

Etiology of Neuroleptic-Induced Dyskinesias

THE DOPAMINE SUPERSENSITIVITY HYPOTHESIS

The dopamine supersensitivity hypothesis proposes that the CNS nigrostriatal dopamine system develops increased sensitivity to dopamine as a consequence of chronic dopamine postsynaptic receptor blockade induced by neuroleptic drugs. In the face of chronic D2 receptor blockade, postsynaptic dopamine receptors are increasingly recruited. Eventually increased dopamine receptor number alters dopamine neurotransmission and results in EPS. Additionally, if D2 blockade is lessened, as when neuroleptic drugs are withdrawn or the dose reduced, increased dopamine neurotransmission occurs across a greater number of D2 receptors, resulting in withdrawal dyskinesias. The relationship between CNS D2 blockade, antipsychotic action, and EPS is illustrated in the following figure 1.

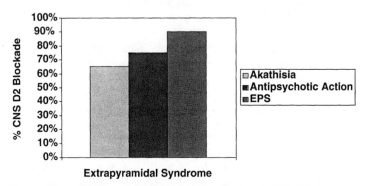

Figure 19.1 Relationship between blockade of CNS D2 receptors as measured by positron emission tomography, antipsychotic action, and EPS.

THE NEUROTOXICITY HYPOTHESIS

The neurotoxicity hypothesis suggests that tardive dyskinesia is due to neurotoxic effects from oxidative free-radical byproducts of dopamine and other catecholamine metabolism. The basal ganglia have a high rate of oxidative metabolism. Cell membrane lipid peroxidation can occur as a result of the increased catecholamine turnover induced by neuroleptic drugs. Cumulative cell damage in the basal ganglia eventually results in tardive dyskinesia. This hypothesis provides a theoretical reason for the treatment of tardive dyskinesia with vitamin E (alpha-tocopherol), which scavenges free radicals and may prevent cumulative oxidative damage to neurons.

Treatment of Neuroleptic-Induced Dyskinesias

One approach to the treatment of neuroleptic-induced dyskinesias is to try and prevent them from developing by preferentially using atypical antipsychotics whenever possible and for the shortest time periods necessary to reduce cumulative lifetime exposure. If a neuroleptic or atypical antipsychotic-induced dyskinesia does develop, consider the following actions and options.

• Discontinue or lower the dose of the antipsychotic. Presently, all reports of neuroleptic-induced dyskinesias in children and adolescents suggest that dyskinesias are not irreversible in youngsters (like they may be in adults) when neuroleptics are discontinued.

- Discontinue all anticholinergic agents. Anticholinergic agents may exacerbate a vulnerability to drug-induced dyskinesias.
- Monitor the dyskinesia by obtaining serial AIMS examinations.
- Notify parents and/or guardians of the dyskinesia.
- If neuroleptic/antipsychotic medications must be continued despite the emergence of a dyskinesia, document the reason in the medical chart and complete an informed consent discussion with parents/guardians. Use the lowest effective dose of neuroleptic/antipsychotic medication and for the shortest duration possible.
- Benzodiazepines such as clonazepam in divided daily doses between 0.25–1.0 mg may help treat the dyskinesia.
- Beta-blockers such as propranolol in divided daily doses of 20–160 mg/day may help treat the dyskinesia.
- Vitamin E in doses of 300–1200 mg/day may help treat the dyskinesia by preventing oxidative damage to neurons.

NEUROLEPTIC MALIGNANT SYNDROME

Neuroleptic malignant syndrome (NMS) is a potentially lethal condition associated with the use of neuroleptic medications. It can occur after a single dose but most frequently occurs within 2 weeks after initiation of neuroleptic therapy or following an increase in daily dose. Males and younger individuals appear to be most at risk. The use of high-potency first-generation neuroleptics such as haloperidol or combination treatment with a high-potency neuroleptic and lithium may increase risk. However, NMS with the use of low-potency agents such as chlorpromazine has also been reported. NMS has been reported in infants, preschool children, school-age children, adolescents, and adults.

NMS should be considered a medical emergency. Symptoms of NMS develop rapidly and emergently. The cardinal symptoms include severe muscular rigidity ("lead pipe rigidity"), altered mental status and consciousness, stupor, catatonia, hyperreflexia, autonomic nervous system instability (i.e., labile pulse and blood pressure, diaphoresis, incontinence), and fever. Occasionally, myoglobinemia is present. Most patients have elevated creatine phosphokinase (CPK) levels. Leukocytosis and abnormal liver function studies (i.e., serum glutamic oxaloacetic transaminase [SGOT] and serum glutamic phosphotransaminase [SGPT]) may occur. NMS may persist for up to 2 weeks or longer after neuroleptic medication is discontinued.

Mortality rates from NMS are high and appear inversely correlated with age. The lethality for children younger than 12 years appears to be higher than for adolescents and adults. Mortality rates between 13% and 27% are reported for pediatric cases. Adult mortality rates range between 5% and 20%. In the last decade mortality rates from NMS appear to be declining, presumably due to earlier recognition of the disorder, earlier emergency medical intervention for the disorder, and the increasing use of safer atypical antipsychotics.

The treatment of NMS is emergent and generally requires medical intensive care for the full-blown disorder.

Table 19.1 Symptoms of Neuroleptic Malignant Syndrome

- Mental status changes including confusion, hypomania, or a euphoric state
- Muscular rigidity ("lead pipe rigidity")
- Feeling intoxicated or dizzy
- Drowsiness
- Clumsiness
- Restlessness
- Muscle twitching
- Rapid muscle contraction and relaxation in the jaw, causing abnormal movements of the face and jaw
- Rapid muscle contraction and relaxation in the ankle, causing abnormal movements of the foot
- Sustained rapid eye movement
- Hyperreflexia
- Sweating
- Fever
- Shivering
- Diarrhea
- Stupor
- Loss of consciousness
- Catatonia
- Death

- Immediately discontinue all neuroleptic or antipsychotic drugs.
- Institute supportive measures for fever and hydration.
- Monitor cardiac and renal status.
- Consider somatic therapies:
  - Bromocriptine
  - Dantrolene
  - Amantadine
- Anticholinergic drugs and diphenhydramine are generally not effective for NMS.

CENTRAL SEROTONIN SYNDROME

Drugs that increase CNS serotonin neurotransmission and affect the 5HT1A receptor may cause central serotonin syndrome (CSS). Symptoms may begin after an increase in serotonin drug monotherapy, but generally occur immediately or soon after combining medications that have a serotonergic mechanism of action. For example, combining an SSRI with lithium and trazodone for sleep at night brings together three drugs with serotonergic action and increases risk for CSS. Central serotonin syndrome may present after overdose and intoxication with a serotonergic agent such as an SSRI. Drugs with the potential to cause the serotonin syndrome are presented in the following table.

Central serotonin syndrome is manifested by cognitive, neuromuscular, and autonomic symptoms. CSS exists on a spectrum of severity with symptoms ranging from mild to severe. Mild symptoms include tremor, incoordination, and confusion. Moderate symptoms include shivering, sweating, hyperreflexia, and agitation. Severe symptoms include fever, myoclonus, and diarrhea. The symptoms of CSS and their relative frequency are presented in the following table.

Table 19.2 Medications Associated with Serotonin Syndrome

Mechanism	Drug
Metabolic serotonin precursor	L-tryptophan
Inhibit serotonin metabolism	MAOIs
Increase serotonin release	Amphetamines
	Lithium
	MDMA (ecstasy)
Inhibit serotonin reuptake	Cocaine
	Dextromethorphan
	Merperidine
	SSRIs
	Tricyclic antidepressants
	Trazodone
	Venlafaxine
Serotonin receptor agonists	Buspirone
	Lysergic acid diethylamide (LSD)
Dopamine agonists	L-dopa

Table 19.3 Symptom Frequency in the Serotonin Syndrome

Symptom	Percent of Total Cases
Cognitive–Behavioral	
Confusion/disorientation	54%
Agitation/irritability	35%
Coma/unresponsiveness	28%
Anxiety	16%
Hypomania	15%
Lethargy	15%
Seizures	14%
Hallucinations	6%
Dizziness	6%
Neuromuscular	
Myoclonus	57%
Hyperreflexia	55%
Muscle rigidity	49%
Tremor	49%
Ataxia/incoordination	38%
Shivering/chills	25%
Babinski's sign (bilateral)	14%
Nystagmus	13%
Autonomic Nervous System	
Hyperthermia	46%
Diaphoresis	46%
Sinus tachycardia	41%
Hypertension	33%
Tachypnea	28%
Dilated pupils	26%
Nonreactive pupils	18%
Flushed skin	14%
Hypotension	14%
Diarrhea	12%
Abdominal cramps	5%
Salivation	5%

The central serotonin syndrome can be life threatening, though less life threatening than unrecognized NMS. The optimal treatment is to discontinue the offending agent or agents, offer supportive measures, and wait for the symptoms to resolve. If the offending medication is discontinued, the condition often resolves on its own within a 24-hour period. If serotonergic medications are not promptly discontinued, the condition can progress rapidly and become fatal.

If serotonin syndrome has occurred as a result of an acute overdose, activated charcoal may be beneficial soon after the ingestion. Supportive care is the mainstay of treatment.

- Hyperthermia should be treated with aggressive external cooling measures such as ice, mist, fans, and a cooling blanket.
- Rigidity, seizures, and agitation are treated with benzodiazepines.
- Severe symptoms have been successfully treated with cyproheptadine (a 5HT2 antagonist) 4–8 mg po every 1–4 hours (max 32 mg/day) or 0.25 mg/kg/day divided every 1–4 hours in children.
  - Cyproheptadine is available in 4 mg tablets and a syrup (2 mg/5 mL); no parenteral product is available.

Once the symptoms resolve, there does not appear to be a need for continued medical monitoring.

The greater the enhancement of serotonin levels, the greater the chances of producing the central serotonin syndrome. Therefore, it is recommended that serotonergic agents be used concurrently with each other only with caution and close clinical monitoring.

20. Anxiety Disorders

Anxiety may be generally defined as emotional uneasiness accompanied by physiological arousal associated with the anticipation of danger. Anxiety is usually diffuse and lacking in specificity; it is considered a normal human emotion, in contrast to many other forms of psychopathology. Fear is an adaptive reaction to real or imagined danger and threats to one's well-being. Fears and worries are common in nonreferred children and adolescents. Normal anxieties evolve and change over time as the child develops and matures.

In contrast, phobias involve excessive, specific, persistent fear of a stimulus that is then avoided or endured with significant distress. Phobic reactions are disproportionate to the demands of the situation, impervious to logical reasoning, and often occur outside the normal developmental period of a fear. Phobias lead to avoidance of the specific stimulus, which then may cause impairment in daily functioning. For example, phobic stimuli can include social situations, public speaking, the dark, thunderstorms, insects, or blood. In contrast to anxiety, phobias are clearly abnormal.

Research has investigated the developmental patterns of normal fear and anxiety in children and adolescents. Across the child and adolescent years, normal anxieties evolve and change.

Because childhood fears and anxieties are common and play an adaptive and protective role in development, the distinction between normal and abnormal childhood anxiety is not always clear. The extent to which anxiety impairs normal everyday functioning is an important factor in making this distinction. Fears and worries that begin to cause daily impairment in functioning should be considered excessive. The timing of the worry in development is also important. Acute separation fears from an attachment figure are normal for a 3-year-old but abnormal in a 13-year-old.

The distinction between anxious symptoms and anxiety syndromes or disorders is important. Symptoms of anxiety are normal and a part of everyday life; everyone gets anxious at some point or another. In contrast, disorders are defined as clusters of symptoms that exist together over time, have a discrete

411

Table 20.1 Normal Fears and Worries in Children and Adolescents

Age	Fear/Worry
Infant	Stimuli in the immediate environment
1–3 years old	Strangers/heights/unfamiliar places
3–5 years old	Being alone/dark/animals/imaginary creatures
School age	Bodily injury/natural disaster/supernatural phenomenon/evaluation by authority figures/social situations
Adolescents	Performance anxiety/social anxiety/ anticipatory anxiety/identity consolidation/ sexuality

onset and longitudinal course, cause subjective distress and impairment in functioning, and may have a familial heritability. Anxiety syndromes and disorders are clearly abnormal in daily life.

There are many different types of anxiety disorders. Some include phobias, although not all anxiety disorders are phobic in nature. Anxiety disorders are seen in psychiatric, neurological, surgical, medical, and pediatric practices. They present with a range of cognitive, behavioral, and physiological symptoms. Considerable impairment is associated with early-onset childhood and adolescent anxiety disorders. Anxiety and phobic disorders are associated with low self-esteem, social isolation, inadequate social skills, and problems in academic functioning. Youngsters with anxiety disorders often have multiple physical symptoms such as headaches and gastrointestional symptoms. In some children early-onset anxiety disorders tend to remit over time, but they also tend to recur over the course of development. In other children anxiety disorders take a chronic course and may predispose to other psychopathology in later life. This chapter reviews separation anxiety, panic disorder with and without agoraphobia, generalized anxiety disorder, and social anxiety disorder. Specific phobia is not discussed. Obsessive–compulsive disorder and posttraumatic stress disorder are reviewed in chapters 21 and 22, respectively.

PREVALENCE AND EPIDEMIOLOGY

In general, anxiety disorders are considered to be one of the most common psychiatric disorders in children and adolescents. In community samples anxiety disorders occur in 5–18% of children. In preadolescent children the prevalence of anxiety diagnoses ranges between 0.3% to almost 13%. In adolescents, depending on the disorder, prevalence lies between 0.6% and 7%. In nonreferred youngsters, specific phobias, generalized anxiety disorder, and separation anxiety disorder are the most common disorders. In samples of children referred to pediatrics, between 8% and 15% may meet criteria for an anxiety disorder. Girls tend to have more anxiety diagnoses than boys, except for obsessive–compulsive disorder.

COMORBIDITY

Anxiety disorders in children and adolescents frequently co-occur with other psychiatric disorders. Comorbidity with other anxiety disorders or depression is very common. Between 14% and 39% of nonreferred children and adolescents residing in the community with a diagnosable anxiety disorder have another simultaneous psychiatric disorder. In clinically referred samples up to 50% of anxious youngsters may have another comorbid disorder. In addition to comorbidity with anxiety and depression, anxiety disorders may also occur with attention-deficit/hyperactivity disorder and conduct disorders.

ASSESSMENT

All children referred for anxiety disorders should have a comprehensive clinical psychiatric evaluation. The assessment might include a structured or semistructured psychiatric diagnostic interview to confirm anxiety diagnoses and other comorbid psychiatric disorders. Diagnostic interviews include semistructured instruments such as the Schedule for Affective Disorders and Schizophrenia for School-Age Children (K-SADS). Examples of highly structured diagnostic interviews include the Diagnostic Interview for Children and Adolescents (DICA) and the NIMH Diagnostic Interview Schedule for Children (DISC).

Once it has been established that the youngster may be experiencing anxiety symptoms beyond what one would expect for the child's developmental age, a more careful review of symptoms should be undertaken. A comprehensive clinical assessment must pay attention to a number of specific issues. These include the following:

- Whether anxiety is stimulus specific, spontaneous, and/or anticipatory
- The degree of impairment in daily life caused by anxiety
- Stimuli that precipitate anxiety
- Reinforcers of anxiety symptoms
- Developmental history of anxiety symptoms, including infant temperament, attachment fears, stranger anxiety, and childhood fears
- Family history of anxiety disorders in biological relatives
- Family functioning
- School functioning
- Social functioning

The medical workup for a child or adolescent with an anxiety disorder should include routine pediatric evaluation. Specific medical factors and conditions that may mimic anxiety disorders should be considered. These include:

- Medications
- Herbal supplements and remedies
- Drugs of abuse

ANXIETY DISORDERS

- Over-the-counter medications
- Hypoglycemia
- Hyperthyroidism
- Cardiac arrhythmias
- Caffeine-induced anxiety
- Pheochromocytoma
- Migraine headache
- Seizure disorder

The clinician should be aware of several assessment issues in youngsters. For example, children and young adolescents may not recognize that their anxiety is excessive and have difficulty reporting on their internal feeling state. Young children may demonstrate anxious symptoms in their behavior (e.g., crying, temper tantrums, somatic complaints, irritability).

Once an anxiety disorder diagnosis has been established by clinical psychiatric assessment, rating scales can help assess the severity of anxiety. Some established rating scales for the assessment of anxiety severity in children and adolescents are listed in the following table.

SEPARATION ANXIETY DISORDER

The central clinical feature of separation anxiety disorder (SAD) is tremendous fear, worry, and anxiety regarding separation from home or primary attachment figures. The anxiety must be inappropriate for the child's age and developmental level. For example, separation fears are a common and normal part of development in 6-month to 6-year-old children. To make the diagnosis, SAD should last at least 4 weeks and cause impairment to the child's daily functioning.

The following table presents the DSM-IV–TR criteria for SAD.

Prevalence
- The reported prevalence of SAD is 2.4–5.4%.

Course of illness and outcome
- In some children SAD will eventually remit with complete recovery.
- In other children SAD may have a variable course, with acute exacerbations during times of stress or transition.
- Predictors of poor outcome in SAD include
  ○ A later age of onset (> 6 years old)
  ○ Comorbidity with other psychiatric disorders
  ○ Family psychopathology, especially anxiety disorders in parents
  ○ Missing more than 1 year of school because of SAD or school refusal
- Severe childhood SAD may predict later life psychopathology such as other anxiety or depressive disorders.
- Somatic complaints such as headaches and stomachaches may lead to multiple medical evaluations.

Table 20.2 Rating Scales for Anxiety in Children and Adolescents

Rating Scale	Type of Scale	What Is Assessed?	Age Range (years)	Reliability	Validity	Sensitivity to Change
Anxiety Sensitivity Index	Self-report	Anxiety severity	6–17	++	+	Possibly
Child Behavior Checklist (CBCL)	Parent-rated	Severity of anxiety and depression	6–18	++	—	Yes
Fear Survey Schedule for Children—Revised	Self-report	Fear	7–18	++	—	No
Hamilton Anxiety Rating Scale	Clinician-rated	Psychological and physiological anxiety severity	Adolescents	++	++	Yes
Multidimensional Anxiety Scale for Children	Self-report	Anxiety severity	8–19	++	++	Yes
Pediatric Anxiety Rating Scale	Clinician-rated	Anxiety severity	6–17	+	++	Yes
Revised Children's Manifest Anxiety Scale	Self-report	Anxiety severity	6–19	++	+	Yes
Screen for Child Anxiety Related Emotional Disorders—Revised	Self-report	DSM-IV anxiety disorder severity	8–18	++	++	Yes
Social Anxiety Scale for Adolescents	Self-report	Social phobia severity	13–18	++	++	Not reported
Social Anxiety Scale for Children	Self-report	Social phobia severity	6–12	++	++	Not reported
Social Phobia Anxiety Inventory	Self-report	Social phobia severity	Older adolescents	++	++	Not reported
Social Phobia Anxiety Inventory for Children	Self-report	Social phobia severity	8–14	++	++	Not reported
State–Trait Anxiety Inventory	Self-report	State and trait anxiety	Older adolescents	++	+	Not reported
State–Trait Anxiety Inventory for Children	Self-report	State and trait anxiety	9–12	+	++	Yes
Youth Self Report	Self-report	Severity of anxiety and depression	11–18	++	+	Not reported

Source: Brooks SJ and Kutcher S. Diagnosis and measurement of anxiety disorder in adolescents: A review of commonly used instruments. *J Child Adolesc Psychopharmacol* 13(3):351–400, 2003.
++ = good; + = fair; — = no data.

ANXIETY DISORDERS

415

Table 20.3 Diagnostic Criteria for Separation Anxiety Disorder

A. Developmentally inappropriate and excessive anxiety concerning separation from home or from those to whom the individual is attached, and three or more of the following:
  (1) Recurrent excessive distress when separation from home or major attachment figures occurs or is anticipated
  (2) Persistent and excessive worry about losing, or about harm befalling, a major attachment figure
  (3) Persistent and excessive worry that an untoward event will lead to separation from a major attachment figure
  (4) Persistent reluctance or refusal to go to school or elsewhere because of fear of separation
  (5) Persistently and excessively fearful or reluctant to be alone or without major attachment figures at home or in other settings
  (6) Repeated nightmares involving the theme of separation
  (7) Repeated complaints of physical symptoms (such as headaches or stomachaches) when separation from major attachment figures occurs or is anticipated
B. The duration of disturbance is at least 4 weeks
C. The onset is before age 18 years
D. The disturbance causes clinically significant distress or impairment in social, academic, or other important areas of functioning
E. Exclusion criteria: The disturbance does not occur exclusively during the course of a Pervasive Developmental Disorder, Schizophrenia, other Psychotic Disorder, or is not better accounted for by Panic Disorder With Agoraphobia

American Psychiatric Association. *Desk Reference to the Diagnostic Criteria from DSM-IV–TR.* Washington, DC, American Psychiatric Association, pp. 76–77, 2000. Reprinted with permission.

PANIC DISORDER WITH AND WITHOUT AGORAPHOBIA

Panic disorder refers to the experience of unexpected panic attacks accompanied by anxious apprehension about their recurrence or modifications in daily behavior as a result of worry about panic attacks. A panic attack is a discrete period of intense fear and anxiety that is characterized by the presence of other somatic or cognitive symptoms. Panic attacks are characterized by their rapid onset and crescendo of anxiety symptoms, reaching peak intensity within 10 minutes of onset.

Panic disorder may or may not be accompanied by symptoms of agoraphobia, which is anxiety about being in places or situations in which escape might be difficult or embarrassing if one should experience a panic attack. Typical feared situations include being outside alone without a companion, being in a crowd, standing in line, traveling through a tunnel or across a bridge, being in shopping malls or in movie theaters. Agoraphobic symptoms increasingly restrict the patient's movements and cause impairment in daily life.

Diagnosing children with panic disorder has been somewhat controversial; it is clear, however, that adolescents can have panic attacks.

The following table presents the DSM-IV–TR criteria for panic disorder with or without agoraphobia.

Prevalence
• The estimated prevalence of panic disorder, with or without agoraphobia, in community samples of adolescents is 0.6–4.7%.
• Some cases of panic disorder have been described in prepubertal children.
• The prevalence of panic disorder rises markedly in adolescence.

Table 20.4 Diagnostic Criteria for Panic Disorder

A. A discrete period of intense fear or discomfort, in which four or more of the following symptoms developed abruptly and reached a peak within 10 minutes:
   (1) Palpitations, pounding heart, or accelerated heart rate
   (2) Sweating
   (3) Trembling or shaking
   (4) Sensations of shortness of breath or smothering
   (5) Feelings of choking
   (6) Chest pain or discomfort
   (7) Nausea or abdominal distress
   (8) Feeling dizzy, unsteady, lightheaded, or faint
   (9) Derealization (feelings of unreality)
   (10) Depersonalization (being detached from oneself)
   (11) Fear of losing control or going crazy
   (12) Fear of dying
   (13) Paresthesias (numbness or tingling sensations)
   (14) Chills or hot flushes
B. Panic attacks are recurrent and unexpected
C. At least one of the attacks has been followed by 1 month (or more) of one (or more) of the following:
   (1) Persistent concern about having additional attacks
   (2) Worry about the implications of the attack or its consequences
   (3) A significant change in behavior related to the attacks
D. The panic attacks are not the due to the direct physiological effects of a substance or medical condition.
E. Panic Disorder Without Agoraphobia
F. Panic Disorder With Agoraphobia:
   (1) Presence of anxiety about being in places or situations from which escape might be difficult or embarrassing or in which help might not be available in the event of experiencing panic anxiety.
   (2) Situations are avoided because of worries about having a panic attack.
   (3) Exclusion criteria: The anxiety or phobic avoidance is not better accounted for by another mental disorder such as Social Phobia, Specific Phobia, Obsessive–Compulsive Disorder, Posttraumatic Stress Disorder, or Separation Anxiety Disorder.

American Psychiatric Association. *Desk Reference to the Diagnostic Criteria from DSM-IV–TR.* Washington, DC, American Psychiatric Association, pp. 209–213, 2000. Reprinted with permission.

Course of illness and outcome
- The modal age of onset for panic disorder is 14 years old.
- Little longitudinal research is presently available to facilitate an understanding of the outcome of children and adolescents with onset of panic disorder early in life. It appears likely that if untreated, panic attacks and panic disorder may persist into adulthood.

GENERALIZED ANXIETY DISORDER

Generalized anxiety disorder (GAD) is characterized by diffuse worry that is excessive and out of proportion to the situation, and uncontrollable, meaning that the worried individual finds it difficult to contain the anxiety and stop worrying. The distinction between developmentally appropriate worry and GAD therefore rests not on the object of worry, but on the persistence and unrealistic nature of the anxieties. To be diagnosed as having GAD, a youth needs to display a pattern of excessive worry that interferes with daily functioning for at least 6 months.

Typically children and adolescents worry about

- Competence and performance
- Approval

- The appropriateness of past behavior
- The future
- Social situations
- Sexuality and sexual identity

The following table presents the DSM-IV–TR criteria for GAD.

Table 20.5 Diagnostic Criteria for Generalized Anxiety Disorder (includes Overanxious Disorder of Childhood)

A. Excessive anxiety, worry, and apprehensive expectation, occurring more days than not for at least 6 months, about a number of events or activities.
B. The person finds it difficult to control the worry.
C. The anxiety and worry are associated with three or more of the following symptoms. At least some symptoms are present for more days than not for the past 6 months.

Note: Only one additional symptom is required for children.

(1) Restlessness or feeling on edge
(2) Being easily fatigued
(3) Difficulty concentrating or mind going blank
(4) Irritability
(5) Muscle tension
(6) Sleep disturbance
D. The focus of anxiety is not confined to features of another Axis I disorder.
E. The anxiety and worry cause clinically significant distress or impairment in social, occupational, or other important areas of functioning.
F. The disturbance is not due to the direct physiological effects of a substance or (e.g., a drug of abuse, a medication) a general medical condition (e.g., hyperthyroidism), and does not occur exclusively during a Mood Disorder, a Psychotic Disorder, or a Pervasive Developmental Disorder.

American Psychiatric Association. *Desk Reference to the Diagnostic Criteria from DSM-IV–TR.* Washington, DC, American Psychiatric Association, pp. 222–223, 2000. Reprinted with permission.

Prevalence
- The reported prevalence estimates for GAD range between 2.7% and 4.6% for children and adolescents.

Course of illness and outcome
- GAD appears to be a chronic and persistent disorder; adults with GAD report being anxious most of their lives, with the onset of disabling anxiety commonly reported in childhood.
- GAD typically follows a chronic but fluctuating course; symptoms generally worsen in times of stress.

SOCIAL PHOBIA

Social phobia is a persistent fear of one or more social situations involving exposure to unfamiliar persons or to the scrutiny of others. Exposure to the feared situation provokes anxiety, fear of embarrassment, and occasional panic attacks. In children, selective mutism is now generally considered a form of social phobia, and sometimes school refusal may be a result of it. Commonly feared situations include speaking in front of others, attending social gatherings, dealing with authority figures such as teachers or coaches, performing in public, and speaking to strangers. Children and adolescents may have little insight into their social fears and may not recognize them as excessive or unreasonable. The following table presents the DSM-IV–TR criteria for social phobia.

Table 20.6 Diagnostic Criteria for Social Phobia (Social Anxiety Disorder)

A. A marked and persistent fear of one or more social or performance situations in which the person is exposed to unfamiliar people or to possible scrutiny by others. The individual fears that he or she will act in a way that will be humiliating or embarrassing. Note: In children, there must be evidence of the capacity for age-appropriate social relationships with familiar people and the anxiety must occur in peer settings, not just in interactions with adults.
B. Exposure to the feared social situation almost invariably provokes anxiety, which may take the form of a panic attack. Note: In children, the anxiety may be expressed by crying, tantrums, freezing, or shrinking from social situations with unfamiliar people.
C. The person recognizes that the fear is excessive. Note: In children, this feature may be absent.
D. The feared social or performance situations are avoided or else are endured with intense anxiety or distress.
E. The avoidance, anxious anticipation, or distress in the feared social or performance situation significantly interferes with daily life functioning.
F. In individuals under age 18 years, the duration is at least 6 months.
G. The social or performance anxiety is not due to the direct physiological effects of a substance (e.g., a drug of abuse, a medication) or a general medical condition, and is not better accounted for by another mental disorder.

American Psychiatric Association. *Desk Reference to the Diagnostic Criteria from DSM-IV–TR.* Washington, DC, American Psychiatric Association, pp. 215–216, 2000. Reprinted with permission.

Prevalence
• Social phobia has been estimated to occur in 1% of children and adolescents.
• As children age into adolescence and young adulthood, prevalence rates rise.
• In clinical samples the prevalence rate of social phobia has been reported to be as high as 14.9%.

Course of illness and outcome
• The average age of onset of social phobia in clinically referred youngsters is between 11 and 12 years old.
• Although research is limited, unrecognized and untreated social phobia may have significant and long-lasting negative effects on academic and occupational achievement, self-esteem, and interpersonal interactions.

TREATMENT OPTIONS FOR ANXIETY DISORDERS

Treatment options for pediatric anxiety disorders currently emphasize cognitive–behavioral therapy (CBT) approaches as initial therapeutic interventions for youngsters with separation anxiety, school refusal, generalized anxiety disorder, selective mutism, mild or infrequent panic attacks, and social anxiety disorders. In general, these directive approaches are more effective than nondirective therapies based on general psychodynamic therapy principles. Psychologists with at least a master's degree are generally the type of professional who are most trained in the delivery of CBT. Pharmacotherapy is considered adjunctive to CBT for more severe or disabling anxiety disorders. The

ANXIETY DISORDERS

exceptions to this statement are obsessive–compulsive disorder (discussed in chapter 21) and frequent or severe panic disorder, both of which require additional early pharmacotherapy intervention. In this section, CBT interventions are discussed first, followed by psychopharmacological treatment studies.

Psychosocial Therapies

Currently there are 13 controlled studies of CBT for anxiety disorders in children and adolescents. Across all CBT studies, between 50% and 80% of treated children improve and no longer meet criteria for an anxiety disorder after completion of CBT. This approach emphasizes time-limited interventions generally averaging 10–16 weeks of treatment. The learning of new skills and coping techniques for individual anxiety management and mastery are crucial to successful CBT treatment. Assessment of a priori and objectively defined outcome measures occurs in most CBT therapies. Many CBT techniques are supported by empirical evidence for their efficacy in pediatric anxiety disorders.

Treatment includes individual, group, and family CBT formats. Group CBT is an ideal psychosocial intervention for social phobia. The group setting provides a natural arena for anxiety exposure and the application and practice of CBT treatment techniques. In family CBT, parents are an important part of the treatment plan; parents may have many anxieties, fears, and worries that require management if the child with anxiety is to succeed in treatment.

Cognitive–behavioral strategies emphasize the following techniques.

• Gradual exposure to the feared situation
• Systematic desensitization using relaxation strategies
• Contingency management (e.g., positive reinforcement, shaping of behaviors, extinction)
• Cognitive strategies (e.g., problem solving, coping techniques, positive self-talk)
• Modeling and demonstration of appropriate behaviors
• Family interventions
  ○ Parent anxiety management
  ○ Teaching parents to function as co-therapists in the home environment (i.e., the CBT therapist transfers skills to the parents, who then transfer skills to the anxious child in the home environment).
• Involvement of the school and classroom teacher in the behavioral therapy
• Expectations that the child will succeed
• Monitoring of progress using a priori defined outcome measures

In summary, individual, group, and family CBT are effective and well tolerated psychosocial therapies for pediatric anxiety disorders. They appear more effective than nonspecific psychodynamic therapy for early-onset anxiety disorders.

Psychopharmacology in Pediatric Anxiety Disorders

Pharmacological interventions for pediatric anxiety disorders should be considered for anxiety disorders with the following characteristics.

- Symptoms not responding to 6–8 weeks of CBT with a family component
- Comorbid psychiatric disorders such as ADHD, depression, psychosis, or bipolar illness
- Obsessive–compulsive disorder (discussed in chapter 21)
- Severe symptoms with prominent daily impairment or avoidance
- Severe physiological symptoms of anxiety
- Impairment caused by anxiety in ≥ 3 areas of the patient's life (home, school, occupational, interpersonal, social)

Pertinent medication studies

Medications for pediatric anxiety disorders are only just beginning to be rigorously studied. In general, SSRI antidepressants are the medications of first choice for anxiety disorders in youngsters, with or without combined CBT. Fluvoxamine, fluoxetine, paroxetine, and sertraline are presently the best-studied medications for pediatric anxiety disorders. Benzodiazepines are rarely used to treat chronic anxiety in the young because of concerns about abuse potential and drug diversion. Benzodiazepines are best used for acute situational anxiety before medical or dental procedures. Tricyclic antidepressants such as imipramine have been found helpful for pediatric anxiety disorders. However, they have an unfavorable side effect profile and risk of lethality in overdose, compared with SSRI antidepressants. Buspirone is a nonbenzodiazepine anxiolytic with effectiveness in adults with anxiety disorders. A large buspirone clinical trial in pediatric anxiety is currently underway, but results are not presently available.

Antihistamines, chloral hydrate, antipsychotics, sedatives, clonidine, and beta-blockers have either not been formally investigated or lack efficacy in pediatric anxiety disorders. These agents are generally not recommended for anxiety disorders that are not complicated by other comorbid psychiatric disorders. The following table summarizes research in this area.

CHOOSING AND INITIATION A MEDICATION

- SSRI antidepressants are agents of first choice in pediatric anxiety disorders.
- Benzodiazepines are used only on a time-limited basis for preprocedural anxiety and worry associated with medical and dental interventions.
- Imipramine may be used when pediatric anxiety is complicated by comorbid ADHD, enuresis, or insomnia.

Medication treatment initiation

Dose ranges for the commonly used medications to treat anxiety disorders in children and adolescents are given in the following table.

Before treatment

- Obtain baseline (off-drug) rating scales of anxiety symptoms and severity for the purpose of comparing with on-drug symptoms and treated severity.
- Obtain baseline (off-drug) rating scales of symptoms before drug therapy actually begins.

Table 20.7 Controlled Studies of Medications in Pediatric Anxiety Disorders[a]

Study (year)	Drug	Disorder	N	Age Range (years)	Dose (mg/day)	Duration (weeks)	Outcome
Berney et al. (1981)	Clomipramine	SR	51	9–14	40–75		No drug differences
Bernstein et al. (1990)	Alprazolam	SR	24	7–18	Avg 1.4	8	No drug differences
Bernstein et al. (2000)	Imipramine	SR	47	12–18	Avg 180	8	Imi + behavior therapy superior to Imi + placebo
Black & Uhde (1994)	Fluoxetine	SM	15	6–11	12–27	12	Significant improvement on drug compared to placebo
Gittleman-Klein & Klein (1971)	Imipramine	SR	35	6–14	100–200	6	Imi + behavior therapy superior to Imi + placebo
Graee et al. (1994)	Clonazepam	SAD	15	7–13	0.5–2	4	No drug differences
Klein et al. (1992)	Imipramine	SR	21	6–15	100–200	6	No drug differences
RUPP Anxiety Study Group (2001)	Fluvoxamine	GAD, SP, SAD	128	6–16	50–250	8	Significant improvement on drug compared to placebo. Effect size = 1.1
Rynn et al. (2001)	Sertraline	GAD	22	5–17	50	9	Significant improvement on drug compared to placebo
Simeon et al. (1992)	Alprazolam	OAD	30	8–16	0.5–3.5	4	No drug differences
Wagner et al. (2004)	Paroxetine	SP	322	8–17	10–50	16	Paroxetine is effective compared to placebo

[a]Excludes obsessive–compulsive disorder and posttraumatic stress disorder.
GAD = generalized anxiety disorder; OAD = overanxious disorder (now called GAD); SAD = separation anxiety disorder; SM = selective mutism (now part of social phobia); SP = social phobia; SR = school refusal (not a diagnosis but part of SAD, GAD, and/or social phobia)

Table 20.8 Suggested Pediatric Dose Ranges for Anxiety Disorders

Medication	Children (dose per day)	Adolescents (dose per day)
Buspirone	10–30 mg	10–60 mg
Citalopram	5–20 mg	10–40 mg
Clonazepam	0.125–0.5 mg	0.5–2 mg
Escitalopram	2.5–10 mg	5–20 mg
Fluoxetine	5–20 mg	10–50 mg
Fluvoxamine	50–150 mg	100–300 mg
Imipramine	2–5 mg/kg/day	2–5 mg/kg/day
Lorazepam	0.5–2 mg	2–4 mg
Paroxetine	5–20 mg	10–50 mg
Sertraline	25–100 mg	50–250 mg

Source: Labellarte MJ and Ginsburg GS. Anxiety disorders. In: Martin A, Scahill L, Charney DS, and Leckman JF (Eds.), Pediatric Psychopharmacology Principles and Practice New York: Oxford University Press, pp. 497–510, 2003.

- ○ Parents frequently misreport symptoms of their child's anxiety as medication side effects. Comparing parent reported on-drug symptoms with a pre-drug evaluation allows a more accurate picture of true medication side effects to be appreciated.
- Educate parents/guardians and the child about the expected benefits of drug treatment, possible side effects, use of the medication, and duration of medication treatment.
  - ○ Written materials about the drug and disorder are helpful for parents/guardians and older children.
- Determine if the child has any contraindications to anxiolytic therapy.

Initiating treatment
- Selective serotonin reuptake inhibitors
  - ○ SSRIs may cause behavioral activation, agitation, jittery feelings, and increase risk for suicidal ideation and behaviors in children and adolescents.
    - ■ These agents, and all antidepressants used in pediatric psychopharmacology, now carry a black box warning cautioning about the possibility of these side effects.
    - ■ Weekly follow-up over the first month after initiating treatment with an SSRI and every-other-week monitoring in the second month are now recommended. While on continuation therapy, follow-up every 3 months, as necessary, is advised.
  - ○ Initiate SSRI at the lowest possible dose.
    - ■ Weight-based dosing is not available for SSRIs.
  - ○ Titrate dose every 5–7 days until the daily dose is within the therapeutic range.
  - ○ Fluoxetine may be given once daily even in young children because if its active metabolites and long half-life.
  - ○ If activation, jitteriness, or insomnia occurs as a side effect, give the majority of the SSRI dose in the morning.

- ○ If sedation is a prominent side effect, give the majority of the SSRI dose in the evening.
- ○ If no response occurs within 2–4 weeks, titrate the SSRI dose into the medium to high range for no less than 2 weeks.
  - ▪ If no response occurs, switch to a different anxiolytic medication.
- ○ High doses of SSRIs other than fluoxetine may require twice daily dosing in young children because of increased metabolism and a shorter half-life compared to adults.
- • Imipramine
  - ○ Baseline and on-drug EKGs are required; EKG parameters for youngsters on tricyclic antidepressants include the following.
    - ▪ Pulse < 125 bpm
    - ▪ QTc < 460 msec
    - ▪ On-drug QTc increase < 30% of baseline QTc
    - ▪ PR interval < 200 msec
  - ○ Baseline and on-drug vital signs are necessary
  - ○ Imipramine dosing is weight based; the final daily dose for imipramine is 2–5 mg/kg/day in divided doses.
  - ○ Initiate imipramine at 25 mg for young children and 50 mg for adolescents in the evening.
  - ○ Titrate by 25–50 mg every 5–7 days.
    - ▪ Use a twice to three times daily dose schedule for prepubertal children.
    - ▪ Use a twice daily dose schedule for young teenagers.
    - ▪ Use a once daily dose schedule given in the evening for older teenagers (Tanner Stage 5) and young adults.
- • Buspirone
  - ○ No pre-drug workup is necessary.
  - ○ Initiate at 5 mg three times daily.
  - ○ Titrate every 5–7 days to a maximum dose of 30 mg in prepubertal children or 60 mg in adolescents.
- • Benzodiazepines
  - ○ Used only for the short-term (1–14 days) relief of acute situational anxiety in child and adolescent psychopharmacology
  - ○ Not used for chronic anxiety in children and adolescents.
  - ○ Initiate at the lowest dose; titrate to the lowest effective dose while monitoring sedative side effects.
  - ○ The use of longer-acting benzodiazepines with a long half-life, such as clonazepam, will protect against subtle daily benzodiazepine withdrawal effects in youngsters.

Duration of Treatment
- • Time to treatment effects vary with the type of medication.
  - ○ SSRIs may take 2–6 weeks
  - ○ Imipramine may take 2–6 weeks
  - ○ Buspirone may take 2–4 weeks
  - ○ Benzodiazepines have almost immediate effects on anxiety.

- Duration of treatment
  - ○ Not well established.
  - ○ Should be of long enough duration and effective enough in reducing anxiety symptoms that, when combined with psychosocial therapies such as CBT, the child is able to learn new mastery and coping techniques to help him or her eventually manage anxiety without medications.
  - ○ After anxiety medication is discontinued, the child should be monitored periodically for the possible return of anxiety. Youngsters who have had an anxiety disorder are at risk for the emergence of a second anxiety disorder later in life, especially during times of stress or transition.

ANXIETY DISORDERS

21. Obsessive–Compulsive Disorder

Obsessive–compulsive disorder (OCD) is an anxiety disorder that can occur in children and adolescents as well as in adults, and is not as rare as previously thought. More benign obsessional thinking and mild worry are common in community populations of children and adolescents and do not warrant a psychiatric diagnosis. Compulsions must be distinguished from the more benign habit disorders of young children. In OCD, obsessions are defined as intrusive, repetitive thoughts, ideas, images, or impulses that are anxiety provoking and excessive. They are typically recognized as being unwanted and are disturbing to the individual. Compulsions are ritualized actions designed to thwart distressing anxiety and worry. When obsessions and/or compulsions are frequent, consume more than 60 minutes in a single day, and cause impairment on a daily basis, OCD may be present. The diagnostic criteria for OCD are given in Table 21.1.

Common obsessions and compulsions are listed below.

Despite similarities between children, adolescents, and adults in OCD symptoms, some developmental differences in phenotypic expression may be present. For example, children and adolescents may have higher rates of obsessions about fears of catastrophic events (e.g., death of a loved one, illness) than adults. Sexual obsessions appear underrepresented in children. In terms of compulsions, hoarding rituals are more often observed in children and adolescents than in adults.

PREVALENCE

OCD was initially thought to be a rare disorder. More recent epidemiological studies indicate that it may be more common than suggested by previous research.

- In adults the prevalence of OCD is about 1%.
- In children and adolescents the prevalence of OCD is between 1% and 2%.
- The gender ratio is about equal between males and females with pediatric onset OCD.

O
C
D

427

Table 21.1 Diagnostic Criteria for Obsessive–Compulsive Disorder

A. Either obsessions or compulsions:
 Obsessions as defined by (1), (2), (3), and (4):
 (1) Recurrent and persistent thoughts, impulses, or images that are experienced, at some time during the disturbance, as intrusive and inappropriate and that cause marked anxiety or distress.
 (2) The thoughts, impulses, or images are not simply excessive worries about real-life problems.
 (3) The person attempts to ignore or suppress such thoughts, impulses, or images, or to neutralize them with some other thought or action.
 (4) The person recognizes that the obsessional thoughts, impulses, or images are a product of his or her own mind (not imposed from without as in thought insertion).
 Compulsions as defined by (1) and (2):
 (1) Repetitive behaviors (e.g., hand washing, ordering, checking) or mental acts (e.g., praying, counting, repeating words silently) that the person feels driven to perform in response to an obsession, or according to rules that must be applied rigidly.
 (2) The behaviors or mental acts are aimed at preventing or reducing distress or preventing some dreaded event or situation; however, these behaviors or mental acts either are not connected in a realistic way with what they are designed to neutralize or prevent or are clearly excessive.
B. At some point doing the course of the disorder, the person has recognized that the obsessions or compulsions are excessive or unreasonable. Note: This does not apply to children.
C. The obsessions or compulsions cause marked distress, are time consuming (take more than 1 hour a day), or significantly interfere with the person's normal routine, occupational (or academic) functioning, or usual social activities or relationships.
D. If another psychiatric disorder is present, the content of the obsessions or compulsions is not restricted to it.
E. The disturbance is not due to the direct physiological effects of a substance (e.g., a drug of abuse, a medication) or a general medical condition.

American Psychiatric Association. *Desk Reference to the Diagnostic Criteria from DSM-IV–TR.* Washington, DC, American Psychiatric Association, pp. 217–218, 2000. Reprinted with permission.

Table 21.2 Common Obsessions and Compulsions in Children and Adolescents

Obsessions	Compulsions
Concern over dirt and germs	Cleaning rituals
Fears of an ill fate befalling loved ones	Repeating actions
Exactness or symmetry	(doing and undoing)
Religious scrupulousness	Checking rituals
Bodily functions	Ordering rituals
Lucky numbers	Counting rituals
Somatic preoccupations	Washing rituals
Preoccupation with fears over	Hoarding
possible catastrophes	
Sexual preoccupations	
Aggressive preoccupations	

COMORBIDITY

OCD rarely occurs as a single diagnosis in children and adolescents. Lifetime comorbidity rates approach 80% in persons with OCD. Psychiatric disorders that co-occur with OCD in children and adolescents are:

• Depression in 8–73%.
• Anxiety disorders in 13–70%.
• Disruptive behavioral disorders (ODD, CD, ADHD) in 3–57%.
• Tic disorders in 13–26%.

Other types of comorbidity with OCD may occur.

• Trichotillomania (persistent hair pulling to the point of alopecia)
• Eating disorders
• Body dysmorphic disorder
• Psychotic disorders
• Anxious and perfectionistic temperamental traits

COURSE OF ILLNESS AND OUTCOME

The onset of OCD is generally subacute and insidious. Sometimes environmental precipitants can be found that seem to trigger onset. Often no precipitant can be identified. Although OCD can start in adulthood, the mean age of onset in children is around 10 years. Symptoms generally start slowly, build over time, and then wax and wane. Children and adolescents typically come to clinical attention many years after the start of OCD, suggesting a long lag time between disease onset and clinical referral.

Impairment from OCD can be severe, yet selective. Often the symptoms are hidden from nonfamily members. Academic achievement and extracurricular activities may not be affected. However, at home the child with OCD may involve the entire family in his or her rituals and obsessions, leading to severe impairment in the home environment and family dysfunction. Social relationships with friends may be affected by OCD, leading to increasing isolation of the child.

The longitudinal outcome of OCD is variable. Outcome can range from complete remission after an episode to a relentless, chronic course. In one 40-year longitudinal study of adults with OCD, Skoog and Skoog (1999) found:

• OCD onset < 20 years old in 29%
• An intermittent OCD course with remission between episodes in 56%
• An unremitting, chronic OCD course in 27%
• Complete remission after a single episode (episode lasting ≤ 5 years) in 17%
• In adolescents, a 69% recovery rate after 2 years was reported (Berg et al., 1989).
• Often, residual symptoms of anxiety, OCD, and/or depression remain for many years and continue to influence daily life functioning and cause impairment

ASSESSMENT

The assessment of children and adolescents with OCD includes a comprehensive psychiatric evaluation that reviews current and past obsessive–compulsive symptoms and comorbid psychiatric disorders. An adequate evaluation obtains information from multiple sources, including the child, parents, and reports on school functioning and interpersonal relationships. Symptoms of OCD must be distinguished from common childhood repetitive, perfectionistic, or habit behaviors that are normal for children at various stages of development. Habits and rituals (e.g., bedtime rituals) are most common for young children ages 2–5 years. Anxiety is a common reaction to life stress at any age. Repetitive rituals that are pleasurable, readily suppressible, and do not interfere with daily

O
C
D

functioning are not considered symptoms of OCD. In contrast, pathological obsessions and compulsions are recurrent, bothersome, and interfere with daily functioning. Children and adolescents are often embarrassed by, and secretive about, their OCD symptoms and hide them from others.

Assessment of the child should include:

• Identification of specific symptoms and their frequency, context, and associated degree of impairment
• The child or adolescent's efforts to resist the obsessions and compulsions
• The child or adolescent's insight into the symptoms
• History of any associated tic disorders
• Comorbid depression and/or anxiety symptoms
• The context, onset, and longitudinal course of symptoms

Once a clinical diagnosis of OCD has been established, rating scale instruments such as the Yale–Brown Obsessive–Compulsive Scale or the Child's Version of the Leyton Obsessional Inventory may be used to ascertain symptom severity and track symptoms over time. The following table summarizes OCD rating scales.

Assessment of the family should include:

• The degree to which parents and siblings have become entangled in the child's symptoms
• Family dysfunction caused by the OCD symptoms
• Biological family history of OCD, tic disorders, Tourette's disorder, ADHD, anxiety disorders, and depression

Medical history should include:

• A history of upper respiratory tract infections, including those caused by group A beta-hemolytic streptococcus infection (e.g., pediatric autoimmune neuropsychiatric disorders associated with streptococcus [PANDAS]).
  ○ Most important for the child with an explosive, abrupt onset or exacerbation of OCD and/or tics in the context of a sore throat or upper respiratory infection.

TREATMENT

OCD is a spectrum disorder. The nature and severity of symptoms, the degree of comorbid psychopathology, and the impact of the disorder on child and family functioning vary significantly in youngsters with OCD. Mild obsessions or compulsions that are not a source of distress may only warrant monitoring over time without specific treatment intervention. When treatment is clinically indicated, two treatment modalities, cognitive–behavioral therapy (CBT) and selective serotonin reuptake inhibitors (SSRIs), have been systematically studied in pediatric OCD and shown empirically to have specific efficacy for the core symptoms of OCD. Although not sufficient alone for the treatment of OCD, adjunctive family therapy is often useful clinically to help the family better

Table 21.3 Rating Scales for Obsessions and Compulsions in Children and Adolescents

Rating Scale	Type of Scale	What Is Assessed?	Age Range (years)	Reliability	Validity	Sensitivity to Change
Yale–Brown Obsessive Compulsive Scale	Clinician rated	Severity of OCD symptoms	Child, adolescent	++	++	Yes
Leyton Obsessional Inventory—Child Version	Self-report	Severity of OCD symptoms over the past 2 weeks	Child, adolescent	++	++	No
Obsessive–Compulsive Scale of the Child Behavior Checklist	Parent report	Severity of OCD symptoms	Child, adolescent	++	++	No

++ = good; + = fair

OCD

understand their child's symptoms and disentangle themselves from the child's obsessions and compulsions at home.

Cognitive-Behavioral Therapy

Although research is lacking as to how to predict which individuals will benefit most from CBT, clinical experience suggests that relatively mild to moderate OCD symptoms, older child age, the absence of comorbid psychiatric disorders, a stable family, at least average intelligence, and good insight will increase the chances of a successful CBT therapy. A 13–20 week course of CBT is usually adequate, with "booster sessions" as needed. Therapy works best if delivered by a master's- or Ph.D.-level therapist specifically trained in CBT.

Component analysis of CBT in adult OCD suggests that both exposure to the anxiety-provoking stimulus and response prevention are active ingredients of treatment. Exposure reduces phobic anxiety and response prevention reduces the performance of rituals. Relaxation training, breathing-control training, positive reinforcement using contingency behavioral techniques, and cognitive restructuring help the patient tolerate the anxious feelings induced by exposure. Exposure with response prevention (ERP) is more effective in OCD than CBT alone. Response rates for ERP coupled with CBT range between 60% and 90% for uncomplicated cases of OCD.

Psychopharmacology

Along with ADHD, early-onset OCD is the most well studied disorder in pediatric psychopharmacology. At least 19 scientific studies report that serotonergic medications are effective in the short- and medium-term treatment of OCD. Several studies report that efficacy can be maintained over at least 1 year of treatment. Across all medication studies, response rates range between 42% and 53%. The placebo response rate for pediatric OCD ranges between 8% and 37%. Pharmacological interventions for pediatric OCD are effective. However, response rates remain modest and residual symptoms often remain.

Pharmacological interventions should be considered for OCD with the following characteristics.

- Severe and impairing symptoms
- High comorbidity with other psychiatric disorders
- Symptoms that do not respond to a 4–6-week trial of ERP and CBT.
- Patients with moderate to severe symptoms who are not motivated for ERP/CBT therapy.

Systematic dose–response data are not available for pediatric OCD. However, in randomized controlled clinical studies and as ascertained from expert clinician consensus, several drug management criteria are generally agreed upon for OCD.

- Use robust doses of SSRI agents. Generally OCD responds better to higher rather than lower doses of medications. Dose ranges of commonly used drugs to treat OCD and the average dose used in clinical trial data are given in the table below.

Table 21.4 Dose Range for clomipramine and SSRIs Used in Pediatric OCD

Drug	Child Starting Dose (mg)	Adolescent Starting Dose (mg)	Typical Dose Range (mg)	Average Dose in Controlled Studies (mg)
Clomipramine	12.5–25	25	50–200 or 3 mg/kg/day	150
Fluoxetine	5–10	10–20	10–80	25
Sertraline	12.5–25	25–50	50–250	178
Fluvoxamine	12.5–25	25–50	50–300	165
Paroxetine	5–10	10	10–60	32
Citalopram	5–10	10–20	10–60	——

Source: Geller DA and Spencer T. Obsessive–compulsive disorder. In: Martin A, Scahill L, Charney DS, and Leckman JF (Eds.), *Pediatric Psychopharmacology Principles and Practice.* New York: Oxford University Press, pp. 511–525, 2003.

• An adequate trial of an SSRI consists of at least 10–12 weeks of drug treatment at maximal tolerated dose. Gradual improvement may accrue beyond the first 12 weeks of treatment. Treatments of shorter duration may fail.

PERTINENT MEDICATION STUDIES IN PEDIATRIC OCD

Controlled studies conducted in pediatric OCD patients indicate that serotonergic medications are effective in the treatment of OCD. These agents include SSRI antidepressants such as fluoxetine, fluvoxamine, paroxetine, citalopram, and sertraline. Fluoxetine, sertraline, and fluvoxamine are FDA approved for manufacturer's advertising in pediatric OCD. SSRIs are now considered the pharmacological treatment of choice for pediatric OCD. A tricyclic antidepressant, clomipramine, is also effective for the pharmacological treatment of early-onset OCD. Because of an increased rate of side effects, including possible cardiovascular treatment-emergent adverse events, clomipramine should not be considered a first-line choice in the medication treatment of OCD.

Medications are not a "cure" for OCD. Because of modest response rates, residual symptoms often remain. Children and parents must be educated about response rates for medications in OCD. Because of residual symptoms, medication interventions are often combined with ERP/CBT therapies in OCD.

March and colleagues (2004) recently reported results from the Pediatric OCD Treatment Study (POTS). In this study 112 children and adolescents were randomly assigned to receive CBT for 12 weeks, sertraline for 12 weeks, the combination, or placebo. Results showed that combination treatment was superior to CBT alone and sertraline alone. All active treatments were significantly superior to placebo. CBT alone and sertraline alone did not differ from each other. The rate of clinical remission was 53.6% for the combination arm, 39.3% for CBT alone, 21.4% for sertraline alone, and 3.6% for placebo treatment. This study suggests that combination treatment of pediatric OCD with CBT and an SSRI is effective.

O
C
D

Table 21.5 Controlled Studies of Medications in Pediatric Obsessive–Compulsive Disorder

Study (year)	Drug	Study Type	N	Age Range (years)	Dose (mg/day)	Duration (weeks)	Outcome
DeVeaugh-Geiss et al. (1992)	Clomipramine	RCT	60	10–17	200	8	Effective
Geller et al. (2001)	Fluoxetine	RCT	103	7–17	20–60	7	Effective
Geller et al. (2002)	Paroxetine	RCT	203	7–17	10–50	10	Effective
Leonard et al. (1991)	Clomipramine	Discontinuation design	26	8–19	50–225	12	Effective
Liebowitz et al. (2002)	Fluoxetine	RCT	43	8–17	20–80	16	Effective
March et al. (1998)	Sertraline	RCT	187	6–17	25–200	12	Effective
March et al. (2004)	Sertraline	RCT	112	7–17	150–250	12	Effective
Riddle et al. (1992)	Fluoxetine	CO	14	8–15	20	8	Effective
Riddle et al. (2001)	Fluvoxamine	RCT	120	8–17	50–200	10	Effective

RCT = randomized controlled trial; CO = crossover design

434

COURSE OF TREATMENT

Selecting an initial agent
- SSRIs are the initial treatment of choice.
- There is no evidence that one SSRI is superior to another in the treatment of OCD.
- Fluoxetine, fluvoxamine, paroxetine, and sertraline all have at least one RCT supporting their safety and efficacy in pediatric OCD; support for citalopram comes only from open-label studies at the present time.
- Clomipramine should be reserved for patients who have failed an adequate trial (maximal dose for at least 10–12 weeks) of an SSRI, or who have comorbid ADHD.

Before treatment
- Complete a thorough psychiatric evaluation and document any comorbid psychiatric diagnoses that will be a focus of treatment in addition to OCD.
- Obtain results of a physical exam completed within the 6–12 months prior to initiating therapy.
- Obtain a baseline level of OCD symptom severity using an established rating scale.
- Obtain baseline ratings of drug side effects to compare against on-drug reported side effects.
- Educate the family about the nature of OCD, expected benefits of drug treatment, possible side effects, use of the medication, and expected duration of treatment.
- Determine if the child has any contraindications to SSRI therapy.

Initiating treatment
- Selective serotonin reuptake inhibitors
  - Initiate at lowest possible dose and titrate every 5–7 days until dose is in the therapeutic range.
  - In OCD response generally requires moderate to high doses maintained for at least 10–12 weeks.
  - SSRIs and other antidepressants used in pediatric psychopharmacology may cause increased agitation, disinhibition, akathisia, and jittery feelings, and may exacerbate risk for suicidal behaviors. Antidepressants now carry a black box warning about these risks. Close physician follow-up after initiating antidepressant treatment is now recommended.
- Clomipramine
  - A baseline and on-drug EKG is required for tricyclic antidepressant use in children and adolescents; EKG parameters for youngsters on tricyclic antidepressants include the following:
    - Pulse < 125 bpm
    - QTc < 460 msec
    - On-drug QTc increase < 30% of baseline QTc
    - PR interval < 200 msec
  - Baseline and on-drug vital signs are necessary for children and adolescents receiving tricyclic antidepressants.

○ Clomipramine dosing is weight based; the final daily dose for clomipramine should not exceed 3 mg/kg/day or 200 mg (whichever is lower) administered in divided doses.

○ Initiate clomipramine at 25 mg for young children or 50 mg for adolescents in the evening.

○ Titrate by 25–50 mg every 5–7 days until therapeutic dose range is achieved.
  ■ Use a twice to three times daily dose schedule for prepubertal children.
  ■ Use a twice daily dose schedule for young teenagers.

○ Use a once daily dose schedule given in the evening for older teenagers (Tanner Stage 5) and young adults.

Duration of treatment

• The optimal duration of treatment for children with OCD is presently unknown.

• Expert consensus suggests 9–18 months of treatment after symptom resolution or stabilization to prevent relapse of the index episode.

• Medications should be discontinued gradually (about 25% every 1–2 months) with careful psychiatric monitoring for any return of OCD.

• OCD is a chronic condition in some patients; when OCD medication is discontinued the child should be monitored periodically for the possible return of OCD.

STRATEGIES FOR OCD TREATMENT RESISTANCE

If the patient with OCD does not respond to an adequate dose of medication after an adequate duration of therapy, consider the following:

• Psychiatrically reevaluate for the presence of comorbid psychiatric disorders such as ADHD, depression, other anxiety disorders, and/or substance abuse.
  ○ Treat comorbid conditions in addition to OCD.

• Failure to respond to an initial medication trial for OCD does not predict failure to respond to another drug. If little clinical response is seen after 10–12 weeks of an initial SSRI trial or if the initial drug is not well tolerated, switch to another SSRI or consider a clomipramine trial.

• For patients who achieve a partial response after several SSRI trials, consider augmentation strategies with a second agent.
  ○ The atypical antipsychotic agent risperidone can be used adjunctively with SSRIs to achieve a more robust response in OCD.
  ○ Clonazepam can be used adjunctively with SSRIs to increase response; the clinician should monitor for any sedation or behavioral disinhibition caused by clonazepam.
  ○ An SSRI such as sertraline is sometimes combined with clomipramine in treatment-resistant cases of severe OCD. Careful attention to potential pharmacokinetic interactions with drug metabolism is recommended. Elevated clomipramine plasma levels (and risks of cardiovascular side effects) by SSRI interference with CYP isoenzyme metabolic pathways are possible.
    ■ Sertraline and citalopram are least likely to elevate tricyclic plasma levels due to less potential CYP isoenzyme interactions.

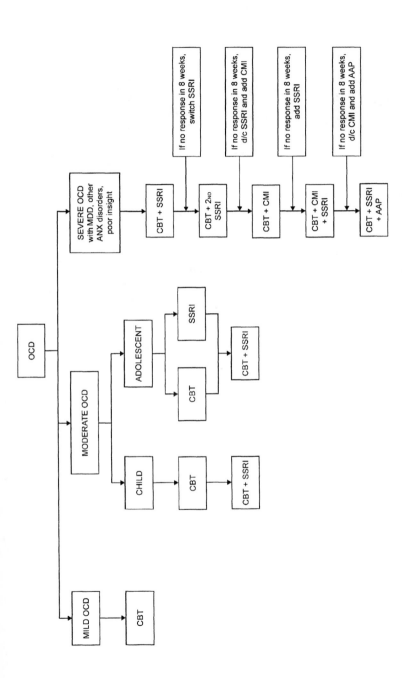

Figure 21.1 A treatment algorithm for obsessive–compulsive disorder (OCD) in children and adolescents.
CBT = cognitive–behavioral therapy; SSRI = selective serotonin reuptake inhibitor; MDD = major depressive disorder; ANXI = anxiety disorder; CMI = clomipramine; AAP = atypical antipsychotic. Adapted from Geller DA and Spencer T. Obsessive–compulsive disorder. In Martin A, Scahill L, Charney DS, and Leckman JF (Eds.). *Pediatric Psychopharmacology Principles and Practice.* New York: Oxford University Press, pp. 511–525, 2003.

OCD

437

MEDICATION TREATMENT ALGORITHMS

Systematic approaches to the treatment of child and adolescent OCD may be found in treatment algorithms. One such algorithm is presented in the following figure. Although algorithms for pediatric OCD have not been tested in clinical research trials, they are based on empirical evidence and are a useful means of organizing an approach to the young patient with OCD.

PEDIATRIC AUTOIMMUNE NEUROPSYCHIATRIC DISORDERS ASSOCIATED WITH STREPTOCOCCAS (PANDAS)

Some children may develop OCD symptoms after group A beta-hemolytic streptococcal infection. In contrast to the insidiously slow onset of the psychiatric disorder of OCD, streptococcal-associated OCD often has an explosive, abrupt onset in the context of a sore throat or flu-like illness. As the full name implies pediatric autoimmune neuropsychiatric disorders associated with streptococcas (PANDAS) involve an autoimmune response in which there is cross-reaction of group A beta-hemolytic streptococcal bacteria and CNS basal ganglia structures such as the caudate nucleus, putamen, and globus pallidus. Often tics may be present along with OCD symptoms. This mechanism may be important for 10–20% of children and adolescents developing OCD.

If PANDAS are suspected, the child should be assessed for evidence of group A beta-hemolytic streptococcal infection.

• A throat culture, antistreptolysin O (ASO) and anti-DNAase B titer should be obtained.
• Interepisode antibody levels are recommended to demonstrate a later rise associated with an intercurrent streptococcal infection and subsequent increase in OCD or tic symptoms.

Treatment consists of antibiotic therapy for the streptococcal infection and psychiatric treatment for the OCD or tic disorder.

22. Posttraumatic Stress Disorder

The essential feature of posttraumatic stress disorder (PTSD) and acute stress disorder (ASD) is the development of a characteristic cluster of psychological, behavioral, and physiological symptoms following exposure to a severe stressor or traumatic incident that arouses "intense fear, helplessness, and/or horror." Exposure can occur through direct experience or through learning about a traumatic event that caused or threatened death or serious injury to oneself or others. Traumatic events can include witnessing violence or a disaster, being the victim of a natural disaster, violence, torture, rape, sexual abuse and/or physical abuse, or learning that others have been subjected to these events. Events can be one-time disasters such as an earthquake or hurricane, or multiple ongoing and chronic traumas as occur in war or during prolonged physical/sexual abuse.

Endorsement of some PTSD symptoms is adaptive following exposure to a trauma and does not imply psychopathology. When the danger persists, symptoms of PTSD can be adaptive and promote individual survival. When the danger passes, symptoms generally abate over time. However, in some traumatized individuals symptoms of traumatic stress do not fade away once the danger has passed. These persons may be at risk for the development of PTSD.

Adaptation to traumatic stress differs depending on whether the trauma is a one-time event or is chronic and persisting over time. PTSD is a complicated condition involving dysregulation of multiple neurobiological systems and cognitive, affective, and behavioral domains of functioning. Partial PTSD symptomatology may be disabling, and the full symptom complex may take time to develop fully.

That psychological reactions occur to severe stress has been known for thousands of years. In the past hundred years the study of human reactions to extreme stress has been confined mostly to war and combat situations under the names of "shell shock," "battle fatigue," or "combat neurosis." After the Vietnam war PTSD research intensified and expanded to include extreme trauma that may occur to civilians, such as rape or being burned in a fire. Initially studied only in adults, PTSD is now being increasingly investigated in children and adolescents.

The clinical presentation of PTSD in children and adolescents is heterogeneous, often with multiple and varied symptoms. The cardinal features of PTSD include initial exposure to a traumatic event and the subsequent development of three characteristic symptom clusters. The *A criterion* includes exposure to trauma and the experiencing of, witnessing of, or being confronted with a traumatic event. The *B criterion* involves reexperiencing the traumatic event after it is over and includes persistent, unwanted, and intrusive memories of the trauma, sudden reminders of the event, or flashbacks associated with the trauma. The *C criterion* involves avoidance of reminders associated with the trauma. Included here are the individual's efforts to avoid thoughts, feelings, or memories of the event. Hyperarousal, the *D criterion*, may manifest as anger outbursts, irritability, sleep disturbance, hypervigilance and scanning of the environment for signs of danger, or an exaggerated startle reaction. There are three PTSD subtypes, including an acute type, a chronic type, and a delayed type. Symptoms must be persistent for at least 1 month. Child-specific PTSD symptoms include repetitive play, generalized nightmares, and "trauma-specific reenactment."

Acute stress disorder (ASD) was added as a new diagnostic category in DSM-IV. Diagnosis requires at least three dissociative symptoms, one reexperiencing symptom, avoidance of reminders of the trauma and marked anxiety or hyperarousal. ASD must occur within 4 weeks of exposure to the trauma and last 2 days to 4 weeks.

PREVALENCE

Exposure to catastrophic trauma is not as rare as once thought.

• The estimated lifetime prevalence of PTSD in the general population ranges between 1% and 14%.
• Between 6% and 7% of the U.S. population is exposed annually to extreme stressors, ranging from natural disasters, to crime, to motor vehicle accidents, and/or to acts of terrorism.
• In 2000, approximately 879,000 children were found to have suffered from maltreatment such as neglect, physical abuse, and/or sexual abuse.
• By age 18 years up to 6% of children and adolescents in samples of lower-middle-class households met criteria for a lifetime diagnosis of PTSD.
• Random samples of urban youth exposed to community violence yield PTSD rates as high as 35%.
• In high-risk populations (e.g., incarcerated youth) prevalence rates ranging between 3% and 100% have been reported.
• PTSD occurs across all cultural and ethnic groups.
• Some studies indicate that whereas girls may develop more severe PTSD symptoms when exposed to traumatic events than boys, boys are more likely than girls to be exposed to such events.

Table 22.1 Diagnostic Criteria for Posttraumatic Stress Disorder

A. The person has been exposed to a traumatic event in which both of the following were present:
   (1) The person experienced, witnessed, or was confronted with an event or events that involved actual or threatened death or serious injury, or a threat to the physical integrity of self or others
   (2) The person's response involved intense fear, helplessness, or horror. Note: In children, this may be expressed instead by disorganized or agitated behavior.
B. The traumatic event is persistently reexperienced in one (or more) of the following ways:
   (1) Recurrent and intrusive distressing recollections of the event, including images, thoughts, or perceptions. Note: In young children, repetitive play may occur in which themes or aspects of the trauma are expressed.
   (2) Recurrent distressing dreams of the event. Note: In children, there may be frightening dreams without recognizable content.
   (3) Acting or feeling as if the traumatic event were recurring (includes a sense of reliving the experience, illusions, hallucinations, and dissociative flashback episodes. Note: In young children, trauma-specific reenactment may occur.
   (4) Intense psychological distress at exposure to internal or external cues that symbolize or resemble an aspect of the traumatic event
   (5) Physiological reactivity on exposure to internal or external cues that symbolize or resemble an aspect of the traumatic event
C. Persistent avoidance of stimuli associated with the trauma and numbing of general responsiveness (not present before the trauma), as indicated by three or more of the following:
   (1) Efforts to avoid thoughts, feelings, or conversations associated with the trauma
   (2) Efforts to avoid activities, places, or people that arouse recollections of the trauma
   (3) Inability to recall an important aspect of the trauma
   (4) Markedly diminished interest or participation in significant activities
   (5) Feelings of detachment or estrangement from others
   (6) Restricted range of affect
   (7) Sense of a foreshortened future
D. Persistent symptoms of increased arousal (not present before the trauma), as indicated by two or more of the following:
   (1) Difficulty falling or staying asleep
   (2) Irritability or outbursts of anger
   (3) Difficulty concentrating
   (4) Hypervigilance
   (5) Exaggerated startle response
E. Duration of the disturbance is more than 1 month.
F. The disturbance causes clinically significant distress or impairment in social, occupational, or other important areas of functioning.
Specify if:
   Acute: if duration of symptoms is less than 3 months.
   Chronic: if duration of symptoms is 3 months or more.
   Delayed Onset: if onset of symptoms is at least 6 months after the stressor.

American Psychiatric Association. *Desk Reference to the Diagnostic Criteria* from *DSM-IV-TR*. Washington, DC, American Psychiatric Association, pp. 218–220, 2000. Reprinted with permission.

COMORBIDITY

Children, adolescents, and adults with PTSD commonly meet diagnostic criteria for other psychiatric disorders. Indeed, PTSD rarely, if ever, occurs in the absence of other psychiatric conditions. Comorbid disorders often found in persons with PTSD include the following.

• Depression
• Substance abuse
• Other anxiety disorders
• ADHD
• Conduct disorder

Table 22.2 Diagnostic Criteria for Acute Stress Disorder

A. The person has been exposed to a traumatic event in which both of the following were present:
   (1) The person experienced, witnessed, or was confronted with an event or events that involved actual or threatened death or serious injury, or a threat to the physical integrity of self or others
   (2) The person's response involved intense fear, helplessness, or horror
B. Either while experiencing or after experiencing the distressing event, the individual has three (or more) of the following dissociative symptoms:
   (1) A subjective sense of numbing, detachment, or absence of emotional responsiveness
   (2) A reduction in awareness of his or her surroundings (e.g., "being in a daze")
   (3) Derealization
   (4) Depersonalization
   (5) Dissociative amnesia (i.e., inability to recall an important aspect of the trauma)
C. The traumatic event is persistently reexperienced in at least one of the following ways: recurrent images, thoughts, dreams, illusions, flashback episodes, or a sense of reliving the experience; or distress on exposure to reminders of the traumatic event.
D. Marked avoidance of stimuli that arouse recollections of the trauma (e.g., thoughts, feelings, conversations, activities, places, people).
E. Marked symptoms of anxiety or increased arousal (e.g., difficulty sleeping, irritability, poor concentration, hypervigilance, exaggerated startle response, motor restlessness).
F. The disturbance causes clinically significant distress or impairment in social, occupational, or other important areas of functioning.
G. The disturbance lasts for a minimum of 2 days and a maximum of 4 weeks and occurs within 4 weeks of the traumatic event.
H. The disturbance is not due to the direct physiological effects of a substance (e.g., a drug of abuse, a medication) or a general medical condition, is not better accounted for by Brief Psychotic Disorder, and is not merely an exacerbation of a preexisting psychiatric disorder.

American Psychiatric Association. *Desk Reference to the Diagnostic Criteria from DSM-IV–TR*. Washington, DC, American Psychiatric Association, pp. 221–222, 2000. Reprinted with permission.

- Borderline personality disorder (in traumatized adolescents)
- Psychotic symptoms may occur in severely traumatized children and adolescents.

COURSE OF ILLNESS AND OUTCOME

Few studies have examined the longitudinal course of pediatric PTSD. Most studies document a variable course with trauma-associated symptoms varying over time. In some individuals symptoms decrease, but for others they endure or increase. PTSD symptoms often persist over many years in some severely traumatized children and adolescents. At times, PTSD can have a delayed onset. Studies have documented the emergence of PTSD 5–8 years after the end of the original trauma. Often PTSD symptoms recede with time, but other symptoms such as anxiety or depression may endure.

Several factors have been identified that appear to affect an individual's response to trauma and help determine the longitudinal course of PTSD.

- Characteristics of the traumatic event
  - Man-made events are thought to be more traumatic than naturally occurring events.
  - Community-wide events may prompt more support (and less chance of developing PTSD) than traumatic events that happen to only one individual (and may be borne alone).

- Exposure
  - Physical proximity to the event is thought to increase risk; those individuals further away and more distant from the site of the trauma appear to be at less risk.
  - A dose–response relationship to the trauma and increased risk for PTSD have been reported; the more closely exposed the individual is to the trauma and the longer the time exposed to the event, the higher the risk.
  - Physical injury to the individual as a result of trauma increases risk.
  - Interpersonal closeness to a victim increases risk for PTSD to a child.
  - Multiple forms of exposure to the traumatic event, such as being physically injured and witnessing the injury of a loved one increases risk.
- Personal and family characteristics
  - Preexisting emotional and behavioral problems and a history of prior trauma increase risk for poor outcomes.
  - Parental PTSD reactions may increase the risk for child PTSD development.
  - Poor parental functioning and a priori parental psychopathology increase risk for the traumatized child.

ASSESSMENT

Clinical assessment of the traumatized child or adolescent should involve both the child and his or her parents. Children may not spontaneously report their symptoms, and adults may underestimate the degree of trauma to the child. Thus assessment must include gathering information from both the child and the parents.

Assessment of trauma involves the completion of a comprehensive clinical psychiatric evaluation. Particular emphasis should be placed upon

- Assessment of the youngster's current safety
- Description and history of exposure to the current trauma
- History of prior trauma and adaptation
- Comorbid psychiatric conditions
- Parental and family functioning
- Sources of comfort and support available to the patient

Once a diagnosis of PTSD or ASD has been established by clinical psychiatric evaluation, PTSD rating scales can help assess the severity of symptoms. Some established rating scales for the assessment of PTSD symptom severity in children and adolescents are given in the following table.

TREATMENT OPTIONS

There currently exists a paucity of empirical treatment studies in childhood PTSD. As such, no empirically based approach to treatment is available to guide clinical practice. A variety of modalities is used to treat PTSD and ASD, including individual psychodynamic psychotherapy, cognitive–behavioral therapy (CBT), family therapy, group psychotherapy, school-based interventions,

Table 22.3 Rating Scales for PTSD in Children and Adolescents

Rating Scale	Type of Scale	What Is Assessed?	Age Range (years)	Reliability	Validity
Checklist for PTSD Symptoms in Infants and Young Children	Clinician rated	PTSD symptoms	0–3	—	—
Child PTSD Symptom Scale	Child interview	PTSD symptoms	Not Specified	+ +	+ +
Child Stress Reaction Checklist	Parent, teacher, or staff report	PTSD symptoms	Not Specified	+ +	+ +
Children's PTSD Inventory	Self-report	PTSD diagnostic criteria	Not Specified	+ +	+
Posttraumatic Symptom Inventory for Children	Child interview	PTSD symptoms	4–8	+ +	+
PTSD Checklist/Parent Report	Parent report	PTSD symptoms	Not Specified	+ +	+ +
PTSD Reaction Index	Self-report	PTSD symptoms	Not Specified	+ +	+ +
When Bad Things Happen Scale	Self-report	PTSD symptoms	≥ 9	+ +	+ +

+ + = good; + = fair

444

and psychopharmacology. Little research presently documents the effectiveness of treatment, and no comparative treatment studies of childhood PTSD are available to guide the clinician in choosing one specific treatment modality over another. Psychosocial interventions are currently considered the mainstay of therapeutic treatment for the traumatized child or adolescent. Psychopharmacology is considered adjunctive when trauma symptoms are severe and/or become disabling.

Psychosocial Interventions

PSYCHOEDUCATION

The initial step in PTSD treatment for the traumatized child or adolescent is the provision of education about the disorder. Psychoeducational interventions should provide the child, parents, and caregivers with information about the following.

• A description of PTSD symptoms and diagnosis
• The nature of the human stress response
• Treatment targets and goals
• Rationales for each treatment intervention
• Expected course of PTSD symptoms
• The possibility of comorbid psychiatric disorders in need of intervention

INDIVIDUAL PSYCHODYNAMIC PSYCHOTHERAPY

• The goal of traditional individual psychodynamic psychotherapy is to transform the child's self-concept from victim to survivor in a safe and empathic professional setting in which painful and overwhelming emotions and experiences can be safely explored.
• A target of psychotherapy is the patient's avoidance of PTSD associated experiences. Avoidance of memories and feelings about the trauma is a core symptom of PTSD. Avoidance may prevent the initiation of treatment and impede progress once treatment has begun. This process must be handled in a sensitive manner so as to avoid overwhelming the patient with intense unpleasant emotions.
• Another target of psychotherapy is an understanding of the patient's inaccurate appraisals and attributions about the traumatic event(s), such as self-blame, guilt, or omen formation.

COGNITIVE–BEHAVIORAL THERAPY

• Desensitization to fear-inducing environmental stimuli that are reminders of trauma, coupled with relaxation techniques and cognitive restructuring, has been used in the clinical treatment of childhood PTSD.

FAMILY THERAPY

• The family plays a major role in the degree of adjustment the child makes to the trauma and should be included in the treatment.

- Helping parents master their own trauma and emotional distress will help them become more emotionally available to the traumatized child.
- Family work should focus on the following:
  ○ Validate the traumatized child's experiences.
  ○ Help the child regain a sense of safety and security.
  ○ Anticipate situations in which the child will require additional support.
  ○ Find ways within the family structure to decrease traumatic reminders and trauma-related stresses.

GROUP THERAPY

- Group therapy is useful when large numbers of children are exposed to a common traumatic event.
- Group therapy should focus on the following:
  ○ Usual responses of human beings to trauma
  ○ Reactions to traumatic reminders
  ○ Reactions to trauma anniversaries
  ○ Coping mechanisms
  ○ Relaxation techniques

SCHOOL-BASED INTERVENTIONS

- School-based PTSD interventions are most useful for large numbers of children exposed to a common traumatic event.
- School-based interventions should focus on the following:
  ○ Correcting misperceptions and fears
  ○ Encouraging normalization and recovery
  ○ Explaining the traumatic event, providing information, and addressing the normal stress response
- School-based interventions should work to identify and refer children in need of more intensive individual and family interventions.

Psychopharmacology

A scientific body of literature is beginning to emerge on the neurobiology of stress and trauma from both preclinical and clinical studies. This research is starting to guide clinical pharmacological practice in PTSD. The physiological systems involved in traumatic stress include the immune system, the neuroendocrine system, and the central nervous system (CNS). These systems may become altered in PTSD. Associated trauma-related symptoms may involve cognition, memory, affect and emotions, and behavior.

At least eight neurobiological systems mediate the mammalian stress response and may be involved in PTSD. These neurobiological systems in the CNS are most relevant to psychopharmacological interventions. A rational approach to the pharmacotherapy of PTSD can be informed by understanding medication effects on these systems. These CNS systems include:

- Adrenergic system
- Dopaminergic system
- Serotonergic system

- Gamma-aminobutyric acid (GABA)/benzodiazepine system
- Opioid system
- N-methyl D-aspartate (NMDA) system
- Neuroendocrine systems
  ○ Hypothalamic–pituitary–adrenal (HPA) system
  ○ Growth hormone
  ○ Thyroid hormone
  ○ Gonadal axis

It should be noted that most of the scientific work on the neurobiology of PTSD accrues from the adult literature; there is a lack of empirical studies in pediatric PTSD. This is also true for psychopharmacological treatments. Most controlled medication studies involve adult PTSD patients and are extrapolated downward to help inform psychopharmacological treatment of traumatized children and adolescents.

Psychopharmacology has two adjunctive roles to play in the treatment of pediatric PTSD:

- Target disabling PTSD symptoms so that daily impairment is diminished and the child may pursue a more normal developmental trajectory.
- Help the traumatized child tolerate emotionally painful material in order to participate in rehabilitative psychosocial therapy.

Medication interventions should be considered for pediatric PTSD with the following characteristics:

- Severe PTSD symptoms that significantly interfere with daily functioning
- Moderate PTSD symptoms with a marked physiological component (autonomic nervous system hyperarousal, sleep disturbance, rage attacks, irritability)
- Disabling PTSD symptoms that do not respond to 6–8 weeks of psychosocial intervention with a family component
- PTSD symptoms that are comorbid with pharmacologically responsive psychiatric disorders such as ADHD, other anxiety disorders, psychotic symptoms, and/or depression.

Only one controlled study has been completed about the effectiveness of pharmacotherapy in pediatric PTSD (Roberts et al., 1999). This study compared imipramine to chloral hydrate in pediatric burn victims. Imipramine was more effective than chloral hydrate in treating ASD. No other controlled medication studies of pediatric PTSD are available. Other studies of medications in pediatric PTSD are given in the following table.

MEDICATION TREATMENT INITIATION

Before treatment
- Ensure that the traumatized child is safe from ongoing traumatic stress. Medication therapy is of little value in treating PTSD if the trauma remains ongoing. For example, treating an abused PTSD child with medications is not

Table 22.4 Studies of Medications in Pediatric PTSD

Study (year)	Drug	Study Type	N	Age Range (years)	Dose (mg/day)	Duration	Outcome
Famularo et al. (1988)	Propranolol	ABA Open	11	Avg 8.5	0.8 mg/kg/dose tid	4 weeks	Improved hyperarousal and aggression
Harmon & Riggs (1996)	Clonidine	Open	7	3–6	0.05–0.2	4 weeks	Improved hyperarousal and aggression
Loof et al. (1995)	Carbamazepine	Open	28	8–17	300–1200; serum levels 10–11.5	2–13 weeks	All patients improved
Domon & Anderson (2000)	Nefazodone	Open	Not reported	Adolescents	200–600	Not reported	Improvement in hyperarousal, aggression, insomnia
Perry (1994)	Clonidine	Open	17	Child	0.1–0.2	Variable	Improved anxiety, hyperarousal, impulsivity
Roberts et al. (1999)	Imipramine	RCT	25	2–19	1 mg/kg hs	1 week	80% with improved symptoms
Seedat et al. (2002)	Citalopram	Open	24	10–18	20–40	8 weeks	Suggested effectiveness

ABA = on-off-ondrug trial; RCT = randomized controlled trial

P
T
S
D

helpful if the child continues to be abused. Establishing the safety of the child is of first importance.

- Educate parents and the child about the expected benefits of drug treatment for the symptoms of traumatic stress, possible side effects, use of the medication, and duration of medication treatment. Explain that medication therapy is adjunctive to psychosocial treatments and is not a "cure" for PTSD.
  - Written materials about the drug and disorder are helpful for parents and older children.
- Obtain baseline (off-drug) rating scales of PTSD/ASD symptoms and severity for the purpose of comparing with on-drug side effects, symptoms, and treated severity.
  - Parents frequently misreport symptoms of the disorder as medication side effects. Comparing parent reported on-drug side effects with a pre-drug evaluation allows a more accurate picture of true medication side effects.
- Determine if the child has any contraindications to medication therapy.

CHOOSING A MEDICATION

Selective serotonin reuptake inhibitors (SSRIs)
In the adult PTSD literature, a number of successful case reports, open-label trials, and randomized controlled trials have documented that SSRIs such as fluoxetine, sertraline, paroxetine, and fluvoxamine are effective (Brady et al., 2000; Marshall et al., 2001). Paroxetine and sertraline are currently FDA approved for adult PTSD. Currently, only a single open-label study using an SSRI, citalopram (Seedat et al., 2002), has been published in pediatric PTSD. Despite the paucity of pediatric evidence, SSRIs are a common first choice for adjunctive pharmacotherapy in childhood PTSD and ASD because of their generally benign safety profile and safety in overdose. Because SSRIs have been proven effective in adult PTSD, it is hoped they will also eventually be shown to be effective in pediatric PTSD.

Treatment
- May be most effective by reducing avoidant and numbing symptoms in PTSD/ASD.
- Optimal results may require high doses of SSRIs for a minimum duration of 8–12 weeks.
- If target symptoms are not reduced by 25–50% after 8–12 weeks of SSRI treatment, consider switching to a different SSRI.
- May be very useful in traumatized children with comorbid depression or panic anxiety.
- Initiate SSRI at the lowest possible dose.
  - Weight-based dosing is not available for SSRIs.
- Titrate dose every 5–7 days until the daily dose is within the therapeutic range.
- For high doses, consider split dosing.
- Dose ranges for commonly used SSRIs in PTSD:
  - Fluoxetine 10–80 mg/day
  - Fluvoxamine 50–300 mg/day

- ○ Paroxetine 5–60 mg/day
- ○ Sertraline 25–200 mg/day
- ○ Citalopram 5–60 mg/day
- ○ Escitalopram 5–20 mg/day
- SSRIs may cause behavioral activation, agitation, jittery feelings, and increase risk for suicidal ideation and behaviors in children and adolescents. These agents, and all antidepressants used in pediatric psychopharmacology, now carry a black box warning cautioning about the possibility of these side effects. Weekly follow-up over the first month after initiating treatment with an SSRI and every-other-week monitoring in the second month are now recommended. While on continuation therapy, follow-up every 3 months, as necessary, is advised.

Adrenergic agents

Alpha-adrenergic agents such as clonidine and guanfacine and beta-blockers such as propranolol have been used adjunctively in pediatric and adult PTSD. The catecholamines norepinephrine and epinephrine are involved in sympathetic nervous system arousal, anxiety, aggression, mood regulation, thinking, and memory. Reduction of autonomic nervous system overarousal with adrenergic agents may be effective in the treatment of hyperarousal, impulsivity, explosive aggression, and irritability seen in PTSD and ASD.

Treatment

- Baseline and on-drug monitoring of pulse and blood pressure are necessary because clonidine, guanfacine, and propranolol are hypotensive agents.
  - ○ Pulse should not fall below 50 bpm.
  - ○ SBP should not fall below 80 mmHg.
  - ○ DBP should not fall below 50 mmHg.
- A baseline and on-drug EKG
  - ○ Should be completed during beta-blocker treatment; the clinician should be alert to the development of bradycardia arrhythmias.
  - ○ May be considered for clonidine.
  - ○ Not necessary for guanfacine treatment.
- Children with a medical history of cardiovascular disease, stroke, or syncope should not receive adrenergic hypotensive agents.
- Adrenergic agents may be most useful in PTSD complicated by insomnia, overarousal, hyperactivity, and explosive aggression.

Clonidine

- Initiate with a low dose and titrate to effect.
  - ○ Begin at 0.05 mg hs for 3–4 days; titrate by 0.05 mg every 3–4 days until therapeutic dose range is reached.
  - ○ For younger children give clonidine in three or four divided daily doses.
  - ○ For teenagers give clonidine in two or three divided daily doses.
  - ○ The dose range for clonidine in the treatment of PTSD has not been established; the usual dose range for clonidine in child and adolescent psychopharmacology is 0.05 to 0.35 mg/day.

Guanfacine
- Initiate with a low dose and titrate to effect.
  - Begin at 0.5 mg hs for 3–4 days; titrate by 0.5 mg every 3–4 days until therapeutic dose range is reached.
  - Guanfacine has a longer half-life than clonidine and can be given less frequently.
    - For younger children, give guanfacine in two or three divided daily doses.
    - For teenagers, give guanfacine in two divided daily doses.
  - The dose range for guanfacine in the treatment of PTSD has not been established; the usual dose range for guanfacine in child and adolescent psychopharmacology is 0.5–4.0 mg/day.

Propranolol
- Initiate with a low dose and titrate to effect.
  - Begin at 10 mg hs for young children and 20 mg hs for teenagers. Titrate upward by 10–20 mg every 3–4 days until therapeutic dose range is reached.
  - Give in two to four divided daily doses.
  - The dose range for propranolol in the single pediatric study assessing effects in childhood PTSD was 20–160 mg/day.
  - The weight-based average dose range was 0.8–2.5 mg/kg tid.

Withdrawal
- Adrenergic agents may cause a withdrawal reaction if abruptly discontinued. They must be titrated downward by approximately 20% of the total daily dose every 3–4 days when being discontinued.
- The psychiatrist must educate guardians and patients about the dangers of medication noncompliance with adrenergic agents, especially when high doses are prescribed.

Tricyclic antidepressants (TCAs)
In the only controlled study completed to date in the pharmacological treatment of pediatric PTSD, imipramine 1 mg/kg administered as a single evening dose was superior to chloral hydrate 25 mg/kg in the hospital treatment of pediatric burn victims with PTSD symptoms. The symptoms of hyperarousal and intrusive memories appeared to respond best to imipramine therapy. Other tricyclic antidepressants have not been investigated for PTSD/ASD in child and adolescent psychopharmacology.

Treatment
- Pulse and blood pressure monitoring are necessary when treating with a tricyclic antidepressant such as imipramine.
  - BP should not exceed 140/90.
  - BP should not be less than 80/50.
  - TCAs may cause an anticholinergic-mediated tachycardia; pulse should not exceed 125 bpm.
- Initiate imipramine
  - At 25 mg hs for children
  - At 50 mg hs for teenagers

• Titrate by 25 mg every 3–4 days until 1 mg/kg/hs. *Note*: This dose is much lower than the dose of imipramine in the treatment of depression and anxiety disorders (2–5 mg/kg in divided doses).

Atypical Antipsychotics

• Although currently there are no studies of risperidone, olanzapine, quetiapine, ziprasidone, or aripiprazole in pediatric PTSD, these agents are occasionally used when psychotic symptoms or extreme aggression are present.
• Low doses are generally used in the clinical treatment of pediatric PTSD. Initiate treatment at the lowest possible dose and titrate every 5–7 days until desired effect.
• Dose ranges used in clinical practice include the following:
  ○ Risperidone 0.25–2.0 mg in 2–4 divided daily doses
  ○ Olanzapine 2.5–10 mg in two divided daily doses
  ○ Quetiapine 100–400 mg in two or three divided daily doses
  ○ Ziprasidone 20–120 mg in two daily divided doses
  ○ Aripiprazole 2–10 mg in one dose

Nefazodone

• One case report suggests its effectiveness in pediatric PTSD with adolescents (Domon & Anderson, 2000). Studies in young children with PTSD/ASD have not been completed.
• May be most helpful for prominent symptoms of hyperarousal, anger, aggression, insomnia, and concentration problems.
• In the one case series completed in adolescents, the average effective dose for PTSD was 200 mg bid.
• Has been associated with hepatic toxicity.
  ○ It is recommended that baseline LFTs be obtained and followed every 3 months during treatment. It should be noted that nefazodone is not currently labeled for use in the pediatric age range.

Carbamazepine

• One open-label study suggests effectiveness in pediatric PTSD (Loof et al., 1995).
• May be most useful in PTSD complicated by a seizure disorder. It also appears helpful in decreasing PTSD symptoms of avoidance, numbing, hyperarousal, and sleep dysregulation.
• For children under 6 years of age initiate carbamazepine at 10–20 mg/kg/day bid or tid and titrate weekly until the therapeutic dose range is reached.
• For older children initiate at 100 mg bid and titrate weekly until the therapeutic dose range is reached.
• For teenagers initiate at 200 mg bid and titrate weekly until the therapeutic dose range is reached.
• Based on the single available open-label study, the dose range of carbamazepine for pediatric PTSD is 300–1200 mg/day given in divided doses.
• Trough serum levels between 4 and 12 μg/ml should be achieved.

- Because of a rare risk of agranulocytosis and aplastic anemia reported with carbamazepine use, baseline and on-drug hematological monitoring is required.
- Because of reports of liver toxicity, baseline and on-drug liver function tests are recommended.
- Because of reports of hyponatremia associated with carbamazepine use, baseline and on-drug electrolytes, BUN, creatinine, and urinalysis should be monitored.
- Because carbamazepine is a tricyclic compound, EKG changes, including the possibility of QTc prolongation, may occur with use. Baseline and on-drug EKG monitoring is recommended. EKG guidelines are the same as those for tricyclic antidepressants.

23. Mental Retardation, Autism, and Other Pervasive Developmental Disorders

"Developmental disorders" encompass both children and adolescents with mental retardation as well as those with more pervasive developmental disorders such as autism and autism spectrum disorders. Both mental retardation and pervasive developmental disorders are considered in this chapter.

MENTAL RETARDATION

Mental retardation (MR) is a behavioral syndrome characterized by impairments in a present level of intellectual and adaptive skills. MR is not a single entity but includes a heterogeneous group of individuals with a broad spectrum of levels of functioning, disabilities, and strengths. There exists no single disease entity, with a single cause or mechanism, that explains the clinical diversity of persons with MR. Likewise, the natural course and prognosis of persons with MR may vary widely. MR is not necessarily lifelong; as persons with MR grow up, they may learn enough skills to function adequately. The diagnosis requires deficits in adaptive functioning as a result of MR, so these individuals, especially those with mild MR, may shed the diagnosis later in life. However, for others MR may be a chronic condition with sustained deficits in daily life skills and functioning that require supported living.

Diagnostic Features

The American Association on Mental Retardation (1992) developed a tridimensional definition that is widely accepted:

> Mental retardation refers to substantial limitations in present functioning. It is characterized by significantly subaverage functioning, existing concurrently with related limitations in 2 or more of the following applicable adaptive skill areas: communication, self-care,

home living, social skills, community use, self-direction, health and safety, functional academics, leisure, and work. Mental retardation manifests before age 18.

This definition is clinically useful because it subclassifies MR according to the intensity and nature of needed supports. It emphasizes the need for a comprehensive assessment in multiple relevant domains of individual functioning, including the importance of diagnosing comorbid mental health disorders in the assessment of MR.

The DSM-IV criteria for mental retardation are given in the following table. Note that MR is classified by severity, as assessed by standardized and individually administered psychological tests of intellectual functioning.

Table 23.1 Diagnostic criteria for Mental Retardation

A. Significantly subaverage intellectual functioning: an IQ of approximately 70 or below on an individually administered IQ test (for infants, a clinical judgment of significantly subaverage intellectual functioning)
B. Concurrent deficits or impairments in present adaptive functioning (i.e., the person's effectiveness in meeting the standards expected for his or her age by his or her cultural group) in at least two of the following areas: communication, self-care, home living, social/interpersonal skills, use of community resources, self-direction, functional academic skills, work, leisure, health, and safety
C. The onset is before 18 years.

Code based on degree of severity reflecting level of intellectual impairment:
317   Mild Mental Retardation: IQ level 50–55 to approximately 70
318.0 Moderate Mental Retardation: IQ level 35–40 to 50–55
318.1 Severe Mental Retardation: IQ level 20–25 to 35–40
318.2 Profound Mental Retardation: IQ level below 20 or 25
319   Mental Retardation, Severity Unspecified, when there is a strong presumption of Mental Retardation but the person's intelligence is untestable by standard tests (e.g., for individuals too impaired or uncooperative, or with infants).

American Psychiatric Association. *Desk Reference to the Diagnostic Criteria from DSM-IV–TR.* Washington, DC, American Psychiatric Association, pp. 52, 2000. Reprinted with permission.

The etiology of MR is diverse. The etiology for most mild MR (IQ 50–70) is unknown. As the IQ falls below 50, more organic causes can be identified. Identifiable causes of MR and their estimated frequency include the following.

- Genetic prenatal disorders (32%)
  ◦ Chromosomal aberrations (e.g., Down syndrome)
  ◦ Monogenic mutations (e.g., tuberous sclerosis, fragile X, phenylketonuria)
  ◦ Malformation syndromes due to known microdeletions (e.g., Williams syndrome, Prader–Willi syndrome)
  ◦ Multifactorial "familial MR"
- External prenatal causes (12%)
  ◦ Maternal infection
  ◦ Toxins (e.g., fetal alcohol syndrome)
  ◦ Toxemia, placental insufficiency
  ◦ Hypothyroidism

- Perinatal causes (11%)
  - Infections
  - Delivery problems (e.g., neonatal asphyxia)
  - Other (e.g., hyperbilirubinemia)
- Malformations of unknown causation (8%)
  - Malformations of the CNS (e.g., neural tube defects)
  - Multiple malformation syndromes (e.g., Cornelia de Lange syndrome)
- Postnatal causes (8%)
  - Infections
  - Toxins (e.g., lead poisoning)
  - Psychosocial deprivation
  - Other (e.g., head trauma, CNS tumor)
  - Child abuse and neglect
- Unknown causes (29%)

Prevalence and Epidemiology

The prevalence of MR in the population is approximately 1%. About 85% of persons with MR are thought to have mild MR (IQ 50 to 70–75); about 10% have moderate MR (IQ 35–49); about 4% have severe MR (IQ 20–34); and about 1%, profound MR (IQ < 20). The time of diagnosis varies with age; the more severe the MR, the earlier in development it is diagnosed.

Comorbidity

Medical comorbidity
As retardation becomes more severe, the prevalence of associated medical disorders increases. Seizure disorders occur in 15–30% of persons with IQs below 50, motor handicaps, including cerebral palsy, occur in 20–30%, and sensory impairments (e.g., hearing and vision deficits) occur in 10–20%. Persons with mild MR do not seem to have an increased prevalence of associated medical conditions, as compared to the general population.

Psychiatric comorbidity
Mental disorders are frequently comorbid with MR. Prevalence estimates of psychiatric disorder in persons with MR range between 30% and 70%, which is far higher than in the general population. An early study comparing the prevalence of psychopathology in children with and without MR in an unselected population on the Isle of Wight (Rutter et al., 1976) indicated that the prevalence was 5 or more times higher in children with MR than in those without MR.

- ADHD occurs at about the same rate in persons with MR as in the general population, estimated at between 4% and 12%.
- Conduct disorder and oppositional defiant disorder rates are elevated in persons with mild MR.
  - CD/ODD rates as high as 33% have been reported in this population.

- Depression occurs more frequently in the MR population than in the general population.
  - Rates between 1% and 11% have been reported.
- Schizophrenia may or may not occur more frequently in persons with MR; rates between 1% and 9% have been reported. Because the clinical diagnosis of schizophrenia requires some degree of language competency, schizophrenia is not able to be diagnosed in persons with severe or profound MR.
- About 75% of persons with autism also meet criteria for MR.
- Anxiety disorders are thought to occur in about 25% of persons with MR.

Course of Condition and Outcome

The course of MR is heterogeneous without a single, uniform natural history. The prognosis for a given individual typically reflects the interaction of three levels: biomedical, psychological, and social–environmental.

- Biomedical factors
  - The presence of inborn errors of metabolism or degenerative conditions will affect the lifespan and abilities of an individual.
  - The presence of epilepsy or cerebral palsy may affect a person's functional adaptation.
- Psychological factors
  - Cognitive ability and the balance between cognitive impairments and strengths are important determinants of outcome. In general, the more severe the cognitive impairment, the less autonomous will be the individual and the more supports for daily adaptation will be needed.
  - Communication skills are extremely important and influence adaptation to daily life.
  - Comorbid psychiatric disorders are important factors influencing adaptation and quality of life.
- Social–environmental factors
  - The availability of family support and educational, habilitative, medical, and social services is an important determinant of outcome.

Assessment

Patients with MR are typically referred to mental health professionals because of behavioral or emotional problems. Psychiatrists, primary care physicians, and other mental health professionals are seldom expected to do the initial diagnosis and assessment of MR. The initial cognitive assessment is generally completed by special education personnel and psychologists. The psychiatric evaluation of persons who have MR should follow the general rules of psychiatric assessment. The evaluation must be comprehensive, using multiple reporters to assess the functioning of the patient with MR in many different situations. Because of associated cognitive and language disabilities, physical disabilities, and/or life circumstances, the psychiatrist should expect that the diagnostic evaluation may take more time and effort than the evaluation of persons of normal cognition. The psychiatric evaluation of the person with MR should never be focused solely on a "medication evaluation," but rather assess the patient's strengths and vulnerabilities across all important areas of life functioning. Components of a comprehensive psychiatric evaluation are given in the following table.

Table 23.2 Components of a Comprehensive Psychiatric
Assessment of Children and Adolescents with Mental Retardation

Domain	Information Assessed
Presenting symptoms	Behavioral description of symptoms. Examples
	Management measures used and results
	Precipitants to symptoms
	How behavioral problems commonly begin and end
Assessments	Review of past assessments, including
	Cognition
	Information-processing strengths and weaknesses
	Communication skills
	Adaptive functioning
Medical review	Results from most recent physical examination
	Review of systems
	Review of current medication use
Adaptive skills	Communication
	Social Community integration
	Self-care
	Self-direction
	Functional academic skills
	Work and leisure
	Health
	Safety
Mental health	Past diagnoses
	Current psychosocial treatments
	Psychiatric medication use, dose, side effects, duration of treatment, beneficial effects
Environmental supports	Living situation
	Family supports
	Treatment plan
	Current therapies
Stressors	Family events
	Losses
	Transitions
	Traumatic events
Family	Structure and functioning
	Style: overprotection vs. encouraging patient growth
	Behavioral management techniques and results
	Expectations for the patient
	Family dynamics

Source: American Academy of Child and Adolescent Psychiatry Work Group on Quality Issues. Practice parameters for the assessment and treatment of children, adolescents, and adults with mental retardation and comorbid mental disorders. *J Am Acad Child Adolesc Psychiatry* 38(Suppl):17S, 1999.

Rating scales to assess the presence and severity of comorbid psychopathology and adaptive skills are given in the table below.

Psychoeducational Treatment

Children and adolescents with MR require a comprehensive psychoeducational treatment plan. The goal of treatment is not merely removal of symptoms but helping the patient to achieve the best possible quality of life. Treatment

Table 23.3 Rating Scales for Mental Retardation and Associated Psychopathology in Children and Adolescents

Rating Scale	Type of Scale	What Is Assessed?	Age Range	Reliability	Validity	Sensitivity to Change
Aberrant Behavior Checklist	Parent and/or teacher report	Irritability, lethargy, stereotypy, hyperactivity, speech	5 yrs, to adult	+ +	+ +	Yes
Nisonger Child Behavior Rating Form	Parent and/or teacher report	Prosocial and problem behaviors	Child and adolescent	+ +	+ +	Yes
The Reiss Screen for Maladaptive Behavior—Child and Adolescent Version	Parent	Psychopathology and problem behaviors	Child and adolescent	+ +	+ +	Yes
Vineland Adaptive Behavior Scales	Parent	Adaptive functioning	Child, adolescent, adult	+ +	+ +	No

+ + = good; + = fair

emphasizes the concept of normalization; that is, making available to the mentally retarded patterns and conditions of everyday life that are as close as possible to the norms and patterns of the mainstream of society.

PSYCHOSOCIAL TREATMENTS

Persons with MR may benefit from a wide variety of psychosocial treatments, including behavioral therapy, milieu treatment, and group, family, and individual therapy.

Behavioral therapy
- The goal of behavior therapy is to replace maladaptive behaviors with more appropriate coping through skill building.
- Contingency reinforcement behavioral techniques that provide consequences for maladaptive behaviors and reinforce prosocial behaviors are a mainstay of treatment.
- To be effective, a behavior management program should be generalized and consistent across all settings, such as home and school.

Milieu treatment
- Environment influences emotions and behavior; the provision of work, educational opportunities, and living situation should be commensurate with the patient's needs and abilities.

Group, family, and individual therapy
Persons with MR can benefit from psychotherapy provided they possess sufficient communication skills (verbal or nonverbal) to permit a meaningful interchange with the therapist. Psychotherapy techniques may require modification and adjustment to accommodate the patient's mental age and cognitive strengths and weaknesses.

- Group therapy can help in developing social and communication skills.
- Family therapy can help members recognize the patient's strengths, support pathways to independence, and help identify opportunities for a patient's success.
- Individual therapy can help individuals with MR recognize their strengths and vulnerabilities, understand their own disability, develop realistic self-expectations, and alter patterns of maladaptive behavior.

EDUCATIONAL SUPPORTS

- Public education and related comprehensive services are guaranteed for children and adolescents with MR by the Education for All Handicapped Children Act (PL94-142 of 1975).
  - With later amendments this law is now called the Individuals with Disabilities Education Act (IDEA).
- This law provides for diagnostic, educational, and support services from age 3 to 21 years.

PERVASIVE DEVELOPMENTAL DISORDERS

• Parents have the right to participate in developing an individualized educational program (IEP) for their child.
  ◦ IEP planning now emphasizes inclusion and placement of disabled children and adolescents in age-appropriate classrooms.

Psychopharmacological Treatment

Psychiatric medications are used in persons with MR to target comorbid psychiatric disorders and as adjuncts to a comprehensive psychoeducational treatment plan. They are never used as the only intervention in persons with MR because there is no evidence that medications ameliorate the CNS conditions that cause MR. Thus they do not "cure" mental retardation. Medication effects in persons with MR appear to be no different from those that appear in the absence of MR.

MEDICATION GUIDELINES

Several cautions are in order when medications are used in persons with MR.

• Persons with MR have higher rates of comorbid medical conditions such as epilepsy than the general population; when the treatment is medicinal, there is a risk of drug–drug interactions with psychiatric agents.
• Persons with mild MR appear no more prone to medication adverse events than the general population. However, in persons with IQs < 50–55 a higher rate of treatment-emergent adverse events to medications have been reported. Given their communication disabilities, close clinical monitoring is required to evaluate treatment-emergent drug side effects in persons with MR.
• Persons with MR may be very sensitive to the effects of medications. Medications should be initiated in low doses and titrated slowly especially in this population. When discontinuing medications, they should be tapered gradually.

Guidelines for psychiatric medication use in persons with MR are given in the next table.

Table 23.4 HFCA Guidelines for Psychotropic Medication Use in Persons with Mental Retardation

---

Prior to prescribing psychotropic medication:
• Medical causes of behavioral problems must be ruled out.
• Environmental causes of behavioral problems must be ruled out.
• A detailed description of symptoms is required.
• A detailed differential diagnosis is required.
• Behavioral data should be collected.
• Begin treatment using the least intrusive interventions first.

When medication is prescribed:
• It should be an integral part of an overall individual treatment program.
• It should not diminish the patient's functional status.
• The lowest effective dose must be used.
• A gradual dose reduction should be periodically considered (at least annually) unless clinically contraindicated.
• Adverse drug effects should be monitored.
• Data should be collected documenting that the drug achieves the desired outcome (include patient's quality of life).

HCFA = Health Care Financing Administration
Source: AACAP Work Group on Quality Issues. Practice parameters for the assessment and treatment of children, adolescents, and adults with mental retardation and comorbid mental disorders. *J Am Acad Child Adolescent Psychiatry* 38(12 Suppl):5S–31S, 1999.

Given the high prevalence of medication use in children and adolescents with MR, it is noteworthy that few controlled studies have been completed in the pediatric age range. Controlled medication studies in children and adolescents with MR and various comorbid psychiatric disorders are presented in the following table.

ATTENTION-DEFICIT/HYPERACTIVITY DISORDER

More research has been done on the pharmacotherapy of ADHD in children and adolescents with MR than for other disorders. Studies support the use of stimulants for ADHD in persons with mild to moderate MR. Substantial benefit for motor overactivity, attention span, and impulsivity are reported.

Stimulants
- The overall response rate to stimulants in MR children and adolescents with ADHD is approximately 54%; this is lower than the stimulant response rate for ADHD in the non-MR population, which is about 75%.
- Response to stimulants for ADHD is best when the IQ > 50 and the mental age > 4.5 years.
- When the IQ is below 50, the response to stimulants becomes poor and an increased rate of side effects is reported.
- The therapeutic dose range for stimulants for persons with MR and ADHD is the same as for ADHD in the general population.
  - Methylphenidate dose range: 5–80 mg/day
  - Dextroamphetamine dose range: 2.5–40 mg/day

Alpha-adrenergic agents
- There is one controlled study reporting that clonidine is effective for ADHD in children with MR.
  - The dose range is 0.05–0.10 mg given bid or tid.
- Vital sign monitoring is required in persons prescribed clonidine.

DISRUPTIVE BEHAVIOR

Disruptive behaviors, impulsive aggression, motor hyperactivity, severe oppositional and defiant symptoms, and impulsive self-injurious behaviors are the most frequent reason for the use of psychiatric medication in persons with MR.

Atypical antipsychotics
- Several controlled studies show that risperidone is helpful compared with placebo for disruptive behavior, aggression, hyperactivity, and conduct problems in persons with MR.
  - Generally given in low doses of 0.25–3 mg in two or three divided daily doses for the adjunctive treatment of disruptive behaviors.
- Other atypical antipsychotics such as olanzapine, quetiapine, ziprasidone, and aripiprazole are probably as helpful as risperidone but have not been studied under controlled conditions in the pediatric MR population.

Table 23.5 Controlled Studies of Medications in Children and Adolescents with Subaverage IQ or Mental Retardation

Study (year)	Drug	Disorder	IQ	N	Age Range (years)	Dose	Duration (weeks)	Outcome
Agarwal et al. (2001)	Clonidine	Hyperkinetic disorder (ICD 9)	30–69	10	6–15	4–8 mcg per dose bid or tid	6	Effective for hyperactivity, inattention, and impulsivity
Aman et al. (1991)	Methylphenidate	ADHD	Mean IQ = 52	30	6–12	0.4 mg/kg/day	3	Effective for ADHD symptoms in children with mild MR
Aman et al. (2002)	Risperidone	Disruptive behaviors	36–84	118	5–12	0.02–0.06 mg/kg/day	6	Improvement in conduct problems, aggression, and hyperactivity
Buitelaar et al. (2001)	Risperidone	Disruptive behaviors	50–85	38	Adolescents	1.5–4 mg/day	6	Improvement in disruptive behaviors
Handen et al. (1994)	Methylphenidate	ADHD	48–77	47	6–12	0.6 and 1.2 mg/kg/day	1 per condition	Effective for ADHD symptoms but ↑ side effects
Niederhofer et al. (2003)	Melatonin	Insomnia	< 70	20	14–18	0.1–3 mg/hs	1	Improved sleep
Van Bellinghen & de Troch (2001)	Risperidone	Disruptive behaviors	66–85	13	6–14	Mean dose = 1.2 mg/day	4	Improvement in disruptive behaviors

Beta-blockers
- Beta-blockers such as propranolol or nadolol are sometimes used to treat explosive aggression in persons with MR.
  - Propranolol is prescribed in doses of 20–160 mg in two to four divided daily doses.
  - Nadolol is prescribed in doses between 20–120 mg in two or three daily divided doses.
- Pulse and blood pressure need to be monitored when these agents are used.
- Pre-drug and on-drug EKG monitoring is generally recommended.

ANXIETY DISORDERS

Anxiety disorders are difficult to recognize in children and adolescents with mental retardation. These youngsters have difficulty recognizing and describing anxiety symptoms in themselves. Instead, anxiety may manifest as somatic symptoms, behavioral changes, and/or temper tantrums in this population.

Selective serotonin reuptake inhibitors
- Although no controlled studies exist of SSRIs in the pediatric MR population, clinicians prefer these agents in the treatment of anxiety disorders because of their low rates of toxicity and side effects.
- The dose range of SSRIs for anxiety disorders in children and adolescents with MR is the same as that for anxiety disorders in youth with normal cognition.

Buspirone
- Buspirone has not been studied for anxiety disorders in the pediatric MR population; however, its low rate of side effects and low addiction potential make it an attractive alternative to benzodiazepines.
- The dose range is 15–60 mg in two or three divided daily doses.

Benzodiazepines
- There is concern that rates of behavioral disinhibition, sedation, and cognitive slowing are high in children and adolescents with MR treated with benzodiazepines. *Benzodiazepines are not recommended for use in anxiety disorders in the pediatric MR population.*

DEPRESSION

The diagnosis of depression in young people with MR is difficult because these patients may have a poor ability to report on their internal emotional state. Depression in this population may be recognized by the following signs.

- Low mood, sadness, tearfulness, and/or social withdrawal
- Changes in behavior, such as hostility, irritability, or loss of interest in previously enjoyed activities
- Alterations in sleep patterns
- Alterations in eating patterns

PERVASIVE DEVELOPMENTAL DISORDERS

- Somatic complaints
- Changes in energy level
- Altered school performance
- Changes in physical appearance or speech
- Regression in behavior
- Expression of grim, pessimistic thoughts

Selective serotonin reuptake inhibitors
- Although no controlled studies presently exist investigating SSRIs for depression in youngsters with MR, these agents are the first choice for treatment of serious depression in this population. Because these agents are effective antidepressants in depressed individuals of normal cognition, clinicians hope they will prove effective in persons with mental retardation and depression. That they have a low rate of medically serious side effects also makes them attractive for use in the MR population.
- The dose range for SSRI treatment of depression in children and adolescents with MR is the same as for non-MR depressed youth.

ENURESIS

Behavioral therapy is the treatment of choice for children with MR and enuresis. Medication interventions should not be undertaken without first considering behavioral management strategies. These include the use of positive reinforcement (sticker charts) for dry nights, evening fluid restriction, bladder-stretching exercises, and/or the bell and pad system. However, some MR patients may be unable to cooperate with such strategies and may need medication.

Desmopressin (DDAVP)
- DDAVP is the synthetic analog of vasopressin; it acts by increasing water retention and urine concentration in the renal distal tubules.
- DDAVP is administered intranasally in doses of 20–40 µg using a unit-dose spray pump delivery system.
  ○ The duration of anti-enuretic action is 10–12 hours.
- There is a high rate of relapse when DDAVP is discontinued.

Imipramine
- Imipramine is an effective anti-enuretic agent in young people of normal cognition; however, the available data suggest that children with MR have a less favorable response to imipramine.
- Treatment carries cardiovascular risks and risks of lowering the seizure threshold.

SLEEP DISORDERS

Sleep disorders in persons with MR can cause considerable distress. Often the family is sleep deprived from being up at night with the developmentally delayed child. They are seeking help for the child, not because the child is complaining of sleep deprivation, but because family members are sleep deprived on account of the child's atypical sleep habits. However, it should be noted that sleep problems in developmentally delayed children and adolescents may be a function of their altered neurobiology and may be fundamentally different from sleep problems in children of normal cognition. The developmentally delayed child may not have normal sleep requirements or need as much sleep as nondevelopmentally delayed youngsters.

In the evaluation of the child with MR and sleep problems the clinician should rule out comorbid psychiatric disorders that affect sleep, such as the mood disorders. Sleep problems can exacerbate and be exacerbated by psychiatric problems such as depression or anxiety. If psychiatric disorders are ruled out, the first intervention is the establishment of a bedtime routine, regular schedules for sleep and waking, limiting daytime napping, reduction of environmental disruptions, and reduction of caffeine intake.

Many psychiatric medications cause sedation; these may be useful in helping the child with MR settle for sleep. However, parents should be cautioned that medications do not enhance normal sleep architecture and may wear off late at night, causing subtle withdrawal effects that cause nighttime awakening. Medications to treat sleep problems in this population include the following.

Melatonin
- A hormone found useful in sleep disorders in children with CNS neurological insults and developmental disorders.
- Can be started at 1 mg hs and titrated until effective, up to 10 mg hs.
- As an unregulated product, there exist concerns about the purity and safety of some commercially available preparations.

Clonidine
- As an alpha-adrenergic medication that is highly sedating, clonidine is sometimes used to treat initial insomnia in doses of 0.05–0.20 mg hs.

Imipramine
- Imipramine is a tricyclic antidepressant that causes sedation as a side effect. In doses of 10–75 mg hs it is sometimes used to treat sleep problems in young people with MR.

Antihistamines (diphenhydramine)
- Over-the-counter antihistamines are widely used by parents for sleep problems in children.
- The commonly used dose is 1 mg/kg/hs.

SELF-INJURIOUS BEHAVIOR

Self-injury is defined as external trauma resulting from repetitive acts directed against oneself. Factors that increase risk for self-injurious behavior (SIB) in persons with MR appear to include more severe MR, younger age, and male gender. Within residential institutions the prevalence of SIB ranges between

PERVASIVE DEVELOPMENTAL DISORDERS

10% and 15%. In community living situations the prevalence is much lower, reported as between 1% and 2.5%.

The initial evaluation of the person with MR and SIB should emphasize a functional analysis of behavior. An attempt to identify the antecedents of the behavior should be completed. Common antecedents include dysphoric emotions, such as depression or loneliness, or physical pain. The behavior should be characterized in terms of precipitating factors, frequency, duration, and severity. Finally and most importantly, the consequences of SIB should be identified. Staff responses to SIB may inadvertently reinforce the self-injurious behavior by providing attention, support, and/or allowing the patient to vent frustration. Once a functional analysis of behavior is completed, more appropriate staff interventions may be identified that do not reinforce SIB and provide more appropriate coping mechanisms to the patient.

SIB appears to be poorly responsive to medication. The medications that appear most useful in the pharmacological treatment of SIB in persons with MR appear to be atypical antipsychotics such as risperidone, olanzapine, quetiapine, ziprasidone, and aripiprazole, and SSRI antidepressants. These are generally given in the usual therapeutic dose range.

CHILDHOOD AUTISM AND THE PERVASIVE DEVELOPMENTAL DISORDERS

Diagnostic Features

Autism and the pervasive developmental disorders (PDDs) are characterized by severe and pervasive impairment and deviance in several areas of development. These areas include reciprocal social interaction, communication, and the presence of restricted, stereotyped behavior, interests, and activities. These conditions have an early onset and are usually evident in the first 1–3 years of life. Autism and the PDDs differ from mental retardation and the more specific developmental disorders such as learning disorders in that the behavioral features and patterns of development affect multiple areas, are highly distinctive and deviant, and are not merely a manifestation of developmental delay (i.e., behavior or skills that are normal for a younger developmental age).

Autism and the PDDs are a heterogeneous group of disorders. The current DSM-IV diagnostic taxonomy specifies five related PDD diagnoses: Rett's disorder, childhood disintegrative disorder, Asperger's disorder, PDD not otherwise specified, and autistic disorder.

- Rett's disorder has been diagnosed almost exclusively in females. It is characterized by normal development through the first 5 months of life, followed by deterioration. There is a characteristic pattern of head growth deceleration, loss of previously acquired purposeful hand movements, intermittent hyperventilation, and the appearance of gait and/or truncal ataxia.
- Childhood disintegrative disorder is very rare. After normal development over the first 2 years of life, but before the age of 10, the child with disintegrative disorder has a significant loss of previously acquired skills in at least

two areas, including language, social skills, adaptive behavior, play skills, motor control, or bladder/bowel control.
- Asperger's disorder is characterized by normal cognition, language development, and adaptive behavior. Odd reciprocal social interactions, a restricted range of stereotyped interests, motor clumsiness, and delayed motor milestones identify the disorder.
- PDD NOS is diagnosed when there is a severe and pervasive impairment in the development of reciprocal social interaction. Impaired language skills and stereotyped interests and activities may be present but do not meet full criteria for autistic disorder (PDD NOS is essentially a subthreshold disorder).

The diagnostic criteria for autistic disorder are given in the following table.

Table 23.6 Diagnostic Criteria for Autistic Disorder

A. A total of six (or more) items from (1), (2), and (3), with at least two from (1), and one each from (2) and (3):
- (1) Qualitative impairment in social interaction, as manifested by at least two of the following:
  - (a) Marked impairment in the use of multiple nonverbal behaviors such as eye-to-eye gaze, facial expression, body postures, and gestures to regulate social interaction
  - (b) Failure to develop peer relationships appropriate to developmental level
  - (c) A lack of spontaneous seeking to share enjoyment, interests, or achievements with other people (e.g., by a lack of showing, bringing, or pointing out objects of interest)
  - (d) Lack of social or emotional reciprocity
- (2) Qualitative impairments in communication as manifested by at least one of the following:
  - (a) Delay in, or total lack of, the development of spoken language (not accompanied by an attempt to compensate through alternative modes of communication such as gesture or mime)
  - (b) In individuals with adequate speech, marked impairment in the ability to initiate or sustain a conversation with others
  - (c) Stereotyped and repetitive use of language or idiosyncratic language
  - (d) Lack of varied, spontaneous make-believe play or social imitative play appropriate to developmental level
- (3) Restricted repetitive and stereotyped patterns of behavior, interests, and activities, as manifested by at least one of the following:
  - (a) Encompassing preoccupation with one or more stereotyped and restricted patterns of interest that is abnormal either in intensity or focus
  - (b) Apparently inflexible adherence to specific, nonfunctional routines or rituals
  - (c) Stereotyped and repetitive motor mannerisms (e.g., hand or finger flapping or twisting, or complex whole-body movements)
  - (d) Persistent preoccupation with parts of objects
B. Delays or abnormal functioning in at least one of the following areas, with onset prior to age 3 years: (1) social interaction, (2) language as used in social communication, or (3) symbolic or imaginative play.
C. The disturbance is not better accounted for by Rett's Disorder or Childhood Disintegrative Disorder.

American Psychiatric Association. *Desk Reference to the Diagnostic Criteria from DSM-IV–TR.* Washington, DC, American Psychiatric Association, pp. 59–61, 2000. Reprinted with permission.

Prevalence

- The prevalence of autistic disorder is reported as 1–5 per 10,000 children. More recent epidemiological studies suggest that the prevalence rate for autistic disorder may be rising in the population, up to 7.2 per 10,000 children.
- PDD NOS is much more common, with a prevalence rate reported as 1 per several hundred children.

- Rett's disorder and childhood disintegrative disorder are apparently much rarer.
- The prevalence of Asperger's disorder is unknown.
- In autism and all PDDs except Rett's disorder, there is a male to female predominance of about 4:1.

Comorbidity

Medical comorbidity
- Seizures occur in 25–33% of persons with autism.
- Fragile X syndrome occurs in approximately 1 per 100 persons with autism.
- About 20% of tuberous sclerosis patients also meet criteria for autism; however, tuberous sclerosis is observed in only a small number of cases of autism.
- Medical conditions relating to the etiology of autism occur in 10–25% of cases. These include congenital rubella, cerebral palsy, phenylketonuria, and neurofibromatosis.

Psychiatric comorbidity
- Mental retardation occurs in up to 75% of persons with autism.
  - Autism increases with the degree and severity of mental retardation.
- Symptoms of ADHD (e.g., hyperactivity, attentional deficits, impulsivity) often occur in young people with PDDs. A formal psychiatric diagnosis of ADHD is now allowed by DSM-IV in young people with PDDs, including autistic disorder.
- Features suggesting obsessive–compulsive disorder occur frequently in children and adolescents with autistic disorder and other PDDs; such symptoms may respond to selective serotonin reuptake inhibitors.
- Depression may occur in individuals with autism and other PDDs. Because of language difficulties and odd behaviors, the diagnosis of depression is particularly difficult to make in this population. Depression may be more likely to occur in higher-functioning individuals with autism, Asperger's disorder, or PDD NOS, reflecting higher levels of communicative skills and cognitive ability.
- Although anxiety disorders may occur in this population, the diagnostic may be difficult to make because of communication difficulties in young people with PDD. Anxiety may manifest by symptoms of irritability, repetitive behaviors such as self-stimulation, temper tantrums, and/or sleep difficulties.
- Stereotyped motor movements, habit disorders, and tics are frequently seen in this population.

Course and Outcome

The outcomes of persons with autism have been studied; outcomes for the other PDDs are less well studied. Predictors of better outcome for persons with PDDs include:

- IQ > 60
- The presence of some socially reciprocal language skills by age 5

Outcome also varies by type of PDD.
- Asperger's disorder and PDD NOS have a relatively good prognosis in terms of the ability to eventually live independently.
  - Probably related to better communication and cognitive skills relative to other PDDs.
- Rett's disorder and childhood disintegrative disorder have the worst overall prognosis.
- For autistic disorder as adults:
  - About two-thirds exhibit very significant limitations in the ability to care for basic personal needs.
  - About one-third are able to achieve some level of personal and occupational independence, although they continue to demonstrate residual and disabling social impairments.

An important trend in outcome studies completed since 1980 suggests higher rates of improved outcomes and decreased rates of poor outcomes in persons with autistic disorder. This improvement probably reflects the positive impact of early case identification and early intervention with intensive psychosocial and language treatments that were not available to persons with PDDs living earlier in the 20th century.

Assessment

A diagnosis of PDD implies that multiple important areas of development are affected, making assessments of multiple domains of functioning essential. The assessment of the child or adolescent with autism or another PDD is multifactorial and includes the following.

- A comprehensive psychiatric evaluation assessing the core features of PDD and any comorbid psychiatric disorders or symptoms that may be treatment responsive.
- A cognitive assessment evaluating IQ and the patient's information-processing strengths and weaknesses.
- An evaluation of adaptive functioning using a validated instrument such as the Vineland Adaptive Behavior Scales (Sparrow et al., 1994).
- An assessment of behavioral problems.
- Strengths in the patient and family that can be used as resources to support treatment.
- Available community and educational resources to facilitate psychoeducational treatment.
- A medical evaluation documenting any sensory or motor deficits, neurological problems, hearing and vision screening, and a complete physical examination, vital signs, and measurement of height and weight.
- Laboratory studies screening for fragile X syndrome and amino/organic acid metabolic abnormalities are recommended.
- Rating scales aiding in the diagnosis of autism/PDD or in establishing the severity of symptoms are recommended. Some commonly used rating scales in the assessment of individuals with autism are given below.

PERVASIVE DEVELOPMENTAL DISORDERS

Table 23.7 Rating Scales for Assessing Autism and Associated Psychopathology in Children and Adolescents

Rating Scale	Type of Scale	What Is Assessed?	Age Range	Reliability	Validity	Sensitivity to Change
Aberrant Behavior Checklist	Parent and/or teacher report	Irritability, lethargy, stereotypy, hyperactivity, speech	5 yrs, to adult	+ +	+ +	Yes
Autism Diagnostic Interview— Revised	Semistructured diagnostic interview	Autism diagnostic criteria	Child, adolescent	+ +	+ +	No
Childhood Autism Rating Scale	Rating scale	Severity of autism	Child, adolescent	+ +	+ +	Yes
Children's Yale–Brown Obsessive Compulsive Scale	Parent and/or teacher report	Repetitive behaviors and obsessive–compulsive symptoms	Child, adolescent	+ +	+ +	Yes
Clinical Global Impressions Scale	Clinician report	Overall symptom severity and improvement	Child, adolescent, adult	+ +	+ +	Yes
Gilliam Autism Rating Scale	Parent report	Core and comorbid symptoms	Child, adolescent	+ +	+ +	Yes
PDD Behavior Inventory	Rating scale	Maladaptive and adaptive behaviors	Child, adolescent	+ +	+ +	Yes
Ritvo–Freeman Real Life Rating Scale	Rating scale	Severity of associated psychopathology	Child, adolescent	+	+	Yes

+ + = good; + = fair

Treatment

Research suggests the importance of early case identification and intensive, sustained treatment in improving the long-term outcome in autism and related conditions. Treatment is multidisciplinary, involving many different psychoeducational, service, and mental health providers in the child and family's life over extended periods of time. Treatment planning should be related to assessment of the individual's current levels of functioning and his or her strengths and weaknesses. The primary care provider should function as the child's case manager, advocating for and coordinating needed services and treatments across childhood and adolescence.

PSYCHOSOCIAL TREATMENTS

Psychoeducational Interventions
- Educational: The best available research evidence suggests the importance of intensive, chronic, and appropriate special educational interventions to foster acquisition of basic social, communicative, and cognitive skills. The acquisition of these skills is related to ultimate outcome later in adult life.
  - With the passage of Public Law 94-142, schools are mandated to provider or these services for persons from 3 to 21 years of age.
- Vocational: Adolescents with autism/PDDs require vocational training to develop useful skills toward independence and supported employment.
  - Vocational training provides opportunities to enhance further social development.

Behavioral interventions
- Behavioral modification, environmental structure, and applied behavioral analysis are important aspects of continuing treatment for individuals with these conditions.
- Behavioral modification reinforces desirable behaviors and decreases maladaptive behavior.
- Social skills training can be used to enhance social competence and build social skills.

Family interventions
- Support for the families is an integral part of any treatment plan.
- Parents should be involved in the assessment and treatment process.
- Positive attempts at coping should be encouraged, including education about the disorder and parental involvement with local and national resources that support families with an autistic PDD member.

Psychotherapy
- The usefulness of psychotherapy in autism appears very limited. The core symptoms of autism and other PDDs do not respond to psychotherapy. For individuals with Asperger's disorder or PDD-NOS who have higher cognitive skills, individual psychotherapy may be helpful in serving a supportive function.

PHARMACOLOGICAL TREATMENT

There is no pharmacological intervention to cure autism or other PDDs, nor do medications appear to ameliorate the core symptoms. However, medications may help treat associated psychiatric conditions such as ADHD, depression, or anxiety disorders in young persons with autism/PDDs. The treatment of target symptoms may increase the ability of persons with autism/PDD to profit from psychoeducational and rehabilitative interventions and enhance the possibility of more independent functioning.

Because individuals with autism/PDD are frequently nonverbal, care must be taken in the selection and administration of psychiatric medicines. The guidelines for medication use in persons with mental retardation, presented earlier in this chapter, apply equally well to those with autism/PDD.

Controlled studies of medications in young persons with autism are presented in the following table.

Atypical antipsychotics
Atypical antipsychotics are now the pharmacological treatment of choice for disruptive behavioral problems, aggression, self-injury, conduct problems, and hyperactivity in children and adolescents with autism/PDD. Atypical antipsychotics have now replaced older neuroleptics such as haloperidol in the treatment of these conditions because they appear to have a more favorable side effect profile. Reports have now appeared in which risperidone, olanzapine, and possibly quetiapine are helpful as adjunctive treatments in the care of persons with autistic disorders.

- Risperidone: Numerous open-label studies and one randomized controlled study support the use of risperidone in the adjunctive treatment of disruptive behaviors in children, adolescents, and adults with autism and related PDDs (McCracken et al., 2002).
  ○ The dose range is 1–6 mg given in two to four divided daily doses.
- Olanzapine: Open-label studies and case reports support the use of olanzapine in subjects with PDDs.
  ○ The dose range is 5–20 mg given in two divided daily doses.
- Quetiapine: To date, only one case series of six autistic individuals has reported on the use of quetiapine in autistic children and adolescents. No improvement was found over a dose range of 100–350 mg/day. However, two subjects appeared to benefit from continued quetiapine treatment.
- Clozapine: Use of clozapine is complicated in this population by fears of seizure induction and agranulocytosis associated with use of this drug.
- No data are presently available on the use of ziprasidone or aripiprazole in this population.

Selective serotonin reuptake inhibitors (SSRIs)
Abnormalities in serotonergic functioning have been identified in subjects with autistic disorder and other PDDs. Given that SSRIs are effective in the treatment of obsessive–compulsive disorder (OCD), and given the high prevalence

Table 23.8 Controlled Studies of Medications in Children and Adolescents With Autism and Autistic Spectrum Disorders

Study (year)	Drug	N	Age Range (years)	Dose (mg/day)	Duration (weeks)	Outcome
Anderson et al. (1989)	Haloperidol	45	2–8	0.25–4.0	4	Significant improvement in behavioral symptoms
Belsito et al. (2001)	Lamotrigine	28	3–11	5.0 mg/kg/day	4	No significant improvement relative to placebo
Campbell et al. (1993)	Naltrexone	41	3–8	1 mg/kg/day	3	Improvement in hyperactivity; no improvement in core autistic symptoms
Chez et al. (2002)	L-carnosine	31	3–12	800 mg	8	Improvement in autism symptoms relative to placebo
Fankhauser et al. (1992)	Clonidine transdermal	9	5–33	5 µg/kg/day	4	Improvement in hyperactivity and anxiety
Feldman et al. (1999)	Naltrexone	24	3–8	1 mg/kg/day	2	No improvement in autistic communication
Findling et al. (1997)	Pyridoxine and magnesium	10	Mean age = 6.3	639 mg pyridoxine and 216 mg magnesium oxide	10	No significant improvement relative to placebo
Gordon et al. (1993)	Clomipramine	12	6–18	Mean dose = 152	10	Improvement in anger and OCD behaviors
Handen et al. (2000)	Methylphenidate	13	5–11	0.3 and 0.6 mg/kg/day	2	Symptoms of ADHD improved; autistic symptoms did not improve
Jaselskis et al. (1992)	Clonidine	8	5–11	0.05–2.0	6	Symptoms of hyperactivity improved; autistic symptoms did not improve
King et al. (2001)	Amantadine	39	5–19	5.0 mg/kg/day	3	No significant improvement relative to placebo
Levy et al. (2003)	Human secretin	62	3–8	2 CU/kg	Single infusion	No significant improvement relative to placebo
McCracken et al. (2002)	Risperidone	101	5–17	0.5–3.5	8	Improvement in aggression, tantrums, irritability, and SIB
Quintana et al. (1995)	Methylphenidate	10	7–11	20–40	2	Improvement in hyperactivity; no improvement in autistic symptoms
Unis et al. (2002)	Porcine secretin	85	3–12	0.4 µg/kg	Single infusion	No significant improvement relative to placebo
Willemsen-Swinkels et al. (1996)	Naltrexone	23	3–7	1 mg/kg/day	4	No improvement

of OCD-like symptoms in youngsters with PDDs, there exists considerable interest in the effectiveness of these agents in autism/PDDs. Aggression, self-injury, and anxiety may respond to SSRIs.

- Fluoxetine use is supported by open-label studies and case reports in persons with PDDs.
  - The dose range is 10–80 mg given once daily.
- Sertraline use is supported by open-label reports in this population. Symptoms of anxiety, irritability, and transition-induced behavioral deterioration may respond.
  - The dose range is 25–150 mg given in two divided daily doses.
- Fluvoxamine was not found useful in one controlled study of adults with autism/PDDs and in another controlled study of pediatric patients with PDDs.
  - The dose range used was 25–250 mg/day.
- Paroxetine is poorly studied in the pediatric autism/PDD population.
- Citalopram is poorly studied in the pediatric autism/PDD population.
- Escitalopram has not been studied in the pediatric autism/PDD population.

Clomipramine
- Clomipramine is a tricyclic antidepressant that has been studied and found effective under controlled conditions in pediatric autism. Symptoms of aggression, obsessions, and compulsions respond. However, clomipramine use is complicated by a high rate of treatment-emergent side effects, including constipation, seizures, and dry mouth. The high side effect rate does not make clomipramine a first choice for use in this population.
  - A dose range of 50–150 mg given in two or three divided daily doses is used.
  - Vital sign and EKG monitoring are necessary when using clomipramine.

Stimulants
Many young persons with autism and other PDDs may have associated symptoms of ADHD, including attention deficits, motor hyperactivity, and impulsivity. These symptoms may cause further daily impairment and additionally limit independent functioning over and above the core symptoms of the pervasive developmental disorder. Stimulants have been cautiously evaluated in this population.
- Methylphenidate and dextroamphetamine are effective treatments for symptoms of ADHD in persons with PDDs.
  - Their effects are less than in persons with ADHD without PDDs.
  - Side effects are greater in this population and require careful clinical monitoring.
- Dose range
  - For methylphenidate 0.3–0.6 mg/kg/dose given in two or three daily doses.
  - For dextroamphetamine 0.1–0.4 mg/kg/dose given in two or three daily doses.

Clonidine
There currently are two controlled trials of clonidine in children with autism and other PDDs. One study used clonidine tablets and the other used the

transdermal clonidine patch system (see Table 23.8). Both studies reported benefits in associated psychopathology and behavioral symptoms in this population.

- Vital sign monitoring is necessary with clonidine use.
- The dose range is 0.05–0.35 mg given in two to four divided daily doses.
- Sedation, irritability, and other treatment-emergent side effects may be problematic in children with PDDs.

Not established or ineffective treatments

Given the relatively poor prognosis and severity of early-onset autism and other PDDs, it is not surprising that a wide variety of nutritional, vitamin, psychosocial, and pharmacological interventions have been attempted in this population. Although scientifically uncontrolled clinical observations or case reports may attest to efficacy, the following treatments have either not been studied under controlled conditions, or if they have, been found ineffective.

- Secretin (ineffective in RCTs)
- Megavitamin therapy
- Nutritional supplements
- Psychodynamic psychotherapy
- Play therapy
- Dietary changes
- Steroid treatments
- Immunoglobulins
- Facilitated communication (ineffective in RCTs)
- Auditory training
- Holding therapy
- Sensory integration

PERVASIVE DEVELOPMENTAL DISORDERS

24. Eating Disorders

The two major eating disorders are anorexia nervosa and bulimia nervosa. They are complex psychiatric disorders with considerable psychiatric and medical comorbidities. In clinical practice eating disorders are best understood as multidimensional syndromes that occur along a continuum between the two disorders. Many patients demonstrate a mixture of both anorexic and bulimic behaviors. Excessive weight preoccupation and intensive self-evaluation of weight and body shape are the primary symptoms in both anorexia nervosa and bulimia nervosa. Eating disorders commonly begin with problematic dieting behaviors in adolescence or young adulthood. Psychological, biological, and social vulnerabilities and influences antecedent to the dieting experience then propel the symptoms into a full-blown eating disorder.

Patients with anorexia nervosa and bulimia nervosa often experience other associated psychiatric symptoms and behaviors. Individuals with anorexia nervosa often demonstrate social isolation, and adolescents and adults with the disorder may show a disinterest in sex. Associated psychopathology includes depressive, anxious, obsessional, and compulsive symptoms, perfectionistic traits, and an inflexible cognitive style. These patients often rigidly deny the seriousness of their illness and are highly resistant to treatment. An overwhelming feeling of inadequacy and ineffectiveness is a core symptom of all anorectic patients. Success at dieting and losing weight becomes an impressive accomplishment and boosts their self-confidence.

Patients with bulimia nervosa often experience depressive, anxious, and impulsive symptoms (which may include sexual promiscuity, suicidal behaviors, substance abuse, binge alcohol use, shoplifting, and/or self-injurious behaviors). Patients with bulimia nervosa often recognize their disorder, but shame may prevent them from seeking treatment.

Although psychopharmacology is never the sole or primary treatment for eating disorders, interest has grown in the use of adjunctive medications primarily in bulimia nervosa, but also in anorexia nervosa. Because little research into eating disorders is presently completed in the pediatric population, this chapter draws heavily on the adult literature.

DIAGNOSTIC CRITERIA

Anorexia Nervosa

Four major criteria define anorexia nervosa.

- Weight loss: An adult is considered underweight if he or she weighs less than 85% of a weight that is considered normal for that person's gender, age, and height. Standardized pediatric growth charts should be used for children and adolescents. Some children will not show overt weight loss but will fail to make expected gains in weight during a growth in height.
- Intense fear of gaining weight: Anorexics often deny their fear of gaining weight but demonstrate behaviors that reveal rigorous attempts to prevent weight gain, such as vigorous exercise regimens and/or severe food restriction.
- Body image disturbance: The significance of body weight and shape is severely distorted in these patients. Some anorexics feel globally overweight despite malnutrition. Others feel thin but insist that parts of their body, such as abdomen or thighs, are too fat. The distorted significance of body shape and weight is related to the patient's self-image of being very ineffective in life. Losing weight and dieting are the one area in life in which these patients can experience effectiveness and control.
- Amenorrhea: Defined as the absence of at least three consecutive menstrual cycles, amenorrhea may appear before significant amounts of weight loss have occurred.

There are two types of anorexia nervosa.

- Restricting type: These patients lose weight by severely and drastically reducing their daily food intake; some develop rigorous exercise programs. Most develop elaborate and obsessive rituals around food and may secretly hoard food and carry it around with them. Psychological and medical symptoms develop as a consequence of starvation and malnutrition. Often these associated symptoms become much better when refeeding is accomplished.
- Binge-eating/purging type: These patients also rigorously diet but episodically lose control of their food restriction and binge. Binge eating behaviors result in anxiety and guilt feelings that are temporarily relieved by purging behaviors consisting of self-induced vomiting and/or misuse of laxatives, diuretics, or enemas. Associated impulsive symptoms may occur, such as suicide attempts, self-mutilation, stealing, and substance abuse. Purging-type anorexics are at risk for electrolyte disturbances such as hypokalemic alkalosis with associated hypochloremia and hypokalemia and elevated serum bicarbonate. These patients may develop physical symptoms of weakness, lethargy, and (occasionally) cardiac arrhythmias that may result in sudden cardiac death.

Table 24.1 Diagnostic Criteria for Anorexia Nervosa

A. Refusal to maintain body weight at or above a minimally normal weight for age and height (e.g., weight loss leading to maintenance of body weight less than 85% of that expected; or failure to make expected weight gain during period of growth, leading to body weight less than 85% of that expected).
B. Intense fear of gaining weight or becoming fat, even though underweight.
C. Disturbance in the way in which one's body weight or shape is experienced, undue influence of body weight or shape on self-evaluation, or denial of the seriousness of the current low body weight.
D. In postmenarcheal females, amenorrhea, i.e., the absence of at least three consecutive menstrual cycles. (A woman is considered to have amenorrhea if her periods occur only following hormone, e.g., estrogen, administration.)

Specify type:
Restricting Type: During the current episode of Anorexia Nervosa, the person has not regularly engaged in binge-eating or purging behavior (i.e., self-induced vomiting or the misuse of laxatives, diuretics, or enemas)
Binge-Eating/Purging Type: During the current episode of Anorexia Nervosa, the person has regularly engaged in binge-eating or purging behavior (i.e., self-induced vomiting or the misuse of laxatives, diuretics, or enemas)

American Psychiatric Association. *Desk Reference to the Diagnostic Criteria from DSM*-IV–TR. Washington, DC, American Psychiatric Association, pp. 263, 2000. Reprinted with permission.

Bulimia Nervosa

The diagnostic criteria for bulimia nervosa are more arbitrary and less specific than those given for anorexia nervosa.

Table 24.2 Diagnostic Criteria for Bulimia Nervosa

A. Recurrent episodes of binge eating. An episode of binge eating is characterized by both of the following:
   (1) Eating, in a discrete period of time (e.g., within any 2-hour period), an amount of food that is definitely larger than most people would eat during a similar period of time and under similar circumstances
   (2) A sense of lack of control over eating during the episode (e.g., a feeling that one cannot stop eating or control what or how much one is eating)
B. Recurrent inappropriate compensatory behavior in order to prevent weight gain, such as self-induced vomiting; misuse of laxatives, diuretics, enemas, or other medications; fasting; or excessive exercise.
C. The binge eating and inappropriate compensatory behaviors both occur, on average, at least twice a week for 3 months.
D. Self-evaluation is unduly influenced by body shape and weight.
E. The disturbance does not occur exclusively during episodes of Anorexia Nervosa.

Specify type:
Purging Type: During the current episode of Bulimia Nervosa, the person has regularly engaged in self-induced vomiting or the misuse of laxatives, diuretics, or enemas.
Nonpurging Type: During the current episode of Bulimia Nervosa, the person has used other inappropriate compensatory behaviors, such as fasting or excessive exercise, but has not regularly engaged in self-induced vomiting or the misuse of laxatives, diuretics, or enemas.

American Psychiatric Association. *Desk Reference to the Diagnostic Criteria from DSM*-IV–TR. Washington, DC, American Psychiatric Association, pp. 264–265, 2000. Reprinted with permission.

Binge Eating Disorder

Binge eating disorder is currently classified within the eating disorders not otherwise specified category of DSM-IV. Binge eating disorder is the subject of current

EATING DISORDERS

research in adult eating disorders; it is conceptualized as a category of eating disorder without overt weight and body shape concerns such as those present in anorexia nervosa and bulimia nervosa. Although not currently approved as a specific DSM-IV eating disorder at this time, there are research diagnostic criteria for binge eating disorder that consist of disturbances in one or more of the following domains.

• Eating behaviors such as binge eating
• Somatic symptoms such as obesity
• Psychological problems such as body image dissatisfaction, depression, or self-esteem difficulties

PREVALENCE

Estimates of the incidence or prevalence of eating disorders vary depending on the sample studied and the assessment methods. No prevalence studies of eating disorders have yet to be conducted on large, representative pediatric samples. Thus the following data come from investigations of adults with eating disorders.

• Anorexia nervosa: The lifetime prevalence for women ranges between 0.5% and 3.7%.
  ○ The yearly incidence rates for anorexia nervosa are approximately 14.6 per 100,000 women and 1.8 per 100,000 men.
• Bulimia nervosa: The lifetime prevalence for women ranges between 1.1% and 4.2%.
• Gender ratio: Eating disorders are more commonly seen in females. Estimates of the male–female prevalence ratio range between 1:6 to 1:10. About 19–30% of the adolescent and young-adult patient populations with anorexia nervosa is male.

COURSE OF ILLNESS

Anorexia Nervosa

Anorexia nervosa is a serious, chronic eating disorder with substantial morbidity and mortality. The percentage of individuals with anorexia nervosa who fully recover from their illness is modest. Patients may substantially improve over time with treatment, but most continue to have chronic disturbances with body image, disordered patterns of eating, and other psychopathology. Early mortality is a risk for women with anorexia nervosa.

• The onset of anorexia nervosa is usually between ages 13 and 20 years; about 85% of all anorectic patients develop the illness in adolescence.
• A review of a large number of outcome studies in anorexia nervosa revealed that by 4 years

- About 44% had a good outcome, with weight restored to within 15% of recommended weight for age, gender, and height and regular menstruation established
- About 24% had poor outcomes, with weight never restored to within 15% of ideal weight and no resumption of regular menses
- About 28% had intermediate outcomes.
- Early mortality occurred in about 5%.
- Time to recovery with intensive treatment can be protracted, ranging from 4 to 6 years.
- Even with recovery from anorexia nervosa, most patients continue to have persistent psychiatric problems such as depression, anxiety disorders, personality disorders, and/or substance use disorders.
- Mortality in anorexia nervosa is primarily the result of suicide or cardiac arrest.
  - Mortality rates increase with length of follow-up, reaching 20% in women followed for more than 20 years.
  - The overall mortality rate in anorexia nervosa is approximately 5.6% per decade, which is 12 times the death rate for women in the community and twice the mortality rate for women with other psychiatric disorders.
- Risk factors for poor outcome in anorexia nervosa include the following.
  - Lower initial minimum weight
  - The presence of both anorexia and purging behaviors
  - Failure to respond to previous treatment
  - Disturbed family relationships before illness onset
  - Married status

Bulimia Nervosa

- The onset of bulimia nervosa is usually in adolescence or young adulthood.
- Bulimia nervosa generally has a better prognosis than anorexia nervosa, with lower lifetime mortality and better recovery rates.
  - In community samples over a 1- to 2-year period, spontaneous improvement has been reported, with 25–30% reductions in binge eating, purging, and laxative abuse.
- The overall success rate for bulimia nervosa with treatment has been reported in the range of 50–70%; however, relapse rates are high.
  - Between 30% and 50% of patients resume bingeing and purging behaviors at 6-month follow-up, even after successful treatment.
- In long-term outcome studies after intensive treatment for bulimia, about 60% have a good outcome, 10% have a poor outcome, and 29% have an intermediate outcome.
  - The mortality rate is about 1%.
- Risk factors for poor outcome in bulimia nervosa include the following.
  - Bulimics whose symptoms are severe enough to require hospitalization
  - Electrolyte imbalance caused by purging behaviors
  - Poor motivation for treatment
  - A higher frequency of pretreatment bingeing and purging behaviors
  - High rates of comorbid psychiatric disorders

EATING DISORDERS

Binge Eating Disorder

• Usually has its onset in adulthood and is rarely found among adolescents.
• Is associated with obesity in the majority of cases.
• Is rare in nonreferred community populations, but is common among patients seeking treatments for obesity in hospital-affiliated weight programs.
• A higher proportion of males has binge eating disorders than other eating disorders.

COMORBIDITY

Comorbid psychiatric disorders are common among patients with eating disorders and substantially contribute to ongoing morbidity and impairment.

• Substance abuse/dependence is common among women with eating disorders; appears to be more common among impulsive eating disordered patients with bingeing and purging behaviors and less common among restricting types of anorectics.
  ○ Alcohol abuse has been reported to occur in up to 22.9% of bulimic women.
  ○ Substance abuse has been found in 30–37% of women with bulimia nervosa.
  ○ In patients with anorexia nervosa substance abuse rates are estimated to range from 12% to 18%.
  ○ Bulimic women with anorexia are about 7 times more likely to develop substance abuse problems than restricting anorectic women.
• Depression is common among women with eating disorders. In anorectic patients symptoms of depression may be due to the physiological and psychological effects of starvation. Treatment of depression is generally not recommended until refeeding has occurred. With nutritional stabilization many depressive symptoms will disappear. If depressive symptoms persist despite weight improvement, treatment of associated depressive disorders may be necessary.
  ○ About 50–75% of women with anorexia nervosa or bulimia nervosa meet diagnostic criteria for either major depression or dysthymia.
  ○ About 4–6% meet diagnostic criteria for bipolar disorder.
• The lifetime prevalence of obsessive–compulsive disorder may be as high as 25% among patients with eating disorders.
• Other anxiety disorders also occur at rates greater than population frequencies in patients with anorexia nervosa and bulimia nervosa.
  ○ Social phobias
  ○ Panic attacks
• Personality disorders are found in 42–75% of patients with eating disorders.
  ○ Associations between bulimia and cluster B and C disorders, such as borderline and avoidant personality disorders, are reported.
  ○ Women with anorexia nervosa frequently have associated cluster C disorders, such as avoidant and obsessive–compulsive personality disorders.
  ○ Eating disordered patients with comorbid personality disorders may have high rates of substance abuse problems.

- Sexual abuse has been found in 20–50% of patients with bulimia nervosa and anorexia nervosa. Histories of childhood sexual abuse are reported more frequently in women with eating disorders than in women from the general population.

ASSESSMENT

The clinical assessment of patients with eating disorders requires a comprehensive psychiatric, family, psychosocial, nutritional, and medical approach. The areas of assessment needed to evaluate the patient with eating disorders are given in the following table.

Table 24.3 General Areas of Assessment for Patients with Anorexia Nervosa and Bulimia Nervosa

Weight history	Family functioning and support
Eating behavior	Interpersonal functioning and
Purging behavior	support
Preoccupations and rituals	Academic and occupational
concerning food and weight	functioning
Activity and exercise history	Previous treatment history
Menstrual history	Hospitalizations
Psychiatric history	Outpatient treatment
Depression	Psychiatric medications
Anxiety	Medical history and current findings
Suicidal thoughts/acts	
Self-injury	
Obsessive–compulsive symptoms	
Substance abuse history	
Alcohol abuse history	
Personality disorders	

- Psychiatric evaluation: It is important to remember that most anorectic patients deny their symptoms and are not motivated for treatment. Bulimic patients may minimize their symptoms. It is therefore important to involve family members or close friends in the evaluation process to obtain an accurate assessment of the patient's actual behaviors and symptoms. It is important to find out about purging behaviors because these may lead to an increased risk of medical complications. The clinician should assess the patient for comorbid psychiatric disorders and self-destructive behaviors.
- Often eating disorder rating scales can supplement the psychiatric evaluation. Examples of such scales are given in the following table.
- Family evaluation: Assess the degree of family conflict present and the amount of support available to the patient.
- Interpersonal supports: Assess the degree of social isolation the patient is experiencing. Are friends available who can support the patient?
- Nutritional history: Often it is necessary to obtain a formal nutritional consultation to understand the patient's food preferences and eating patterns, degree of starvation, purging behaviors, and to develop a refeeding plan.
- Medical consultation: A thorough physical exam, EKG, and laboratory studies are needed to ascertain the risk of medical complications resulting from

EATING DISORDERS

Table 24.4 Rating Scales for Eating Disorders in Adolescents and Adults

Rating Scale	Type of Scale	What Is Assessed?	Age Range
Diagnostic Survey for Eating Disorders	Self-report or clinician semistructured interview	Weight history, body image, psychiatric history, medical history	Adolescent and adult
Eating Attitudes Test	Self-report	Symptoms of eating disorder	Adolescent and adult
Eating Disorders Examination (EDE)	Clinician semistructured interview	Eating disorder diagnoses	Adolescent and adult
EDE-Q4	Self-report	Severity of symptoms	Adolescent and adult
Eating Disorders Questionnaire	Self-report	Severity of symptoms	Adolescent and adult
Questionnaire of Eating and Weight Patterns	Self-report	Symptoms of binge eating	Adolescent and adult
Yale–Brown–Cornell Eating Disorder Scale	Clinician interview	Symptoms and associated psychopathology	Adolescents and adult

starvation or purging behaviors and to follow the patient's weight status and physical status during treatment. Physical examination and laboratory abnormalities that may occur in patients with eating disorders are given below.

Table 24.5 Medical Abnormalities in Eating Disorders

Dry, cracking skin from dehydration
Lanugo hair from starvation
Calluses on dorsum of hand from self-induced vomiting
Perioral dermatitis from vomiting
Enlarged parotid glands from vomiting
Teeth enamel erosion and dental caries from vomiting
Periodontitis from vomiting
Bradycardia from starvation
Hypotension from starvation and dehydration
Cardiac arrhythmias from electrolyte imbalance
Hypokalemia resulting from purging
Laboratory abnormalities
  Leukopenia with a relative lymphocytosis
  Anemia
  Hypokalemia
  Hypochloremic metabolic alkalosis
  Hyperamylasemia
  Hypercholesterolemia
  Hypercarotinemia
  EKG Q-T and T-wave changes
  Photon absorptiometry: reduced bone density

MULTIDISCIPLINARY TREATMENT

Eating disorders require a multidisciplinary approach to treatment and the availability of a continuum of care ranging from ambulatory mental health treatment to acute medical hospitalization. Sometimes multidisciplinary treatment takes the form of specialized eating disorder teams. Otherwise, either the primary care provider or the psychiatrist must construct a multidisciplinary team in order to facilitate treatment. A team approach to treatment is most important for the treatment of anorexia nervosa, a disorder with a poor prognosis and a high rate of medical complications. Components of the treatment team include a psychiatrist, therapist, nutritionist, and primary care physician.

The first decision to be made is choosing a site of treatment. Recommended guidelines for inpatient versus outpatient levels of care in the treatment of anorexia nervosa and bulimia nervosa are given in the table below.

Table 24.6 Indications for Levels of Care in Eating Disorders

Acute Inpatient	Outpatient
Anorexia Nervosa • Relapse from previous treatment • Acute length of illness < 6 months • Weight loss of 10–15% from normal weight if relapse • Weight loss of 16–20% if first episode illness • Hypokalemic alkalosis (K^+ < 2.5 meq/L) • Acute EKG change • Sustained body temperature < 97° F • Orthostatic pulse > 20 bpm lying to standing • Orthostatic systolic BP > 20 mmHg lying to standing • Sustained pulse < 40 bpm or > 110 bpm	*Anorexia Nervosa* • Normal weight *or* • Gradual weight loss over ≥ 3 months • Normal serum electrolytes • Normal EKG • High motivation for treatment
Bulimia Nervosa • Frequent purging with electrolyte imbalance • Serum K^+ < 2.5 meq/L • Cardiac failure caused by recurrent ipecac-induced cardiomyopathy	*Bulimia Nervosa* • First episode with no previous treatment history • Relapse after a stable period of abstinence from bingeing and purging • Normal serum electrolytes • Normal weight

Anorexia Nervosa

The components of a treatment plan for patients with anorexia nervosa include the following.

• Nutritional rehabilitation: The goals of nutritional rehabilitation are to restore weight to a minimum of 90% of ideal weight for gender, age, and height, normalize eating patterns, achieve normal perceptions of hunger and satiety, and correct the biological and psychological sequelae of malnutrition and starvation.
  ○ For inpatients the goal is to achieve a 2–3 lb. per week weight gain.
  ○ For outpatients the goal is to achieve a 0.5–1 lb. per week weight gain.
• Psychosocial treatments: The goals of psychosocial treatments in anorexia nervosa are to help patients understand and cooperate with their nutritional rehabilitation, understand and change their dysfunctional attitudes and behaviors related to eating, improve their interpersonal and social functioning, and address comorbid psychopathology that reinforces or maintains dysfunctional eating disorder behaviors.
  ○ Initial psychosocial therapy should emphasize cognitive–behavioral therapy (CBT) approaches, which have been found to be more effective than psychodynamic approaches in the treatment of anorexia nervosa.
• Family therapy: For patients less than 18 years old, the addition of family therapy to the treatment plan has been shown to improve outcome; for patients older than 18 years, family therapy may actually worsen outcome.
• Medical monitoring: Patients with anorexia nervosa require close medical monitoring and supervision.
  ○ Post-void morning weight checks two or three times per week

EATING DISORDERS

488 Pediatric Psychopharmacology: Fast Facts

- Monitoring of core body temperature and vital signs
- Monitoring of food and fluid intake and output, including urine-specific gravity
- Assessing for dehydration
- Evaluating cardiac functioning during starvation and refeeding
- Evaluating serum electrolytes and minerals (such as potassium and phosphorous) during refeeding.

Bulimia Nervosa

Bulimia nervosa is generally associated with less medical comorbidity and has a better prognosis than anorexia nervosa, although relapse rates are high. Treatment for most bulimics takes place in outpatient mental health settings. Components of a treatment plan for bulimia nervosa include the following.

- Nutritional counseling: A focus of nutritional counseling is to monitor the bulimic patient's patterns of binge eating and purging, encourage healthy patterns of exercise, and encourage normal patterns of eating behaviors. Because most bulimics are of normal weight, refeeding and weight gain are not a central focus of treatment.
- Cognitive–behavioral therapy: In the acute 16–20-week treatment of bulimia nervosa, CBT has the most evidence of efficacy. Over 35 controlled studies document the efficacy of CBT in the short-term (16–20 weeks) reduction of bingeing and purging behaviors. In these studies 40–50% of bulimic patients achieve abstinence from bingeing and purging behaviors, and a reduction of bingeing and purging occurs in approximately 70–95% of patients.
  - CBT focuses on restructuring bulimics' dysfunctional beliefs about food, eating, body image, and overall self-efficacy.
- Family therapy: For adolescents < 18 years old with bulimia nervosa, family therapy is often included in the treatment plan.

PSYCHOPHARMACOLOGICAL TREATMENT

Psychopharmacology is always adjunctive to the multidisciplinary treatment plan outlined above for the treatment of eating disorders. Medications appear to have less of a role in the treatment of anorexia nervosa than in bulimia. In the comprehensive treatment of anorexia nervosa, medications are sometimes used to treat associated obsessive–compulsive, depressive, and other anxiety disorders that persist after nutritional stabilization. Treatment with psychiatric medications for psychopathology is not recommended in anorexia nervosa until refeeding and weight restoration have occurred. Many of the symptoms of psychopathology in anorexia are secondary to the physical and psychological effects of starvation and malnutrition and will disappear as the patient regains weight.

Medications, particularly antidepressants, have been found more useful in reducing bingeing and purging behaviors and associated psychopathology that occurs with bulimia nervosa. The most recent pharmacological trials have focused on reducing binge eating and promoting weight loss in obese adult patients with binge eating disorders. Open and controlled medication studies in adults with eating disorders are presented in the following two tables.

Table 24.7 Open Studies of Medications for Adolescent and Adult Eating Disorders

Study (year)	Drug	Disorder	Study Type	N	Age	Dose (mg/day)	Duration (weeks)	Outcome
Kotler et al. (2003)	Fluoxetine	BN	Open	10	Adolescents	60	8	70% improved
Malina et al. (2003)	Olanzeapine	AN	Retrospective	18	Adolescents and adults	2.5–10	3–70	Improvement in obsessions about body image and weight fears
McElroy et al. (2004)	Zonisamide	BED	Open	15	Adults	100–600	12	Improvement
Pallanti et al. (1997)	Citalopram	AN	Open	32	Adults	20	24	Improvement
Powers et al. (2002)	Olanzapine	AN	Open	20	Adolescents and adults	10	10	10 of 14 completers gained weight
Santonastaso et al. (2001)	Sertraline	AN	Open	11	Adolescents and adults	50–100	14	Improvement in associated depression and perfectionism
Strober et al. (1999)	Fluoxetine	AN	Open	66	Adolescents and adults	60	6	No difference

AN = anorexia nervosa; BED = binge eating disorder; BN = bulimia nervosa

EATING DISORDERS

Table 24.8 Controlled Studies of Medications for Adolescents (> 18 years old) and Adult Eating Disorders

Study (year)	Drug	Disorder	Study Type	N	Age	(mg/day)	Dose (weeks)	Duration Outcome
Carruba et al. (2001)	Moclobemide	BN	RCT	52	Adults	600	6	No significant difference
Fassino et al. (2002)	Citalopram	AN	RCT	52	Adults	20	12	Improvement in associated depression, OCD, and impulsivity
Hoopes et al. (2003)	Topiramate	BN	RCT	69	Adults	25–400	10	Effective in reducing number of binges and purges
Hudson et al. (1998)	Fluvoxamine	BED	RCT	85	Adults	50–300	9	Significantly associated with decreased number of binges
Kaye et al. (2001)	Fluoxetine	AN	RCT	35	Adults	10–60	Up to 52	Significantly associated with decreased relapse
McElroy et al. (2000)	Sertraline	BED	RCT	34	Adults	50–200	6	Significantly associated with decreased number of binges
McElroy, Hudson et al. (2003)	Citalopram	BED	RCT	38	Adults	20–60	6	Effective in reducing number of binges
McElroy, Arnold et al. (2003)	Topiramate	BED	RCT	61	Adults	25–600	14	Effective in reducing number of binges
Romano et al. (2002)	Fluoxetine	BN	RCT, discontinuation study	150	Adults	60	Time to relapse	Significantly associated with decreased relapse

AN = anorexia nervosa; BED = binge eating disorder; BN = bulimia nervosa; RCT = randomized controlled trial

Adjunctive Medications in Anorexia Nervosa

There are three approaches to medications in patients with anorexia nervosa: (1) promote weight gain in underweight anorexics; (2) attempt to reduce relapse in treated and stabilized anorectics; and (3) use medications to target symptoms of continuing obsessive–compulsive, depressive, or anxiety disorders that persist despite nutritional rehabilitation of the anorectic patient.

• *Weight gain*: Few medication studies report any success in promoting weight gain in malnourished patients with anorexia nervosa. There exist some early investigations of antidepressants and cyproheptadine that report weight gain compared with placebo in anorectic patients. However, findings are not robust and the risks of medication-induced side effects in malnourished patients are high. Several open-label studies report that olanzapine, an atypical antipsychotic, is associated with weight gain in anorectic patients. However, there are no controlled studies of atypical antipsychotics assessing weight gain compared with placebo in these patients. Presently, medications are not recommended during the refeeding phase of treatment for anorexia nervosa.

• *Relapse reduction*: More success is reported for medication-associated reductions in relapse in already-stabilized anorectic patients. Fluoxetine in doses of 20 mg–60 mg/day or citalopram in doses of 20 mg/day may help prevent relapse and treat associated psychopathology in stable anorectics who are also participating in a comprehensive treatment plan. Other SSRI antidepressants have not yet been investigated in controlled trials for the reduction of relapse in anorexia nervosa.

• *Associated psychopathology*: Symptoms of depression, obsessions, compulsive behaviors, and anxiety disorders may persist after weight stabilization in anorectic patients. Treatment of these persistent disorders follows the same recommendations and dose schedules as for any patient.

Adjunctive Medications in Bulimia Nervosa

Over a dozen randomized controlled trials of antidepressants have been conducted in normal-weight bulimic patients. These antidepressant trials were driven by the clinical observation that depression often accompanies bulimia nervosa. Desipramine, imipramine, amitriptyline, nortriptyline, phenelzine, and fluoxetine have been investigated in doses similar to those used for depression. In almost all trials antidepressants were more effective than placebo in reducing binge eating and improving depression. The effect on binge eating reduction appears to occur independently of the presence of depression. The complete abstinence rate from bingeing and purging occurs in only 20–25% of patients. Thus medications should never be the only treatment given to bulimic patients.

• Fluoxetine (Prozac®) is FDA labeled for use in the treatment of binge eating and purging in moderate to severe bulimia nervosa.
  ○ In the prevention of relapse in bulimia nervosa, higher doses of 60–80 mg/day may be required.

EATING DISORDERS

492 Pediatric Psychopharmacology: Fast Facts

- Tricyclic antidepressants are not recommended in the adjunctive treatment of bulimia nervosa because of their many side effects and toxicity in overdose.
- Monoamine oxidase inhibitors such as phenelzine are not recommended in the adjunctive treatment of bulimia nervosa because of their potential for inducing a hypertensive crisis if combined with tyramine-containing foods.

Recent controlled investigations suggest that the anticonvulsants may be effective in reducing binge eating and purging behaviors in bulimia nervosa and in binge eating disorder. Topiramate is a structurally novel agent approved for the treatment of epilepsy. In clinical trials for epilepsy, topiramate was observed to improve co-occurring binge eating and induce weight loss in patients. Topiramate has been investigated in eating disorders characterized by obesity and binge eating (see Table 24.8); preliminary evidence suggests that it may be effective in short-term treatment.

- Topiramate is initiated at 25 mg in the evening for 3 days, then increased to 50 mg hs on days 4–6, and then increased to 75 or 100 mg hs beginning on day 7.
- If no response to bingeing occurs at this dose for 2 weeks, then increase topiramate by 50 mg a week until a dose of 300 mg/day is reached.
- If no response occurs at 300 mg/day (defined as a 50% reduction in the number of binge/purge episodes), then topiramate may be increased by 75 mg/week to a maximum dose of 600 mg/day.

Zonisamide is another anticonvulsant currently being investigated in eating disorders characterized by obesity and binge eating. Zonisamide is a novel anticonvulsant drug indicated in the adjunctive treatment of partial seizures in adults with epilepsy.

- In open trials zonisamide significantly decreased episode frequency of binge eating in daily doses between 100 mg and 600 mg.
- Zonisamide is initiated at 100 mg/day and titrated by 100 mg every week to a maximum daily dose of 600 mg in adults.

25. Sleep Disorders

Sleep disorders are common problems in infancy, childhood, and adolescence. About 20–30% of children and adolescents experience sleep problems that their parents consider significant. Between 25% and 45% of young people referred for psychiatric or pediatric consultation have difficulty falling asleep or staying asleep. Sleep problems can be associated with behavioral and academic problems in children and adolescents and cause considerable daily impairment.

Numerous psychiatric medications can be used to transiently sedate the restless child with sleep difficulties, suppress unusual arousal events during sleep, or make a sleepy youngster more alert. However, medications tend to be overused for common sleep problems in the pediatric years, leading to short-lived improvements that occur often without an assessment for the presence of an underlying sleep disorder. Therefore, it is clinically important to recognize sleep problems associated with a sleep disorder, psychiatric diagnosis, or medical condition and treat appropriately. Many common sleep problems will improve with supportive or behavioral interventions alone. Sleep disorders associated with a medical condition such as narcolepsy or a psychiatric condition such as depression may require medication therapy.

The categories and criteria for sleep difficulties, as set forth in DSM-IV, include four major groups: (1) dyssomnias, which entail disturbances in the duration, type, and pattern of sleep; (2) parasomnias, which consist of arousal events directly related to the process of sleep and sleep architecture; (3) sleep disorders related to psychiatric disorders; and (4) sleep disorders resulting from general medical conditions or substance abuse. However, sleep difficulties in children tend to have causes that are different from those in adults. Thus this classification appears more useful for adults than for children and adolescents.

Clinically children and adolescents with sleep problems present with symptoms from one or more of four areas:

- Difficulties falling asleep and/or night waking
- Unusual arousal events during sleep
- Excessive daytime sleepiness
- Sleep problems associated with psychiatric or medical conditions

After a brief review of normal sleep architecture, this chapter discusses each of these problem areas in turn.

NORMAL SLEEP ARCHITECTURE

In order to appreciate disorders of sleep, an understanding of normal sleep architecture and how it evolves with development and age is necessary. Sleep stages are determined by three electrophysiological measures: the electroencephalogram (EEG), the electromyogram (EMG), and the electrooculogram (EOG). The patterning of CNS electrical activity, muscle tone, and eye movements allows recognition of different stages and types of sleep. Non-REM sleep is divided into stage 1, 2, 3, and 4. Stages 3 and 4 are often combined and are called delta or slow-wave sleep; slow-wave sleep is the deepest sleep in human beings and is conserved. This means that the length of slow-wave sleep increases in proportion to increasing awake time and is made up after sleep deprivation. Slow-wave sleep occurs predominantly in the first half of the night. Children are often difficult to wake during this stage of sleep, and if awakened, they often appear confused and disoriented. Parasomnias, such as sleepwalking, sleep talking, and night terrors, usually emerge from deep, slow-wave sleep.

Rapid eye movement (REM) sleep has aspects of both deep and light sleep. Dreaming occurs in REM sleep. Muscle tone drops dramatically and CNS subcortical functions are altered, but the cortex is very active. Upon awakening from REM sleep, alertness returns quickly. REM sleep occurs in cycles during the night, lasting approximately 90 minutes each. Most REM sleep takes place in the last half of the night, with the most intense REM cycles occurring just after body temperature reaches a minimum between 4 A.M. and 5 A.M.

Normal sleep patterning in a child is illustrated in the following figure. Most of slow wave sleep occurs in the first 1–3 hours after sleep onset. Arousal events and parasomnias occur here. Most of REM sleep occurs in the second half of the night. Nightmares occur here. Short periods of wakefulness typically occur during the night. Most children learn how to soothe themselves and quickly fall back asleep after these brief arousals.

Developmentally, the number of hours spent in sleep decreases with age. The percentage of time spent in REM sleep also decreases with age.

DIFFICULTIES FALLING ASLEEP OR NIGHT WAKING

Difficulty falling asleep and night awakening are common problems for young children. Between 3% and 14% of nonreferred children living in the community have sleep difficulties. The process of settling, self-soothing, and falling asleep is a learned one for children. After brief nighttime arousals, the child must

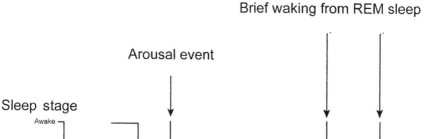

Figure 25.1 **Sleep architecture in a school-age child.**

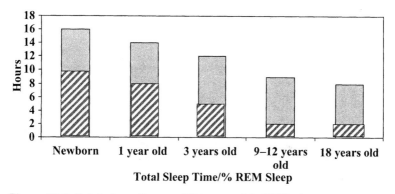

Figure 25.2 **Total sleep time and time spent in REM sleep as a function of age.**

learn to settle into sleep once again. A child who requires parental assistance in order to sleep might not be able to fall back asleep after awakening without a parent present. The most common sources of difficulty with initiating and maintaining sleep in children are maladaptive associations with sleep onset, which sometimes reflect parent–child interactional problems.

Because insomnia in children seems to be more of a psychosocial problem based on the relationship between parent and child, treatment is addressed primarily through psychosocial interventions. The most successful treatments for this common problem are behavioral. Techniques include graduated extinction or stimulus control along with parental education, development of a soothing bedtime routine, and support. Medications are generally not indicated. When sleep medications are prescribed, they should be used only adjunctively, for short periods of time, accompanying a behavioral intervention. Medication should be used in the service of facilitating the learning of new sleep-onset associations and to help the child develop self-soothing skills at bedtime.

Typical pharmacological interventions for problems initiating sleep include the following.

- Diphenhydramine 25–75 mg before bed.
- Melatonin 1–10 mg before bed.
  - Caution is advised with the use of melatonin because the FDA does not regulate the manufacture of this drug.
- Chloral hydrate 25–50 mg/kg 30 minutes before bed.

Older children and adolescents may develop insomnia related to specific fears and worries. Identifying and addressing the sources of fear and worry is an essential first step in treatment. Medication is generally not indicated for insomnia in older children and adolescents, unless the medication is being used to treat a specific disorder that is related to sleep problems, such as an anxiety disorder or depression. Often sleep hygiene techniques are useful in the treatment of insomnia in older children. These techniques are noted in the next table.

Table 25.1 Sleep Hygiene Techniques

Go to sleep at the same time every night.

Get up at the same time every day, including weekends and holidays.

Do not take daytime naps.

Limit the intake of caffeinated beverages after dinner.

Avoid strenuous exercise within 6 hours of bedtime.

Use the bed only for sleeping; do not read, watch TV, or eat in bed.

If sleep does not occur within 20 minutes of lying down in bed, get out of bed and do something quiet (such as reading) until drowsy. Then try again to go to sleep. Repeat as often as necessary.

UNUSUAL AROUSAL EVENTS DURING SLEEP (PARASOMNIAS)

Parasomnias refer to a group of unusual arousal events or behaviors during sleep. These events include night terrors, sleepwalking, sleep talking, nightmares, and nocturnal enuresis.

Night Terrors, Sleepwalking, and Sleep Talking

Night terrors, sleepwalking, and sleep talking are all closely related arousal behaviors emerging from deep slow-wave sleep. At the end of the deep sleep period in the first half of the night, the transition to lighter stages of sleep is often accompanied by unusual arousal events. Many children demonstrate grimacing, awkward movements, or mumbling during this transition. Walking, talking, or full-blown agitated night terrors occasionally accompany these behaviors in some children. Arousal disorders are difficult to predict because occurrences are sporadic.

These events occur most frequently at the ages in childhood when the largest amount of slow-wave sleep occurs. There may be a developmental sequence to the manifestation of delta sleep arousal events. Sleep terrors first appear after 18 months of age, and sleepwalking occurs in older preschool and school-age children. By adolescence arousal disorders generally disappear.

Arousal disorders usually occur in the first 1–3 hours after falling asleep. In night terrors, the sleeping child suddenly sits up in bed, is agitated, confused, and stares with unseeing eyes. Palpitations, irregular respirations, and diaphoresis may be present. The child is inconsolable and difficult to awaken. After 30 seconds to 5 minutes the child abruptly calms and goes back to sleep. In the morning no recollection of the event is available to the child. In sleepwalking, body movements are poorly coordinated and walking is directionless. Sleepwalking is dangerous; the patient may trip, collide with objects, or fall down stairs. These disorders may have a familial basis in families with high amounts of slow-wave sleep.

Treatment is generally supportive. Parents are often very alarmed when they first encounter an arousal event in their child. Education about the nature of sleep, the disorder, and the favorable prognosis as the child matures can be very helpful. A 30–60 minute nap in the afternoon may decrease the child's need for delta sleep at night and decrease the frequency of arousal events. For severe, dangerous, or frequent arousal events, benzodiazepines or tricyclic antidepressants can be helpful. These medications decrease the time spent in slow-wave sleep.

- Diazepam 2.5–5 mg hs.
- Clonazepam 0.5 mg hs.
- Imipramine 10–75 mg hs.

Nightmares

Nightmares are REM-related events that commonly occur in the second half of the night. Nightmares usually start between the ages of 3 and 6 years and affect 10–50% of children in this age group. A child awakening from a nightmare is usually alert and oriented, can lucidly describe details of the event, and has trouble going back to sleep. In the morning the child often can remember the nightmare. Pragmatic and supportive approaches to addressing the sources of the child's fears and anxieties are usually sufficient. Medications are not necessary.

Nocturnal Enuresis

Nocturnal enuresis is a common sleep-related problem in children. It is defined as bedwetting that occurs after bladder control should have been established, usually between the ages of 2 and 3 years. Enuresis may be diagnosed in children after the age of 5 years. About 10–15% of children between the ages of 3 and 11 years wet the bed at night. The prevalence decreases with age, reaching 3% at 12 years old.

Enuresis exists in two forms: primary and secondary. Children with primary enuresis have never been able to achieve bladder control and stop bedwetting for longer than a month. Primary enuresis is associated with a positive family history of bedwetting. Genetic and maturational factors are correlated with primary enuresis. These children usually have a small functional bladder capacity. Patients with secondary enuresis are dry for at least 6 months before bedwetting begins once again. Secondary enuresis is more prevalent than the primary type, and is more prevalent in boys. Secondary enuresis is generally associated with stressful psychological factors rather than maturational factors such as a small bladder capacity. In a minority of children medical disorders such as urinary tract infections, diabetes mellitus, or nocturnal epilepsy may be the cause of secondary enuresis.

Treatment begins with a careful evaluation to rule out medical causes of enuresis. The following domains should be considered in the treatment of the enuretic child.

- Physiological: A small functional bladder capacity is often present in children with primary enuresis.
  - Bladder training exercises are indicated to increase capacity and sphincter control.
  - Most children outgrow primary enuresis as bladder capacity enlarges with age.
- Psychological: Secondary enuresis is often associated with stressful psychological events.
  - Parental counseling and education to explain the disorder and reduce parental responses that increase guilt or shame in the bedwetting child are indicated.
- Behavioral conditioning
  - Bell and pad system is used at night.
  - Bell or buzzer awakens the child after the first drops of urine are passed.
  - The child wakes up, completes toileting, and changes the sheets.
  - Initial success rate is about 75%, but there exists a high relapse rate.
- Pharmacological
  - Imipramine in doses of 1–2.5 mg/kg/hs.
  - DDAVP in doses of 0.1–0.8 mg/hs.
  - There is a high relapse rate when medications are discontinued.

EXCESSIVE DAYTIME SLEEPINESS

Complaints of excessive daytime sleepiness occur frequently in older children and adolescents. The most common cause is inadequate number of hours in bed. The combination of late bedtimes and early morning awakening to go to school often leaves children with inadequate sleep and a growing sleep debt. The treatment is a behavioral contract between parents and child that specifies exact hours in bed, bedtimes for school nights and weekends, and rules for late-night social activities.

Disturbed Nocturnal Sleep

If the child or adolescent is getting an adequate number of hours in bed but continues to experience excessive sleepiness during the day, an occult sleep disorder should be suspected. Causes can include medications such as stimulants and/or asthma drugs. Excessive caffeine intake after dinner may cause insomnia. Strenuous exercise prior to bedtime may disrupt sleep.

Sleep-Disordered Breathing and Sleep Apnea

Sleep-disordered breathing is a common, often unrecognized, source of chronic sleep disruption among children. Sleep-disordered breathing results in multiple brief arousals from sleep during the night, which leave the child sleep deprived the next day. Clues include loud snoring, restless sleep, and intermittent apnea spells. In contrast to adult obstructive sleep apnea syndrome, in children obesity is less of a factor in sleep-disordered breathing. In the young child enlarged tonsils and adenoids and micrognathia are more common sources of this problem. Children at risk for sleep-disordered breathing and sleep apnea include those with maxillofacial abnormalities, cleft palate, micrognathia, children with enlarged tonsils and adenoids, and children with Down's syndrome.

Addressing the source of the breathing obstruction treats sleep-disordered breathing. Referral to an otolaryngologist is generally indicated. Treatment with continuous positive airway pressure (CPAP) or biphasic airway pressure (BiPAP) may be helpful.

Narcolepsy

Narcolepsy is a chronic neurological disorder characterized by excessive daytime sleepiness and abnormal REM sleep events that intrude upon waking consciousness. Prevalence is estimated at between 40–90 per 100,000 adults. The disorder usually first manifests in the second or third decade of life, but childhood onset cases have been reported. About 50% of patients report a positive family history of narcolepsy.

The clinical features of narcolepsy include the following.

- Bouts of irresistible sleep attacks may occur multiple times during the day, each lasting from a few seconds to as long as 30 minutes. Sleep attacks occur in conjunction with REM sleep abnormalities such as cataplexy, sleep paralysis, and/or hypnagogic hallucinations. In children with narcolepsy the prevalence of associated REM sleep abnormalities may be less than in adults with this condition.
- Cataplexy is a brief, sudden, complete or partial loss of muscle tone that frequently is precipitated by strong emotions such as laughter, surprise, or anger.
  ○ About 60–80% of patients with narcolepsy also have cataplexy.
- Sleep paralysis is a temporary loss of muscle control and a resulting inability to move, most often occurring upon awakening in the morning.

- Hypnagogic hallucinations are vivid dream-like hallucinatory perceptions that occur at sleep onset.

The treatment of narcolepsy consists of therapeutic daytime naps, the use of wake-promoting medications to decrease sleep attacks, and the use of medications that diminish REM sleep, such as tricyclic antidepressants.

- Stimulants such as methylphenidate 5–10 mg bid or dextroamphetamine 2.5–5 mg bid are used to treat sleep attacks. Long-acting stimulants may also be used.
- Modafinil is a novel wake-promoting agent that is effective for sleep attacks. Modafinil is given in doses of 100–400 mg/day, usually in two divided doses (A.M. and noon).
- Tricyclic antidepressants such as protriptyline are nonsedating, have a long half-life, and diminish REM sleep. Doses of 15–25 mg/day are recommended for the treatment of cataplexy, sleep paralysis, and hypnagogic hallucinations.

SLEEP PROBLEMS ASSOCIATED WITH PSYCHIATRIC CONDITIONS

Children and adolescents with psychiatric disorders appear to suffer frequently from sleep problems. The regulation of sleep and arousal seem to overlap and have a close association with the control of emotions and behavior in children. Behavioral and emotional problems can cause sleep disruption, and conversely, disrupted sleep may exacerbate emotional and behavioral disorders. Perhaps nowhere else are psychiatric medications as indicated in the treatment of sleep disorders as when sleep difficulties occur as part of a psychiatric disorder. Ideally, the specific mediations used for sleep should also be effective in the treatment of the specific disorder. The following table presents medications used for sleep difficulties in various child and adolescent psychiatric disorders.

Attention-Deficit/Hyperactivity Disorder

Decreased sleep needs, difficulties falling asleep, and awakening early in the morning full of energy and "on the go" are frequent symptoms in children with ADHD. Although stimulants can cause initial insomnia as a medication side effect, sleep difficulties may also be intrinsic to the ADHD disorder itself. Children with ADHD are significantly more restless in sleep, have more extraneous muscle movements, have more snoring, head banging, and nighttime awakening problems than comparison children. Medications including clonidine, imipramine, and melatonin may be helpful in allowing the ADHD child to settle more easily to sleep at night.

Depression

Sleep disturbance is a core symptom in major depressive disorder. Difficulties falling asleep, staying asleep, fragmented sleep, and/or early-morning awakenings

Table 25.2 Pharmacological Treatment of Insomnia Associated with Psychiatric Disorders

Psychiatric Disorder	Medication
Attention-deficit/hyperactivity disorder	Clonidine 0.05–0.2 mg hs
	Imipramine 10–100 mg hs
	Melatonin 1–10 mg hs
Depression	Imipramine 10–100 mg hs
	Amitriptyline 25–100 mg hs
	Trazodone 25–100 mg hs
Bipolar disorder	Risperidone 0.5–2 mg hs
	Olanzapine 2.5–10 mg hs
	Quetiapine 50–100 mg hs
Anxiety disorders	Lorazepam 0.5–1 mg hs for < 2 weeks
	Clonazepam 0.25–0.5 mg hs for < 2 weeks
	Imipramine 10–100 mg hs
	Melatonin 1–10 mg hs
	Diphenhydramine 10–100 mg hs
Posttraumatic stress disorder	Clonidine 0.05–0.2 mg hs
	Imipramine 10–100 mg hs
Psychotic disorders	Risperidone 0.25–2 mg hs
	Olanzapine 2.5–10 mg hs
	Quetiapine 50–100 mg hs
Developmental delay (MR and PDD)	Risperidone 0.25–2 mg hs
	Melatonin 1–10 mg hs

MR = mental retardation; PDD = pervasive developmental delay

frequently occur in persons suffering from depressive disorders. Antidepressants with sedating properties such as trazodone, imipramine, or amitriptyline may help treat sleep difficulties in depressed children and adolescents. SSRI antidepressants may cause jitteriness, arousal, and insomnia as medication side effects. Although they may be effective for depression, they are not generally used as a sleep-inducing medication.

Bipolar Disorder

Bipolar disorder can occur in adolescents; occurrence in childhood is more controversial. Because psychotic symptoms may occur in bipolar disorder, atypical antipsychotics are a mainstay of treatment for this condition; and because many atypical antipsychotics are sedating, they can be used at bedtime to treat sleep difficulties in this disorder.

Anxiety Disorders

Sleep difficulties often accompany anxiety disorders such as generalized anxiety disorder, obsessive–compulsive disorder, and/or posttraumatic stress disorder. Although benzodiazepines are used for sleep difficulties in anxiety disorders, they are only prescribed for short periods of time lasting less than 2 weeks because of concerns of medication tolerance. Other medications include imipramine, which has serotonergic and anxiety-reduction properties as well as being sedating. Diphenhydramine and melatonin may also prove useful for the child with anxiety and sleep difficulties.

Psychotic Disorders

Children with psychotic disorders often complain of hallucinations and night-time anxiety. Atypical antipsychotics given before bedtime are helpful for the sleep problems associated with these conditions.

Developmental Delay

Persons with mental retardation or pervasive developmental disorders often have atypical sleep needs perhaps related to their altered CNS neurobiology. They may need less sleep than persons without developmental delay. Families are greatly concerned when the developmentally delayed child wakes up in the middle of the night and begins to roam around the house, playing with toys and turning on lights without supervision. Often the family members become sleep deprived because of monitoring the child who does not seem to need as much sleep as they. Atypical antipsychotics in low doses or melatonin may be helpful in regulating the child's sleep patterns to be more synchronous with the needs of his or her family.

SLEEP PROBLEMS ASSOCIATED WITH MEDICAL AND NEUROLOGICAL DISORDERS

A wide variety of medical and neurological disorders may include sleep problems as an associated symptom. In the assessment of sleep disorders of childhood and adolescence, the clinician must make sure that routine medical evaluation has ruled out the occurrence of medial and neurological conditions. Some of these conditions are presented in the table below.

Table 25.3 Sleep Disorders Associated with a Medical or Neurological Condition

Medical Disorder	Neurological Disorder
Obstructive airway disease	Degenerative disorders
Sleep-related asthma	Narcolepsy
Gastroesophageal reflux	Sleep-related epilepsy
Obesity	Sleep-related headaches
Thyroid disorders	Kleine–Levin syndrome
	Down's syndrome
	Prader–Willi syndrome

26. Other Important Topics in Pediatric Psychopharmacology

This chapter discusses several important topics in pediatric psychopharmacology that have not been previously presented. These topics include the issue of combined pharmacotherapy in children and adolescents, psychopharmacology and the suicidal patient, an approach to pediatric psychopharmacology in conflicted family situations such as divorce, and psychopharmacology and the substance-abusing youngster.

COMBINED PHARMACOTHERAPY

Combined pharmacotherapy (CPT) is defined as the simultaneous use of two or more psychiatric medications either for the same or for different behavioral and/or emotional disorders or target symptoms. The use of CPT in pediatric psychopharmacology has been steadily increasing over the past 15 years. This increase parallels the overall increase in the use of psychiatric medications in the young that began in the 1990s. There is only limited scientific data on the use of CPT in children and adolescents, and the practice often receives no discussion in textbooks of pediatric psychopharmacology. Given the prevalence of CPT in clinical practice, this section presents a discussion of CPT in pediatric psychopharmacology.

Reasons for Rational Combined Pharmacotherapy

The need for clinicians to use combinations of psychiatric medications arises out of the often less than satisfactory response to monotherapy with single agents in child and adolescent psychopharmacology, an awareness of high rates of comorbid psychopathology in youngsters, and the hope that combined agents will result in synergistic treatment effects in certain psychiatric disorders.

General guidelines to assist the clinician in determining the appropriateness of prescribing CPT include the following (after Wilens et al., 1995).

503

- Significant symptoms of a psychiatric disorder known to be medication responsive, which are only partially responding to treatment with a single agent in an adequate dose and for an adequate treatment duration: For example, adding bupropion to ongoing stimulant treatment to help ADHD symptoms that are only partially responsive to stimulant monotherapy.
- Potential synergistic effects of combined agents: For example, combining mood stabilizers or a mood stabilizer and an atypical antipsychotic for rapid cycling pediatric bipolar disorder may be more effective than treatment with a single agent alone.
- CPT may allow the use of lower doses of each agent compared to monotherapy, thus reducing the potential for adverse effects associated with high doses of a single agent.
- Comorbid diagnoses potentially requiring the use of two or more agents, such as ADHD + depression or psychotic depression.
- Treatment of medication-induced adverse events, such as interventions for extrapyramidal side effects during antipsychotic therapy.
- Overlapping treatment when changing medications to avoid clinical deterioration when stopping one medication and starting another.

Prevalence of Combined Pharmacotherapy

The prevalence rates of pediatric CPT appear to be growing. One study revealed that between 1997 and 1998, 24.7% of the representative physician office visits for youth in which a stimulant was prescribed were also associated with the use of concomitant psychiatric medication (Bhatara et al., 2002). This represented a 5-fold increase over reported rates in 1993–1994 of 4.8% (Olfson et al., 2002; Safer et al., 2003). In ambulatory settings the majority of CPT involves ADHD and a comorbid psychiatric disorder such as depression, anxiety, or conduct problems. As such, stimulants are often co-prescribed with SSRIs or alpha-agonists such as clonidine or guanfacine.

In populations of seriously emotionally disturbed children and adolescents, rates of CPT are often higher. In a study of children in residential care, CPT was present in 60% of subjects. Two to five drugs were often combined in these children. CPT was associated with aggressive behavior rather than the treatment of specific psychiatric diagnoses (Connor et al., 1997). In this seriously emotionally disturbed population, neuroleptics and atypical antipsychotics were often combined with other agents.

Controlled Studies of Combined Pharmacotherapy

There are fewer controlled studies of children and adolescents than adults that support the use of CPT. In adult psychiatric patients methodologically controlled studies support the use of CPT for psychotic depression, treatment-resistant depression, bipolar disorders, and obsessive–compulsive disorder. In contrast, most of the extant controlled CPT studies in youngsters focus on ADHD. These studies include the following.

- Methylphenidate combined with desipramine in the treatment of ADHD and depression (Carlson et al., 1995)
- Methylphenidate combined with thioridazine in the treatment of ADHD (Gittelman-Klein et al., 1976)
- Methylphenidate combined with clonidine in the treatment of ADHD and conduct or oppositional defiant disorder (Connor et al., 2000)
- Methylphenidate combined with clonidine in the treatment of ADHD and tic disorder (Kurlan et al., 2002)
- Clonidine combined with stimulants in the treatment of ADHD and conduct or oppositional defiant disorder (Hazell & Stuart, 2003)
- Divalproex combined with quetiapine in the treatment of adolescent mania (DelBello et al., 2002)

Open trials suggest the utility and safety of combining other agents (see Safer et al., 2003 for review).

- Stimulants with atypical antipsychotics for the treatment of ADHD and conduct disorder
- Clonazepam with clonidine for the treatment of ADHD and tic disorder
- Trazodone with haloperidol for the treatment of chronic tic disorder
- Clomipramine with an SSRI for the treatment of OCD
- Clozapine with lithium for the treatment of mixed psychosis
- Risperidone with an SSRI for the treatment of OCD
- Lithium with imipramine for the treatment of major depression
- Olanzapine with divalproex for the treatment of pediatric bipolar disorder
- Lithium with nortriptyline for the treatment of major depression
- Fluoxetine with clomipramine for the treatment of OCD
- Methylphenidate with fluoxetine for the treatment of ADHD and major depression
- Stimulants with atomoxetine for the treatment of ADHD
- A neuroleptic with an SSRI for the treatment of Tourette's disorder and OCD
- Methylphenidate with lithium for the treatment of ADHD and a mood disorder

Given the widespread use of CPT with a wide variety of different agents in youngsters with many different psychiatric disorders, there clearly exists a need for more controlled research to provide additional empirical evidence supporting this common clinical practice.

Combined Pharmacotherapy in the Clinical Setting

Clinicians should approach CPT cautiously. When combining psychoactive agents, there is risk for increased side effects and drug–drug interactions. These risks multiply as the number of concurrent medications increases. The astute clinician will be aware of common psychotropic drug–drug interactions. For example, some common interactions include the following.

- TCAs interact with SSRIs to increase serotonin levels and risk for serotonin syndrome.
- Fluoxetine inhibits the metabolism of all TCAs, raising TCA plasma levels and possibly inducing cardiovascular toxicity.
- Fluvoxamine is a significant inhibitor of melatonin clearance.
- Carbamazepine induces hepatic metabolism and lowers the plasma levels of all psychotropic agents that undergo hepatic metabolism.
- Cimetidine impairs the metabolism of TCAs.
- Methylphenidate may diminish the metabolism of imipramine.
- Aminophylline and theophylline increase lithium excretion and decrease plasma lithium levels.

Prescribing clinicians should have a systematic approach to the initiation and titration of psychiatric medications in children and adolescents. CPT should not be introduced in a casual or haphazard manner. Rather, CPT should result from a logical process that considers how the addition of a second agent to the treatment plan will enhance medication effectiveness for the disorder under treatment, and also be well tolerated by the patient.

- Only use medications within a coordinated psychoeducational treatment plan.
- Use psychiatric medications to treat psychiatric diagnoses that are known from empirical research to be medication responsive. Do not use medications to treat psychiatric diagnoses that are not medication responsive or to "chase" symptoms by adding more medication to the treatment plan.
- When beginning treatment, use the most benign interventions first.
- When beginning medication treatment, have some quantifiable means of assessing drug effectiveness and safety.
  - Obtain baseline data before drug initiation, against which to compare data once the child is prescribed medication.
  - Obtain data at regular intervals during treatment.
  - Use reliable and validated rating scale instruments to measure drug effectiveness and side effects.
- Institute drug trials systematically.
  - Introduce medication as a single variable into treatment at any one point in time.
  - Once the medication is initiated, if possible, explore the full dose range of the agent (low, medium, high dose) before abandoning the drug as ineffective or adding a second agent. Too often physicians discontinue a medication as "ineffective" after only titrating the dose to a low or moderate dose range. For example, medications such as SSRIs for OCD or panic attacks might require high doses to be effective.
  - Avoid polypharmacy with multiple drugs all given at subtherapeutic doses.
  - Allow for an adequate duration of treatment before concluding that a medication is ineffective. For example, antidepressants may take 2–12 weeks to become fully effective.
  - Follow drug plasma levels when available.

○ Introduce medication trials to youngsters for preplanned periods of time that have a clear beginning and ending, so that drug effectiveness and the need for continuing medication therapy can be clinically assessed over time.

PSYCHOPHARMACOLOGY AND THE SUICIDAL PATIENT

Clinicians who prescribe psychiatric medications to children and adolescents with neuropsychiatric disorders generally evaluate and treat youngsters with complicated and severe symptoms. Some of these young patients become suicidal. This section presents a brief discussion about suicide risk and management issues in children and adolescents.

Suicidal ideation and acts are episodic events that have a discrete onset and duration. Suicidality is generally transient and reversible. Only occasionally is suicidality persistent and irreversible. Intent to cause harm or death to oneself is an essential ingredient of suicidal behavior. Suicidal behavior among children and adolescents involves a continuum from nonsuicidal behavior to suicidal ideas, suicide attempts, and death by suicide.

Epidemiology

Completed suicide rates rise precipitously in the population as children grow into middle and late adolescence. Suicide is relatively uncommon in school-age children but is the third leading cause of adolescent death. About 250,000 adolescents make a suicide attempt in the United States each year. Suicide attempts are far more common than death by suicide. The ratio of attempted to completed suicide in children and adolescents is about 50:1. In samples of children and adolescents with a history of psychiatric hospitalization, suicide attempts occur approximately 9 times more frequently than in the community. Age-related suicide rates include the following.

• The rate of suicide for 5- to 14-year-olds is about 0.8 per 100,000 persons.
• The rate of suicide for 14- to 24-year-olds is about 11.1 per 100,000 persons.

Gender-related suicide rates include the following.

• Women attempt suicide more often than men.
• Men kill themselves by suicide more often than women.

Etiology

Youngsters with depression, bipolar disorder, substance abuse problems, and disruptive behavioral disorders are at increased risk. It is important to note that psychiatric disorders are highly correlated with suicide. About 90% of suicide victims have a diagnosable psychiatric illness. Often a psychiatric disorder is present but unrecognized and untreated at the time of suicide.

As noted in Chapters 5 and 17, initiation of an antidepressant to treat mood disorders, obsessive–compulsive disorders, or anxiety disorders may result in increased suicidal ideation and behaviors in children and adolescents. In October 2004 the FDA completed a study of over 4,400 children and adolescents receiving one of nine antidepressants in 24 randomized controlled pediatric antidepressant studies, largely sponsored by the pharmaceutical industry. The antidepressants investigated included fluoxetine, sertraline, paroxetine, fluvoxamine, citalopram, mirtazapine, venlafaxine, wellbutrin, and nefazodone. The studies included 16 medication trials in depression, 4 in obsessive–compulsive disorder, 2 in generalized anxiety disorder, and 2 in attention-deficit/hyperactivity disorder. No completed suicides were found in any subject in any of the medication trials. However, 78 events of increased suicidal ideation and behaviors were found. This rate was about twice the rate found for placebo and led the FDA to place a black box warning on all antidepressants used for children and adolescents. There may exist a complicated interaction between depression and the activating effects of some antidepressants that results in increased risk for suicidal behaviors in children and adolescents (Federal Drug Administration, 2004).

Other risk factors for suicidality and protective factors are outlined in the following two tables.

Table 26.1 Risk Factors Associated with Suicide in Children and Adolescents

Easy access to irreversible lethal means (e.g., firearms)
Gay, lesbian, or homosexual orientation
History of previous suicide attempt
Hopelessness
Impaired judgment
Impulsivity
Intense aggression
Intention to commit suicide
Physical and/or sexual abuse
Psychiatric disorder (e.g., depression, bipolar, psychosis, substance abuse, conduct)
Social isolation and lack of support
Stressful life events

Table 26.2 Protective Factors in Suicidal Children and Adolescents

Ability to communicate openly with others
Future orientation
Good judgment
High impulse control
Low hopelessness
Low social isolation
Strong and positive family supports

Assessment of the Suicidal Child or Adolescent

The purpose of risk assessment is to determine the degree of immediate danger for a suicidal youngster and to develop and implement an emergency treatment plan to keep the patient safe. The following table outlines issues for suicide risk assessment.

Table 26.3 Issues for Risk Assessment in Suicidal Children and Adolescents

---

Current suicide intent
Past suicide intent
History of previous suicide attempts and lethality
Balance between wish to live and wish to die
Type of suicide method previously used or currently contemplated
Lethality of method (firearms = jumping from a high place > hanging > drowning > suffocation > overdose)
Access to suicide method
Degree of planning versus impulsivity
Likelihood of discovery by others
Underlying risk factors (see previous table)
Preoccupation with death
Antidepressant side effects, including:
- Increased arousal
- Increased activation
- Jitteriness
- Disinhibition
- Hypomanic side effects

It is recommended that the clinician develop a systematic approach to evaluating and interviewing the suicidal youngster. Because suicidal impulses wax and wane, becoming more urgent and then less urgent, continuing reassessment of suicidal intent is necessary for most patients. Close clinical monitoring for increased suicidality is now recommended for youngsters initiating antidepressant therapies, including weekly face-to-face evaluation by the prescribing clinician over the first 4 weeks of treatment, every-other-week evaluation over the 2nd month of treatment, and every 3 months thereafter, as indicated. Clinical experience does not support the fear that asking about suicide will introduce the idea into anyone's mind. Assessment should progress from more general to more specific questions, as presented in the example below:

"How are you feeling?"

"Do you ever get really down about things?"

"Do you ever get so down that it seems like nothing will ever get better?"

"When you get down like that, is it is hard to go on?"

"Have you ever thought about hurting yourself?"

"Do those thoughts last a long time?"

"Do they come back over and over again?"

"Have you ever thought about actually killing yourself?"

"When you think about killing yourself, do you have a plan as to how to do it?

"Did you ever start to kill yourself and then change your mind?"

"How did you attempt to kill yourself before?"

"Are there guns, pills, or poisons in your house?"

"If you do kill yourself, what do you hope to accomplish?"

Treatment of the Suicidal Child or Adolescent

- Immediate safety concerns should drive the treatment plan. If assessment reveals a seriously suicidal youngster, then immediate emergency evaluation and possible inpatient hospitalization are necessary.
- If assessment reveals suicidal ideation but family supports suggest that ambulatory treatment is a possibility, the prescribing clinician is faced with the possible difficulty of giving medication to a potentially self-destructive patient. Some recommendations for management of the ambulatory suicidal patient are given below:
  - If the prescribing physician is a primary care doctor, immediate consultation with child and adolescent psychiatrist is necessary.
  - Psychiatric medication should not be withheld from the suicidal patient if evaluation reveals an underlying medication-responsive psychiatric disorder such as depression, psychosis, or ADHD.
  - The psychiatrist should assess the suicidal youngster frequently and as often as necessary in order to evaluate mental status, suicide potential, and safety.
  - Family members must be involved in the treatment plan. Potential suicidal behavior is an emergency; hence issues of therapist–patient confidentiality do not apply. Family members must be informed of the patient's potential suicidal behaviors and an emergency plan developed with the psychiatrist. This plan includes the following:
    - Location and telephone number of the nearest emergency room.
    - How to communicate with the treating psychiatrist during the evening, night, weekend, and holiday hours.
    - How to transport the patient to the nearest emergency room if the child or adolescent does indeed become suicidal.
    - Helping the family to safely lock away or remove from the home potentially lethal means of suicide, such as firearms, knives, poisons, and pills.
    - Helping the family develop a systematic plan to check in with the patient and discuss feelings and any self-destructive urges at regular intervals.
  - The prescribing physician should prescribe the minimum amount of psychiatric medications that are just enough to last until the next appointment. Medication refills should not be given automatically without psychiatric follow-up.
    - This is to minimize the number of medications available at home should the patient overdose.
  - Parents should take responsibility for the child or teenager's medications in the home environment and keep them in a secure place.

It is important to remember that most suicidal patients communicate their intentions or distress before acting on a suicide plan. People who attempt suicide usually seek comfort or help before they act on their self-destructive impulses. With recognition of symptoms and clinical awareness of any underlying psychiatric disorder, appropriate intervention and treatment can change the minds of most suicidal children and adolescents before self-destructive acts become fatal.

AN APPROACH TO PEDIATRIC PSYCHOPHARMACOLOGY IN CONFLICTED FAMILY SITUATIONS

The pediatric psychopharmacology treatment plan should be developed to the best extent possible in conjunction with both of the child's parents. If there is only a single primary caregiver, then the treatment plan must involve this adult. Active engagement of parents is crucial to the success of all mental health interventions for children and adolescents. A detailed discussion with the parents concerning the recommended treatment plan, medication, and an examination of alternative treatments is necessary as a beginning part of psychopharmacological treatment. Realistic and unrealistic expectations that parents may have about the medication need to be addressed. Once a medication is chosen, the dose schedule, potential side effects, anticipated benefits, and time needed for the medication to become effective are important areas to discuss with parents. Failure to involve the parents in the psychopharmacological decision-making process may threaten treatment compliance and undermine the success of medication interventions.

However, some families may be in conflict over the appropriateness of the recommended treatment plan. For example, divorced parents may disagree about what is best for their child or one spouse may favor psychiatric assessment and treatment, whereas the other spouse disagrees. Parents who are involved in legal proceedings against each other might use the child's evaluation and treatment plan in an adversarial manner with one another. In highly conflicted situations, one parent may bring the child for treatment without the other parent even knowing that a psychiatric evaluation has occurred.

The physician should proceed with caution in the evaluation and medication treatment of referred children and adolescents from homes in which parents are in serious disagreement and conflict. Every effort should be made to involve both parents in the process of evaluation and clinical intervention for their offspring. Failure to involve both parents in the treatment plan will increase the likelihood that therapeutic recommendations for the referred child will ultimately fail, as treatment recommendations become part of a more general pattern of parental animosity toward one another.

Some recommendations for approaching the psychopharmacological treatment of youngsters with parents in conflict are given below.

- At the time of the initial phone call requesting evaluation or services for a child or adolescent, determine if both parents are available and in agreement about the need for referral.
  - If possible, include both parents in the initial assessment of the youngster.
- If parents are in disagreement about the need for services, the following are suggested before the child or adolescent is actually seen in consultation:
  - Request that both parents speak on the telephone to the physician.
  - Assess parents' areas of agreement and disagreement about the need for referral of their child.
  - Try and reach some consensus with parents about the need for assessment of their child or adolescent.

○ Request that both parents be actively involved, if possible, in the assessment and treatment planning process for their child.

○ If necessary, meet with each parent separately.

• If parents remain in marked conflict and disagreement as to the need for evaluation and treatment of the child, then it is not wise to proceed with psychopharmacological assessment until some parental consensus is reached. Referral to a therapist or legal mediator (in the case of contested custody or acrimonious divorce) is necessary before evaluation and treatment of the child can proceed.

PSYCHOPHARMACOLOGY AND THE SUBSTANCE-ABUSING YOUNGSTER

Substance abuse is one of the most common and serious of the mental health disorders. Substance use disorders (SUDs) are increasingly understood to have their developmental beginnings in childhood and adolescence. Between 30% and 50% of SUDs begin before age 18 years. Early onset of SUDs is associated with high rates of psychiatric comorbidity, antisocial behaviors, and high-risk lifestyle behaviors such as increased rates of suicide, school dropout, motor vehicle accidents, and early, promiscuous sexual behaviors.

Current research suggests that the treatment of pediatric SUDs requires a multimodal, comprehensive psychoeducational treatment plan tailored to the specific needs of the individual patient. Psychosocial interventions, specific SUD interventions, and random drug testing are necessary components of the treatment plan. The pharmacotherapy of SUD is an active area of scientific investigation, but few studies have been completed in pediatric populations. Research in adult SUDs suggests effectiveness for medications that substitute for the addiction, are aversive therapies, or diminish craving; these include disulfiram and naltrexone for alcohol disorders, bupropion for nicotine addiction, and/or methadone or buprenorphine for opiate use disorders. However, the use of these aversion or substitution agents is not well supported by the extant research in pediatric psychopharmacology.

The specific treatment of SUDs with psychopharmacological agents in children and adolescents is uncommon. However, the prescribing clinician often encounters youngsters who have an SUD plus a potentially medication-responsive psychiatric disorder, such as ADHD, depression, anxiety, or bipolar disorder. For example, psychiatric disorders have been observed in up to 75–85% of youth with an SUD. Effective treatment of comorbid psychiatric disorders may help reduce the severity of associated SUD. The therapeutic challenge is how to treat comorbid psychopathology in these children and adolescents.

General Treatment Considerations in Youth with Psychiatric Disorder and SUDs

• Maximize family involvement with the treatment plan.
• Consider self-help interventions such as Alcohol Anonymous or Narcotics Anonymous.
• Consider random urine testing for drugs of abuse and alcohol.

- Consider adjunctive psychosocial therapies.
- Consider involvement of family court via a stubborn child petition.
  - Supports the treatment plan with the power of a court-appointed probation officer, should the child or adolescent become noncompliant with recommended treatment interventions.

ATTENTION-DEFICIT/HYPERACTIVITY DISORDER AND SUDs

Adolescents with ADHD may develop a SUD at a higher rate than comparison youths. The treatment of ADHD and a comorbid SUD is complicated because stimulants may be diverted, misused, or abused in such patients. Current treatment recommendations include the following.

- A period of abstinence in the range of 2–4 weeks before initiating medications for ADHD is recommended.
- Behavioral and psychosocial interventions may be used in the interim for ADHD.
- Treat ADHD with noradrenergic agents of low abuse potential, such as:
  - Bupropion
  - Atomoxetine
  - Desipramine
  - Nortriptyline
- If stimulants must be prescribed to the substance-abusing ADHD patient, longer-acting preparations such as Concerta or Adderall XR are less likely to be abused than stimulants with a shorter duration of action.
- Early stimulant therapy for ADHD may actually prevent the occurrence of a later SUD. In a meta-analytic review of the relationship between medication treatment of ADHD and the risk of developing later SUD, Wilens et al. (2003) found that early stimulant treatment of ADHD reduced the risk of a later SUD by a factor of 1.9.
- There is no evidence that early stimulant treatment for ADHD sensitizes the patient to later SUD, according to the findings of a 13-year prospective study of ADHD youngsters (Barkley et al., 2003).

ANXIETY DISORDERS AND SUDs

Pharmacological treatment of patients with anxiety disorders and an SUD is difficult. Benzodiazepines should be avoided. Agents of low abuse potential should be used to treat anxiety.

- SSRI antidepressants
- TCA antidepressants
- Buspirone

DEPRESSION AND SUDs

Patients with depression and an SUD sometimes experience remission of their depressive symptoms after 2–4 weeks of abstinence. Thus it is recommended that pharmacological treatment of depression occur only after a period of abstinence has been achieved and depression continues to be problematic.

OTHER IMPORTANT TOPICS

- SSRIs such as fluoxetine are effective in pediatric depression and have a low abuse potential.
- Bupropion has a low abuse potential and may be effective in substance-abusing adolescents with depression.
- Psychosocial interventions such as cognitive–behavioral or interpersonal therapies with accompanying family involvement are effective in pediatric depression.

BIPOLAR DISORDER AND SUDs

There exists strong and growing scientific evidence that bipolar disorder is associated with SUDs in adolescents. A period of abstinence before the initiation of psychiatric medication is not indicated for the bipolar-disordered teenager with substance abuse. Bipolar disorder is a serious psychiatric illness that requires immediate clinical intervention; emerging evidence indicates that mood stabilizers may treat pediatric bipolar disorder as well as comorbid SUD.

- Lithium has demonstrated effectiveness for pediatric bipolar disorder and for diminishing substance abuse in youth with bipolar disorder. Lithium has a low abuse potential. However, lithium has a narrow therapeutic index and must be carefully clinically monitored.
- Valproic acid has been reported to significantly reduce substance use in bipolar youngsters; it has a low abuse potential.
- Atypical antipsychotics are effective for the manic phase of pediatric bipolar disorder. These agents have a low abuse potential, although they have not yet been shown to actually reduce substance abuse in manic adolescents.

PSYCHOTIC DISORDERS AND SUDs

Psychotic symptoms such as delusions, paranoid thinking, and auditory and/or visual hallucinations often require immediate treatment. It is recommended that atypical antipsychotic medication be started immediately in psychotic youngsters who also have a comorbid SUD. The exception is youth who abuse hallucinogens and have persisting perceptual disturbances even when the hallucinogen is stopped (e.g., hallucinogen-persisting perceptual disorder). There is some evidence that antipsychotics, particularly risperidone, may exacerbate perceptual disorders in these patients.

Appendices

Appendix 1.
Pediatric Psychopharmacology Summary Table: Evidence of Efficacy by Drug and Disorder in Children and Adolescents < 18 Years Old

Drug	ADHD	ODD/CD	SAD	PD	GAD	SP	PTSD	OCD	MDD	BPD	TIC	SCHIZ	DD[a]	Enuresis
Aripiprizole		C					D			D	D	D	D	
Atomoxetine	A	B	B				D				B			
Benzodiazepines					D									
Beta-Blockers		C		D			C			D				
Buspirone	B				D				E				C	
Carbamazepine	C	C							D	D		D	D	
Citalopram			D	D	C	D	D	C	B					
Clonidine	A	B		D			D			D	A		A	
Clozapine		C										B	E	
DDAVP	E	E	E	E	E	E	E	E	E	E	E	E	D	A
Divalproex		A								B		D		
Fluoxetine	C		D	D	D	B	C	A	A	D			D	
Fluvoxamine			B	C	B	B	D	A	C					
Guanfacine	B	D					D				B			
Lamotrigine														
Lithium	E	A							D	D		D	D	E
Mirtazapine						C			D	B			C	
Nefazadone[b]									C					
Neuroleptics	D	A								C	A	A	A	
Olanzapine	D	C								C	D	C	B	
Oxcarbazepine		D								D			D	
Paroxetine			B	D	D	B	D	A	B[c]	D				
Quetiapine	D	D					D	C		B	D	C	D	
Risperidone	D	A					D	A		C	B	B	A	
Sertraline			B	D	B	C	C		B	D				
Stimulants	A	A									E	E		
St. John's wort									C				A	

TCA	A	C	B	C	D	D	A[d]	C	—	B	D	A
Topiramate	C	—	D	D	D	D	D	E[e]	C	E	—	—
Venlafaxine	A	C	—	—	—	—	—	C	D	C	—	—
Wellbutrin	D	C	—	—	—	—	—	D	D	C	—	—
Ziprazidone	D	C	—	D	—	—	—	C	D	C	C	—

ADHD = attention-deficit/hyperactivity disorder; ODD = oppositional defiant behavior; CD = conduct disorder; SAD = separation anxiety disorder; PD = panic disorder; GAD = generalized anxiety disorder; SP = social phobia (selective mutism); PTSD = posttraumatic stress disorder; OCD = obsessive-compulsive disorder; MDD = major depressive disorder; BPD = bipolar disorder; TIC = Tic or Tourette's disorder; SCHIZ = schizophrenia; DD = developmental delay

[a]Medication for associated symptoms of DD. No medicine currently effective for the core symptoms of autism or mental retardation.

[b]Not recommended because of increased rates of hepatic toxicity.

[c]Recommended by FDA to not use paroxetine in children < 18 years old with MDD.

[d]Clomipramine only

[e]Recommended by manufacturer to not use venlafaxine in children < 18 years old with MDD.

KEY:

A: Evidence of empirical support in ≥ two randomized controlled trials
B: Evidence of empirical support in one randomized controlled trial
C: Evidence of empirical support in open trials only
D: Evidence of support in clinical experience only
E: Ineffective or contraindicated
———: No data or not indicated

Sources:

Geller DA, Biederman J, Stewart SE, Mullin B, Martin A, Spencer T, and Faraone SV. Which SSRI? A meta-analysis of pharmacotherapy trials in pediatric obsessive–compulsive disorder. Am J Psychiatry 160(11):1919–1928, 2003.
Green WH. Child and Adolescent Clinical Psychopharmacology (3rd ed.). Philadelphia: Lippincott, Williams & Wilkins, 2001.
Jobson KO and Potter WZ. International psychopharmacology algorithm project report. Psychopharmacol Bull 31:457–459, 1995.
Martin A, Scahill L, Charney DS, & Leckman JF (Eds.). Pediatric Psychopharmacology: Principles and Practice. New York Oxford University Press, 2003.
Research Unit on Pediatric Psychopharmacology Anxiety Study Group. Fluvoxamine for the treatment of anxiety disorders in children and adolescents. NEJM 344(17):1279–1285, 2001.
Riddle MA, Kastelic EA, and Frosch E. Pediatric psychopharmacology. J Child Psychol Psych 42(1):73–90, 2001.
Rosenberg DR, Davanzo PA, and Gershon S. Pharmacotherapy for Child and Adolescent Psychiatric Disorders (2nd ed.). New York: Marcel Dekker, 2002.
Varley CK. Psychopharmacological treatment of major depressive disorder in children and adolescents. JAMA 290(8):1091–1093, 2003.
Werry JS and Aman MG (Eds.). Practitioner's Guide to Psychoactive Drugs for Children and Adolescents (2nd ed.). New York: Plenum Press, 1999.
Wolraich ML. Annotation: The use of psychotropic medications in children: An American view. J Child Psychol Psych 44(2):159–168, 2003.

APPENDIX 1

Appendix 2.
Pharmacodynamics of
Psychiatric Medications
Commonly Used in Children and
Adolescents

- Antidepressants
- Atypical antipsychotics
- Anticonvulsants
- Stimulants

Information about how a drug exerts its effects is obtained, in part, from pharmacodynamic investigation of drug action at specific receptor sites. A high affinity of a compound for a specific receptor gives clues as to the possible effects of the drug in the body. For example, a high affinity for:

- Histamine receptors may suggest sedation or appetite changes as possible drug effects.
- Muscarinic acetylcholine receptors may suggest anticholinergic effects, such as dry mouth, constipation, or blurred vision.
- Alpha-adrenergic receptors may suggest cardiovascular drug effects, such as changes in blood pressure or pulse rate.
- Monoamine reuptake transport proteins may suggest drug action by altering monoamine presynaptic reuptake and raising synaptic monoamine concentrations, with possible enhanced effects on postsynaptic neurotransmission.
- Dopamine receptors in the caudate or putamen, whose neuronal projection fields originate in the A9 substantia nigra region of the nucleus accumbens (midbrain), suggest a propensity for extrapyramidal side effects.

- Dopamine receptors in the mesocortical regions, whose neuronal projection fields originate in the A10 ventral tegmental region of the nucleus accumbens (midbrain), suggest antipsychotic activity.

Little pharmacodynamic information is available for older agents, especially psychiatric medications whose patents have expired and are currently available in generic form. These agents include tricyclic antidepressants, lithium, phenothiazines, and stimulants. More information is available on newer agents, which include the newer second-generation antidepressants and atypical antipsychotics. Data for the following pharmacodynamic discussion was obtained directly from the pharmaceutical manufacturer of the drug, except where referenced.

PHARMACODYNAMICS OF ANTIDEPRESSANTS

- Reversible inhibition of presynaptic monoamine reuptake transporters (except mirtazapine). This enhances the monoamine concentration in the synaptic cleft and facilitates postsynaptic serotonin, norepinephrine, and/or dopamine neurotransmission.
- Mirtazapine does not inhibit monoamine reuptake transporters. Mirtazapine is thought to exert its antidepressant action by blocking 5HT2 and 5HT3 receptors and antagonizing the adrenergic alpha-2-autoreceptors and alpha-2-heteroreceptors, facilitating release of norepinephrine and 5HT1A mediated serotonergic neurotransmission.

PHARMACODYNAMICS OF ATYPICAL ANTIPSYCHOTICS

- It is thought that blockade of dopamine receptors in the mesocortical CNS confers the antipsychotic properties of these agents.
- The simultaneous blockade of serotonin type 2 receptors is thought responsible for the low risk of extrapyramidal side effects seen with atypical antipsychotics. In contrast, haloperidol (a typical neuroleptic) has a high risk of extrapyramidal side effects. It has high affinity for dopamine receptors, but low affinity for serotonin receptors.
- Aripiprazole is a partial dopamine/serotonin agonist/antagonist. It functions as a partial agonist at the dopamine D2 receptor and the serotonin 5HT1A receptor, and as an antagonist at the serotonin 5HT2A receptor.

PHARMACODYNAMICS OF ANTICONVULSANTS

Anticonvulsants are increasingly used in psychiatry as mood stabilizers for bipolar disorder and recurrent mood disorder, and as anti-aggression agents. Topiramate is being investigated in eating disorders, headache, and alcoholism.

Table A2.1 Receptor Binding Affinities of Some Antidepressants: equilibrium inhibition constant (K_i) values (nM) calculated by in vitro measurement of monoamine uptake into rat brain synaptosomes[a]

Antidepressant	5HT Uptake	NE Uptake	DA Uptake	5HT1A	5HT1B	5HT1C	5HT1D	5HT2	5HT2c	Alpha-1	Alpha-2	D2	H1	ACHm
Atomoxetine	77	5	1451	—	—	—	—	> 2000	—	> 2000	> 2000	> 10,000	> 10,000	> 10,000
Bupropion		2200	1500	—	—	—	—	—	—	—	—	—	—	—
Citalopram	1.6	7865	16,540	—	—	—	—	—	2051	1211	—	—	283	1430
Escitalopram	1.1	7841	27,410	—	—	—	—	—	2531	3870	—	—	1973	1242
Fluoxetine	25	777	4200	> 10,000	> 10,000	150	> 10,000	—	72	3800	13,900	12,000	5400	590
Fluvoxamine	2.3	2950	16,790	—	—	—	—	—	5786	1288	—	—	29,250	31,200
Mirtazapine				5.3	4.9	—	5.3	—	8.2	6.5	6.8	5.6	9.3	6.2
Paroxetine	1.1	85	2000	> 10,000	> 10,000	> 10,000	> 10,000	—	9034	4600	17,000	32,000	22,000	108
Sertraline	2.4	817	230	> 10,000	> 10,000	1500	> 10,000	—	2298	380	4100	10,700	24,000	630

[a]A low K_i value indicates high receptor affinity. Affinity is a measure of how potent a drug is at binding to a receptor site. K_i (inhibition constant) represents the concentration of drug necessary to occupy 50% of the available receptors. In physical terms, affinity is a function of how well the three-dimensional structure of the receptor and the drug fit together. 5HT uptake = serotonin reuptake transporter; NE uptake = norepinephrine reuptake transporter; DA uptake = dopamine reuptake transporter; 5HT1A–2C = specific serotonin receptors; α1,2 = adrenergic receptors; D2 = dopamine 2 receptor; H1 = histamine receptor; —— = Information not available

Table A2.2 Antidepressant Affinities for Monoamine Reuptake Transporter Proteins: equilibrium inhibition constant (K$_i$) values (nmol/L) calculated by in vitro measurement of monoamine uptake into rat brain synaptosomes[a]

Antidepressant	Affinity for SERT	Affinity for NET
Amitriptyline	36	102
Citalopram	8.9	7865
Fluoxetine	20	777
Fluvoxamine	14	2950
Nortriptyline	279	21
Paroxetine	0.83	85
Sertraline	3.3	817
Venlafaxine	102	2269

Source: Owens MJ, Morgan WN, Plott SJ, Nemeroff CB. Neurotransmitter receptor and transporter binding profile of antidepressants and their metabolites. *J Pharmacol Exp Ther* 283:1305, 1997.
[a]A low K$_i$ value indicates high receptor affinity.
SERT = human serotonin transporter
NET = human norepinephrine transporter

Zonisamide is under investigation for binge eating disorder. In neurology these agents are used for seizures, neuralgic pain, and migraine headache. The mechanism of action of anticonvulsant medications for psychiatric disorders is largely unknown.

Seizures are thought to be mediated by defective synaptic function, either a reduction of inhibitory synaptic activity or enhancement of excitatory synaptic activity. GABA is the principal inhibitory neurotransmitter in the CNS, and glutamate (NMDA, AMPA, and kainate are glutamate agonists) is the principal excitatory CNS neurotransmitter. Anticonvulsants have antiepileptic actions via three mechanisms.

- Blockade of voltage-gated Na$^+$ channels: During a seizure, individual neurons undergo depolarization and fire action potentials at high frequencies. This pattern of neuronal activity is characteristic of a seizure and is uncommon during physiological neuronal activity. Blockade of voltage-gated Na$^+$ channels by anticonvulsant agents reduces the firing rate of neurons.
- Inhibition of T-type Ca^{2+} channels: The recurrent pacemaker thalamic rhythm in spikes and waves seen in generalized absence seizures can be reduced by inhibiting Ca^{2+} flow into neurons.
- GABA enhancement: The inhibitory actions of GABA may be enhanced by several mechanisms at the level of the individual neuron. These include blocking GABA reuptake into the presynaptic neuron (tiagabine), inhibiting the action of the enzyme that degrades GABA (vigabatrin), and promoting GABA release from the presynaptic neuron (gabapentin). All of these actions increase the availability of GABA at the postsynaptic neuron.
- The anticonvulsant mechanism of action of levetiracetam is presently unknown.

Table A2.3 Receptor Binding Profiles of Atypical Antipsychotic Agents: K_i values (nM)[a]

Antipsychotic	D1	D2	D4	5HT1A	5HT2A	5HT2C	ACHM	Alpha-1	Alpha-2	H1
Aripiprazole	—	0.34	44	1.7	3.4	15	—	57	—	61
Clozapine	85	160	25	—	9.6	23.5	130	5.5	20.4	6
Haloperidol	25	1	5	7930	78	3085	1475	46	360	3630
Olanzepine	31	21	28	—	3.1	11	20	19	230	7
Quetiapine	455	160	> 10,000	256	220	2424	> 10,000	9	180	4.6
Risperidone	75	5.9	11.5	—	0.71	62.5	> 10,000	2.3	10.5	69.6
Ziprasidone	4.4	4.8	4	3.4	0.4	1.3	6.9	10	15	47

[a]A low K_i value indicates high receptor affinity.
—— = Information not available

Table A2.4 Mechanism of Action of Anticonvulsant Medications

Anticonvulsant	Blockade of voltage-gated Na⁺ channels	Inhibition of T-type Ca²⁺ channels	GABA enhancement
Carbamazepine	+	−	−
Gabapentin	−	−	+
Lamotrigine	+	−	?
Levetiracetam	−	−	−
Oxcarbazepine	+	−	−
Tiagabine	−	−	+
Topiramate	+	−	+
Valproate	+	+	+
Vigabatrin	−	−	+
Zonisamide	+	+	−

PHARMACODYNAMICS OF STIMULANTS

Stimulants include immediate-release, intermediate-acting, and long-acting dextroamphetamine, mixed amphetamine salts, and methylphenidate preparations.

• Stimulants reversibly bind to the presynaptic dopamine transporter, inhibiting dopamine reuptake into the presynaptic neuron, and facilitating dopamine neurotransmission at the postsynaptic neuron.
• Stimulants reversibly bind to the presynaptic norepinephrine transporter, inhibiting norepinephrine reuptake into the presynaptic neuron and facilitating norepinephrine neurotransmission at the postsynaptic neuron.
• Amphetamines also facilitate the release of dopamine and norepinephrine from the cytoplasm and from cytoplasmic storage granules in the presynaptic neuron.
  ○ The dextro isomer of amphetamine is 4 to 5 times more potent than the levo isomer in blocking dopamine reuptake and promoting dopamine release.
• In attention-deficit/hyperactivity disorder, the pathophysiological substrate is unknown. One influential model suggests the possibility of norepinephrine deficiency in the posterior attention system, and dopamine deficiency in the prefrontal synapses involved with working memory, or hyperfunctioning of the mesolimbic dopamine system as important in the etiology of ADHD.

Table A2.5 Attentional Systems in the CNS

Attentional System	Neurotransmitter	CNS Structures	Activity
Posterior	Norepinephrine	• Parietal lobe • Frontal lobe • Pulvinar • Thalamus • Superior colliculus	• Disengage from stimuli • Change focus to new stimuli • Engage attention to new stimuli • Arousal
Anterior	Dopamine and norepinephrine	• Prefrontal cortex • Cingulate gyrus	• Analyze data • Prepare for response • Executive cognitive tasks

Table A2.6 Receptor Binding Profiles of Stimulant Agents on Presynaptic DA, NE, and 5HT Reuptake Transporter: K_i values (nM)[a]

Stimulant	DAT	NET	5HTT
Methylphenidate	34	339	> 10,000
Dextroamphetamine	2260	55	> 10,000

[a]A low K_i value indicates high receptor affinity. DAT = dopamine transporter; NET = norepinephrine transporter; 5HTT = serotonin transporter

Appendix 3.
Pediatric Psychopharmacology and the Cardiovascular System

Some medications used in pediatric psychopharmacology may have adverse effects on the cardiovascular system. These agents may have effects on cardiac electroconductivity (as measured by the electrocardiogram [ECG]) and on hemodynamics (as measured by blood pressure). Reports of sudden deaths of children and adolescents treated with psychiatric medications have raised concerns about the possible cardiovascular effects of some psychiatric medications in youngsters. This is especially true of tricyclic antidepressants. At least eight deaths have been reported in children taking tricyclic antidepressants in therapeutic doses (not overdoses). Six deaths occurred in children taking desipramine and two in children prescribed imipramine. Although these deaths have not been proven to be cardiac related, cardiovascular toxicity is suspected. Sudden death can occur by a variety of mechanisms; however, cardiac arrhythmias are the most frequent cause.

The practicing pediatric psychopharmacologist needs a basic understanding of cardiovascular physiology, a working knowledge of how to read an ECG, and the ability to obtain a pulse and blood pressure from patients.

THE ECG

An idealized schematic of the ECG tracing is presented in the figure below.

- Located in the upper-posterior wall of the right atrium, the sinoatrial (SA) node is the heart's dominant pacemaker. The SA node generates a depolarization wave at regular intervals (automaticity) that proceeds outward and initiates atrial depolarization and muscle contraction. The *P wave* on the ECG represents atrial depolarization.
- The *PR interval* on the ECG represents the time of spread of depolarization from the atria to the atrioventricular (AV) node, where ventricular depolarization is initiated.

529

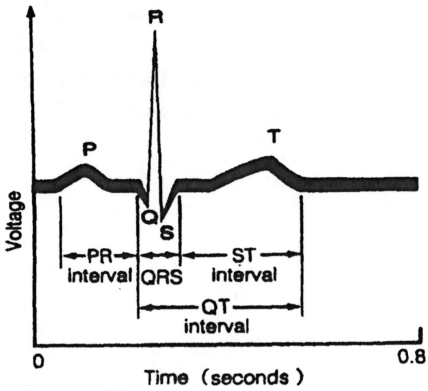

Figure A3.1 The ECG tracing

- The AV node is the beginning of the ventricular conduction system. From the AV node the impulse is carried into the His Bundle and the right and left bundle branches and then into the terminal filaments of the Purkinje fibers, causing ventricular myocardium contraction. The *QRS complex* on the ECG represents depolarization of the ventricular myocardium.
- The initial phase of ventricular repolarization is represented by the *ST interval* on the ECG.
- The *T wave* represents the rapid phase of ventricular repolarization.
- The *QT interval* represents the total time of ventricular depolarization and repolarization.

Reading the ECG

In the usual ECG tracing 1 mV = 10 mm (small boxes), and the paper speed is generally 25 mm/sec. A systematic approach to reading the ECG is advised.

- *Rhythm*: Refers to the origin of the heartbeat and its regularity. Sinus rhythm is identified by a P wave and a PR interval before every QRS complex.

• *Heart rate*: A close estimate of the heart rate can be determined by dividing 300 by the number of small squares on the electrocardiographic paper (at the routine paper speed of 25 mm/second) between two QRS complexes.

Table A3.1 Estimating Ventricular Heart Rate

No. of Small Squares on ECG Paper Between Two QRS Complexes	Heart Rate (beats per minute)
5	300
10	150
15	100
20	75
25	60
30	50

• Intervals
  ○ *PR interval*: The length of the PR interval is inversely related to heart rate and is affected by patient age. A useful guide for the upper limits of normal at various ages is:
    ▪ Newborn: 0.11 sec
    ▪ Child: 0.14 sec
    ▪ Adolescent 0.16 sec
  ○ *QRS interval*: Representing the time of ventricular depolarization, the QRS should be < 0.10 sec. Longer times may represent ventricular conduction delay.
  ○ *QT interval*: Inversely related to heart rate. The QT interval must be corrected for heart rate. The corrected QT interval should be < 0.46 sec.
  ○ *QRS axis*: Electrical forces represented by the QRS complex have a mean magnitude and direction that can be drawn as a vector. A normal QRS axis is down and to the left between 0 and + 90 degrees, as measured by the R/S ratio in leads I and aVF.

ECG Parameters

When using psychiatric agents that are known to affect cardiovascular physiology, such as tricyclic antidepressants, phenothiazines, pimozide, or carbamazepine, a baseline ECG is compared with an on-drug ECG. In children and adolescents, ECG parameters on-drug should be within the following guidelines.

• Sinus rhythm: Every QRS complex is preceded by a P wave and a PR interval.
• Rate: 60–110 beats per minute
• PR interval < 200 msec
• QRS interval < 120 msec and no more than 30% over baseline (before drug initiation)
• QTc interval < 460 msec

A
P
P
E
N
D
I
X

3

Psychiatric Medications and the ECG

The American Heart Association (Gutgesell et al., 1999) reviewed psychiatric drug effects on the ECG for children and adolescents and recommended ECG monitoring when prescribing the following agents:

- Tricyclic antidepressants
- Phenothiazines such as thioridazine
- Butyrophenones such as haloperidol
- Diphenylbutylpiperidines such as pimozide

Effects of other psychiatric drugs on the ECG can include:

- Agents with anticholinergic properties increase heart rate; these include tricyclic antidepressants, phenothiazines, and some anti-parkinsonian medications.
- Agents with sympathomimetic effects increase heart rate; these include stimulants and atomoxetine.
- Agents that decrease sympathomimetic tone may decrease heart rate; these include beta-blockers, clonidine, and guanfacine.
- Agents with quinidine-like properties may slow electrical conduction through the AV node and His Bundle–Purkinje system, which is reflected in a widening of the QRS complex on the ECG >120 msec. Common agents in pediatric psychopharmacology with these effects include tricyclic antidepressants, phenothiazines, pimozide, and carbamazepine.
- Agents may prolong ventricular myocardial repolarization, as reflected in a prolonged QTc $\geq$ 460 msec. If the QTc is prolonged far enough, the next cardiac impulse may fall on a not completely repolarized ventricular myocardium and increase the probability of initiating an unstable ventricular arrythmia, such as torsades de pointes, which is not compatible with life. Medications reported to cause QT prolongation or torsade de pointes are given in the following table.

Table A3.2 Medications Reported to Cause QT Prolongation or Torsade de Pointes

Drug Class	Medication
Psychotropic	Phenothiazine antipsychotics, haloperidol, pimozide, sertindole, ziprasidone, carbamazepine, tricyclic antidepressants, lithium, chloral hydrate
Antiarrhythmic	Disopyramide, procainamide, quinidine, amiodarone, bretylium, sotalol
Antihistamine	Astemizole, terfenadine
Antimicrobial	Erythromycin, trimethoprim-sulfamethoxazole, tetracycline
Gastrointestinal prokinetic	Cisapride
Antimalarial or antiprotozoal	Chloroquine, halofantrine, mefloquine, pentaminidine, quinine
Miscellaneous	Amantadine, probucol, tacrolimus, vasopressin

PULSE AND BLOOD PRESSURE

Some psychiatric medications used in children and adolescents affect hemo-dynamic functioning, with resulting alterations in systolic and diastolic blood pressure and pulse. Slight alterations in blood pressure are usually clinically nonsignificant in healthy children. However, monitoring of the pulse and blood pressure is recommended for several classes of medication. Clinical signs of altered hemodynamic status include exercise-related dizziness, faintness, and syncope (hypotension) or headaches (hypertension). Psychiatric medications that require pulse and blood pressure monitoring include (Gutgesell et al., 1999) the following:

• Phenothiazine antipsychotics
• Clonidine
• Guanfacine
• Tricyclic antidepressants
• Carbamazepine
• Beta-blockers

Normal values for pulse in beats per minute (bpm) by age of the child are presented in the following table.

Table A3.3 Normal Heart Rate (Pulse) in Children and Adolescents

Age (years)	Range (bpm)	Mean (bpm)
4–5	65–135	110
6–8	60–130	100
9–11	60–110	85
12–16	60–110	85
> 16	60–100	80

Source: Gunn VL, Nechyba C. *The Harriet Lane Handbook* (16th ed.). Philadelphia: Mosby, p. 136, 2002.

Normal values for systolic and diastolic blood pressure by age and gender are presented in the following two figures. Blood pressures should not exceed the 95 percentile or fall below the 5 percentile for age and gender.

As a general rule in pediatric psychopharmacology, vital signs should not exceed the following parameters:

• Heart rate: maximum of 130 bpm
• Systolic blood pressure: maximum of 130 mmHg
• Diastolic blood pressure: maximum of 85 mmHg

APPENDIX 3

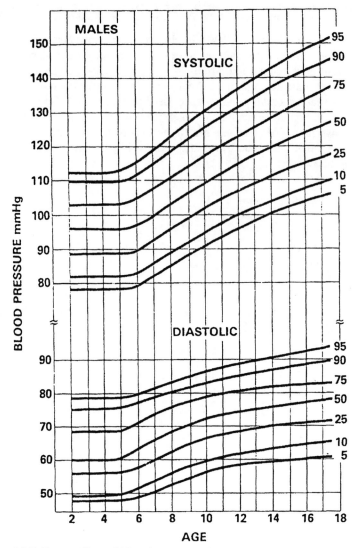

Figure A3.2 Percentiles of blood pressure in seated males by age.

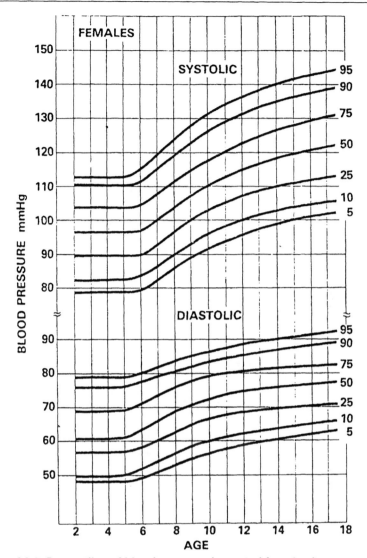

Figure A3.3 Percentiles of blood pressure in seated females by age.

Appendix 4.
Practical Tools for the Clinical Child and Adolescent Psychopharmacologist

Rating scales are useful to the practicing pediatric psychopharmacologist. They provide a concise and time-efficient method for obtaining and organizing useful information about the child from diverse sources such as parents and teachers. Rating scales serve to quantify important behavioral, symptom, medical, and clinical data for comparison purposes as treatment proceeds. Quality of life measures and rating scales measuring functional daily impairment are found here. Other tools found in Appendix 4 help the clinician organize background psychiatric history and the child's developmental history. Another tool provides a means for displaying the child's treatment over time at a glance. Also found in this Appendix are side effects rating scales organized by drug type. Some of these tools are in the public domain. However, others are copyrighted by the author of the tool and require permission to use.

Growth Curves. Boys stature-for-age and weight-for-age percentiles: 2–20 years.

Name_____

Record#_____

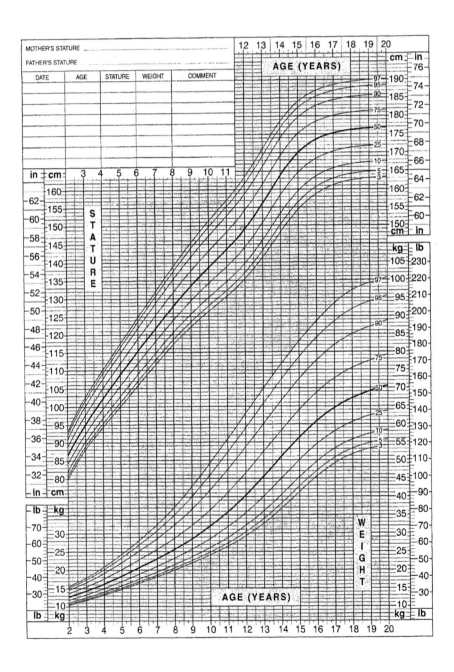

Growth Curves. Girls stature-for-age and weight-for-age percentiles: 2–20 years.

Name_____

Record#_____

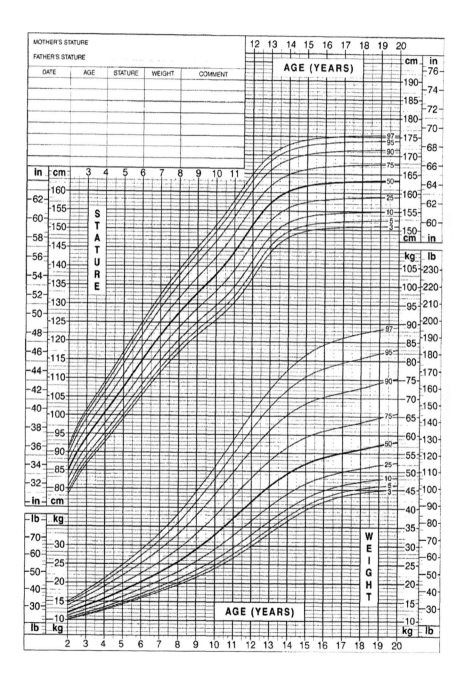

Child and Adolescent Psychopharmacology Clinic
Parent's Questionnaire

INSTRUCTIONS: Please help us better understand your child's needs by completing and returning this questionnaire prior to scheduling your appointment at the clinic.

PATIENT'S NAME:
MENTAL HEALTH HISTORY
A. Briefly describe your child's difficulties, moods, and/or behaviors that you hope medication may help.
B. Briefly list any previous medication trials for the above problems. Please try to remember the name, dose, benefit, and side effects of previous medications (if any):
C. Please list the current treatment plan (if any) to help with the above difficulties. Include therapists, pediatrician, special education services, and/or other services:

INFORMATION REGARDING PRIMARY CARE PHYSICIAN
Physician's full name:
Physician's address:
Physician's phone number:

HEALTH HISTORY
A. Date of child's last physical exam (please forward copy):   /   /
B. List all problems that are a focus of current medical/surgical treatments:
1.
2.
3.
4.
C. Does your child suffer from allergies to *any* food or medicine that causes fever, rash, swelling, or edema?
D. Please list all prescribed medication (including psychotropic medication), medical reason for taking drug, daily dose, and times of dosing:
1.
2.
3.
4.

E. *At any time has your child had:*	NEVER	PAST	PRESENT
1. Asthma			
2. Diabetes, arthritis, or other chronic illness			

3. Epilepsy or seizure disorder			
4. Abnormal EEG *with* or *without* a seizure			
5. Febrile seizures			
6. Congenital heart problems			
7. Heart arrhythmia/irregular heart beat			
8. Fainting			
9. Heart murmur			
10. Broken bones			
11. Severe cuts requiring stitches			
12. Head injury *with loss of consciousness*			
13. Organic brain disease, infection, or brain damage			
14. Lengthy hospitalization (> 1 week)			
15. Speech or language problems			
16. Chronic ear infections			
17. Hearing difficulties			
18. Eye or vision problems			
19. Glaucoma			
20. Headaches			
21. Fine motor/handwriting problems			
22. Gross motor difficulties, clumsiness			
23. Appetite problems (overeating or undereating)			
24. Sleep problems (falling asleep, staying asleep)			
25. Soiling problems			
26. Wetting problems			
27. Other health difficulties. Please describe:			

DEVELOPMENTAL INFORMATION

PREGNANCY AND DELIVERY		
A. Length of pregnancy (e.g., full term or 40 weeks, 32 weeks, etc.)		
B. Length of delivery (number of hours from initial labor pains to birth)		
C. Mother's age when child was born		
D. Child's birth weight		
E. *Did any of the following conditions occur during pregnancy/delivery?*	**NO**	**YES**
1. Bleeding		
2. Excessive weight gain (more than 30 pounds)		
3. Toxemia/preeclampsia		
4. Rh factor incompatibility		
5. Frequent nausea or vomiting		
6. Serious illness or injury		
7. Took prescription medication (a) If so, name of medication:		
8. Took illegal drugs		
9. Used alcoholic beverages (a) If so, approximate number of drinks per week:		
10. Smoked cigarettes (a) If so, approximate number of cigarettes per day (e.g., 10):		
11. Was given medication to ease labor pains (a) If true, name of medication:		
12. Delivery was induced		
13. Forceps were used during delivery		
14. Had a breech delivery		
15. Had a cesarean section delivery		
16. Other problems, please describe:		

APPENDIX 4

F. *Did any of the following conditions affect your child during delivery or within the first few days after birth?*		
1. Injured during delivery		
2. Cardiopulmonary distress during delivery		
3. Delivered with cord around neck		
4. Had trouble breathing following delivery		
5. Needed oxygen		
6. Was cyanotic, turned blue		
7. Was jaundiced, turned yellow		
8. Had an infection		
9. Had seizures		
10. Was given medications		
11. Born with a congenital defect		
12. Was in hospital more than 7 days		

INFANT HEALTH AND TEMPERAMENT		
A. *During the first 12 months, was your child:*	**NO**	**YES**
1. Difficult to feed		
2. Difficult to get to sleep		
3. Colicky		
4. Difficult to put on schedule		
5. Alert		
6. Cheerful		
7. Affectionate		
8. Sociable		
9. Easy to comfort		
10. Difficult to keep busy		
11. Overactive, in constant motion		
12. Very stubborn, challenging		

EARLY DEVELOPMENTAL MILESTONES		
A. *At what age did your child first accomplish the following:*	**NO**	**YES**
1. Sitting without help		
2. Crawling		
3. Walking alone, without assistance		
4. Using single words (e.g., *mama, dada, ball*)		
5. Putting two or more words together (e.g., *mama up*)		
6. Bowel training, day and night		
7. Bladder training, day and night		
B. At what age did you first become concerned about your child?		
C. At what age did you first seek mental health or pediatric evaluation/service for your child's problem?		

Source: Copyright Daniel F. Connor

Pediatric Psychopharmacology Clinic Patient Medication Log

Patient Name:

D.O.B:

Date of Initial Evaluation:

Medical Record #:

Allergy:

Diagnosis (#) Axis I: _____, _____,

Axis II: _____, _____,

Axis III: _____, _____,

Axis IV: _____, _____,

CGI-Severity: _____   CGAS: _____

VISIT DATE	MEDICATIONS	DOSE SCHEDULE	BLOOD LEVEL	WGT (KG) HGT (CM)	PULSE BP	SIDE EFFECTS	RATING SCALE SCORES	CGI-IMPROVSCORE	SCRIPTS[a]	COMMENTS

[a] number of medication perscriptions and refills provided patient.

Antipsychotic Side Effects Profile

Name:	
Date of Birth:	
Case #:	
Sex:	
Date:	
Medicine:	
Dose:	

Instructions: Please complete profile once weekly by self/parent/nurse. Rate the past week. Rate each behavior from "0" (absent) to "9" (serious). *Circle only one number beside each item.* A "0" means that you have not seen this behavior in yourself/child during this past week. A "9" means that you have noticed it and believe it to be either *very serious* or occurring *very frequently.* Hand carry to next appointment (do not mail).

Side Effect:	Absent							Serious		
Sedation/fatigue/drowsiness	0	1	2	3	4	5	6	7	8	9
Diminished facial expression	0	1	2	3	4	5	6	7	8	9
Diminished emotional expression	0	1	2	3	4	5	6	7	8	9
Social withdrawal	0	1	2	3	4	5	6	7	8	9
Decreased mental alertness	0	1	2	3	4	5	6	7	8	9
Decreased energy	0	1	2	3	4	5	6	7	8	9
Increased appetite	0	1	2	3	4	5	6	7	8	9
Weight gain	0	1	2	3	4	5	6	7	8	9
Weight loss	0	1	2	3	4	5	6	7	8	9
Restlessness	0	1	2	3	4	5	6	7	8	9
Pacing	0	1	2	3	4	5	6	7	8	9
Agitation	0	1	2	3	4	5	6	7	8	9
Irritability	0	1	2	3	4	5	6	7	8	9
Muscle stiffness/rigidity	0	1	2	3	4	5	6	7	8	9
Finger/hand tremors	0	1	2	3	4	5	6	7	8	9
Drooling	0	1	2	3	4	5	6	7	8	9
Dry mouth	0	1	2	3	4	5	6	7	8	9
Easy bruising	0	1	2	3	4	5	6	7	8	9
Fever	0	1	2	3	4	5	6	7	8	9
Sore throat	0	1	2	3	4	5	6	7	8	9
Sweating	0	1	2	3	4	5	6	7	8	9
Constipation	0	1	2	3	4	5	6	7	8	9
Diarrhea	0	1	2	3	4	5	6	7	8	9
Sexual side effects	0	1	2	3	4	5	6	7	8	9

Tics, nervous movements, or twitches	0	1	2	3	4	5	6	7	8	9
Muscle spasms	0	1	2	3	4	5	6	7	8	9
Deviation of eyes	0	1	2	3	4	5	6	7	8	9
Continuous involuntary muscle movements in face, tongue, lips, fingers, toes	0	1	2	3	4	5	6	7	8	9
Seizures	0	1	2	3	4	5	6	7	8	9
Sensitivity to sunlight	0	1	2	3	4	5	6	7	8	9
Anxiety	0	1	2	3	4	5	6	7	8	9
School refusal/avoidance	0	1	2	3	4	5	6	7	8	9
If female: menstrual irregularities	0	1	2	3	4	5	6	7	8	9
If female: breast pain/fluid	0	1	2	3	4	5	6	7	8	9
Other	0	1	2	3	4	5	6	7	8	9

Comments:

Total number side effects endorsed: _____

MEAN severity score =

Source: Copyright Daniel F. Connor.

Atomoxetine Side Effects Profile

Name:	
Date of Birth:	
Case #:	
Sex:	
Date:	
Medicine:	
Dose:	

Instructions: Please complete profile once weekly by self/parent/nurse. Rate the past week. Rate each behavior from "0" (absent) to "9" (serious). *Circle only one number beside each item*. A "0" means that you have not seen this behavior in yourself/child during this past week. A "9" means that you have noticed it and believe it to be either *very serious* or occurring *very frequently*. Hand carry to next appointment (do not mail).

Side Effect:	Absent									Serious
Stomachaches	0	1	2	3	4	5	6	7	8	9
Constipation	0	1	2	3	4	5	6	7	8	9
Diarrhea	0	1	2	3	4	5	6	7	8	9
Vomiting	0	1	2	3	4	5	6	7	8	9
Decreased appetite	0	1	2	3	4	5	6	7	8	9
Decreased weight	0	1	2	3	4	5	6	7	8	9
Dizziness	0	1	2	3	4	5	6	7	8	9
Sedation/fatigue	0	1	2	3	4	5	6	7	8	9
Irritability	0	1	2	3	4	5	6	7	8	9
Rash	0	1	2	3	4	5	6	7	8	9
Other	0	1	2	3	4	5	6	7	8	9

Comments:

Total number side effects endorsed: _____

MEAN severity score = _____

Source: Copyright Daniel F. Connor.

Antidepressant Side Effects Profile

Name:	
Date of Birth:	
Case #:	
Sex:	
Date:	
Medicine:	
Dose:	

Instructions: Please complete profile once weekly by self/parent/nurse. Rate the past week. Rate each behavior from "0" (absent) to "9" (serious). *Circle only one number beside each item.* A "0" means that you have not seen this behavior in yourself/child during this past week. A "9" means that you have noticed it and believe it to be either *very serious* or occurring *very frequently.* Hand carry to next appointment (do not mail).

Side Effect:	Absent								Serious	
Blurred vision	0	1	2	3	4	5	6	7	8	9
Dry mouth	0	1	2	3	4	5	6	7	8	9
Confusion	0	1	2	3	4	5	6	7	8	9
Dizziness	0	1	2	3	4	5	6	7	8	9
Fainting	0	1	2	3	4	5	6	7	8	9
Irregular heartbeat	0	1	2	3	4	5	6	7	8	9
Fast heartbeat	0	1	2	3	4	5	6	7	8	9
Constipation	0	1	2	3	4	5	6	7	8	9
Diarrhea	0	1	2	3	4	5	6	7	8	9
Difficulty urinating	0	1	2	3	4	5	6	7	8	9
Skin rash	0	1	2	3	4	5	6	7	8	9
Shakiness	0	1	2	3	4	5	6	7	8	9
Sore throat	0	1	2	3	4	5	6	7	8	9
Fever	0	1	2	3	4	5	6	7	8	9
Sedation/sleepiness	0	1	2	3	4	5	6	7	8	9
Headache	0	1	2	3	4	5	6	7	8	9
Stomachache	0	1	2	3	4	5	6	7	8	9
Nausea	0	1	2	3	4	5	6	7	8	9
Weight gain	0	1	2	3	4	5	6	7	8	9
Weight loss	0	1	2	3	4	5	6	7	8	9
Leg spasms at night	0	1	2	3	4	5	6	7	8	9
Sexual side effects	0	1	2	3	4	5	6	7	8	9
Sweating	0	1	2	3	4	5	6	7	8	9

APPENDIX 4

Vomiting	0	1	2	3	4	5	6	7	8	9
Increased appetite	0	1	2	3	4	5	6	7	8	9
Decreased appetite	0	1	2	3	4	5	6	7	8	9
Hallucinations	0	1	2	3	4	5	6	7	8	9
Seizures	0	1	2	3	4	5	6	7	8	9
Numbness or tingling in toes/fingers	0	1	2	3	4	5	6	7	8	9
Sensitivity to sunlight	0	1	2	3	4	5	6	7	8	9
Anxiety	0	1	2	3	4	5	6	7	8	9
Sleep disturbance	0	1	2	3	4	5	6	7	8	9
Nightmares	0	1	2	3	4	5	6	7	8	9
Other	0	1	2	3	4	5	6	7	8	9

Comments:

Total number side effects endorsed: _____

MEAN severity score = _____

Source: Copyright Daniel F. Connor.

Benzodiazepine Side Effects Profile

Name:	
Date of Birth:	
Case #:	
Sex:	
Date:	
Medicine:	
Dose:	

Instructions: Please complete profile once weekly by self/parent/nurse. Rate the past week. Rate each behavior from "0" (absent) to "9" (serious). *Circle only one number beside each item.* A "0" means that you have not seen this behavior in yourself/child during this past week. A "9" means that you have noticed it and believe it to be either *very serious* or occurring *very frequently.* Hand carry to next appointment (do not mail).

Side Effect:	Absent									Serious
Sedation/fatigue/drowsiness	0	1	2	3	4	5	6	7	8	9
Decreased mental alertness	0	1	2	3	4	5	6	7	8	9
Decreased memory	0	1	2	3	4	5	6	7	8	9
Impaired concentration	0	1	2	3	4	5	6	7	8	9
Agitation	0	1	2	3	4	5	6	7	8	9
Irritability/rage	0	1	2	3	4	5	6	7	8	9
Hallucinations	0	1	2	3	4	5	6	7	8	9
Seizures	0	1	2	3	4	5	6	7	8	9
Fever	0	1	2	3	4	5	6	7	8	9
Insomnia	0	1	2	3	4	5	6	7	8	9
Shakiness/tremor	0	1	2	3	4	5	6	7	8	9
Sweating	0	1	2	3	4	5	6	7	8	9
Slurred speech	0	1	2	3	4	5	6	7	8	9
Difficulty walking	0	1	2	3	4	5	6	7	8	9
Headache	0	1	2	3	4	5	6	7	8	9
Upset stomach	0	1	2	3	4	5	6	7	8	9
Dry mouth	0	1	2	3	4	5	6	7	8	9
Other	0	1	2	3	4	5	6	7	8	9

Is there any possibility that you are pregnant?   No ____   Yes ____

Comments:

Total number side effects endorsed: _____
MEAN severity score = _____
Source: Copyright Daniel F. Connor.

Buspirone Side Effects Profile

Name:	
Date of Birth:	
Case #:	
Sex:	
Date:	
Medicine:	
Dose:	

Instructions: Please complete profile once weekly by self/parent/nurse. Rate the past week. Rate each behavior from "0" (absent) to "9" (serious). *Circle only one number beside each item.* A "0" means that you have not seen this behavior in yourself/child during this past week. A "9" means that you have noticed it and believe it to be either *very serious* or occurring *very frequently.* Hand carry to next appointment (do not mail).

Side Effect:	Absent									Serious
Headaches	0	1	2	3	4	5	6	7	8	9
Drowsiness	0	1	2	3	4	5	6	7	8	9
Lethargy	0	1	2	3	4	5	6	7	8	9
Feeling faint	0	1	2	3	4	5	6	7	8	9
Feeling dizzy	0	1	2	3	4	5	6	7	8	9
Sleeplessness	0	1	2	3	4	5	6	7	8	9
Nausea	0	1	2	3	4	5	6	7	8	9
Vomiting	0	1	2	3	4	5	6	7	8	9
Diarrhea	0	1	2	3	4	5	6	7	8	9
Heart racing	0	1	2	3	4	5	6	7	8	9
Sweating	0	1	2	3	4	5	6	7	8	9
Tremor	0	1	2	3	4	5	6	7	8	9
Numbness of hands or feet	0	1	2	3	4	5	6	7	8	9
Tingling in hands or feet	0	1	2	3	4	5	6	7	8	9
Sadness	0	1	2	3	4	5	6	7	8	9
Irritability	0	1	2	3	4	5	6	7	8	9
Excitability	0	1	2	3	4	5	6	7	8	9
Confusion	0	1	2	3	4	5	6	7	8	9
Nervousness	0	1	2	3	4	5	6	7	8	9
Other	0	1	2	3	4	5	6	7	8	9

Comments:

Total number side effects endorsed: _____

MEAN severity score = _____

Source: Copyright Daniel F. Connor.

Carbamazepine Side Effects Profile

Name:	
Date of Birth:	
Case #:	
Sex:	
Date:	
Medicine:	
Dose:	

Instructions: Please complete profile once weekly by self/parent/nurse. Rate the past week. Rate each behavior from "0" (absent) to "9" (serious). *Circle only one number beside each item.* A "0" means that you have not seen this behavior in yourself/child during this past week. A "9" means that you have noticed it and believe it to be either *very serious* or occurring *very frequently.* Hand carry to next appointment (do not mail).

Side Effect:	Absent								Serious	
Dry mouth	0	1	2	3	4	5	6	7	8	9
Drowsiness	0	1	2	3	4	5	6	7	8	9
Unsteady gait	0	1	2	3	4	5	6	7	8	9
Blurred vision	0	1	2	3	4	5	6	7	8	9
Double vision	0	1	2	3	4	5	6	7	8	9
Tremor	0	1	2	3	4	5	6	7	8	9
Headaches	0	1	2	3	4	5	6	7	8	9
Dizziness	0	1	2	3	4	5	6	7	8	9
Tinnitus	0	1	2	3	4	5	6	7	8	9
Skin rash	0	1	2	3	4	5	6	7	8	9
Nausea	0	1	2	3	4	5	6	7	8	9
Vomiting	0	1	2	3	4	5	6	7	8	9
Diarrhea	0	1	2	3	4	5	6	7	8	9
Constipation	0	1	2	3	4	5	6	7	8	9
Stomach pains	0	1	2	3	4	5	6	7	8	9
Decreased appetite	0	1	2	3	4	5	6	7	8	9
Leg cramps	0	1	2	3	4	5	6	7	8	9
Muscle aches	0	1	2	3	4	5	6	7	8	9
Fever and chills	0	1	2	3	4	5	6	7	8	9
Cough/cold symptoms	0	1	2	3	4	5	6	7	8	9
Other	0	1	2	3	4	5	6	7	8	9

Comments:

Total number side effects endorsed: _____
MEAN severity score = _____
Source: Copyright Daniel F. Connor.

Clonidine/Guanfacine Side Effects Profile

Name:	
Date of Birth:	
Case #:	
Sex:	
Date:	
Medicine:	
Dose:	

Instructions: Please complete profile once weekly by self/parent/nurse. Rate the past week. Rate each behavior from "0" (absent) to "9" (serious). *Circle only one number beside each item.* A "0" means that you have not seen this behavior in yourself/child during this past week. A "9" means that you have noticed it and believe it to be either *very serious* or occurring *very frequently*. Hand carry to next appointment (do not mail).

Side Effect:	Absent									Serious
Sedation/sleepiness	0	1	2	3	4	5	6	7	8	9
Headache	0	1	2	3	4	5	6	7	8	9
Dizziness	0	1	2	3	4	5	6	7	8	9
Fainting	0	1	2	3	4	5	6	7	8	9
Stomachache	0	1	2	3	4	5	6	7	8	9
Nausea	0	1	2	3	4	5	6	7	8	9
Vomiting	0	1	2	3	4	5	6	7	8	9
Depression/moody	0	1	2	3	4	5	6	7	8	9
Dry mouth	0	1	2	3	4	5	6	7	8	9
Dry eyes	0	1	2	3	4	5	6	7	8	9
Constipation	0	1	2	3	4	5	6	7	8	9
Diarrhea	0	1	2	3	4	5	6	7	8	9
Nightmares	0	1	2	3	4	5	6	7	8	9
Sleep difficulties	0	1	2	3	4	5	6	7	8	9
Tingling in toes/fingers	0	1	2	3	4	5	6	7	8	9
Anxiety	0	1	2	3	4	5	6	7	8	9
Feeling faint when exercising	0	1	2	3	4	5	6	7	8	9
Other	0	1	2	3	4	5	6	7	8	9

Comments:

Total number side effects endorsed: _____

MEAN severity score = _____

Source: Copyright Daniel F. Connor.

Lamotrigine Side Effects Profile

Name:	
Date of Birth:	
Case #:	
Sex:	
Date:	
Medicine:	
Dose:	

Instructions: Please complete profile once weekly by self/parent/nurse. Rate the past week. Rate each behavior from "0" (absent) to "9" (serious). *Circle only one number beside each item.* A "0" means that you have not seen this behavior in yourself/child during this past week. A "9" means that you have noticed it and believe it to be either *very serious* or occurring *very frequently.* Hand carry to next appointment (do not mail).

Side Effect:	Absent								Serious	
Rash	0	1	2	3	4	5	6	7	8	9
Dizziness	0	1	2	3	4	5	6	7	8	9
Unsteady walking	0	1	2	3	4	5	6	7	8	9
Sedation	0	1	2	3	4	5	6	7	8	9
Headaches	0	1	2	3	4	5	6	7	8	9
Blurred/double vision	0	1	2	3	4	5	6	7	8	9
Nausea	0	1	2	3	4	5	6	7	8	9
Vomiting	0	1	2	3	4	5	6	7	8	9
Stomachaches	0	1	2	3	4	5	6	7	8	9
Sensitivity to light	0	1	2	3	4	5	6	7	8	9
Tremor/shaking	0	1	2	3	4	5	6	7	8	9
Other	0	1	2	3	4	5	6	7	8	9

Comments:

Total number side effects endorsed: _____

MEAN severity score = _____

Source: Copyright Daniel F. Connor.

Lithium Side Effects Profile

Name:	
Date of Birth:	
Case #:	
Sex:	
Date:	
Medicine:	
Dose:	

Instructions: Please complete profile once weekly by self/parent/nurse. Rate the past week. Rate each behavior from "0" (absent) to "9" (serious). *Circle only one number beside each item.* A "0" means that you have not seen this behavior in yourself/child during this past week. A "9" means that you have noticed it and believe it to be either *very serious* or occurring *very frequently.* Hand carry to next appointment (do not mail).

Side Effect:	Absent								Serious	
Anxiety	0	1	2	3	4	5	6	7	8	9
Fatigue/drowsiness	0	1	2	3	4	5	6	7	8	9
Lethargy/no energy	0	1	2	3	4	5	6	7	8	9
Tension	0	1	2	3	4	5	6	7	8	9
Impaired mental alertness	0	1	2	3	4	5	6	7	8	9
Impaired concentration	0	1	2	3	4	5	6	7	8	9
Blurred vision	0	1	2	3	4	5	6	7	8	9
Decreased memory	0	1	2	3	4	5	6	7	8	9
Muscle weakness	0	1	2	3	4	5	6	7	8	9
Hand/finger tremor	0	1	2	3	4	5	6	7	8	9
Diminished coordination	0	1	2	3	4	5	6	7	8	9
Increased thirst	0	1	2	3	4	5	6	7	8	9
Increased frequency of urination	0	1	2	3	4	5	6	7	8	9
Metallic taste	0	1	2	3	4	5	6	7	8	9
Nausea	0	1	2	3	4	5	6	7	8	9
Stomachaches	0	1	2	3	4	5	6	7	8	9
Diarrhea	0	1	2	3	4	5	6	7	8	9
Vomiting	0	1	2	3	4	5	6	7	8	9
Irregular/fast heartbeat	0	1	2	3	4	5	6	7	8	9
Acne	0	1	2	3	4	5	6	7	8	9
Rash	0	1	2	3	4	5	6	7	8	9
Increased appetite	0	1	2	3	4	5	6	7	8	9
Decreased appetite	0	1	2	3	4	5	6	7	8	9

Weight gain	0	1	2	3	4	5	6	7	8	9
Weight loss	0	1	2	3	4	5	6	7	8	9
Seizure	0	1	2	3	4	5	6	7	8	9
Other	0	1	2	3	4	5	6	7	8	9

Is there any possibility that you are pregnant? No ____ Yes ____

Comments:

Total number side effects endorsed: _____

MEAN severity score = _____

Source: Copyright Daniel F. Connor.

Monoamine Oxidase Inhibitor Side Effects Profile

Name:	
Date of Birth:	
Case #:	
Sex:	
Date:	
Medicine:	
Dose:	

Instructions: Please complete profile once weekly by self/parent/nurse. Rate the past week. Rate each behavior from "0" (absent) to "9" (serious). *Circle only one number beside each item.* A "0" means that you have not seen this behavior in yourself/child during this past week. A "9" means that you have noticed it and believe it to be either *very serious* or occurring *very frequently*. Hand carry to next appointment (do not mail).

Side Effect:	Absent									Serious
Trouble sleeping	0	1	2	3	4	5	6	7	8	9
Feeling dizzy	0	1	2	3	4	5	6	7	8	9
Feeling weak/faint	0	1	2	3	4	5	6	7	8	9
Feeling tense/nervous	0	1	2	3	4	5	6	7	8	9
Restlessness	0	1	2	3	4	5	6	7	8	9
Irritability	0	1	2	3	4	5	6	7	8	9
Heart racing	0	1	2	3	4	5	6	7	8	9
Heart pounding	0	1	2	3	4	5	6	7	8	9
Pressure in head	0	1	2	3	4	5	6	7	8	9
Nausea	0	1	2	3	4	5	6	7	8	9
Vomiting	0	1	2	3	4	5	6	7	8	9
Headaches	0	1	2	3	4	5	6	7	8	9
Sweating	0	1	2	3	4	5	6	7	8	9
Trouble keeping balance	0	1	2	3	4	5	6	7	8	9
Dry mouth	0	1	2	3	4	5	6	7	8	9
Blurred vision	0	1	2	3	4	5	6	7	8	9
Constipation	0	1	2	3	4	5	6	7	8	9
Diarrhea	0	1	2	3	4	5	6	7	8	9
Abdominal fullness	0	1	2	3	4	5	6	7	8	9
Stomach pains	0	1	2	3	4	5	6	7	8	9
Delays when urinating	0	1	2	3	4	5	6	7	8	9
Itchiness/dry skin	0	1	2	3	4	5	6	7	8	9
Rash	0	1	2	3	4	5	6	7	8	9

Light hurting eyes	0	1	2	3	4	5	6	7	8	9
Increased/decreased appetite (circle)	0	1	2	3	4	5	6	7	8	9
Drowsy	0	1	2	3	4	5	6	7	8	9
Tremor	0	1	2	3	4	5	6	7	8	9
Sexual: _____	0	1	2	3	4	5	6	7	8	9
Other: _____	0	1	2	3	4	5	6	7	8	9

Comments:

Total number side effects endorsed: _____

MEAN severity score = _____

Source: Copyright Daniel F. Connor.

A
P
P
E
N
D
I
X

4

Modafinil Side Effects Profile

Name:	
Date of Birth:	
Case #:	
Sex:	
Date:	
Medicine:	
Dose:	

Instructions: Please complete profile once weekly by self/parent/nurse. Rate the past week. Rate each behavior from "0" (absent) to "9" (serious). *Circle only one number beside each item.* A "0" means that you have not seen this behavior in yourself/child during this past week. A "9" means that you have noticed it and believe it to be either *very serious* or occurring *very frequently.* Hand carry to next appointment (do not mail).

Side Effect:	Absent								Serious
Headache	0	1	2	3	4	5	6	7	8	9
Nausea	0	1	2	3	4	5	6	7	8	9
Nervousness	0	1	2	3	4	5	6	7	8	9
Anxiety	0	1	2	3	4	5	6	7	8	9
Insomnia	0	1	2	3	4	5	6	7	8	9
Depression	0	1	2	3	4	5	6	7	8	9
Rash	0	1	2	3	4	5	6	7	8	9
Diarrhea	0	1	2	3	4	5	6	7	8	9
Dry mouth	0	1	2	3	4	5	6	7	8	9
Decreased appetite	0	1	2	3	4	5	6	7	8	9
Runny nose	0	1	2	3	4	5	6	7	8	9
Sore throat	0	1	2	3	4	5	6	7	8	9
Dizziness	0	1	2	3	4	5	6	7	8	9
Other	0	1	2	3	4	5	6	7	8	9

Comments:

Total number side effects endorsed: _____

MEAN severity score = _____

Source: Copyright Daniel F. Connor.

Oxcarbazepine Side Effects Profile

Name:	
Date of Birth:	
Case #:	
Sex:	
Date:	
Medicine:	
Dose:	

Instructions: Please complete profile once weekly by self/parent/nurse. Rate the past week. Rate each behavior from "0" (absent) to "9" (serious). *Circle only one number beside each item.* A "0" means that you have not seen this behavior in yourself/child during this past week. A "9" means that you have noticed it and believe it to be either *very serious* or occurring *very frequently.* Hand carry to next appointment (do not mail).

Side Effect:	Absent								Serious	
Dizziness	0	1	2	3	4	5	6	7	8	9
Sedation/fatigue	0	1	2	3	4	5	6	7	8	9
Blurred/double vision	0	1	2	3	4	5	6	7	8	9
Nausea	0	1	2	3	4	5	6	7	8	9
Vomiting	0	1	2	3	4	5	6	7	8	9
Unsteady walking	0	1	2	3	4	5	6	7	8	9
Stomachaches	0	1	2	3	4	5	6	7	8	9
Tremor/shaking	0	1	2	3	4	5	6	7	8	9
Rash	0	1	2	3	4	5	6	7	8	9
Other	0	1	2	3	4	5	6	7	8	9

Comments:

Total number side effects endorsed: _____

MEAN severity score = _____

Source: Copyright Daniel F. Connor.

Stimulant Side Effects Profile

Name:	
Date of Birth:	
Case #:	
Sex:	
Date:	
Medicine:	
Dose:	

Instructions: Please complete profile once weekly by self/parent/nurse. Rate the past week. Rate each behavior from "0" (absent) to "9" (serious). *Circle only one number beside each item.* A "0" means that you have not seen this behavior in yourself/child during this past week. A "9" means that you have noticed it and believe it to be either *very serious* or occurring *very frequently.* Hand carry to next appointment (do not mail).

Side Effect:	Absent								Serious	
Insomnia or trouble sleeping	0	1	2	3	4	5	6	7	8	9
Nightmares	0	1	2	3	4	5	6	7	8	9
Stares a lot or daydreams	0	1	2	3	4	5	6	7	8	9
Talks less with others	0	1	2	3	4	5	6	7	8	9
Disinterested in others	0	1	2	3	4	5	6	7	8	9
Decreased appetite	0	1	2	3	4	5	6	7	8	9
Irritable	0	1	2	3	4	5	6	7	8	9
Stomachaches	0	1	2	3	4	5	6	7	8	9
Headaches	0	1	2	3	4	5	6	7	8	9
Drowsiness	0	1	2	3	4	5	6	7	8	9
Sad/unhappy	0	1	2	3	4	5	6	7	8	9
Prone to crying	0	1	2	3	4	5	6	7	8	9
Anxious	0	1	2	3	4	5	6	7	8	9
Bites his/her nails	0	1	2	3	4	5	6	7	8	9
Euphoric/usually happy	0	1	2	3	4	5	6	7	8	9
Dizziness	0	1	2	3	4	5	6	7	8	9
Tics, nervous movements, or twitches	0	1	2	3	4	5	6	7	8	9
Weight loss	0	1	2	3	4	5	6	7	8	9
Other	0	1	2	3	4	5	6	7	8	9

Comments:

Total number side effects endorsed: _____

MEAN severity score = _____

Source: Copyright Daniel F. Connor.

Topiramate Side Effects Profile

Name:	
Date of Birth:	
Case #:	
Sex:	
Date:	
Medicine:	
Dose:	

Instructions: Please complete profile once weekly by self/parent/nurse. Rate the past week. Rate each behavior from "0" (absent) to "9" (serious). *Circle only one number beside each item.* A "0" means that you have not seen this behavior in yourself/child during this past week. A "9" means that you have noticed it and believe it to be either *very serious* or occurring *very frequently.* Hand carry to next appointment (do not mail).

Side Effect:	Absent								Serious	
Dizziness	0	1	2	3	4	5	6	7	8	9
Unsteady walking	0	1	2	3	4	5	6	7	8	9
Speech problems	0	1	2	3	4	5	6	7	8	9
Difficulty finding words	0	1	2	3	4	5	6	7	8	9
Memory problems	0	1	2	3	4	5	6	7	8	9
Concentration problems	0	1	2	3	4	5	6	7	8	9
Sedation/fatigue	0	1	2	3	4	5	6	7	8	9
Decreased sweating	0	1	2	3	4	5	6	7	8	9
Feeling hot all the time	0	1	2	3	4	5	6	7	8	9
Confusion	0	1	2	3	4	5	6	7	8	9
Blurred/double vision	0	1	2	3	4	5	6	7	8	9
Rash	0	1	2	3	4	5	6	7	8	9
Decreased appetite	0	1	2	3	4	5	6	7	8	9
Weight decrease	0	1	2	3	4	5	6	7	8	9
Nervousness	0	1	2	3	4	5	6	7	8	9
Increased saliva	0	1	2	3	4	5	6	7	8	9
Constipation	0	1	2	3	4	5	6	7	8	9
Urinary accidents	0	1	2	3	4	5	6	7	8	9
Sore throat	0	1	2	3	4	5	6	7	8	9
Cold symptoms	0	1	2	3	4	5	6	7	8	9
Other	0	1	2	3	4	5	6	7	8	9

Comments:

Total number side effects endorsed: _____
MEAN severity score = _____
Source: Copyright Daniel F. Connor.

APPENDIX 4

Valproic Acid/Divalproex Side Effects Profile

Name:	
Date of Birth:	
Case #:	
Sex:	
Date:	
Medicine:	
Dose:	

Instructions: Please complete profile once weekly by self/parent/nurse. Rate the past week. Rate each behavior from "0" (absent) to "9" (serious). *Circle only one number beside each item.* A "0" means that you have not seen this behavior in yourself/child during this past week. A "9" means that you have noticed it and believe it to be either *very serious* or occurring *very frequently.* Hand carry to next appointment (do not mail).

Side Effect:	Absent								Serious	
Tremor	0	1	2	3	4	5	6	7	8	9
Drowsiness	0	1	2	3	4	5	6	7	8	9
Unsteady gait	0	1	2	3	4	5	6	7	8	9
Headaches	0	1	2	3	4	5	6	7	8	9
Dizziness	0	1	2	3	4	5	6	7	8	9
Double vision	0	1	2	3	4	5	6	7	8	9
Numbness of hands or feet	0	1	2	3	4	5	6	7	8	9
Tingling in hands or feet	0	1	2	3	4	5	6	7	8	9
Swelling of hands or feet	0	1	2	3	4	5	6	7	8	9
Muscle weakness	0	1	2	3	4	5	6	7	8	9
Nausea	0	1	2	3	4	5	6	7	8	9
Vomiting	0	1	2	3	4	5	6	7	8	9
Decreased appetite	0	1	2	3	4	5	6	7	8	9
Stomach pains	0	1	2	3	4	5	6	7	8	9
Heartburn	0	1	2	3	4	5	6	7	8	9
Diarrhea	0	1	2	3	4	5	6	7	8	9
Constipation	0	1	2	3	4	5	6	7	8	9
Weight gain	0	1	2	3	4	5	6	7	8	9
Change in taste	0	1	2	3	4	5	6	7	8	9
Hair loss	0	1	2	3	4	5	6	7	8	9
Bruising	0	1	2	3	4	5	6	7	8	9

Rash	0	1	2	3	4	5	6	7	8	9
Irregularity of periods	0	1	2	3	4	5	6	7	8	9
Bloated abdomen	0	1	2	3	4	5	6	7	8	9
Other	0	1	2	3	4	5	6	7	8	9

Comments:

Total number side effects endorsed: _____

MEAN severity score = _____

Source: Copyright Daniel F. Connor.

APPENDIX 4

Abnormal Involuntary Movement Scale (AIMS)

_____

Name

_____

Hospital Number

_____

Date

_____

Rater

Scoring Code: 0 = None, normal
                1 = Minimal, may be upper limit
                2 = Mild
                3 = Moderate
                4 = Severe

Instructions: Complete examination procedure before making ratings. For movement ratings, rate highest severity observed. See instructions.

FACIAL AND ORAL MOVEMENTS	**1. Muscles of facial expression** e.g., movements of forehead, eyebrows, periorbital area;. include frowning, blinking, grimacing of upper face	*(Circle One)* 0 1 2 3 4
	2. Lips and perioral area e.g., puckering, pouting, smacking	0 1 2 3 4
	3. Jaw e.g., biting, clenching, chewing, mouth opening, lateral movement	0 1 2 3 4
	4. Tongue Rate only increase in movement both in and out of mouth, NOT inability to sustain movement.	0 1 2 3 4
EXTREMITY MOVEMENTS	**5. Upper** (arms, wrists, hands, fingers) Include choreic movements (rapid, objectively purposeless, irregular, spontaneous) and athetoid movements (slow, irregular, complex, serpentine). DO NOT include tremor (repetitive, regular, rhythmic)	0 1 2 3 4
	6. Lower (legs, knees, ankles, toes) e.g., lateral knee movement, foot tapping, heel dropping, foot squirming, inversion and eversion of foot	0 1 2 3 4
TRUNK MOVEMENTS	**7. Neck, shoulders, hips** e.g., rocking, twisting squirming, pelvic gyrations; include diaphragmatic movements	0 1 2 3 4
TOTAL SCORE	**8. Sum of items 1–7**	

GLOBAL JUDGMENTS	**9. Seventy of abnormal movements**
	 Based on highest single score of items 1–7 above.
	     None, normal
	     Minimal
	     Mild
	     Moderate
	     Severe
		
		 0
		 1
		 2
		 3
		 4

APPENDIX 4

	10. Incapacitation due to abnormal movements	
	None, normal	0
	Minimal	1
	Mild	2
	Moderate	3
	Severe	4
	11. Patient's awareness of abnormal movements	
	No awareness	0
	Aware, no distress	1
	Aware, mild distress	2
	Aware, moderate distress	3
	Aware, severe distress	4
DENTAL STATUS	**12. Current problems with teeth and/or dentures?**	No 0 Yes 1
	13. Does patient usually wear dentures?	No 0 Yes 1

INSTRUCTIONS FOR PERFORMING AIMS EXAM

Observe patient unobtrusively at rest (e.g., in waiting room) either before or after completing the examination.

Use a hard, firm chair without arms for the exam.

1. Ask patient whether there is anything in his/her mouth (e.g., gum, candy) and if there is, to remove it.
2. Ask patient about the *current* condition of his/her teeth. Ask patient if he/she wears dentures. Do teeth or dentures bother patients *now*?
3. Ask patient whether he/she notices any movements in mouth, face, hands, or feet. If yes, ask to describe and to rate to what extent they *currently* bother patient or interfere with his/her activities.
4. Have patient sit in chair with hands on knees, legs slightly apart, and feet flat on floor.
5. Ask the patient to sit with hands hanging unsupported; if male, between legs, if female and wearing a dress, hanging over knees. (Observe hands and other body areas.)
6. Ask patient to open mouth. (Observe tongue at rest within mouth.) Do this twice.
7. Ask patient to protrude tongue. (Observe abnormalities of tongue in movement.) Do this twice.
*8. Ask patient to tap thumb, with each finger, as rapidly as possible for 10–15 seconds; separately with right hand, then with left hand. (Observe facial and leg movements.)
9. Flex and extend patient's left and right arms (one at a time.) Note any rigidity and rate on separate scale, if applicable.
10. Ask patient to stand up. (Observe in profile; observe all body areas again, hips included.)
*11. Ask patient to extend both arms outstretched in front with palms down. (Observe trunk, legs, and mouth.)
*12. Have patient walk a few paces, turn, and walk back to chair. (Observe hands and gait.) Do this twice.

* Activated movements

PROPOSED SCORING CONVENTIONS FOR AIMS EXAM[a]

1. Score all involuntary hyperkinetic movements other than tremor (but including tic-like and dystonic movements), regardless of presumptive etiology. For example, score movements of Huntington's disease or Tourette's syndrome.
2. In scoring movement severity, consider the three dimensions of quality, frequency, and amplitude.
3. Do not follow the original AIMS instruction to subtract 1 point from movements seen only on activation. Instead, score by considering the composite amplitude and frequency of movements that are qualitatively consistent with tardive dyskinesia.
4. Consider frequency in distinguishing tremor from choreiform movements. Parkinsonian tremor generally occurs at three to six cycles per second, whereas tardive dyskinesia movements are rarely faster than two per second.
5. Use a score of 1 (minimal, may be extreme of normal) when movements are of marginal quality, amplitude, or frequency.
6. Generally do not rate mirror movements that are nonspecific. If it is unclear whether the movements seen are mirror movements, rate them 1.
7. On AIMS item 1, muscles of facial expression, rate only movements of the upper face (forehead and periorbital areas).
8. In distinguishing lip from jaw movements (a) consider the cranial nerve responsible for the movement noted. Rate movements involving the lower distribution of the facial nerve (e.g., puckering or smacking) as lip movements; rate movements brought about by the lower two-thirds of the trigeminal nerve (e.g., grinding or chewing) as jaw movements. (b) Do not rate lip movements if they are passive secondary to tongue or jaw movement. If both upper and lower lips move, the movements are not considered passive.
9. If necessary, rate tongue movements with the patient's mouth closed, by observing movements of the larynx. As Lane and others propose, "A sufficient condition for giving tongue movement a score of three is if the tongue breaks the imaginary plane considering upper and lower teeth."
10. Score toe tapping and other restless extremity movements (other than tremor) if they appear to be involuntary rather than classical akathisia movements. If the voluntariness of such movements is uncertain, rate them 1, regardless of amplitude or frequency.
11. Note that severity can be assessed in two complementary ways: by the global severity score (item 9), which equals the highest single score in the seven body areas (items 1–7), and by the total severity score (item 8), which is the sum of items 1–7.

Source: Psychopharmacol Bull 21(4):1077, 1985. In the public domain.
[a] Munetz MR, Benjamin S. How to examine patients using the Abnormal Involuntary Movement Scale. *Hosp Commun Psych* 39:1172–1177, 1988.

Clinical Global Impressions (CGI)

CGI Severity of Illness (CGI-S)
Considering your total clinical experience with children and adolescents, how ill is the patient at this time?

0 = Not assessed
1 = Normal (shows no signs of illness)
2 = Borderline ill
3 = Mildly (slightly) ill

4 = Moderately ill
5 = Markedly ill
6 = Severely ill
7 = Among the most extremely ill patients

CGI of Change (CGI-C) or CGI Global Improvement—Rate total improvement whether or not, in your judgment, it is due entirely to study drug treatment.

0 = Not assessed
1 = Very much improved
2 = Much improved
3 = Minimally improved

4 = No change
5 = Minimally worse
6 = Much worse
7 = Very much worse

Efficacy Index—Rate this item on the basis of drug effect only.

		Side Effects		
THERAPEUTIC EFFECT	None	Do Not Interfere with Functioning	Significantly Interfere with Functioning	Outweighs Therapeutic Benefit
MARKED—Vast Improvement	01	02	03	04
MODERATE—Decided Improvement	05	06	07	08
MINIMAL—Slight Improvement	09	10	11	12
UNCHANGED OR WORSE	13	14	15	16
Not Assessed	00	00	00	00

Adapted from CGI. *Psychopharm Bull* 21(4):839, 1985. In the public domain.

APPENDIX 4

Global Assessment Children's Scale
(CGAS)
For children 4–16 years of age

Adaptation of the Adult Global Assessment Scale
(From Axis V of the DSM)

Rate the subject's most impaired level of general functioning for the specified time period by selecting the *lowest* level that describes his/her functioning on a hypothetical continuum of health-illness. Use intermediary levels (e.g., 35, 58, 62).

Rate actual functioning regardless of treatment or prognosis. The examples of behavior provided are only illustrative and are not required for a particular rating.

Specified time period: 1 month

100–91   **Superior functioning** in all areas (at home, at school and with peers), involved in a range of activities and has many interests (e.g., has hobbies or participates in extracurricular activities or belongs to an organized group such as Scouts). Likeable, confident, "everyday" worries never get out of hand. Doing well in school. No symptoms.

90–81   **Good functioning in all areas.** Secure in family, school, and with peers. There may be transient difficulties and "everyday" worries that occasionally get out of hand (e.g., mild anxiety associated with an important exam, occasionally "blow-ups" with siblings, parents, or peers).

80–71   **No more than slight impairment in functioning** at home, at school, or with peers. Some disturbance of behavior or emotional distress (e.g., parental separations, deaths, birth of a sib), but these are brief and interference with functioning is transient. Such children are only minimally disturbing to others and are not considered deviant by those who know them.

70–61   **Some difficulty in a single area, but generally functioning pretty well** (e.g., sporadic or isolated antisocial acts, such as occasionally playing hooky or engaging in petty theft; consistent minor difficulties with schoolwork; mood changes of brief duration; fears and anxieties that do not lead to gross avoidance behavior; self-doubts). Has some meaningful interpersonal relationships. Most people who do not know the child well would not consider him/her deviant, but those who do know him/her well might express concern.

60–51   **Variable functioning with sporadic difficulties or symptoms in several but not all social areas.** Disturbance would be apparent to those who encounter the child in a dysfunctional setting or time but not to those who see the child in other settings.

50–41　**Moderate degree of interference in functioning in most social areas or severe impairment of functioning in one area,** such as might result from, for example, suicidal preoccupations and ruminations, school refusal and other forms of anxiety, obsessive rituals, major conversion symptoms, frequent anxiety attacks, frequent episodes of aggressive or other antisocial behavior, with some preservation of meaningful social relationships.

40–31　**Major impairment in functioning in several areas and unable to function in one of these areas,** i.e., disturbed at home, at school, with peers, or in the society at large, e.g., persistent aggression without clear instigation; markedly withdrawn and isolated behavior due to either mood or thought disturbance; suicidal attempts with clear lethal intent. Such children are likely to require special schooling and/or hospitalization or withdrawal from school (but this is not a sufficient criterion for inclusion in this category).

30–21　**Unable to function in almost all areas,** e.g., stays at home, in ward or in bed all day without taking part in social activities OR severe impairment in communication (e.g., sometimes incoherent or inappropriate).

20–11　**Needs considerable supervision** to prevent hurting others or self, e.g., frequently violent, repeated suicide attempts OR to maintain personal hygiene OR gross impairment in all forms of communication, e.g., severe abnormalities in verbal and gestural communication, marked social aloofness, stupor, etc.

10–1　**Needs constant supervision** (24-hour care) due to severely aggressive or self-destructive behavior or gross impairment in reality testing, communication, cognition, affect, or personal hygiene.

Adapted from Shaffer D, Gould M, Bird H, and Fisher P. Global Assessment Children's Scale, *Psychopharmacol Bull* 21(4):747, 1985. In the public domain.

APPENDIX 4

Brief Psychiatric Rating Scale for Children (BPRS-C)

Directions: Place an X in the appropriate box to represent level of severity of each symptom.

Patient: _____

Rater: _____

Date: _____

	Not Present	Very Mild	Mild	Moderately Severe	Severe	Extremely Severe
1. Uncooperativeness—negative, uncooperative, resistant, difficult to manage						
2. Hostility—angry or suspicious affect, belligerence, accusations, condemnations of others						
3. Manipulativeness—lying, cheating, exploitive of others						
4. Depressive mood—sad, tearful, depressive demeanor						
5. Feelings of inferiority—lacking self-confidence, self-depreciatory, feeling of personal inadequacy						
6. Suicidal ideation—thoughts, threats, or attempts of suicide						
7. Peculiar fantasies—recurrent, odd, unusual, or autistic ideations						
8. Delusions—ideas of reference, persecutory or grandiose delusions						
9. Hallucinations—visual, auditory, or other hallucinatory experiences or perceptions						
10. Hyperactivity—excessive energy expenditure, frequent changes in posture, perpetual motion						
11. Distractibility—poor concentration, shortened attention span, reactivity to peripheral stimuli						
12. Speech or voice pressure—loud, excessive, or pressured speech						

	Not Present	Very Mild	Mild	Moderately Severe	Severe	Extremely Severe
13. Underproductive speech—minimal, sparse inhibited verbal response pattern, or weak, low voice						
14. Emotional withdrawal—unspontaneous relations to examiner, lack of peer interaction, hypoactivity						
15. Blunted affect—deficient emotional expression, blankness, flatness of affect						
16. Tension—nervousness, fidgetiness, nervous movements of hands or feet						
17. Anxiety—clinging behavior, separation anxiety, preoccupation with anxiety topics, fears, or phobias						
18. Sleep difficulties—inability to fall asleep, intermittent awakening, shortened sleep time						
19. Disorientation—confusion over persons, places, or things						
20. Speech deviance—inferior level of speech development, underdeveloped vocabulary, mispronunciations						
21. Stereotypy—rhythmic, repetitive, manneristic movements or posture						

Source: Psychopharmacol Bull 21(4):753–770, 1985. In the public domain.

Pediatric Symptom Checklist (PSC)

Emotional and physical health go together in children. Because parents are often the first to notice a problem with their child's behavior, emotions, or learning, you may help your child get the best care possible by answering these questions.

Please indicate which statements best describe your child.

Please mark under the heading that best describes your child:

		Never	Sometimes	Often
1. Complains of aches and pains	1	_____	_____	_____
2. Spends more time alone	2	_____	_____	_____
3. Tires easily, has little energy	3	_____	_____	_____
4. Fidgety, unable to sit still	4	_____	_____	_____
5. Has trouble with teacher	5	_____	_____	_____
6. Less interested in school	6	_____	_____	_____
7. Acts as if driven by a motor	7	_____	_____	_____
8. Daydreams too much	8	_____	_____	_____
9. Distracted easily	9	_____	_____	_____
10. Is afraid of new situations	10	_____	_____	_____
11. Feels sad, unhappy	11	_____	_____	_____
12. Is irritable, angry	12	_____	_____	_____
13. Feels hopeless	13	_____	_____	_____
14. Has trouble concentrating	14	_____	_____	_____
15. Less interested in friends	15	_____	_____	_____
16. Fights with other children	16	_____	_____	_____
17. Absent from school	17	_____	_____	_____
18. School grades dropping	18	_____	_____	_____
19. Is down on him- or herself	19	_____	_____	_____
20. Visits the doctor, but doctor finds nothing wrong	20	_____	_____	_____
21. Has trouble sleeping	21	_____	_____	_____
22. Worries a lot	22	_____	_____	_____
23. Wants to be with you more than before	23	_____	_____	_____
24. Feels he or she is bad	24	_____	_____	_____
25. Takes unnecessary risks	25	_____	_____	_____
26. Gets hurt frequently	26	_____	_____	_____
27. Seems to be having less fun	27	_____	_____	_____
28. Acts younger than children his or her age	28	_____	_____	_____
29. Does not listen to rules	29	_____	_____	_____
30. Does not show feelings	30	_____	_____	_____
31. Does not understand other people's feelings	31	_____	_____	_____

		Never	Sometimes	Often
32. Teases others	32	_____	_____	_____
33. Blames others for his or her troubles	33	_____	_____	_____
34. Takes things that do not belong to him or her	34	_____	_____	_____
35. Refuses to share	35	_____	_____	_____

Total score _____ (never = 0, sometimes = 1, often = 2)

Does your child have any emotional or behavioral problems for which she or he needs help? ( ) N ( ) Y

Are there any services that you would like your child to receive for these problems? ( ) N ( ) Y

If yes, what service? _____

Source: Jellinek MS, Murphy JM, Little M, et al. Use of the Pediatric Symptom Checklist (PSC) to screen for psychosocial problems in pediatric primary care. A national feasibility study. *Arch Ped Adolesc Med* 153(3):254–260, 1999. PSC available at *www.brightfutures.org*

APPENDIX 4

The SNAP-IV Teacher and Parent Rating Scale

Name: _____ Gender:_____ Age:_____ Grade:_____

Ethnicity (circle one that best applies): African-American   Asian   Caucasian   Hispanic

Other:_____

Completed by:_____ Type of class:_____ Class size:_____

For each item, check the descriptor that best describes this child:

	Not At All	Just A Little	Quite A Bit	Very Much
1. Often fails to give close attention to details or makes careless mistakes in schoolwork or tasks	_____	_____	_____	_____
2. Often has difficulty sustaining attention in tasks or play activities	_____	_____	_____	_____
3. Often does not seem to listen when spoken to directly	_____	_____	_____	_____
4. Often does not follow through on instructions and fails to finish schoolwork, chores, or duties	_____	_____	_____	_____
5. Often has difficulty organizing tasks and activities	_____	_____	_____	_____
6. Often avoids, dislikes, or reluctantly engages in tasks requiring sustained mental effort	_____	_____	_____	_____
7. Often loses things necessary for activities (e.g., toys, school assignments, pencils, or books)	_____	_____	_____	_____
8. Often is distracted by extraneous stimuli	_____	_____	_____	_____
9. Often is forgetful in daily activities	_____	_____	_____	_____
10. Often has difficulty maintaining alertness, orienting to requests, or executing directions	_____	_____	_____	_____
11. Often fidgets with hands or feet or squirms in seat	_____	_____	_____	_____
12. Often leaves seat in classroom or in other situations in which remaining seated is expected	_____	_____	_____	_____
13. Often runs about or climbs excessively in situations in which it is inappropriate	_____	_____	_____	_____
14. Often has difficulty playing or engaging in leisure activities quietly	_____	_____	_____	_____
15. Often is "on the go" or acts as if "driven by a motor"	_____	_____	_____	_____
16. Often talks excessively	_____	_____	_____	_____
17. Often blurts out answers before questions have been completed	_____	_____	_____	_____

18. Often has difficulty awaiting turn
19. Often interrupts or intrudes on others
    (e.g., butts into conversations/games)
20. Often has difficulty sitting still, being
    quiet, or inhibiting impulses in the
    classroom or at home

21. Often loses temper
22. Often argues with adults
23. Often actively defies or refuses adult
    requests or rules
24. Often deliberately does things that
    annoy other people
25. Often blames others for his or her
    mistakes or misbehavior
26. Often is touchy or easily annoyed by
    others
27. Often is angry and resentful
28. Often is spiteful or vindictive
29. Often is quarrelsome
30. Often is negative, defiant, disobedient,
    or hostile toward authority figures

31. Often makes noises (e.g., humming
    or odd sounds)
32. Often is excitable, impulsive
33. Often cries easily
34. Often is uncooperative
35. Often acts "smart"
36. Often is restless or overactive
37. Often disturbs other children
38. Often changes mood quickly and
    drastically
39. Often easily frustrated if demands are
    not met immediately
40. Often teases other children and
    interferes with their activities

41. Often is aggressive to other children
    (e.g., picks fights or bullies)
42. Often is destructive with property of
    others (e.g., vandalism)
43. Often is deceitful (e.g., steals, lies,
    forges, copies the work of others, or
    "cons" others)
44. Often and seriously violates rules
    (e.g., is truant, runs away, or
    completely ignores class rules)
45. Has persistent pattern of violating the
    basic rights of others or major
    societal norms

46. Has episodes of failure to resist aggressive impulses (to assault others or to destroy property) _____ _____ _____ _____
47. Has motor or verbal tics (sudden, rapid, recurrent, nonrhythmic motor or verbal activity) _____ _____ _____ _____
48. Has repetitive motor behavior (e.g., hand waving, body rocking, or picking at skin) _____ _____ _____ _____
49. Has obsessions (persistent and intrusive inappropriate ideas, thoughts, or impulses) _____ _____ _____ _____
50. Has compulsions (repetitive behaviors or mental acts to reduce anxiety or distress) _____ _____ _____ _____

51. Often is restless or seems keyed up or on edge _____ _____ _____ _____
52. Often is easily fatigued _____ _____ _____ _____
53. Often has difficulty concentrating (mind goes blank) _____ _____ _____ _____
54. Often is irritable _____ _____ _____ _____
55. Often has muscle tension _____ _____ _____ _____
56. Often has excessive anxiety and worry (e.g., apprehensive expectation) _____ _____ _____ _____

57. Often has daytime sleepiness (unintended sleeping in inappropriate situations) _____ _____ _____ _____
58. Often has excessive emotionality and attention-seeking behavior _____ _____ _____ _____
59. Often has need for undue admiration, grandiose behavior, or lack of empathy _____ _____ _____ _____
60. Often has instability in relationships with others, reactive mood, and impulsivity _____ _____ _____ _____

61. Sometimes for at least a week has inflated self-esteem or grandiosity _____ _____ _____ _____
62. Sometimes for at least a week is more talkative than usual or seems pressured to keep talking _____ _____ _____ _____
63. Sometimes for at least a week has flight of ideas or says that thoughts are racing _____ _____ _____ _____
64. Sometimes for at least a week has elevated, expansive, or euphoric mood _____ _____ _____ _____
65. Sometimes for at least a week is excessively involved in pleasurable but risky activities _____ _____ _____ _____

66. Sometimes for at least 2 weeks has depressed mood (sad, hopeless, discouraged)

67. Sometimes for at least 2 weeks has irritable or cranky mood (not just when frustrated)

68. Sometimes for at least 2 weeks has markedly diminished interest or pleasure in most activities

69. Sometimes for at least 2 weeks has psychomotor agitation (even more active than usual)

70. Sometimes for at least 2 weeks has psychomotor retardation (slowed down in most activities)

71. Sometimes for at least 2 weeks is fatigued or has loss of energy

72. Sometimes for at least 2 weeks has feelings of worthlessness or excessive, inappropriate guilt

73. Sometimes for at least 2 weeks has diminished ability to think or concentrate

74. Chronic low self-esteem most of the time for at least a year

75. Chronic poor concentration or difficulty making decisions most of the time for at least a year

76. Chronic feelings of hopelessness most of the time for at least a year

77. Currently is hypervigilant (overly watchful or alert) or has exaggerated startle response

78. Currently is irritable, has anger outbursts, or has difficulty concentrating

79. Currently has an emotional (e.g., nervous, worried, hopeless, tearful) response to stress

80. Currently has a behavioral (e.g., fighting, vandalism, truancy) response to stress

81. Has difficulty getting started on classroom assignments

82. Has difficulty staying on task for an entire classroom period

83. Has problems in completion of work on classroom assignments

84. Has problems in accuracy or neatness
of written work in the classroom

85. Has difficulty attending to a group
classroom activity or discussion

86. Has difficulty making transitions to
the next topic or classroom period

87. Has problems in interactions with
peers in the classroom

88. Has problems in interactions with
staff (teacher or aide)

89. Has difficulty remaining quiet
according to classroom rules

90. Has difficulty staying seated
according to classroom rules

Abbreviated Parent Questionnaire

PATIENT NAME _____

PARENT'S OBSERVATIONS

Information obtained _____ by _____
               Month   Day   Year

	Degree of Activity			
Observation	**Not at all**	**Just a little**	**Pretty much**	**Very much**
1. Restless or overactive				
2. Excitable, impulsive				
3. Disturbs other children				
4. Fails to finish things he or she starts—short attention span				
5. Constantly fidgeting				
6. Inattentive, easily distracted				
7. Demands must be met immediately—easily frustrated				
8. Cries often and easily				
9. Mood changes quickly and drastically				
10. Temper outbursts, explosive and unpredictable behavior				

COMMENTS

_____

_____

_____

_____

Source: Psychopharmacol Bull 21(4):816–831, 1985. In the public domain.

APPENDIX 4

Children's Depression Rating Scale—Revised
(CDRS-R)

Patient Name: _____

Date Completed: _____

Patient Number: _____

Instructions: The CDRS-R consists of 17 items. Fourteen of these items are rated on the basis of the subject's responses to a series of standardized questions. This semistandard interview can be administered to children ages 6–12, their parents, teachers, case workers, or other sources of information in approximately 30 minutes. The first 14 items are rated on the basis of this interview. The remaining 3 items of the CDRS-R are rated by the clinician on the basis of the *child's* nonverbal behavior. These 3 items are not rated when interviewing a subject other than the child.

The 17 items of the CDRS-R are scaled from 1 to 5 for sleep, appetite, and tempo of speech items and from 1 to 7 for the remaining 14 items. A rating of 1 indicates no abnormality, whereas a rating of 3 indicates mild symptomatolgy; a rating of 5 or more on all items indicates definite psychopathological symptomatology.

I. Schoolwork

Do you like school or dislike school? What parts do you like? What parts do you dislike?	1 Performance consistent with ability
What kind of grades do you get in school? Are they different now from what they were last year?	2
Do your parents or your teacher(s) think you ought to be doing better? What do they say? Do you agree or disagree with them?	3 Decrease in school performance
If grades are a problem, ask: Do you have trouble paying attention? Why? Do you take longer to finish your assignments than other kids? Do you daydream?	4 5 Major interference in most subjects
Do other children bother you? Does the teacher often ask you to listen to what he/she is saying?	6
If not in school, ask about ability to concentrate on a TV program or game.	7 No motivation to perform

II. Capacity to Have Fun

What do you like to do for fun? (Note interest, involvement, enthusiasm.) Discuss individual activities named.	1 Interest and activities realistically appropriate for age, personality, and social environment. Shows no appreciable change with present illness. Any feelings of boredom are transient. 2
How often do you have fun? (Note whether activities available daily, weekly, seasonally, or very infrequently.)	3 Describes some activities that are realistically available several times a week but not on a daily basis. Shows interest but not enthusiasm. 4
Are you ever bored? How often?	5 Is easily bored. Complains of "nothing to do." Participates in structured activities with a "going through the motions" attitude. May express interest primarily in activities that are (realistically) unavailable on a daily or weekly basis.
(If very inactive) What do you like to watch on TV? Discuss favorite TV shows. (Determine if active or passive viewer.)	6 7 Has no initiative to become involved in any activities. Primarily passive. Watches others play or watches TV but shows little interest. Requires coaxing and/or pushing to get involved in activity. Shows no enthusiasm or real interest. Has difficulty naming activities.

III. Social Withdrawal

Do you have friends to play with? Are they at school or home? What games or things do you do? How often do you play with them?	1 Enjoys friendships with peers at school and home. 2 3 May not actively seek out friendships but waits for others to initiate a relationship or may occasionally reject opportunities to play without a describable alternative.
Have you ever had a really close friend? Do you have one now?	
Do your friends ever call for you and you just don't feel like going out to play? How often?	4 5 Frequently avoids or refuses opportunities for desirable interaction with others and/or sets up situations where rejection is inevitable.
Have you ever lost friends? What happened?	6 7 Does not currently relate to other children. States he or she has "no friends" or actively rejects new or former friends.
Do children ever pick on you? How? What do they do? Is there anyone who will stick up for you?	

IV. Sleep

Do you have trouble sleeping?	1 No (or occasional) difficulty (goes to sleep within an hour or less).
Do you take a long time to go to sleep? (Differentiate from resisting going to bed.) How long? How often?	2 3 Frequently has mild difficulty with sleep.
Do you wake up in the middle of the night? Do you go right back to sleep or stay awake? How often does this happen?	4 5 Moderate difficulty with sleep nearly every night (if applicable, indicate time of difficulty).
Do you ever wake up before you need to in the morning? How early? Do you go back to sleep or stay awake? What do you do? How often (or when) does this happen?	a. Initial b. Middle c. Early

V. Appetite or Eating Patterns

Do you like to eat?	1 No problems or change in eating pattern.
At mealtime, are you hungry for some meals, most meals, all meals? Not hungry (if not hungry, record when and how often not hungry)?	2 3 Mild change from usual eating habits within onset of current behavioral problems. 4
Does your mother complain about your eating?	5 Is not hungry most of the time or has excessive food intake since onset of current behavioral problems or marked increase in appetite. (If applicable, circle one)
Have you gained or lost weight? (If yes) How can you tell?	Increased Appetite Decreased Appetite

VI. Excessive Fatigue
(Consider age and activities of child)

Do you feel tired during the day? Even when you have had enough sleep? (During boring school subjects does not count.) After school?	1 No unusual complaints of "feeling tired" during the day. 2 3 Complaints of fatigue that seem somewhat excessive and not related to boredom.
How often do you feel tired after school?	4 5 Daily complaints of feeling tired.
Do you ever feel so tired you go and take a nap even if you don't have to? How often does this happen?	6 7 Complaints of feeling tired most of the day. May voluntarily take long naps without feeling refreshed. Interferes with play activities.

VII. Physical Complaints

Do you ever get stomachaches, headaches, leg pains?	1 Occasional complaints.
	2
Do you get other aches and pains? What are they like? How often do they occur?	3 Complaints appear mildly excessive.
	4
	5 Complains daily. Some interference with the ability of the child to function.
When you get _____ aches, how long do they last? Does anything make them go away? Do they keep you from playing? How often do they do this?	6
	7 Preoccupied with aches and pains; interferes with play activities several times a week.

VIII. Irritability

What things make you get grouchy or mad?	1 Rare
	2 Occasional
How mad do you get?	3 Several times a week for short periods
Do you ever feel in a mood where everything bothers you? How long do these moods last? How often do these moods occur?	4
	5 Several times a week for longer periods
	6
	7 Constant

IX. Guilt

Do you ever feel like it's your fault or blame yourself if something bad happens?	1 Does not express any undue feelings of guilt. Appears appropriate to precipitating event. 2
Do you ever feel bad or sorry about certain things you have done or wished you had done? What are they? (Note act and whether guilt is proportional to deed.)	3 Exaggerates guilt and/or shame out of proportion to the event described. 4 5 Feels guilty over things not under his or her control. Guilt is definitely pathological.
Do you know what the word *guilty* means? Do certain things make you feel guilty?	6 7 Severe delusions of guilt.

X. Self-Esteem

Do you like the way you look? Can you describe yourself? (With a young child, ask about hair, eyes, face, clothes, etc.) Would you want to change the way you look? What way?	1 Describes self in primarily positive terms. 2
Do you think you are smart or stupid?	3 Describes self with one important area where the child feels deficit.
Do you think you are better or worse than other kids?	4
Do most kids like you? Do any not like you? Why? Do you get called names? What are they? Do other kids put you down?	5 Describes self in preponderance of negative terms or gives bland answers to questions.
What things are you good at? Not so good? What?	6 7 Refers to self in derogatory terms. Reports that other children refer to him/her frequently by using derogatory nicknames, and child puts self down.
Do you ever feel very down on yourself?	
Would you like to change anything about yourself?	

APPENDIX 4

592 Pediatric Psychopharmacology: Fast Facts

XI. Depressed Feelings

What things make you feel unhappy?	1 Occasional feelings of unhappiness that quickly disappear.
When you feel unhappy, how long does it last? An hour? A few hours? A whole day? How often do you feel like this? Every week? Every two weeks? (Note: for younger children, one hour may be equivalent of _____ days or more in older children.)	2
	3 Describes sustained periods of unhappiness that appear excessive for events described.
Do other people know when you are sad?	4
Do you feel sad just at certain times, like when your mother is away?	5 Feels unhappy most of the time without a major precipitating cause.
When you feel unhappy, how miserable do you feel? Do you ever feel so bad it hurts? How often does it feel bad? (Reactivity is an indicator of degree of depressed feelings.)	6
	7 Feels unhappy all of the time, accompanied by psychic pain (e.g., "I can't stand it").

XII. Morbid Ideation

Have you ever had a pet die? A friend? A relative? Do you think about it now? How often?	1 None
	2
Do you ever think about someone dying in your family? Who? Describe. How often do you think about it?	3 Has some morbid thoughts, all of which relate to a reality event but seem excessive.
	4
Do you ever worry about anyone else? Who?	5 Preoccupied with morbid thoughts several times a week. Morbid thoughts extend beyond external realilty.
Do you ever think that you might die? Tell me about it.	6
How often do you have these kinds of thoughts?	7 Preoccupied with death themes or morbid thoughts that are elaborate, extensive, or bizarre on a daily basis.

XIII. Suicidal Ideation

Do you know what the word *suicide* means?	1 Understands the word *suicide* but does not apply term to self.
Have you ever thought of doing it? (If yes) When? How have you thought of doing it?	2 Sharp denial of suicidal thoughts. 3 Has thoughts about suicide, usually when angry.
Have you ever said you would like to kill yourself even if you didn't mean it? Describe.	4 5 Has recurrent thoughts of suicide. 6
(If appropriate) Have you ever tried to kill yourself?	7 Has made suicide attempt within the last month or is actively suicidal.

XIV. Weeping

Do you ever cry very much?	1 Normal for age.
Do you sometimes feel like crying even if you don't cry? What sort of things make you feel this way? How often do these occur?	2 Suggestive statements that child cries, or feels like crying, more frequently than peers. 3 Child cries slightly more than peers. 4
Do you think you feel like crying more than your friends?	5 Cries or feels like crying frequently (several times a week). Admits to crying without knowing reason why.
Do you ever feel like crying for no reason?	6 7 Cries nearly every day.

XV. Depressed Affect

1 Definitely not depressed. Facial expression and voice animated during interview.

2 Mild suppression of affect. Some loss of spontaneity.

3 Overall loss of spontaneity. Looks distinctly unhappy during parts of the interview. May still be able to smile when discussing nonthreatening areas.

4

5 Moderate restriction of affect throughout most of interview. Has longer and frequent periods of looking distinctly unhappy.

6

7 Severe. Looks sad, withdrawn. Minimal verbal interaction throughout interview. Cries or may appear tearful.

XVI. Tempo of Speech

1 Normal

2 Slow

3 Slow: delays interviews

4

5 Severe: low; marked interference with interview

XVII. Hypoactivity

1 None

2

3 Mild. Some body movements.

4

5 Moderate. Definite motor retardation.

6

7 Severe. Motionless throughout interview.

Summary Score = _____

Adapted from Poznanski EO, Freeman LN, and Mokros HB. Children's depression rating scale—revised. *Psychopharmacol Bull* 21(4):979–989, 1985. In the public domain.

Yale–Brown Obsessive Compulsive Scale (Y-BOCS)

Patient's Name	Date of 1st report
Therapy	Date of this report

Instructions: Complete Y-BOCS Symptom Checklist [facing page] before administering Y-BOCS (below). In administering Y-BOCS, make specific reference to patient's principal obsessions and compulsions.

	None	Mild	Moderate	Severe	Extreme
1. TIME SPENT ON OBSESSIONS	0	1	2	3	4
2. INTERFERENCE FROM OBSESSIONS	0	1	2	3	4
3. DISTRESS OF OBSESSIONS	0	1	2	3	4
	Definitely Resists				Completely yields
4. RESISTANCE	0	1	2	3	4
	Complete control	Much control	Moderate control	Little control	No control
5. CONTROL OVER OBSESSIONS	0	1	2	3	4

OBSESSION SUBTOTAL (Items 1–5) [ ]

	None	Mild	Moderate	Severe	Extreme
6. TIME SPENT ON COMPULSIONS	0	1	2	3	4
7. INTERFERENCE FROM COMPULSIONS	0	1	2	3	4
8. DISTRESS OF COMPULSIONS	0	1	2	3	4
	Definitely resists				Completely yields
9. RESISTANCE	0	1	2	3	4
	Complete control	Much control	Moderate control	Little control	No control
10. CONTROL OVER COMPULSIONS	0	1	2	3	4

COMPULSION SUBTOTAL (Items 6–10) [ ]

Total Y-BOCS Score (Items 1–10) [ ]

Y-BOCS Symptom Checklist

Instructions: Generate a *Target Symptoms List* from the attached *Y-BOCS Symptom Checklist* by asking the patient about specific obsessions and compulsions. Check all that apply. Distinguish between current and past symptoms. Mark principal symptoms with a "p." These will form the basis of the *Target Symptoms List.* Items marked "*" may or may not be OCD phenomena.

AGGRESSIVE OBSESSIONS

Current Past

_____ _____ Fear might harm self
_____ _____ Fear might harm others
_____ _____ Violent or horrific images
_____ _____ Fear of blurting out obscenities or insults
_____ _____ Fear of doing something else embarrassing*
_____ _____ Fear will act on unwanted impulses (e.g., to stab friend)
_____ _____ Fear will steal things
_____ _____ Fear will harm others because not careful enough (e.g., hit/run motor vehicle accident)
_____ _____ Fear will be responsible for something else terrible happening (e.g., fire, burglary)
_____ _____ Other _____

CONTAMINATION OBSESSIONS

_____ _____ Concerns or disgust with bodily waste or secretions (e.g., urine, feces, saliva)
_____ _____ Concern with dirt or germs
_____ _____ Excessive concern with household items (e.g., cleansers, solvents)
_____ _____ Excessive concern with animals (e.g., insects)
_____ _____ Bothered by sticky substances or residues
_____ _____ Concerned will get ill because of contaminant
_____ _____ Concerned will get others ill by spreading contaminant (Aggressive)
_____ _____ No concern with consequences of contamination other than how it might feel
_____ _____ Other _____

SEXUAL OBSESSIONS

_____ _____ Forbidden or perverse sexual thoughts, images, or impulses
_____ _____ Content involves children or incest
_____ _____ Content involves homosexuality*
_____ _____ Sexual behavior towards others (Aggressive)*
_____ _____ Other _____

HOARDING/SAVING OBSESSIONS

(distinguish from hobbies and concern with objects of monetary or sentimental value)

_____ _____ _____

RELIGIOUS OBSESSIONS (Scrupulosity)

_____ _____ Concerned with sacrilege and blasphemy
_____ _____ Excess concern with right/wrong, morality
_____ _____ Other _____

OBSESSION WITH NEED FOR SYMMETRY OR EXACTNESS

_____ _____ Accompanied by magical thinking (e.g., concerned that another will have accident unless things are in the right place)

MISCELLANEOUS OBSESSIONS

_____ _____ Need to know or remember
_____ _____ Fear of saying certain things
_____ _____ Fear of not saying just the right thing
_____ _____ Fear of losing things
_____ _____ Intrusive (nonviolent) images
_____ _____ Intrusive nonsense sounds, words, or music
_____ _____ Bothered by certain sounds/noises*
_____ _____ Lucky/unlucky numbers
_____ _____ Colors with special significance
_____ _____ Superstitious fears
_____ _____ Other _____

SOMATIC OBSESSIONS

Current Past

_____ _____ Concern with illness or disease*
_____ _____ Excessive concern with body part or aspect of appearance (e.g., dysmorphophobia)*
_____ _____ Other _____

CLEANING/WASHING COMPULSIONS

_____ _____ Excessive or ritualized handwashing
_____ _____ Excessive or ritualized showering, bathing, toothbrushing, grooming, or toilet routine
_____ _____ Involves cleaning of household items or other inanimate objects
_____ _____ Other measures to prevent or remove contact with contaminants
_____ _____ Other _____

CHECKING COMPULSIONS

_____ _____ Checking locks, stove, appliances, etc.
_____ _____ Checking that did not/will not harm others
_____ _____ Checking that did not/will not harm self
_____ _____ Checking that nothing terrible did/will happen
_____ _____ Checking that did not make mistake
_____ _____ Checking tied to somatic obsessions
_____ _____ Other _____

A
P
P
E
N
D
I
X

4

REPEATING RITUALS

_____ _____ Rereading or rewriting

_____ _____ Need to repeat routine activities (e.g., in/out door, up/down from chair)

_____ _____ Other _____

COUNTING COMPULSIONS

_____ _____ _____

ORDERING/ARRANGING COMPULSIONS

_____ _____ _____

HOARDING/COLLECTING COMPULSIONS

(distinguish from hobbies and concern with objects of monetary or sentimental value [e.g., carefully reads junk mail, piles up old newspapers, sorts through garbage, collects useless objects])

_____ _____ _____

MISCELLANEOUS COMPULSIONS

_____ _____ Mental rituals (other than checking/counting)

_____ _____ Excessive listmaking

_____ _____ Need to tell, ask, or confess

_____ _____ Need to touch, tap, or rub*

_____ _____ Rituals involving blinking or staring*

_____ _____ Measures (not checking) to prevent: harm to self _____; harm to others _____; terrible consequences ___

_____ _____ Ritualized eating behaviors*

_____ _____ Superstitious behaviors

_____ _____ Trichotillomania*

_____ _____ Other self-damaging or self-mutilating behaviors*

_____ _____ Other _____

Children's Aggression Scale—Parent Version

Child: _____ Gender: M F DOB: _____/_____/_____

Age:_____ Grade: _____ ID_____ School: _____

Respondent _____ Relation to child:_____

I. VERBAL AGGRESSION: This section will focus on incidents in which there was no physical contact or fighting.

DURING THE PAST YEAR, HOW OFTEN HAS YOUR CHILD:

1. snapped or yelled at children living in the home?	Never	Once/month or less	Once/week or less	2–3 times/ week	most days
2. snapped or yelled at adults living the home?	Never	Once/month or less	Once/week or less	2–3 times/ week	most days
3. snapped or yelled at peers/friends who do not live in the home?	Never	Once/month or less	Once/week or less	2–3 times/ week	most days
4. snapped or yelled at adults who do not live in the home?	Never	Once/month or less	Once/week or less	2–3 times/ week	most days
5. cursed or sworn at children who live in the home?	Never	Once/month or less	Once/week or less	2–3 times/ week	most days
6. cursed or sworn at adults who live in the home?	Never	Once/month or less	Once/week or less	2–3 times/ week	most days
7. cursed or sworn at peers/friends who do not live in the home?	Never	Once/month or less	Once/week or less	2–3 times/ week	most days
8. cursed or sworn at adults who do not live in the home?	Never	Once/month or less	Once/week or less	2–3 times/ week	most days
9. verbally threatened to hit a child who lives in the home?	Never	Once/month or less	Once/week or less	2–3 times/ week	most days
10. verbally threatened to hit an adult who lives in the home?	Never	Once/month or less	Once/week or less	2–3 times/ week	most days
11. verbally threatened to hit peers/friends who do not live in the home?	Never	Once/month or less	Once/week or less	2–3 times/ week	most days
12. verbally threatened to hit adults who do not live in home?	Never	Once/month or less	Once/week or less	2–3 times/ week	most days

II. AGGRESSION AGAINST OBJECTS AND ANIMALS

DURING THE PAST YEAR, HOW OFTEN HAS YOUR CHILD:

13. slammed a door, kicked a chair, or thrown or broken objects when angry?	Never	Once/month or less	Once/week or less	2–3 times/ week	most days
14. vandalized or destroyed someone else's property?	Never	Once/month or less	Once/week or less	2–3 times/ week	most days
15. taunted or teased or annoyed a pet or other animal?	Never	Once/month or less	Once/week or less	2–3 times/ week	most days
16. injured or tortured a pet or other living animal?	Never	Once/month or less	Once/week or less	2–3 times/ week	most days

III. PHYSICAL AGGRESSION

A. PROVOKED INTO PHYSICAL AGGRESSION: This section will focus on instances where another person provoked or "picked" a fight with your child (i.e., when the other person made the first physical contact).

DURING THE PAST YEAR, HOW OFTEN HAS YOUR CHILD;

17. fought with another child who lives in the home when provoked?	Never	Once/month or less	Once/week or less	2–3 times/ week	most days

18. fought with an adult who lives in the home when provoked?	Never	Once/month or less	Once/week or less	2–3 times/ week	most days
19. fought with peers/friends when provoked?	Never	Once/month or less	Once/week or less	2–3 times/ week	most days
20. fought with other adults who do not live in the home when provoked?	Never	Once/month or less	Once/week or less	2–3 times/ week	most days
21. How often did these fights result in mild physical injury (e.g., bumps and bruises)	Never	Once or twice	3–5 times	5–10 times	more than 10 times
22. How often did these fights result in serious physical injury (e.g., stitches, broken bones, requiring a doctor's attention)?	Never	Once or twice	3–5 times	5–10 times	more than 10 times

Please describe: _____

B. INITIATED PHYSICAL AGGRESION: This section will focus on those fights your child initiated or started (i.e., when he/she made the first physical contact).

DURING THE PAST YEAR, HOW OFTEN HAS YOUR CHILD:

23. started a physical fight with a child who lives in the home?	Never	Once/month or less	Once/week or less	2–3 times/ week	most days
24. started a physical fight with an adult who lives in the home?	Never	Once/month or less	Once/week or less	2–3 times/ week	most days
25. started a physical fight with peers/ friends who do not live in the home?	Never	Once/month or less	Once/week or less	2–3 times/ week	most days
26. started a physical fight with adults who do not live in the home?	Never	Once/month or less	Once/week or less	2–3 times/ week	most days
27. How often did these fights result in mild physical injury (e.g., bumps and bruises)?	Never	Once or twice	3–5 times	5–10 times	more than 10 times
28. How often did these fights result in serious physical injury (e.g., stitches, broken bones, requiring a doctor's attention)?	Never	Once or twice	3–5 times	5–10 times	more than 10 times

Please describe: _____

IV. USE OF WEAPONS

DURING THE PAST YEAR, HOW OFTEN HAS YOUR CHILD:

29. carried a weapon (e.g., knife, gun)	Never	Once or twice	3–5 times	5–10 times	more than 10 times
30. threatened another with a weapon?	Never	Once or twice	3–5 times	5–10 times	more than 10 times
31. injured another with a weapon?	Never	Once or twice	3–5 times	5–10 times	more than 10 times
32. Did this behavior occur within the context of a gang?	YES	NO			

Scoring Instructions: Never = 0, once/month or less = 1, once a week or less = 2, 2–3 times/week = 3, most days = 4

From: Halperin JM, McKay KE, & Newcorn JH. Development, reliability, and validity of the Children's Aggression Scale—Parent Version. *J Am Acad Child Adolesc Psychiatry* 41(3):245–252, 2002. Reproduced with permission from the author.

OVERT AGGRESSION SCALE

NAME:_____

DATE COMPLETED:_____

PATIENT NUMBER:_____

INSTRUCTIONS: PLEASE COMPLETE AS A SUMMARY OF THE PAST WEEK. THERE MAY BE MANY SUCH INCIDENTS PER WEEK. CHECK ALL CATEGORIES OF AGGRESSION THAT OCCURRED IN THE LAST WEEK. FOR EACH CATEGORY OF AGGRESSIVE BEHAVIOR, CHECK HOW OFTEN IT OCCURRED IN THE LAST WEEK.

Behaviors	(0) Never	(1–2) Sometimes	(3–4) Often	(5–10) Usually	(>10) Always
Verbal aggression					
1. Makes loud noises, shouts angrily					
2. Yells mild personal insults					
3. Curses viciously, uses foul language, makes moderate threats to others or self					
4. Makes clear threats of violence towards others or self, or requests help to control					
Physical aggression against object					
1. Slams doors, makes a mess, scatters clothing					
2. Throws objects, kicks furniture without breaking it, marks the wall					
3. Breaks objects, smashes windows					
4. Sets fires, throws objects dangerously					
Physical aggression against self					
1. Picks or scratches skin, hits self on arms or body, pinches self, pulls hair					
2. Bangs head, hits fist into objects, throws self onto floor or into objects					
3. Small cuts or bruises, minor burns					
4. Mutilates self, makes deep cuts, bites that bleed, internal injury, fracture, loss of consciousness, loss of teeth					
Physical aggression against others					
1. Makes threatening gestures, swings at people, grabs at clothes					
2. Strikes, kicks, pushes, pulls hair					
3. Attacks others, causing physical injury (bruises, sprains, welts)					
4. Attacks others while causing severe physical injury (broken bones, deep lacerations)					

Adapted from Yudofsky SC, Silver JM, Jackson W, Endicott J, Williams D. The overt aggression scale for the objective rating of verbal and physical aggression. Am J Psychiatry 143(1):35–39, 1986; Sorgi P, Ratey J, Knoedler DW, Markert RJ, Reichman M. Rating aggression in the clinical setting: A retrospective adaptation of the overt aggression scale. J Neuropsychiatry 3(2):S52–S56, 1991; Kay SR, Wolkenfeld F, Murrill LM. Profiles of aggression among psychiatric patients II. Covariates and predictors. J Nerv Ment Disease 176(9):547–557, 1988. Used with permission from the author.

The Nisonger Child Behavior Rating Form

PARENT VERSION

Child's Name: _____   Child's Date of Birth: _____/_____/_____
                                                          month   day   year

Rater's Name: _____   Date of Rating: _____/_____/_____
                                                   month   day   year

Relation of Rater to Child: parent [1]   other [9]: _____
                                                          (please specify)

I. Please describe any special circumstances or mediating factors that may have affected the child's behavior in the recent past (the last month or two) or prevented you from making complete ratings.

II. **POSITIVE SOCIAL.** Please describe the child's behavior as it was at home over the last month.

IN THE LAST MONTH, THIS CHILD HAS:	Not True [0]	Somewhat or Sometimes True [1]	Very or Often True [2]	Completely or Always True [3]
1. Accepted redirection				
2. Expressed ideas clearly				
3. Followed rules				
4. Initiated positive interactions				
5. Participated in group activities				
6. Resisted provocation, was tolerant				
7. Shared with or helped others				
8. Stayed on task				
9. Was cheerful or happy				
10. Was patient, able to delay				

III. **PROBLEM BEHAVIOR.** For each item that describes the child's behavior as it was over the last month, circle the:

0.... if the behavior **did not** occur or **was not a problem**
1.... if the behavior occurred **occasionally** or was a **mild problem**
2.... if the behavior occurred **quite often** or was a **moderate problem**
3.... if the behavior occurred **a lot** or was a **severe problem**

For each problem that occurred, circle only the score that best describes the behavior.

PLEASE DO NOT SKIP ANY QUESTIONS. IF YOU DO NOT KNOW THE ANSWER OR HAVE NOT HAD A CHANCE TO OBSERVE THE CHILD FOR A GIVEN TIME, CIRCLE THE ZERO.

1. Apathetic or unmotivated 0 1 2 3
2. Argues with parents, teachers, or other adults 0 1 2 3
3. Clings to adults, too dependent 0 1 2 3
4. Cruelty or meanness to others 0 1 2 3
5. Crying, tearful episodes 0 1 2 3
6. Hits or slaps own head, neck, hands, or other
   body parts 0 1 2 3
7. Defiant, challenges adult authority 0 1 2 3
8. Knowingly destroys property 0 1 2 3
9. Difficulty concentrating 0 1 2 3
10. Disobedient 0 1 2 3
11. Rocks body or head back and forth repetitively 0 1 2 3
12. Doesn't feel guilty after misbehaving 0 1 2 3
13. Easily distracted 0 1 2 3
14. Easily frustrated 0 1 2 3
15. Overly sensitive 0 1 2 3
16. Exaggerates abilities or achievements 0 1 2 3
17. Explosive, easily angered 0 1 2 3
18. Has rituals such as head rolling or floor pacing 0 1 2 3
19. Fails to finish things he/she starts 0 1 2 3
20. Feelings easily hurt 0 1 2 3
21. Feels others are against him/her 0 1 2 3
22. Harms self by scratching skin or pulling hair 0 1 2 3
23. Feels worthless or inferior 0 1 2 3
24. Fidgets, wiggles, or squirms 0 1 2 3
25. Shy around others; bashful 0 1 2 3
26. Gets in physical fights 0 1 2 3
27. Irritable 0 1 2 3
28. Repeatedly flaps or waves hands, fingers or objects
   (such as pieces of string) 0 1 2 3
29. Isolates self from others 0 1 2 3
30. Lying or cheating 0 1 2 3
31. Nervous or tense 0 1 2 3
32. Gouges self, puts things in ears, nose, etc.,
   or eats inedible things 0 1 2 3
33. Overactive, doesn't sit still 0 1 2 3
34. Overly anxious to please others 0 1 2 3
35. Overly excited, exuberant 0 1 2 3
36. Physically attacks people 0 1 2 3
37. Refuses to talk 0 1 2 3

APPENDIX 4

38. Repeats the same sound, word, or phrase over and over .	0	1	2	3
39. Restless, high energy level	0	1	2	3
40. Runs away from adults, teachers, or other authority figures	0	1	2	3
41. Says no one likes him/her	0	1	2	3
42. Secretive, keeps things to self	0	1	2	3
43. Repeatedly bites self hard enough to leave tooth marks or break skin	0	1	2	3
44. Self-conscious or easily embarrassed	0	1	2	3
45. Shifts rapidly from topic to topic when talking	0	1	2	3
46. Short attention span	0	1	2	3
47. Shy or timid behavior	0	1	2	3
48. Steals	0	1	2	3
49. Odd repetitive behaviors (e.g., stares, grimaces, rigid postures)	0	1	2	3
50. Stubborn, has to do things own way	0	1	2	3
51. Sudden changes in mood	0	1	2	3
52. Sulks, is silent and moody	0	1	2	3
53. Physically harms or hurts self on purpose	0	1	2	3
54. Talks back to teacher, parents, or other adults	0	1	2	3
55. Talks too much or too loud	0	1	2	3
56. Temper tantrums	0	1	2	3
57. Threatens people	0	1	2	3
58. Threatens to harm self	0	1	2	3
59. Engages in meaningless, repetitive body movements	0	1	2	3
60. Too fearful or anxious	0	1	2	3
61. Underactive, slow	0	1	2	3
62. Unhappy or sad	0	1	2	3
63. Violates rules	0	1	2	3
64. Withdrawn, uninvolved with others	0	1	2	3
65. Worrying	0	1	2	3
66. Argues with other children or peers	0	1	2	3

Developed by M. G. Aman, M. J. Tassé, J. Rojahn, and D. Hammer, 1995.

Aman, M.G., Tassé, M.J., Rojahn, J., & Hammer, D. (1996). The Nisonger CBRF: A child behavior rating form for children with developmental disabilities. *Research in Developmental Disabilities, 17*, 41–57.

Tassé, M.J., Aman, M.G., Hammer, D., & Rojahn, J. (1996). The Nisonger Child Behavior Rating Form: Age and gender effects and norms. *Research in Developmental Disabilities, 17*, 59–75.

The Nisonger Child Behavior Rating Form

> ## TEACHER VERSION

Child's Name: _____   Child's Date of Birth: ____/____/_____
month day year

Rater's Name: _____   Date of Rating: ____/____/_____
month day year

Relation of Rater to Child: teacher [2]   aide [3]   other [9]: _____
(please specify)

Type of class? (check one)   Regular [1]   DH [2]   MH [3]   SBH [4]   HI [5]

LD [6]   OH [7]   VI [8]   Other [9]: _____

How long have you had this child in your class?   less than 3 months [1]
(check one)   3 to 6 months [2]
                                                  more than 6 months [3]

I. Please describe any special circumstances or mediating factors that may have affected the child's behavior in the recent past (the last month or two) or prevented you from making complete ratings.

II. **POSITIVE SOCIAL.** Please describe the child's behavior as it was in the classroom over the last month.

IN THE LAST MONTH, THIS CHILD HAS:	Not True [0]	Somewhat or Sometimes True [1]	Very or Often True [2]	Completely or Always True [3]
1. Accepted redirection				
2. Expressed ideas clearly				
3. Followed rules				
4. Initiated positive interactions				
5. Participated in group activities				
6. Resisted provocation, was tolerant				
7. Shared with or helped others				
8. Stayed on task				
9. Was cheerful or happy				
10. Was patient, able to delay				

APPENDIX 4

III. **PROBLEM BEHAVIOR.** For each item that describes the child's behavior as it was over the last month, circle the:

> 0.... if the behavior **did not** occur or **was not a problem**
> 1.... if the behavior occurred **occasionally** or was a **mild problem**
> 2.... if the behavior occurred **quite often** or was a **moderate problem**
> 3.... if the behavior occurred **a lot** or was a **severe problem**

For each problem that occurred, circle only the score that best describes the behavior.

PLEASE DO NOT SKIP ANY QUESTIONS. IF YOU DO NOT KNOW THE ANSWER OR HAVE NOT HAD A CHANCE TO OBSERVE THE CHILD FOR A GIVEN TIME, CIRCLE THE ZERO.

1. Apathetic or unmotivated	0	1	2	3
2. Argues with parents, teachers, or other adults	0	1	2	3
3. Clings to adults, too dependent	0	1	2	3
4. Cruelty or meanness to others	0	1	2	3
5. Crying, tearful episodes	0	1	2	3
6. Hits or slaps own head, neck, hands, or other body parts	0	1	2	3
7. Defiant, challenges adult authority	0	1	2	3
8. Knowingly destroys property	0	1	2	3
9. Difficulty concentrating	0	1	2	3
10. Disobedient	0	1	2	3
11. Rocks body or head back and forth repetitively	0	1	2	3
12. Doesn't feel guilty after misbehaving	0	1	2	3
13. Easily distracted	0	1	2	3
14. Easily frustrated	0	1	2	3
15. Overly sensitive	0	1	2	3
16. Exaggerates abilities or achievements	0	1	2	3
17. Explosive, easily angered	0	1	2	3
18. Has rituals such as head rolling or floor pacing	0	1	2	3
19. Fails to finish things he/she starts	0	1	2	3
20. Feelings easily hurt	0	1	2	3
21. Feels others are against him/her	0	1	2	3
22. Harms self by scratching skin or pulling hair	0	1	2	3
23. Feels worthless or inferior	0	1	2	3
24. Fidgets, wiggles, or squirms	0	1	2	3
25. Shy around others; bashful	0	1	2	3
26. Gets in physical fights	0	1	2	3
27. Irritable	0	1	2	3
28. Repeatedly flaps or waves hands, fingers or objects (such as pieces of string)	0	1	2	3
29. Isolates self from others	0	1	2	3
30. Lying or cheating	0	1	2	3

31. Nervous or tense	0	1	2	3
32. Gouges self, puts things in ears, nose, etc., or eats inedible things	0	1	2	3
33. Overactive, doesn't sit still	0	1	2	3
34. Overly anxious to please others	0	1	2	3
35. Overly excited, exuberant	0	1	2	3
36. Physically attacks people	0	1	2	3
37. Refuses to talk	0	1	2	3
38. Repeats the same sound, word, or phrase over and over	0	1	2	3
39. Restless, high energy level	0	1	2	3
40. Runs away from adults, teachers, or other authority figures	0	1	2	3
41. Says no one likes him/her	0	1	2	3
42. Secretive, keeps things to self	0	1	2	3
43. Repeatedly bites self hard enough to leave tooth marks or break skin	0	1	2	3
44. Self-conscious or easily embarrassed	0	1	2	3
45. Shifts rapidly from topic to topic when talking	0	1	2	3
46. Short attention span	0	1	2	3
47. Shy or timid behavior	0	1	2	3
48. Steals	0	1	2	3
49. Odd repetitive behaviors (e.g., stares, grimaces, rigid postures)	0	1	2	3
50. Stubborn, has to do things own way	0	1	2	3
51. Sudden changes in mood	0	1	2	3
52. Sulks, is silent and moody	0	1	2	3
53. Physically harms or hurts self on purpose	0	1	2	3
54. Talks back to teacher, parents, or other adults	0	1	2	3
55. Talks too much or too loud	0	1	2	3
56. Temper tantrums	0	1	2	3
57. Threatens people	0	1	2	3
58. Threatens to harm self	0	1	2	3
59. Engages in meaningless, repetitive body movements	0	1	2	3
60. Too fearful or anxious	0	1	2	3
61. Underactive, slow	0	1	2	3
62. Unhappy or sad	0	1	2	3
63. Violates rules	0	1	2	3
64. Withdrawn, uninvolved with others	0	1	2	3
65. Worrying	0	1	2	3
66. Argues with other children or peers	0	1	2	3

Developed by M. G. Aman, M. J. Tassé, J. Rojahn, and D. Hammer, 1995.

Aman, M.G., Tassé, M.J., Rojahn, J., & Hammer, D. (1996). The Nisonger CBRF: A child behavior rating form for children with developmental disabilities. *Research in Developmental Disabilities, 17*, 41–57.

Tassé, M.J., Aman, M.G., Hammer, D., & Rojahn, J. (1996). The Nisonger Child Behavior Rating Form: Age and gender effects and norms. *Research in Developmental Disabilities, 17*, 59–75.

Agreement and Instructions

We are happy to provide copies of the Nisonger Child Behavior Rating Form (NCBRF) to clinicians and researchers. However, in doing so, we ask that users of the scale abide by the following guidelines.

1. Please do not alter the appearance, wording, or scoring system without prior agreement of the developers, Michael Aman (aman.1@osu.edu) or Marc Tassé (marc.tasse@cdl.unc.edu).

2. For consistency world-wide, we ask that all users employ colored paper to differentiate the two versions of the NCBRF. The Parent version *and score sheet* should be copied onto **blue** paper. The teacher version and score sheet should be copied onto **pink** paper. This is very important, because the scoring systems differ slightly for the two versions. The color coding helps users to employ the correct score sheet.

3. We ask that researchers who employ the NCBRF for research studies cite the two developmental papers in any papers or publications. The original articles describing the NCBRF are as follows:

   Aman, M.G., Tassé, M.J., Rojahn, J., & Hammer, D. (1996). The Nisonger CBRF: A child behavior rating form for children with developmental disabilities. *Research in Developmental Disabilities, 17*, 41–57.
   Tassé, M.J., Aman, M.G., Hammer, D., & Rojahn, J. (1996). The Nisonger Child Behavior Rating Form: Age and gender effects and norms. *Research in Developmental Disabilities, 17*, 59–75.

4. We suggest that workers who receive electronic versions of the NCBRF contact us for an original copy of all materials, including the original publications, the actual rating scales and score sheets (to ensure that formatting is correct), background information on the NCBRF, and–if needed–more extensive normative data.

We thank you for observing these requests.

Michael Aman, Ph.D.
Ohio State University

and

Marc Tassé
University of North Carolina

Pediatric Quality of Life Enjoyment and Satisfaction Questionnaire (PQ-LES-Q)* Jean Endicott, Ph.D**

This questionnaire is designed to help assess the degree of enjoyment and satisfaction experienced during the past week.

Name _____ ID# __ __ __ __ __ __ Date: __ __ / __ __ / __ __

Sex: 1 - Male,   2 - Female   Age: ___ ___

Study # ___ ___   Group: ___ ___ ___

*The Pediatric Q-LES-Q is designed to be used with children and adolescents. The content of the Short Form of the Quality of Life Enjoyment and Satisfaction Questionnaire was modified to be appropriate for ages 6 to 17.

**The PQ-LES-Q was developed with the assistance of a group of clinicians, including several child psychiatrists. It is available from Jean Endicott, Ph.D., Department of Research Assessment and Training, Unit 123, 1051 Riverside Drive, New York, New York 10032.

(Under Copyright).

INSTRUCTIONS: This survey asks for your views about your general health, well-being, and feelings about your life. Please answer EVERY question by circling the number for your response. If you are not sure about how to answer a question, please give the best answer you can. Remember, there are no right or wrong answers.

Over the past week, how have things been with . . .	Very Poor	Poor	Fair	Good	Very Good
1) . . . your health?	1	2	3	4	5
2) . . . your mood or feelings?	1	2	3	4	5
3) . . . school or learning?	1	2	3	4	5
4) . . . helping out at home?	1	2	3	4	5
5) . . . getting along with friends?	1	2	3	4	5
6) . . . getting along with your family?	1	2	3	4	5
7) . . . play or free time?	1	2	3	4	5
8) . . . getting things done?	1	2	3	4	5
9) . . . your love or affection?	1	2	3	4	5
10) . . . getting or buying things?	1	2	3	4	5
11) . . . the place where you live?	1	2	3	4	5
12) . . . paying attention?	1	2	3	4	5
13) . . . your energy level?	1	2	3	4	5
14) . . . feelings about yourself?	1	2	3	4	5
15) . . . Overall, how has your life been?	1	2	3	4	5

Appendix 5.
Parent Support Resources

General Mental Health Resources for Children and Adolescents

American Academy of Child and Adolescent Psychiatry
3615 Wisconsin Avenue, N.W.
Washington, DC 20016-3007
Fax: 202-966-2891
Web: www.aacap.org

American Academy of Pediatrics
141 Northwest Point Boulevard
Elk Grove Village, Illinois 60007-1098
Phone: 847-434-4000
Fax: 847-434-8000
Web: www.aap.org

National Institute of Mental Health
NIMH Public Inquiries
6001 Executive Bloulevard
Room 8184 MSC 9663
Bethesda, Maryland 20892
Phone: 301-443-4513
Web: http://www.nimh.nih.gov/

National Alliance for the Mentally Ill (NAMI)
Colonial Place Three
2107 Wilson Bloulevard, Suite 300
Arlington, VA 22201-3042
Phone: 703-524-7600
HelpLine: 800-950-6264
Web: www.nami.org

U.S. Food and Drug Administration
Web: www.fda.gov

Attention-Deficit/Hyperactivity Disorder

Children and Adults with Attention-Deficit/Hyperactivity Disorder (CHADD)
8181 Professional Place
Suite 201
Landover, Maryland 20785
Phone: 301-306-7090 or 800-233-4050
Fax: 301-306-7090
Web: www.chadd.org

National Attention Deficit Disorder Association (ADDA)
1788 Second Street
Suite 200
Highland Park, Illinois 60035
Phone: 847-432-ADDA
Fax: 847-432-5874
Web: www.add.org

Bipolar Disorder

Bipolar Disorders Information Center
http://www.mhsource.com/bipolar/

Depression

Depression in Children and Adolescents
http://www.psycom.net/depression.central.children.html

Independent Herbal and Alternative Medication Internet Sites

- The Office of Dietary Supplements at NIH:
  http://ods.od.nih.gov/databases/ibids.html
- University of Pittsburg Complementary Medicine
  www.pitt.edu/~cbw/database.html
- The American Botanical Council:
  www.herbalgram.org
- National Center for Complementary and Alternative Medicine Clearinghouse:
  http://nccam.nih.gov/health/clearinghouse/index.htm

Learning Disabilities

National Center for Learning Disabilities
381 Park Avenue, South
Suite 1401
New York, New York 10016

Phone: 212-545-7510
Fax: 212-545-9665
Web: www.ncld.org

Mental Retardation

Kids Health Mental Retardation
http://www.kidshealth.org/kid/health_problems/birth_defect/mental_retardation.html

Obsessive–Compulsive Disorder

Obsessive-Compulsive Foundation, Inc.
337 Notch Hill Road
North Branford, CT 06471
Phone: 203-315-2190
Fax: 203-315-2196
E-mail: info@ocfoundation.org
Web: http://www.familymanagement.com/facts/english/facts60.html

Tic Disorders and Tourette's Disorder

Tourette Syndrome Association, Inc.
42-40 Bell Boulevard
Bayside, New York 11361-2820
Phone: 718-224-2999
Fax: 718-279-9596
E-mail: tourette@ix.netcom.com
Web: http://www.aacap.org/publications/factsfam/tics.htm

Bibliography

INTRODUCTION TO PEDIATRIC PSYCHOPHARMACOLOGY

Bradley C. The behavior of children receiving benzedrine. *American Journal of Orthopsychiatry* 9:577–585, 1937.

Connor DF. Preschool attention deficit hyperactivity disorder: A review of prevalence, diagnosis, neurobiology, and stimulant treatment. *J Dev Behav Pediatr* 23:S1–S9, 2002.

Connor DF, Ozbayrak KR, Harrison RJ, et al. Prevalence and patterns of psychotropic and anticonvulsant medication use in children and adolescents referred to residential treatment. *J Child Adolesc Psychopharmacol* 8(1):27–38, 1998.

Connor DF, Ozbayrak KR, Kusiak KA, et al. Combined pharmacotherapy in children and adolescents in a residential treatment center. *J Am Acad Child Adolesc Psychiatry* 36(2):248–254, 1997.

Green WH. *Child and Adolescent Clinical Psychopharmacology* (3rd ed.). Philadelphia: Lippincott, Williams & Wilkins, 2001.

Greenhill LL, Jensen PS, Abikoff H, et al. Developing strategies for psychopharmacological studies of preschool children. *J Am Acad Child Adolesc Psychiatry* 42(4): 406–414, 2003.

Hoagwood K, Kelleher KJ, Feil M, et al. Treatment services for children with ADHD: A national perspective. *J Am Acad Child Adolesc Psychiatry* 39:198–206, 2000.

Jensen PS, Bhatara VS, Vitiello B, et al. Psychoactive medication prescribing practices for U.S. children: Gaps between research and clinical practice. *J Am Acad Child Adolesc Psychiatry* 38:557–565, 1999.

Jensen PS, Edelman A, Nemeroff R. Pediatric psychopharmacoepidemiology: Who is prescribing? And for whom, how, and why? In: Martin A, Scahill L, Charney DS, Leckman JF (Eds.), *Pediatric Psychopharmacology Principles and Practice*. New York: Oxford University Press, pp. 701–724, 2003.

Laughren TP. Regulatory issues. In: Martin A, Scahill L, Charney DS, and Leckman JF (Eds.), *Pediatric Psychopharmacology Principles and Practice*. New York: Oxford University Press, pp. 725–736, 2003.

Nurcombe B, Partlett DF. *Child Mental Health and the Law*. New York: Free Press, pp. 220–272, 1994.

615

Pincus HA, Tanielian TL, Marcus SC, et al. Prescribing trends in psychotropic medications: Primary care, psychiatry, and other medical specialties. *JAMA* 279:526–531, 1998.

Popper C. Medical unknowns and ethical consent: Prescribing psychotropic medications for children in the face of uncertainty. In: Popper C (Ed.), *Psychiatric Pharmacosciences of Children and Adolescents*. Washington, DC: American Psychiatric Press, pp. 127–161, 1987.

Rappley MD, Mullan PB, Alvarez FJ, et al. Diagnosis of attention deficit/hyperactivity disorder and use of psychotropic medication in very young children. *Arch Pediatr Adolesc Med* 153:1039–1045, 1999.

Riddle MA, Labellarte MJ, Walkup JT. Pediatric psychopharmacology: Problems and prospects. *J Child Adolesc Psychopharmacol* 8:87–97, 1998.

Rivera-Calimlim L, Griesbach PH, Perlmutter R. Plasma chlorpromazine concentrations in children with behavioral disorders and mental illness. *Clin Pharmacol Ther* 26:114–121, 1979.

Roberts R, Rodriguez W, Murphy D, et al. Pediatric drug labeling: Improving the safety and efficacy of pediatric therapeutics. *JAMA* 290(7):905–911, 2003.

Safer DJ, Zito JM, Dos Reis S. Concomitant psychotropic medications for youths. *Am J Psychiatry* 160(3):438–449, 2003.

Schouten R, Duckworth KS. Medicolegal and ethical issues in the pharmacologic treatment of children. In: Werry J and Aman M (Eds.), *Practitioner's Guide to Psychoactive Drugs for Children and Adolescents* (2nd ed.). New York: Plenum Press, pp. 165–181, 1999.

Shaffer D, Fisher P, Dulcan M, et al. The second version of the NIMH diagnostic interview schedule for children (DISC-2). *J Am Acad Child Adolesc Psychiatry* 35:865–877, 1996.

Short EJ, Manos MJ, Findling RL, et al. A prospective study of stimulant response in preschool children: Insights from ROC analyses. *J Am Acad Child Adolesc Psychiatry* 43(3):251–259, 2004.

Zito JM, Safer DJ. Recent child pharmacoepidemiological findings. *J Child Adolesc Psychopharmacol* 15(1):5–9, 2005.

Zito JM, Safer DJ, dosReis S, et al. Trends in the prescribing of psychotropic medications to preschoolers. *JAMA* 283:1025–1030, 2000.

Zito JM, Safer DJ, Riddle MA, et al. Prevalence variations in psychotropic treatment of children. *J Child Adolesc Psychopharmacol* 8:99–105, 1998.

BASIC PHARMACOLOGY

Blanco JG, Harrison PL, Evans WE, et al. Human cytochrome P450 maximal activities in pediatric versus adult liver. *Drug Metab Dispos* 28:379–382, 2000.

Kauffman RE, Kearns GL. Pharmacokinetic studies in paediatric patients: Clinical and ethical considerations. *Clin Pharmacokinet* 23:10–29, 1992.

Osterheld JR. A review of developmental aspects of cytochrome P450. *J Child Adolesc Psychopharmacol* 8:161–174, 1998.

Osterheld JR, Flockhart DA. Pharmacokinetics II: Cytochrome P450-mediated drug interactions. In: Martin A, Scahill L, Charney DS, Leckman JF (Eds.), *Pediatric Psychopharmacology Principles and Practice*. New York: Oxford University Press, pp. 54–66, 2003.

Paxton JW, Dragunow M. Pharmacology. In: Werry J and Aman M (Eds.), *Practitioner's Guide to Psychoactive Drugs* (2nd ed.). New York: Plenum Press, pp. 23–50, 1999.

Vinks AA, Walson PD. Pharmacokinetics I: Developmental principles. In: Martin A, Scahill L, Charney DS, and Leckman JF (Eds.), *Pediatric Psychopharmacology Principles and Practice*. New York: Oxford University Press, pp. 44–53, 2003.

GENERAL PRINCIPLES OF TREATMENT

Achenbach TM. *Manual for the Child Behavior Checklist/4–18 and 1991 profile.* Burlington, VT: University of Vermont Department of Psychiatry, 1991.

Chess S, Thomas A. *Temperament in Clinical Practice.* New York: Guilford Press, 1986.

Conners CK. *Conners Rating Scales—Revised: Technical Manual.* North Tonawanda, NY: Multihealth Systems, 1997.

Connor DF. *Aggression and Antisocial Behavior in Children and Adolescents: Research and Treatment.* New York: Guilford Press, pp. 308–313, 2002.

Connor DF, Fisher SG. An interactional model of child and adolescent mental health clinical case formulation. *Clin Child Psychol Psychiatry* 2(3):353–368, 1997.

Hendren RL, Hamarman S. Clinical assessment of children and adolescents treated pharmacologically. In: Martin A, Scahill L, Charney DS, Leckman JF (Eds.), *Pediatric Psychopharmacology Principles and Practice*. New York: Oxford University Press, pp. 391–403, 2003.

Lachar D, Gruber CP. *Manual for Personality Inventory for Children—Revised.* Los Angeles: Western Psychological Services, 1991.

Moss NE, Racusin GR. Psychological assessment of children and adolescents. In: Lewis M (Ed.), *Child and Adolescent Psychiatry: A Comprehensive Textbook* (3rd ed.). Philadelphia: Lippincott, Williams & Wilkins, pp. 555–572, 2002.

Naglieri JA, LeBuffe PA, Pfeiffer SI. *Devereux Scales of Mental Disorders Manual.* San Antonio, TX: Psychological Corporation, 1994.

Pruett KD, Martin A. Thinking about prescribing: The psychology of psychopharmacology. In: Martin A, Scahill L, Charney DS, Leckman JF (Eds.), *Pediatric Psychopharmacology Principles and Practice*. New York: Oxford University Press, pp. 417–425, 2003.

Reynolds CR, Kamphaus RW. *The Behavior Assessment System for Children.* Circle Pines, MN: American Guidance Service, 1992.

Zametkin AJ, Yamada EM. Monitoring and measuring drug effects. I. Physical effects. In: Werry JS, Aman MG (Eds.), *Practitioner's Guide to Psychoactive Drugs for Children and Adolescents* (2nd ed.). New York: Plenum Press, pp. 69–97, 1999.

STIMULANTS

American Academy of Child and Adolescent Psychiatry. Practice parameters for the assessment and treatment of attention-deficit hyperactivity disorder. *J Am Acad Child Adolesc Psychiatry* 36(10 Suppl):85S–121S, 1997.

American Academy of Child and Adolescent Psychiatry. Practice parameters for the use of stimulant medications in the treatment of children, adolescent, and adults. *J Am Acad Child Adolesc Psychiatry* 41(2 Suppl):26S–49S, 2002.

American Academy of Pediatrics: Committee on Children with Disabilities and Committee on Drugs. Medication for children with attentional disorders. *Pediatrics* 98: 301–304, 1996.

BIBLIOGRAPHY

Barkley RA, DuPaul GJ, and Connor DF. Stimulants. In: Werry JS, Aman MG (Eds.), *Practitioner's Guide to Psychoactive Drugs for Children and Adolescents* (2nd ed.). New York: Plenum, Press, pp. 213–247, 1999.

Cantwell DP, Swanson J, Connor DF. Case study: Adverse response to clonidine. *J Am Acad Child Adolesc Psychiatry* 36(4):539–544, 1997.

Connor DF. Other medications in the treatment of child and adolescent ADHD. In: Barkley RA (Ed.), *Attention-Deficit Hyperactivity Disorder: A Handbook for Diagnosis and Treatment* (2nd ed.). New York: Guilford, Press, pp. 564–581, 1998.

Connor DF, Glatt SJ, Lopez ID, Jackson D, Melloni, Jr. RH. Psychopharmacology and aggression. I. A meta-analysis of stimulant effects on overt/covert aggression-related behaviors in ADHD. *J Am Acad Child Adolesc Psychiatry* 41:253–261, 2002.

Connor DF, Steingard RJ. New formulations of stimulants for attention-deficit hyperactivity disorder: Therapeutic potential. *CNS Drugs* 18(14):1011–1030, 2004.

Dulcan MK, Lizarralde C (Eds.). *Helping Parents, Youth, and Teachers Understand Medications for Behavioral and Emotional Problems* (2nd ed.). Washington DC: American Psychiatric Press, pp. 75–80, 2003.

Elia J, Borcherding BG, Rapoport JL, Keysor CS. Methylphenidate and dextroamphetamine treatments of hyperactivity: Are there true nonresponders? *Psychiatry Res* 36(2):141–155, 1991.

Ford RE, Greenhill L, Posner K. Stimulants. In: Martin A, Scahill L, Charney DS, Leckman JF (Eds.), *Pediatric Psychopharmacology Principles and Practice*. New York: Oxford University Press, pp. 255–263, 2003.

Green WH. *Child and Adolescent Clinical Psychopharmacology* (3rd ed.). Philadelphia: Lippincott, Williams & Williams, 2001.

Greenhill LL, Halperin JM, Abikoff H. Stimulant medications. *J Am Acad Child Adolesc Psychiatry* 38(5):503–512, 1999.

Greenhill LL, Osman BB (Eds.). *Ritalin: Theory and Practice* (2nd ed.). New York: Mary Ann Liebert, 1999.

Klein-Schwartz W, McGrath J. Poison centers' experience with methylphenidate abuse in pre-teens and adolescents. *J Am Acad Child Adolesc Psychiatry* 42(3):288–294, 2003.

Multimodal Treatment of ADHD (MTA) Group. 14-month randomized clinical trial of treatment strategies for attention deficit hyperactivity disorder. *Arch Gen Psychiatry* 56:1073–1086, 1999.

Rosenberg DR. Psychostimulants. In: Rosenberg DR, Davanzo PA, Gershon S (Eds.), *Pharmacotherapy for Child and Adolescent Psychiatric Disorders* (2nd ed.). New York: Marcel Dekker, pp. 113–167, 2002.

Short EJ, Manos MJ, Findling RL, et al. A prospective study of stimulant reponse in preschool children: Insights from ROC analyses. *J Am Acad Child Adolesc Psychiatry* 43:251–259, 2004.

Spencer T, Biederman J, Wilens T. Pharmacotherapy of attention deficit hyperactivity disorder. *Child Adolesc Psychiatr Clin N Am* 9(1):77–97, 2000.

Spencer T, Biederman J, Wilens T, Harding M, O'Donnell D, Griffin S. Pharmacotherapy of attention-deficit hyperactivity disorder across the life cycle. *J Am Acad Child Adolesc Psychiatry* 35(4):409–432, 1996.

Spencer T, Wilens T, Biederman J, Faraone SV, Ablon JS, Lapey K. A double-blind, crossover comparison of methylphenidate and placebo in adults with childhood-onset attention-deficit hyperactivity disorder. *Arch Gen Psychiatry* 52(6):434–443, 1995.

Waslick B, Greenhill F. Attention-deficit/hyperactivity disorder. In: Weiner JM (Ed.), *Textbook of Child and Adolescent Psychiatry* (2nd ed.). Washington, DC: American Psychiatric Press, pp. 398–410, 1997.

Wilens, TE. *Straight Talk about Psychiatric Medications for Kids.* New York: Guilford Press, 2001.

Zito J, Safer D, dosReis S, Gardiner J, Magder LS, Soeken K, Boles M, Lynch F, Riddle MA. Psychotropic practice patterns for youth: A 10-year perspective. *Arch Peds Adolesc Med* 157:17–25, 2003.

ANTIDEPRESSANTS

American Academy of Child and Adolescent Psychiatry. Practice parameters for the assessment and treatment of children and adolescents with depressive disorder. *J Am Acad Child Adolesc Psychiatry* 37(10 Suppl):63S–83S, 1998.

Appelberg BG, Syvalahti EK, Koskinen TE, et al. Patients with severe depression may benefit from buspirone augmentation of selective serotonin reuptake inhibitors: Results from a placebo-controlled, randomized, double-blind, placebo wash-in study. *J Clin Psychiatry* 62(6):448–452, 2001.

Beasley CM Jr, Koke SC, Nilsson ME, Gonzales JS. Adverse events and treatment discontinuations in clinical trials of fluoxetine in major depressive disorder: An updated meta-analysis. *Clin Ther* 22(11):1319–1330, 2000.

Beasley CM Jr, Nilsson ME, Koke SC, Gonzales JS. Efficacy, adverse events, and treatment discontinuations in fluoxetine clinical studies of major depression: A meta-analysis of the 20-mg/day dose. *J Clin Psychiatry* 61(10):722–728, 2000.

Birmaher B, Brent D. Depressive disorders. In: Martin A, Scahill L, Charney DS, Leckman JF (Eds.), *Pediatric Psychopharmacology Principles and Practice.* New York: Oxford University Press, pp. 466–483, 2003.

Birmaher B, Ryan ND, Williamson DE, et al. Childhood and adolescent depression: A review of the past 10 years. Part I. *J Am Acad Child Adolesc Psychiatry* 35:1427–1439, 1996.

Birmaher B, Waterman GS, Ryan ND, et al. Randomized, controlled trial of amitriptyline versus placebo for adolescents with "treatment-resistant" major depression. *J Am Acad Child Adolesc Psychiatry* 37(5):527–535, 1998.

Braconnier A, Le Coent R, Cohen D, DEROXADO Study Group. Paroxetine versus clomipramine in adolescents with severe major depression: A double-blind, randomized, multicenter trial. *J Am Acad Child Adolesc Psychiatry* 42(1):22–29, 2003.

Brent J. Monoamine oxidase inhibitors and the serotonin syndrome. In: Haddad LM, Shannon MW, Winchester JF (Eds.), *Clinical Management of Poisoning and Drug Overdose* (3rd ed.). Philadelphia: W.B. Saunders, pp. 459–463, 1998.

Brown WA, Harrison W. Are patients who are intolerant to one serotonin selective reuptake inhibitor intolerant to another? *J Clin Psychiatry* 56:30–34, 1995.

Casat CD, Pleasants DZ, Van Wyck, et al. A double-blind trial of bupropion in children with attention deficit disorder. *Psychopharmacol Bull* 23(1):120–122, 1987.

Cook EH, Wagner KD, March JS, et al. Long-term sertraline treatment of children and adolescents with obsessive–compulsive disorder. *J Am Acad Child Adolesc Psychiatry* 40(10):1175–1181, 2001.

Cornelius JR, Bukstein OG, Birmaher B, et al. Fluoxetine in adolescents with major depression and an alcohol use disorder: An open-label trial. *Addict Behav* 26(5): 735–739, 2001.

Dalack GW, Glassman AH, Rivelli S, et al. Mood, major depression, and fluoxetine response in cigarette smokers. *Am J Psychiatry* 152(3):398–403, 1995.

Davis WB, Bentivoglio P, Racusin R, et al. Bupropion sustained release in adolescents with comorbid attention-deficit/hyperactivity disorder and depression. *J Am Acad Child Adolesc Psychiatry* 40(3):307–314, 2001.

DeGatta MF, Garcia MJ, Acosta A, et al. Monitoring of serum levels of imipramine and desipramine and individuation of dose in enuretic children. *Ther Drug Monit* 6:438–443, 1984.

Emslie GJ, Heiligenstein JH, Hoog SL, et al. Fluoxetine treatment for prevention of relapse of depression in children and adolescents: A double-blind, placebo-controlled study. *J Am Acad Child Adolesc Psychiatry* 43(11):1397–1405, 2004.

Emslie GJ, Heiligenstein JH, Wagner KD, et al. Fluoxetine for acute treatment of depression in children and adolescents: A placebo-controlled, randomized clinical trial. *J Am Acad Child Adolesc Psychiatry* 41(10):1205–1215, 2002.

Emslie GJ, Rush AJ, Weinberg WA, et al. A double-blind, randomized, placebo-controlled trial of fluoxetine in children and adolescents with depression. *Arch Gen Psychiatry* 54(11):1031–1037, 1997.

Findling RL, Preskorn SH, Marcus RN, Magnus RD, D'Amico F, Marathe P, Reed MD. Nefazodone pharmacokinetics in depressed children and adolescents. *J Am Acad Child Adolesc Psychiatry* 39(8):1008–1016, 2000.

Geller DA, Biederman J, Stewart SE, et al. Impact of comorbidity on treatment response to paroxetine in pediatric obsessive–compulsive disorder: Is the use of exclusion criteria empirically supported in randomized clinical trials? *J Child Adolesc Psychopharmacol* 13(Suppl 1):S19–29, 2003.

Geller B, Cooper TB, Chestnut EC, et al. Child and adolescent nortriptyline single dose kinetics predict steady state plasma levels and suggested dose: Preliminary data. *J Clin Psychopharmacol* 5:154–158, 1985.

Geller B, Cooper TB, Graham DL, et al. Double-blind placebo-controlled study of nortriptyline in depressed adolescents using a "fixed plasma level" design. *Psychopharmacol Bull* 26(1):85–90, 1990.

Geller DA, Hoog SL, Heiligenstein JH, et al. Fluoxetine Pediatric OCD Study Team. Fluoxetine treatment for obsessive–compulsive disorder in children and adolescents: A placebo-controlled clinical trial. *J Am Acad Child Adolesc Psychiatry* 40(7):773–779, 2001.

Geller DA, Wagner KD, Emslie G, et al. Paroxetine treatment in children and adolescents with obsessive–compulsive disorder: A randomized, multicenter, double-blind, placebo-controlled trial. *J Am Acad Child Adolesc Psychiatry* 43(11):1387–1396, 2004.

Green WH. *Child and Adolescent Clinical Psychopharmacology* (3rd ed.). Philadelphia: Lippincott, Williams & Wilkins, 2001.

Gundersen K, Geller B. Antidepressants II: Tricyclic agents. In: Martin A, Scahill L, Charney DS, and Leckman JF (Eds.), *Pediatric Psychopharmacology Principles and Practice*. New York: Oxford University Press, pp. 284–294, 2003.

Gutgessel H, Atkins D, Barst R, et al. AHA scientific statement: Cardiovascular monitoring of children and adolescents receiving psychiatric drugs. *J Am Acad Child Adolesc Psychiatry* 38:1047–1050, 1999.

Joffe RT, et al. Response to an open trial of a second SSRI in major depression. *J Clin Psychiatry* 57:114–115, 1996.

Keller MB, Ryan ND, Strober M, et al. Efficacy of paroxetine in the treatment of adolescent major depression: A randomized, controlled trial. *J Am Acad Child Adolesc Psychiatry* 40(7):762–772, 2001.

Klein RG, Mannuzza S, Koplewicz HS, Tancer NK, Shah M, Liang V, Davies M. Adolescent depression: Controlled desipramine treatment and atypical features. *Depress Anxiety* 7(1):15–31, 1998.

Kramer AD, Feiguine RJ. Clinical effects of amitriptyline in adolescent depression: A pilot study. *J Am Acad Child Psychiatry* 20(3):636–644, 1981.

Kutcher S, Boulos C, Ward B, et al. Response to desipramine treatment in adolescent depression: A fixed-dose, placebo-controlled trial. *J Am Acad Child Adolesc Psychiatry* 33(5):686–694, 1994.

Kye CH, Waterman GS, Ryan ND, et al. A randomized, controlled trial of amitriptyline in the acute treatment of adolescent major depression. *J Am Acad Child Adolesc Psychiatry* 35(9):1139–1144, 1996.

Liebowitz MR, Turner SM, Piacentini J, et al. Fluoxetine in children and adolescents with OCD: A placebo-controlled trial. *J Am Acad Child Adolesc Psychiatry* 41(12): 1431–1438, 2002.

March JS, Biederman J, Wolkow R, et al. Sertraline in children and adolescents with obsessive–compulsive disorder: A multicenter randomized controlled trial. *JAMA* 280(20):1752–1756, 1998.

March J S, Silva S, Petrycki S, Curry J, Wells K, Fairbank J, Burns B, Domino M, McNulty S, Vitiello B, Severe J. Fluoxetine, cognitive–behavioral therapy, and their combination for adolescents with depression: Treatment for Adolescents with Depression Study (TADS) randomized controlled trial. *JAMA* 292(7):807–820, 2004.

The Medical Letter. Duloxetine (*Cymbalta*): A new SNRI for depression. *Med Letter* 46 (1193):81–82, 2004.

Milin RP, Simeon J, Spenst WP. Paroxetine in the treatment of children and adolescents with major depression. Poster NR67:104–105, presented at the 46th annual meeting of the American Academy of Child and Adolescent Psychiatry, Chicago, IL, October 19–21, 1999.

Mills KC. Serotonin syndrome: A clinical update. *Crit Care Clin* 13(4):763–783, 1997.

Pediatric OCD Treatment Study (POTS) Team. Cognitive–behavioral therapy, sertraline, and their combination for children and adolescents with obsessive–compulsive disorder: The Pediatric OCD Treatment Study (POTS) randomized controlled trial. *JAMA* 292(16):1969–1976, 2004.

Preskorn SH, Bupp SJ, Weller EB, et al. Plasma levels of imipramine and metabolites in 68 hospitalized children. *J Am Acad Child Adolesc Psychiatry* 28:373–375, 1989.

Prince JB, Wilens TE, Biederman J, et al. A controlled study of nortriptyline in children and adolescents with attention deficit hyperactivity disorder. *J Child Adolesc Psychopharmacol* 10(3):193–204, 2000.

Riddle MA, Reeve EA, Yaryura-Tobias JA, et al. Fluvoxamine for children and adolescents with obsessive–compulsive disorder: A randomized, controlled, multicenter trial. *J Am Acad Child Adolesc Psychiatry* 40(2):222–229, 2001.

Riddle MA, Scahill L, King RA, et al. Double-blind, crossover trial of fluoxetine and placebo in children and adolescents with obsessive–compulsive disorder. *J Am Acad Child Adolesc Psychiatry* 31(6):1062–1069, 1992.

Rosenbaum JF, Fava M, Hoog SL, et al. Selective serotonin reuptake inhibitor discontinuation syndrome: A randomized clinical trial. *Biol Psychiatry* 44(2):77–87, 1998.

Rynn MA, Siqueland L, Rickels K. Placebo-controlled trial of sertraline in the treatment of children with generalized anxiety disorder. *Am J Psychiatry* 158(12):2008–2014, 2001.

Schatzberg AF, Haddad P, Kaplan EM, et al. Possible biological mechanisms of the serotonin reuptake inhibitor discontinuation syndrome: Discontinuation Consensus Panel. In: Shader RI (Ed.), *Manual of Psychiatric Therapeutics* (3rd ed.). Philadelphia: Lippincott, Williams & Wilkins, pp. 240–270, 2003.

Simeon JG, Dinicola VF, Ferguson HB, et al. Adolescent depression: A placebo-controlled fluoxetine treatment study and follow-up. *Prog Neuropsychopharmacol Biol Psychiatry* 14(5):791–795, 1990.

Soares JC, Gershon S. Prospects for the development of new treatments with a rapid onset of action in affective disorders. *Drugs* 52:477–482, 1996.

B
I
B
L
I
O
G
R
A
P
H
Y

TADS (Treatment for Adolescents with Depression) Study, March et al. Fluoxetine, cognitive–behavioral therapy, and their combination for adolescents with depression: Treatment for Adolescents with Depression Study (TADS) randomized controlled trial. *JAMA* 292(7):807–820, 2004.

Thase ME, Greenhouse JB, Frank E, et al. Treatment of major depression with psychotherapy or psychotherapy–pharmacotherapy combinations. *Arch Gen Psychiatry* 54:1009, 1997.

Varley CK, McClellan J. Case study: Two additional sudden deaths with tricyclic antidepressants. *J Am Acad Child Adolesc Psychiatry* 36:390–394, 1997.

Wagner KD, Ambrosini P, Rynn M, et al. and the Sertraline Pediatric Depression Study Group. Efficacy of sertraline in the treatment of children and adolescents with major depressive disorder: Two randomized controlled trials. *JAMA* 290(8):1033–1041, 2003.

Wagner KD, Berard R, Stein MB, et al. A multicenter, randomized, double-blind, placebo-controlled trial of paroxetine in children and adolescents with social anxiety disorder. *Arch Gen Psychiatry* 61(11):1153–1162, 2004.

Wagner KD, Robb AS, Findling RL, et al. A randomized, placebo-controlled trial of citalopram for the treatment of major depression in children and adolescents. *Am J Psychiatry* 161(6):1079–1083, 2004.

Walkup JT, Ritter-Welzant J, Kastelic E, et al. Antidepressants III: Other agents. In: Martin A, Scahill L, Charney DS, and Leckman JF (Eds.), *Pediatric Psychopharmacology Principles and Practice*. New York: Oxford University Press, pp. 295–308, 2003.

Wilens TE, Biederman J, Baldessarini RJ, et al. Cardiovascular effects of therapeutic doses of tricyclic antidepressants in children and adolescents. *J Am Acad Child Adolesc Psychiatry* 35:1491–1501, 1996.

Wilens TE, Spencer TJ, Biederman J, et al. Case study: Nefazodone for juvenile mood disorders. *J Am Acad Child Adolesc Psychiatry* 36(4):481–485, 1997.

MOOD STABILIZERS

Akiskal HS. Validating 'hard' and 'soft' phenotypes within the bipolar spectrum: continuity or discontinuity? *J Affect Disord.* 73(1–2):1–5, 2003.

Akiskal HS, Bourgeois ML, Angst J, et al. Re-evaluating the prevalence of and diagnostic composition within the broad clinical spectrum of bipolar disorders. *J Affect Disord* 59:S5–S30, 2000.

American Psychiatric Association. *Diagnostic and Statistical Manual of Mental Disorders.*(4th ed., text rev.). Washington, DC: Author, 2000.

Angst J. The emerging epidemiology of hypomania and bipolar II disorder. *J Affect Disord* 50:143–151, 1998.

Baldessarini RJ, Suppes T, Tondo L. Lithium withdrawal in bipolar disorder: Implications for clinical practice and experimental therapeutics research. *Am J Ther* 3(7):492–496, 1996.

Benazzi F. Gender differences in bipolar II and unipolar depressed outpatients: A 557-case study. *Ann Clin Psychiatry* 11:55–59, 1999.

Benedetti A, Lattanzi L, Pini S, et al. Oxcarbazepine as add-on treatment in patients with bipolar manic, mixed, or depressive episode. *J Affect Disord* 79(1–3):273–277, 2004.

Bowden C. The effectiveness of divalproate in all forms of mania and the broader bipolar spectrum: Many questions, few answers. *J Affect Disord* 79(Suppl 1):S9–S14, 2004.

Bowden C, Calabrese J, Sachs G, et al. A placebo-controlled 18-month trial of lamotrigine and lithium maintenance treatment in recently manic or hypomanic patients with bipolar I disorder. *Arch Gen Psychiatry* 60:392–400, 2003.

Bowden CL, Gitlin MJ, Keck PE, et al. Practice guideline for the treatment of patients with bipolar disorder (revision). *Am J Psychiatry* 159(Suppl):18, 2002.

Cabras PL, Hardoy MJ, Hardoy, MC, et al. Clinical experience with gabapentin in patients with bipolar or schizoaffective disorder: Results of an open-label study. *J Clin Psychiatry* 60(4):245–248, 1999.

Calabrese JR, Bowden C, Sachs G, et al. A placebo-controlled 18-month trial of lamotrigine and lithium maintenance treatment in recently depressed patients with bipolar I disorder. *J Clin Psychiatry* 64:1013–1024, 2003.

Calabrese JR, Hirschfeld RMA, Reed M, et al. Impact of bipolar disorder on a U.S. community—sample. *J Clin Psychiatry* 64:425–32, 2003.

Centorrino F, Albert MJ, Berry MJ, et al. Oxcarbazepine: Clinical experience with hospitalized psychiatric patients. *Bipolar Disord* 5(5):370–374, 2003.

Delbello MP, Schwiers ML, Rosenberg HL, et al. A double-blind, randomized, placebo-controlled study of quetiapine as adjunctive treatment for adolescent mania. *J Am Acad Child Adolesc Psychiatry* 41(10):1216–1223, 2002.

Denicoff KD, Smith-Jackson EE, Disney ER, et al. Comparative prophylactic efficacy of lithium, carbamazepine, and the combination in bipolar disorder. *J Clin Psychiatry* 58:470–478, 1997.

DeVane CL, Nemeroff CB. 2000 *Guide to Psychotropic Drug Interactions.* New York: MBL Communications 2000.

Findling RL, McNamara NK, Gracious BL, et al. Combination lithium and divalproex sodium in pediatric bipolarity. *J Am Acad Child Adolesc Psychiatry* 42(8):895–901, 2003.

Frankenburg FR, Tohen M, Cohen BM, et al. Long-term response to carbamazepine: A retrospective study. *J Clin Psychopharmacol* 8:130–132, 1988.

Frye MA, Ketter TA, Kimbrell TA, et al. A placebo-controlled study of lamotrigine and gabapentin monotherapy in refractory mood disorders. *J Clin Psychopharmacol* 20(6):607–614, 2000.

Geller B, Cooper TB, Sun K, et al. Double-blind and placebo-controlled study of lithium for adolescent bipolar disorders with secondary substance dependency. *J Am Acad Child Adolesc Psychiatry* 37(2):171–178, 1998.

Ghaemi SN, Katzow JJ, Desai SP, et al. Gabapentin treatment of mood disorders: A preliminary study. *J Clin Psychiatry* 59(8):426–429, 1998.

Goodwin FK, Jamison KR. *Manic–Depressive Illness.* New York: Oxford University Press, 1990.

Grinspoon L (Ed.). *Psychiatry Update: The American Psychiatric Association Annual Review, Vol. II.* Washington, DC: American Psychiatric Press, pp. 271–292, 1983.

Hantouche EG, Akiskal HS, Lancrenon S, et al. Systematic clinical methodology for validating bipolar-II disorder: Data in mid-stream from a French national multi-site study (EPIDEP). *J Affect Disord* 50:163–173, 1998.

Hirschfeld RMA. Bipolar spectrum disorder: Improving its recognition and diagnosis. *J Clin Psychiatry* 62(Suppl 14):4–9, 2001.

Hirschfeld RMA, Calabrese JR, Weissman MM, et al. Screening for bipolar disorder in the community. *J Clin Psychiatry* 64:53–59, 2003.

Judd LL, Akiskal HS, Schettler PJ, et al. The long-term natural history of the weekly symptomatic status of bipolar I disorder. *Arch Gen Psychiatry* 59:530–537, 2002.

Judd LL, Akiskal HS, Schettler PJ, et al. A prospective investigation of the natural history of the long-term weekly symptomatic status of bipolar II disorder. *Arch Gen Psychiatry* 60(3):261–269, 2003.

Kafantaris V, Coletti DJ, Dicker R, et al. Lithium treatment of acute mania in adolescents: A placebo-controlled discontinuation study. *J Am Acad Child Adolesc Psychiatry* 43(8):984–993, 2004.

BIBLIOGRAPHY

Kleindienst N, Greil W. Differential efficacy of lithium and carbamazepine in the prophylaxis of bipolar disorder: Results of the MAP study. *Neuropsychobiology* 42(Suppl 1):2–10, 2000.

Kowatch RA, Suppes T, Carmody TJ, et al. Effect size of lithium, divalproex sodium, and carbamazepine in children and adolescents with bipolar disorder. *J Am Acad Child Adolesc Psychiatry* 39(6):713–720, 2000.

Licht RW, Vestergaard P, Kessing LV, Larsen JK, Thomsen PH. Psychopharmacological treatment with lithium and antiepileptic drugs: Suggested guidelines from the Danish Psychiatric Association and the Child and Adolescent Psychiatric Association in Denmark. *Acta Psychiatr Scand Suppl* 419:1–22, 2003.

Lish JD, Dime-Meenan S, Whybrow PC, et al. The National Depressive and Manic–Depressive Association (DMDA) survey of bipolar members. *J Affect Disord* 31:281–294, 1994.

Martin R, Kuzniecky R, Ho S, et al. Cognitive effects of topiramate, gabapentin, and lamotrigine in healthy young adults. *Neurology* 52:321–327, 1999.

Maxmen JS, Ward NG. *Psychotropic Drugs Fast Facts* (3rd ed.). New York: Norton, 2002.

McClellan J, Werry J. Practice parameters for the assessment and treatment of adolescents with bipolar disorder. *J Am Acad Child Adolesc Psychiatry* 36(Suppl 10): 157–176, 1997.

Muzina DJ, Calabrese JR. Recent placebo-controlled acute trials in bipolar depression: Focus on methodology. *Int J Neuropsychopharmocol* 6(3):285–291, 2003.

Physician's Desk Reference (58th ed.). Montvale, NJ: Medical Economics, 2004.

Product Information Depakote, 2002. Abbott Laboratories, Abbott Park, IL.

Product Information Eskalith, 2002. GlaxoSmithKline, Pittsburg, PA.

Product Information Lamictal, 2002. GlaxoSmithKline, Pittsburg, PA.

Product Information Tegretol, 2002. Novartis Pharmaceuticals, East Hanover, NJ.

Rana M, Khanzode L, Karnik N, et al. Divalproex sodium in the treatment of pediatric psychiatry disorders. *Expert Rev Neurotherapeutics* 5(2):165–176, 2005.

Rasgon N. The relationship between polycystic ovary syndrome and antiepileptic drugs: a review of the evidence. *J Clin Psychopharmacol* 24(3):322–334, 2004.

Schatzberg AF, Cole JO, DeBattista C. *Manual of Clinical Psychopharmacology* (4th ed.). Washington, DC: American Psychiatric Press, 2003.

Schatzberg AF, DeBattista C. Current psychotropic dosing and monitoring guidelines. *Primary Psychiatry* 9:59–77, 2002.

Suppes T, Dennehy EB, Swann AC, et al. Report of the Texas Consensus Conference Panel on medication treatment of bipolar disorder 2000. *J Clin Psychiatry* 63(4): 288–299, 2002.

Tohen M, Vieta E, Calabrese J, et al. Efficacy of olanzapine and olanzapine–fluoxetine combination in the treatment of bipolar I depression. *Arch Gen Psychiatry* 60(11): 1079–1088, 2003.

Tohen M, Zarate CA Jr, Hennen J, et al. The McLean–Harvard First-Episode Mania study: Prediction of recovery and first recurrence. *Am J Psychiatry* 160:2099–2107, 2003.

Tunnessen WW Jr, Hertz CG. Toxic effects of lithium in newborn infants: A commentary. *J Pediatr* 81(4):804–807, 1972.

Varanka TM, Weller RA, Weller EB, Fristad MA. Lithium treatment of manic episodes with psychotic features in prepubertal children. *Am J Psychiatry* 145(12):1557–1559, 1988.

Wagner KD. Management of bipolar disorder in children and adolescents. *Psychopharmacol Bull* 36:151–159, 2002.

Weissman MM, Bruce LM, Leaf PJ, et al. Affective disorders. In: Robins LN and Regier DA, (Eds.), *Psychiatric Disorders in America: The Epidemiological Catchment Area Study*. New York: Free Press, pp. 53–80, 1991.

Weller EB, Weller RA, Fristad MA. Lithium dosage guide for prepubertal children. *J Am Acad Child Adolesc Psychiatry* 25:92–95, 1986.

Zomberg GL, Pope HG Jr. Treatment of depression in bipolar disorder: New directions for research. *J Clin Psychopharmocol* 13:397–408, 1993.

ANTIPSYCHOTICS

Aman MG, De Smedt G, Derivan A, et al. Double-blind, placebo-controlled study of risperidone for the treatment of disruptive behaviors in children with subaverage intelligence. *Am J Psychiatry* 159:1337–1346, 2002.

Blair J, Scahill L, State M, et al. Electrocardiographic changes in children and adolescents treated with ziprasidone: A prospective study. *J Am Acad Child Adolesc Psychiatry* 44(1):73–79, 2005.

Buitelaar JK, van der Gaag RJ, Cohen-Kettenis P, et al. A randomized controlled trial of risperidone in the treatment of aggression in hospitalized adolescents with subaverage cognitive abilities. *J Clin Psychiatry* 62(4):239–248, 2001.

DelBello MP, Schwiers ML, Rosenberg HL, et al. A double-blind, randomized, placebo-controlled study of quetiapine as adjunctive treatment for adolescent mania. *J Am Acad Child Adolesc Psychiatry* 41(10):1216–1223, 2002.

Findling RL, Blumer J, Kaufman R, et al. Aripiprazole in pediatric conduct disorder: A pilot study [poster]. Presented at the 16th Congress of the European College of Neuropsychopharmacology, Prague, Czech Republic, September 20–24, 2003.

Findling RL, McNamara NK, Branicky LA, et al. A double-blind pilot study of risperidone in the treatment of conduct disorder. *J Am Acad Child Adolesc Psychiatry* 39:509–561, 2000.

Findling RL, McNamara NK, Gracious BL. Antipsychotic agents: Traditional and atypical. In: Martin A, Scahill L, Charney DS, Leckman JF (Eds.), *Pediatric Psychopharmacology Principles and Practice*. New York: Oxford University Press, pp. 328–340, 2003.

Fisman S, Steele M. Use of risperidone in pervasive developmental disorders: a case series. J Child Adolesc Psychopharmacol 6:177–190, 1996.

Frazier JA, Cohen LG, Jacobsen L, et al. Clozapine pharmacokinetics in children and adolescents with childhood-onset schizophrenia. *J Clin Psychopharmacol* 23(1): 87–91, 2003.

Frazier JA, Gordon CT, McKenna K, et al. An open trial of clozapine in 11 adolescents with childhood-onset schizophrenia. *J Am Acad Child Adolesc Psychiatry* 33(5): 658–663, 1994.

Green WH. Antipsychotic drugs. In: Green WH. *Child and Adolescent Clinical Psychopharmacology* (3rd ed.). Philadelphia: Lippincott, Williams & Wilkins, pp. 89–149, 2001.

Grothe DR, Calis KA, Jacobsen L, et al. Olanzapine pharmacokinetics in pediatric and adolescent inpatients with childhood-onset schizophrenia. *J Clin Psychopharmacol* 20(2):220–225, 2000.

Kumra S, Frazier JA, Jacobsen LK, et al. Childhood-onset schizophrenia: A double-blind clozapine–haloperidol comparison. *Arch Gen Psychiatry* 53(12):1090–1097, 1996.

Kumra S, Jacobsen LK, Lenane M, et al. Childhood-onset schizophrenia: An open-label study of olanzapine in adolescents. *J Am Acad Child Adolesc Psychiatry* 37(4):377–385, 1998.

McConville BJ, Arvanitis LA, Thyrum PT, et al. Pharmacokinetics, tolerability, and clinical effectiveness of quetiapine fumarate: An open-label trial in adolescents with psychotic disorders. *J Clin Psychiatry* 61(4):252–260, 2000.

McConville BJ, Carrero L, Sweitzer D, et al. Long-term safety, tolerability, and clinical efficacy of quetiapine in adolescents: An open-label extension trial. *J Child Adolesc Psychopharmacol* 13(1):75–82, 2003.

McCracken JT, McGough J, Shah B, et al. Risperidone in children with autism and serious behavioral problems. *N Engl J Med* 347(5):314–321, 2002.

Misra M, Papakostas GI, Klibanski A. Effects of psychiatric disorders and psychotropic medications on prolactin and bone metabolism. *J Clin Psychiatry* 65:1607–1618, 2004.

Montgomery J, Winterbottom E, Jessani M, et al. Prevalence of hyperprolactinemia in schizophrenia: Association with typical and atypical antipsychotic treatment. *J Clin Psychiatry* 65:1491–1498, 2004.

Mukaddes NM, Abali O. Quetiapine treatment of children and adolescents with Tourette's disorder. *J Child Adolesc Psychopharmacol* 13(3):295–299, 2003.

Physician's Desk Reference (57th ed.). Montvale, NJ: Thompson PDR, pp. 991–995, 2003.

Remschmidt H, Schulz E, Martin PDM. An open trial of clozapine in thirty-six adolescents with schizophrenia. *J Child Adolesc Psychopharmacol* 4:31–41, 1994.

Sallee FR, Kurlan R, Goetz CG, et al. Ziprasidone treatment of children and adolescents with Tourette's syndrome: A pilot study. *J Am Acad Child Adolesc Psychiatry* 39(3):292–299, 2000.

Scahill L, Leckman JF, Schultz RT, et al. A placebo-controlled trial of risperidone in Tourette syndrome. *Neurology* 60(7):1130–1135, 2003.

Shader RI. Approaches to the treatment of schizophrenia. In: Shader RI (Ed.), *Manual of Psychiatric Therapeutics* (3rd ed.). Philadelphia: Lippincott, Williams & Wilkins, pp. 285–314, 2003.

Snyder S. Forty years of neurotransmitters: A personal account. *Arch Gen Psychiatry* 59(11):983–984, 2002.

Van Bellinghen M, de Troch C. Risperidone in the treatment of behavioral disturbances in children and adolescents with borderline intellectual functioning: A double-blind, placebo-controlled pilot trial. *J Child Adolesc Psychopharmacology* 11(1):5–13, 2001.

DRUGS TO TREAT EXTRAPYRAMIDAL SYMPTOMS AND SYNDROMES

Adler LA, Rotrosen J, Edson R, et al. Vitamin E treatment for tardive dyskinesia. Veterans Affairs Cooperative Study #394 Study Group. *Arch Gen Psychiatry* 56(9):836–841, 1999.

Arana GW, Santos AB. Anticholinergics and amantadine. In: Kaplan HI, Sadock BJ (Eds.), *Comprehensive Textbook of Psychiatry* (Vol. 2, 6th ed.). Baltimore: Williams & Wilkins, 1995, pp. 1919–1923.

Boyer WF, Bakalar NH, Lake CR. Anticholinergic prophylaxis of acute haloperidol-induced acute dystonic reactions. *J Clin Psychopharmacol* 7:164–166, 1987.

Caksen H, Odabas D, Anlar O. Use of biperiden hydrochloride in a child with severe dyskinesia induced by phenytoin. *J Child Neuro* 18(7):494–496, 2003.

Camp-Bruno JA, Winsberg BG, Green-Parsons AR, et al. Efficacy of benztropine therapy for drooling. *Dev Med Child Neurol* 31:309–319, 1989.

Dahiya U, Noronha P. Drug-induced acute dystonic reactions in children: Alternatives to diphenhydramine therapy. *Postgrad Med* 75:286–290, 1984.

Eranti VS, Gangadhar BN, Janakiramaiah N. Haloperidol-induced extrapyramidal reaction: Lack of protective effect by vitamin E. *Psychopharmacol* 140(4):418–420, 1998.

Gilbert DL, Sethuraman G, Sine L, et al. Tourette's syndrome improvement with pergolide in a randomized, double-blind, crossover trial. *Neurology* 54(6):1310–1315, 2000.

Goff DC, Arana GW, Greenblatt DJ, et al. The effect of benztropine on haloperidol-induced dystonia, clinical efficacy and pharmacokinetics: A prospective, double-blind trial. *J Clin Psychopharmacol* 11:106–112, 1991.

Gracious BL, Krysiak TE, Yongstrom EA. Amantadine treatment of psychotropic-induced weight gain in children and adolescents: Case series. *J Child Adolesc Psychopharmacol* 12(3):249–257, 2002.

Hoon AH Jr, Freese PO, Reinhardt EM, et al. Age-dependent effects of trihexyphenidyl in extrapyramidal cerebral palsy. *Pediatr Neurol* 25(1):55–58, 2001.

Keepers GA, Clappison VJ, Casey DE. Initial anticholinergic prophylaxis for neuroleptic-induced extrapyramidal syndromes. *Arch Gen Psychiatry* 40(10):1113–1117, 1983.

Kiloh LG, Smith JS, Williams SE. Antiparkinson drugs as causal agents in tardive dyskinesia. *Med J Aust* 2:591–593, 1973.

King BH, Wright DM, Handen BL, et al. Double-blind, placebo-controlled study of amantadine hydrochloride in the treatment of children with autistic disorder. *J Am Acad Child Adolesc Psychiatry* 40(6):658–665, 2001.

Lohr JB, Cadet JL, Lohr MA, et al. Vitamin E in the treatment of tardive dyskinesia: The possible involvement of free radical mechanisms. *Schizophr Bull* 14(2):291–296, 1988.

Lohr JB, Caligiuri MP. A double-blind, placebo-controlled study of vitamin E treatment of tardive dyskinesia. *J Clin Psychiatry* 57(4):167–173, 1996.

Marcus R, Coulston AM. Fat-soluble vitamins. In: Hardman JG, Limbird LE, and Gilman AG (Eds.), *Goodman and Gilman's the Pharmacological Basis of Therapeutics* (10th ed.). New York: McGraw-Hill, pp. 1773–1791, 2001.

Meythaler JM, Brunner RC, Johnson A, et al. Amantadine to improve neurorecovery in traumatic brain injury-associated diffuse axonal injury: A pilot double-blind randomized trial. *J Head Trauma Rehabil* 17(4):300–313, 2002.

Orrego JJ, Chandler WF, Barkan AL. Pergolide as primary therapy for macroprolactinomas. *Pituitary* 3(4):251–256, 2000.

Passler MA, Riggs RV. Positive outcomes in traumatic brain injury-vegetative state: Patients treated with bromocriptine. *Arch Phys Med Rehabil* 82(3):311–315, 2001.

Passos VQ, Souza JJ, Musolino NR, Bronstein MD. Long-term follow-up of prolactinomas: Normoprolactinemia after bromocriptine withdrawal. *J Clin Endocrinol Metab* 87(8): 3578–3582, 2002.

Pezzoli G, Martignoni E, Pacchetti C, et al. Pergolide compared with bromocriptine in Parkinson's disease: A multicenter, crossover, controlled study. *Mov Disord* 9(4):431–436, 1994.

Pranzatelli MR, Mott SH, Pavlakis SG, et al. Clinical spectrum of secondary parkinsonism in childhood: A reversible disorder. *Pediatr Neurol* 10(2):131–140, 1994.

Russo RN, O'Flaherty S. Bromocriptine for the management of autonomic dysfunction after severe traumatic brain injury. *J Paediatr Child Health* 36(3):283–285, 2000.

Shader RI. *Manual of Psychiatric Therapeutics* (3rd ed.). Philadelphia: Lippincott, Williams & Wilkins, 2003, p. 31.

Shahar E, Andraws J. Extra-pyramidal parkinsonism complicating organophosphate insecticide poisoning. *Eur J Paediatr Neurol* 5(6):261–264, 2001.

Teoh L, Allen H, Kowalenko N. Drug-induced extrapyramidal reactions. *J Paediatr Child Health* 38(1):95–97, 2002.

Trasmonte J, Dayner J, Barron TF. Neuroleptic malignant syndrome in an adolescent head trauma patient. *Clin Pediatr (Phila)* 38(10):611–613, 1999.

B
I
B
L
I
O
G
R
A
P
H
Y

van Maldegem BT, Smit LM, Touw DJ, et al. Neuroleptic malignant syndrome in a 4-year-old girl associated with alimemazine. *Eur J Pediatr* 161(5):259–261, 2002.

Walters AS, Mandelbaum DE, Lewin DS, et al. Dopaminergic therapy in children with restless legs/periodic limb movements in sleep and ADHD. Dopaminergic Therapy Study Group. *Pediatr Neurol* 22(3):182–186, 2000.

ANXIOLYTICS

Barnett SR, Riddle MA. Anxiolytics: Benzodiazepines, buspirone, and others. In: Martin A, Scahill L, Charney DS, Leckman JF (eds.). *Pediatric Psychopharmacology Principles and Practice.* New York: Oxford University Press, pp. 341–352, 2003.

Bender BG, McCormick DR, Milgrom H. Children's school performance is not impaired by short-term administration of diphenhydramine or loratadine. *J Pediatr* 138(5): 656–660, 2001.

Bernstein GA, Garfinkel BD, Borchardt CM. Comparative studies of pharmacotherapy for school refusal. *J Am Acad Child Adolesc Psychiatry* 29(5):773–781, 1989.

Buitelaar JK, van der Gaag RJ, van der Hoeven J. Buspirone in the management of anxiety and irritability in children with pervasive developmental disorders: Results of an open-label study. *J Clin Psychiatry* 59(2):56–59, 1998.

Charney DS, Mihic SJ, Harris RA. Hypnotics and sedatives. In: Hardman JG, Limbird LE, Gilman AG (Eds.), *Goodman and Gilman's the Pharmacological Basis of Therapeutics* (10th ed.). New York: McGraw-Hill, pp. 399–428, 2001.

Coffey BJ. Anxiolytics for children and adolescents: Traditional and new drugs. *J Child Adolesc Psychopharmacol* 1(1):57–83, 1990.

Coffey BJ, Shader RI, Greenblatt DJ. Pharmacokinetics of benzodiazepines and psychostimulants in children. *J Clin Psychopharmacol* 3(4):217–225, 1983.

Coldwell SE, Awamura K, Milgrom P, et al. Side effects of triazolam in children. *Pediatr Dent* 21(1):18–25, 1999.

DeVane CL, Ware MR, Lydiard RB. Pharmacokinetics, pharmacodynamics, and treatment issues of benzodiazepines: Alprazolam, adinazolam, and clonazepam. *Psychopharmocol Bull* 27:463–473, 1991.

Everitt IJ, Barnett P. Comparison of two benzodiazepines used for sedation of children undergoing suturing of a laceration in an emergency department. *Pediatr Emerg Care* 18(2):72–74, 2002.

Fisher C, Kahn E, Edwards A, et al. A psychophysiological study of nightmares and night terrors. *Arch Gen Psychiatry* 28(2):252–259, 1973.

Graae F, Milner J, Rizzotto L, et al. Clonazepam in childhood anxiety disorders. *J Am Acad Child Adolesc Psychiatry* 33(3):372–376, 1994.

Green WH. *Child and Adolescent Clinical Psychopharmacology* (3rd ed.). Philadelphia: Lippincott, Williams & Williams, pp. 269–291, 2001.

Greenblatt DJ. Benzodiazepine hypnotics: Sorting the pharmacokinetic facts. *J Clin Psychiatry* 52(Suppl):4–10, 1991.

Gunn VL, Nechyba C. *The Harriet Lane Handbook* (16th ed.). Philadelphia: Mosby, pp. 633–634, 2002.

Hanna GL, Feibusch EL, Albright KJ. Buspirone treatment of anxiety associated with pharyngeal dysphagia in a four-year old. *J Child Adolesc Psychopharmacol* 7(2): 137–143, 1997.

Hymon S, Arana G. *Handbook of Psychiatric Drug Therapy,* Boston: Little, Brown, 1987.

Kay GG. The effects of antihistamines on cognition and performance. *J Allergy Clin Immunol* 105(6 Pt 2):S622–S627, 2000.

Kranzler HR. Use of buspirone in an adolescent with overanxious disorder. *J Am Acad Child Adolesc Psychiatry* 27(6):789–790, 1988.

Kutcher SP. *Child and Adolescent Psychopharmacology*. Philadelphia: Saunders, pp. 129–145, 1997.

Kutcher SP, Reiter S, Gardner DM, et al. The pharmacotherapy of anxiety disorders in children and adolescents. *Psychiatr Clin North Am* 15:41–67, 1992.

Lucas AR, Pasley FC. Psychoactive drugs in the treatment of emotionally disturbed children: Haloperidol and diazepam. *Compr Psychiatry* 10:376–386, 1969.

Malhotra S, Santosh PJ. An open trial of buspirone in children with attention-deficit/ hyperactivity disorder. *J Am Acad Child Adolesc Psychiatry* 37(4):364–371, 1998.

McCall JE, Fischer CG, Warden G, et al. Lorazepam given the night before surgery reduces preoperative anxiety in children undergoing reconstructive burn surgery. *J Burn Care Rehabil* 20(2):151–154, 1999.

Nash LT, Hack S. The pharmacological treatment of anxiety disorders in children and adolescents. *Expert Opin Pharmacother* 3(5):555–571, 2002.

Owens JA, Rosen CL, Mindell JA. Medication use in the treatment of pediatric insomnia: Results of a survey of community-based pediatricians. *Pediatrics* 111(5 Pt 1): E628–635, 2003.

Pfeffer CR, Jiang H, Domeshek LJ. Buspirone treatment of psychiatrically hospitalized prepubertal children with symptoms of anxiety and moderately severe aggression. *J Child Adolesc Psychopharmacol* 7(3):145–155, 1997.

Pfefferbaum B, Overall JE, Boren HA, et al. Alprazolam in the treatment of anticipatory and acute situational anxiety in children with cancer. *J Am Acad Child Adolesc Psychiatry* 26(4):532–535, 1987.

Philpot EE. Safety of second generation antihistamines. *Allergy Asthma Proc* 21(1): 15–20, 2000.

Popper CW. Psychopharmacologic treatment of anxiety disorders in children and adolescents. *J Clin Psychiatry* 54:52–63, 1993.

Popuviciu L, Corfariu O. Efficacy and safety of midazolam in the treatment of night terrors in children. *J Clin Pharmacol* 16:97S–102S, 1983.

Riddle MA, Bernstein GA, Cook EH, et al. Anxiolytics, adrenergic agents, and naltrexone. *J Am Acad Child Adolesc Psychiatry* 38(5):546–556, 1999.

Rosenberg DR. Anxiolytics. In: Rosenberg DR, Davanzo PA, Gershon S (Eds.), *Pharmacotherapy for Child and Adolescent Psychiatric Disorders* (2nd ed.). New York: Marcel Dekker, pp. 489–541, 2002.

Rothschild AJ, Shindul-Rothschild VA, Murray M, et al. Comparison of the frequency of behavioral disinhibition on alprazolam, clonazepam, or no benzodiazepine in hospitalized psychiatric patients. *J Clin Psychopharmacol* 20:7–11, 2000.

Salazar DE, Frackiewicz EJ, Dockens R, et al. Pharmacokinetics and tolerability of buspirone during oral administration to children and adolescents with anxiety disorder and normal healthy adults. *J Clin Pharmacol* 41(12):1351–1358, 2001.

Shader RI, Greenblatt DJ. Use of benzodiazepines in anxiety disorders. *NEJM* 238: 1398–1405, 1993.

Simeon JG. Use of anxiolytics in children. *Encephale* 19(2):71–74, 1993.

Simeon JG, Ferguson HB, Knott V, et al. Clinical, cognitive, and neurophysiological effects of alprazolam in children and adolescents with overanxious and avoidant disorders. *J Am Acad Child Adolesc Psychiatry* 31(1):29–33, 1992.

Simons FE. H1-antihistamines in children. *Clin Allergy Immunol* 17:437–464, 2002.

Steingard RJ, Goldberg M, Lee D, et al. Adjunctive clonazepam treatment of tic symptoms in children with comorbid tic disorders and ADHD. *J Am Acad Child Adolesc Psychiatry* 33:394–399, 1994.

Vinson DR, Drotts DL. Diphenhydramine for the prevention of akathisia induced by prochlorperazine: A randomized controlled trial. *Ann Emerg Med* 37(2):125–131, 2001.

Werry JS, Aman MG. Anxiolytics, sedatives, and miscellaneous drugs. In: Werry JS and Aman MG (Eds.), *Practitioner's Guide to Psychoactive Drugs for Children and Adolescents* (2nd ed.). New York: Plenum Press, pp. 433–469, 1999.

Zweir KJ, Rao U. Buspirone use in an adolescent with social phobia and mixed personality disorder (cluster A type). *J Am Acad Child Adolesc Psychiatry* 33(7): 1007–1011, 1994.

ADRENERGIC AGENTS

Agarwal V, Sitholey P, Kumar S, et al. Double-blind, placebo-controlled trial of clonidine in hyperactive children with mental retardation. *Ment Retard* 39(4):259–267, 2001.

Buitelaar JK, van der Gaag J, Swaab-Barneveld H, Kuiper M. Pindolol and methylphenidate in children with attention deficit hyperactivity disorder: Clinical efficacy and side effects. *J Am Acad Child Adolesc Psychiatry* 37:587–595, 1996.

Buitelaar JK. Miscellaneous compounds: Beta-blockers and opiate antagonists. In: Martin A, Scahill L, Charney DS, Leckman JF (Eds.), *Pediatric Psychopharmacology Principles and Practice*. New York: Oxford University Press, pp. 353–362, 2003.

Cantwell DP, Swanson J, Connor DF. Case study: Adverse response to clonidine. *J Am Acad Child Adolesc Psychiatry* 36:539–544, 1997.

Chappell PB, Riddle MA, Scahill L, et al. Guanfacine treatment of comorbid attention-deficit hyperactivity disorder and Tourette's syndrome: Preliminary clinical experience. *J Am Acad Child Adolesc Psychiatry* 34(9):1140–1146, 1995.

Connor DF. Beta blockers for aggression: A review of the pediatric experience. *J Child Adolesc Psychopharmacol* 3(2):99–114, 1993.

Connor DF, Barkley RZ, Davis HT. A pilot study of methylphenidate, clonidine, or the combination in ADHD comorbid with aggressive oppositional defiant or conduct disorder. *Clin Pediatr (Phila)* 39(1):15–25, 2000.

Connor DF, Fletcher KE, Swanson JM. A meta-analysis of clonidine for symptoms of attention-deficit hyperactivity disorder. *J Am Acad Child Adolesc Psychiatry* 38(12):1551–1559, 1999.

Connor DF, Ozbayrak KR, Benjamin S, et al. A pilot study of nadolol for overt aggression in developmentally delayed individuals. *J Am Acad Child Adolesc Psychiatry* 36(6):826–834, 1997.

Distler A, Kirch W, Luth B. Antihypertensive effect of guanfacine: A double-blind cross-over trial compared with clonidine. *Br J Clin Pharmacol* 10(Suppl 1): 49S–53S, 1980.

Famularo R, Kinscherff R, Fenton T. Propranolol treatment for childhood posttraumatic stress disorder, acute type. *Am J Dis Child* 142:1244–1247, 1988.

Freeman KO, Connelly NR, Schwatz D, et al. Analgesia for paediatric tonsillectomy and adenoidectomy with intramuscular clonidine. *Paediatr Anaesth* 12(7):617–620, 2002.

Gaffney GR, Perry PJ, Lund BC, Bever-Stille KA, Kuperman S. Risperidone versus clonidine in the treatment of children and adolescents with Tourette's syndrome. *J Am Acad Child Adolesc Psychiatry* 41(3):330–336, 2002.

Gerra G, Zaimovic A, Rustichelli P, et al. Rapid opiate detoxification in outpatient treatment: Relationship with naltrexone compliance. *J Subst Abuse Treat* 18(2):185–191, 2000.

Hackmann T, Friesen M, Allen S, et al. Clonidine facilitates controlled hypotension in adolescent children. *Anesth Analg* 96(4):976–981, 2003.

Hazell PL, Stuart JE. A randomized controlled trial of clonidine added to psychostimulant medication for hyperactive and aggressive children. *J Am Acad Child Adolesc Psychiatry* 42(8):886–894, 2003.

Horrigan JP, Barnhill LJ. Guanfacine for treatment of attention-deficit hyperactivity disorder in boys. *J Child Adolesc Psychopharmacol* 5:215–223, 1995.

Hunt RD, Arnsten AFT, Asbell MD. An open trial of guanfacine in the treatment of attention-deficit hyperactivity disorder. *J Am Acad Child Adolesc Psychiatry* 34: 50–54, 1995.

Kuperman S, Stuart MA. Use of propranolol to decrease aggressive outbursts in younger patients. *Psychosomatics* 28:315–319, 1987.

McGrath JC, Klein-Schwartz W. Epidemiology and toxicity of pediatric guanfacine exposures. *Ann Pharmacother* 36(11):1698–1703, 2002.

Newcorn JH, Schulz KP, Halperin JM. Adrenergic agonists: Clonidine and guanfacine. In: Martin A, Scahill L, Charney DS, Leckman JF (Eds.), *Pediatric Psychopharmacology Principles and Practice*. New York: Oxford University Press, pp. 264–273, 2003.

Nichols MH, King WD, James LP. Clonidine poisoning in Jefferson County, Alabama. *Ann Emerg Med* 29(4):511–517, 1997.

Niederhofer H, Staffen W, Mair A. A placebo-controlled study of lofexidine in the treatment of children with tic disorders and attention deficit hyperactivity disorder. *J Psychopharmacol* 17(1):113–119, 2003.

Popper CW. Combining methylphenidate and clonidine: Pharmacologic questions and news reports about sudden death. *J Child Adolesc Psychopharmacol* 5:157–166, 1995.

Rosenberg DR. Adrenergic agents in child and adolescent psychiatry. In: Rosenberg DR, Davanzo PA, and Gershon S (Eds.), *Pharmacotherapy for Child and Adolescent Psychiatric Disorders* (2nd ed.), New York: Marcel Dekker, pp. 543–595, 2002.

Scahill L, Chappell PB, Kim YS, et al. A placebo-controlled study of guanfacine in the treatment of children with tic disorders ant attention deficit hyperactivity disorder. *Am J Psychiatry* 158(7):1067–1074, 2000.

Swanson JM, Connor DF, Cantwell D. Combining methylphenidate and clonidine: Ill-advised/and negative rebuttal [Debate Forum]. *J Am Acad Child Adolesc Psychiatry* 38:614–622, 1999.

Tourette's Syndrome Study Group. Treatment of ADHD in children with tics: A randomized controlled trial. *Neurology* 58(4):527–536, 2002.

Wilens TE, Spencer TJ. Combining methylphenidate and clonidine: A clinically sound medication option/and affirmative rebuttal [Debate Forum]. *J Am Acad Child Adolesc Psychiatry* 38:614–622, 1999.

Williams DT, Mehl R, Yudofsky S, et al. The effect of propranolol on uncontrolled rage outbursts in children and adolescents with organic brain dysfunction. *J Am Acad Child Adolesc Psychiatry* 21:129–135, 1982.

OTHER MEDICATIONS

American Academy of Child and Adolescent Psychiatry. Work Group on Quality Issues. Practice parameters for the assessment and treatment of children and adolescents with enuresis. *J Am Acad Child Adolesc Psychiatry* 43:1540–1550, 2004.

Biederman J. Modafinil improves ADHD symptoms in children in a randomized, double-blind, placebo-controlled study. Annual Meeting of the American Psychiatric Association, San Francisco, May 17–22, 2003.

Bolduc S, Upadhyay J, Payton J, et al. The use of tolterodine in children after oxybutynin failure. *BJU Int* 91(4):398–403, 2003.

Buitelaar JK. Miscellaneous compounds: Beta-blockers and opiate antagonists. In: Martin A, Scahill L, Charney DS, Leckman JF (Eds.), *Pediatric Psychopharmacology Principles and Practice.* New York: Oxford University Press, pp. 357–360, 2003.

Bymaster FP, Katner JS, and Nelson DL. Atomoxetine increases extracellular levels of norepinephrine and dopamine in prefrontal cortex of rat: A potential mechanism for efficacy in attention deficit/hyperactivity disorder. *Neuropsychopharmacol* 27(5): 699–711, 2002.

Campbell M, Anderson LT, Small AM, et al. Naltrexone in autistic children: A double-blind and placebo-controlled study. *Psychopharmacol Bull* 26:130–135, 1990.

Campbell M, Anderson LT, Small AM, et al. Naltrexone in autistic children: Behavioral symptoms and attentional learning. *J Am Acad Child Adolesc Psychiatry* 32:1283–1291, 1993.

Caione P, Arena F, Biraghi M, et al. Nocturnal enuresis and daytime wetting: A multicentric trial with oxybutynin and desmopressin. *Eur Urol* 31(4):459–463, 1997.

Diokno AC, Appell RA, Sand PK, et al. Prospective, randomized, double-blind study of the efficacy and tolerability of the extended-release formulation of oxybutynin and tolterodine for overactive bladder: Results of the OPERA trial. *Mayo Clin Proc* 78(6): 687–695, 2003.

Eggert P, Kuhn B. Antidiuretic hormone regulation in patients with primary nocturnal enuresis. *Arch Dis Child* 73:508–511, 1995.

Feldman HM, Kolman BK, Gonzaga AM. Naltrexone and communication skills in young children with autism. *J Am Acad Child Adolesc Psychiatry* 38:587–593, 1999.

Goessl C, Sauter T, Michael T, et al. Efficacy and tolerability of tolterodine in children with detrusor hyperreflexia. *Urology* 55(3):414–418, 2000.

Guilleminault C, Pelayo R. Narcolepsy in children: A practical guide to its diagnosis, treatment and follow-up. *Paediatr Drugs* 2(1):1–9, 2000.

Heil SH, Holmes HW, Bickel WK, et al. Comparison of the subjective, physiological, and psychomotor effects of atomoxetine and methylphenidate in light drug users. *Drug Alcohol Depend* 67(2):149–156, 2002.

Hjalmas K, Hellstrom A-L, Mogren K, et al. The overactive bladder in children: A potential future indication for tolterodine. *BJU Int* 87(6):569–577, 2002.

Kolmen BK, Feldman HM, Handen BL, et al. Naltrexone in young autistic children: Replication study and learning measures. *J Am Acad Child Adolesc Psychiatry* 36(11): 1570–1578, 1997.

Kratochvil CJ, Heiligenstein JH, Dittmann R, et al. Atomoxetine and methylphenidate treatment in children with ADHD: A prospective, randomized, open-label trial. *J Am Acad Child Adolesc Psychiatry* 41(7):776–784, 2002.

Longstaffe S, Moffatt, ME, Whalen JC. Behavioral and self-concept changes after six months of enuresis treatment: A randomized, controlled trial. *Pediatrics* 105(4 Pt 2): 935–940, 2000.

MacDonald JR, Hill JD, Tarnopolsky MA. Modafinil reduces excessive somnolence and enhances mood in patients with myotonic dystrophy. *Neurology* 59(12):1876–1880, 2002.

Michelson D, Adler L, Spencer T, et al. Atomoxetine in adults with ADHD: Two randomized, placebo-controlled studies. *Biol Psychiatry* 53(2):112–120, 2003.

Michelson D, Allen AJ, Busner J, et al. Once-daily atomoxetine treatment for children and adolescents with attention deficit hyperactivity disorder: A randomized, placebo-controlled study. *Am J Psychiatry* 159(11):1896–1901, 2002.

Michelson D, Faries D, Wernicke J, et al. Atomoxetine in the treatment of children and adolescents with attention-deficit/hyperactivity disorder: A randomized, placebo-controlled, dose-response study. *Pediatrics* 108(5):E83, 2001.

Neveus T. Oxybutynin, desmopressin, and enuresis. *J Urol* 166(6):2459–2462, 2001.

Olsson B, Szamosi J. Multiple dose pharmacokinetics of a new once daily extended release tolterodine formulation versus immediate release tolterodine. *Clin Pharmacokinet* 40(3):227–235, 2001.

Reinberg Y, Crocker J, Wolpert J, et al. Therapeutic efficacy of extended release oxybutynin chloride, and immediate release and long acting tolterodine tartrate in children with diurnal urinary incontinence. *J Urol* 170(3):317–319, 2003.

Robertson P Jr., Hellriegel ET. Clinical pharmacokinetic profile of modafinil. *Clin Pharmacokinet* 42(2):123–137, 2003.

Rugino TA, Copley TC. Effects of modafinil in children with attention-deficit/hyperactivity disorder: An open-label study. *J Am Acad Child Adolesc Psychiatry* 40(2):230–235, 2001.

Rugino TA, Samsock TC. Modafinil in children with attention-deficit hyperactivity disorder. *Pediatr Neurol* 29(2):136–142, 2003.

Sandman CA. The opiate hypothesis in autism and self-injury. *J Child Adolesc Psychopharmacol* 1:237–248, 1990.

Sandman CA, Hetrick WP, Taylor DV, et al. Naltrexone reduces self-injury and improves learning. *Exp Clin Psychopharmacol* 1:1–17, 1993.

Sathyan G, Hu W, Gupta SK. Lack of effect of food on the pharmacokinetics of an extended-release oxybutynin formulation. *J Clin Pharmacol* 41(2):187–192, 2001.

Schulman SL, Stokes A, Salzman PM. The efficacy and safety of oral desmopressin in children with primary nocturnal enuresis. *J Urol* 166(6):2427–2431, 2001.

Spencer T, Biederman J, Wilens T, et al. Effectiveness and tolerability of a tomoxetine in adults with attention deficit hyperactivity disorder. *Am J Psychiatry* 155(5):693–695, 1998.

Swanson JM. Modafinil in children with ADHD: A randomized, placebo-controlled study. Annual Meeting of the American Psychiatric Association, San Francisco, May 17–22, 2003.

Taylor FB, Russo J. Efficacy of modafinil compared to dextroamphetamine for the treatment of attention deficit hyperactivity disorder in adults. *J Child Adolesc Psychopharmacol* 10(4):311–320, 2000.

U.S. Modafinil in Narcolepsy Multicenter Study Group. Randomized trial of modafinil as a treatment for the excessive daytime somnolence of narcolepsy. *Neurology* 54:1166–1175, 2000.

Willemsen-Swinkels SH, Buitelaar JK, van Engeland H. The effects of chronic naltrexone treatment in young autistic children: A double-blind placebo-controlled crossover study. *Biol Psychiatry* 39:1023–1031, 1996.

Witcher JW, Long A, Smith B, et al. Atomoxetine pharmacokinetics in children and adolescents with attention deficit hyperactivity disorder. *J Child Adolesc Psychopharmacol* 13(1):53–63, 2003.

Wolfish NM, Barkin J, Gorodzinsky F, et al. The Canadian Enuresis Study and Evaluation: Short- and long-term safety and efficacy of an oral desmopressin preparation. *Scand J Urol Nephrol* 37(1):22–27, 2003.

Wong YN, Simcoe D, Hartman LN, et al. A double-blind, placebo-controlled, ascending-dose evaluation of the pharmacokinetics and tolerability of modafinil tablets in healthy male volunteers. *J Clin Pharmacol* 39(1):30–40, 1999.

B
I
B
L
I
O
G
R
A
P
H
Y

HERBAL AND ALTERNATIVE MEDICINES

Brenner R, Azbel V, Madhusoodanan S, et al. Comparison of an extract of hypericum (LI 160) and sertraline in the treatment of depression: A double-blind, randomized pilot study. *Clin Ther* 22(4):411–419, 2000.

Coplan J, Souders MC, Mulberg AE, et al. Children with autistic spectrum disorders. II: Parents are unable to distinguish secretin from placebo under double-blind conditions. *Arch Dis Child* 88:737–739, 2003.

Corbett B, Kahn K, Czapansky-Bulman D. A double-blind, placebo-controlled crossover study investigating the effect of porcine secretin in children with autism. *Clin Pediatr* 40(6):327–331, 2001.

Dodge NN, Wilson GA. Melatonin for treatment of sleep disorders in children with developmental disabilities. *J Child Neurol* 16(8):581–584, 2001.

Emsley R, Myburgh C, Oosthuizen P, et al. Randomized, placebo-controlled study of ethyl-eicosapentaenoic acid as supplemental treatment in schizophrenia. *Am J Psychiatry* 159(9):1596–1598, 2002.

Findling RL, McNamara NK, O'Riordan MA, et al. An open-label study of St. John's wort in juvenile depression. *J Am Acad Child Adolesc Psychiatry* 42(8):908–914, 2003.

Fugh-Berman A. Alternative medicine. In: Braunwald E, Fauci AS, Hauser SL, Longo DL, Kasper DL, Jameson JL (Eds.), *Harrison's Principles of Internal Medicine* (15th ed.). New York: McGraw-Hill, pp. 49–54, 2001.

Knuppel L, Linde K. Adverse effects of St. John's wort: A systematic review. *J Clin Psychiatry* 65:1470–1479, 2004.

Lanski SL, Greenwald M, Perkins A, et al. Herbal therapy use in a pediatric emergency department population: Expect the unexpected. *Pediatrics* 111(5):981–985, 2003.

Lecrubier Y, Clerc G, Didi R, et al. Efficacy of St. John's wort extract WS 5570 in major depression: A double-blind, placebo-controlled trial. *Am J Psychiatry* 159(8):1361–1366, 2002.

Levy SE, Souders MC, Wray J, et al. Children with autistic spectrum disorders. I: Comparison of placebo and single dose of human synthetic secretin. *Arch Dis Child* 88:731–736, 2003.

Linde K, Ramirez G, Mulrow CD, et al. St John's wort for depression: An overview and meta-analysis of randomized clinical trials. *Br Med J* 313:253–258, 1996.

Marangell LB, Marinez JM, Zboyan HA, et al. A double-blind, placebo-controlled study of the omega-3 fatty acid docosahexaenoic acid in the treatment of major depression. *Am J Psychiatry* 160(5):996–998, 2003.

Markowitz JS, Donovan JL, DeVane CL, et al. Effect of St John's wort on drug metabolism by induction of cytochrome P450 enzyme. *JAMA* 290(11):1500–1504, 2003.

Paavonen EJ, Neiminen-von Wendt T, Vanhala R, et al. Effectiveness of melatonin in the treatment of sleep disturbances in children with Asperger disorder. *J Child Adolesc Psychopharmacol* 13(1):83–95, 2003.

Pittler MH, Ernest E. Efficacy of kava extract for treating anxiety: Systematic review and meta-analysis. *J Clin Psychopharmacol* 20:84–89, 2000.

Rey JM, Walter G, Horrigan JP. Complementary and alternative medicine in pediatric psychopharmacology. In: Martin A, Scahill L, Charney DS, and Leckman JF (Eds.), *Pediatric Psychopharmacology Principles and Practice*. New York: Oxford University Press, pp. 365–376, 2003.

Roberts W, Weaver L, Brian J, et al. Repeated doses of porcine secretin in the treatment of autism: A randomized, placebo-controlled trial. *Pediatrics* 107:E71, 2001.

Ross C, Davies P, Whitehouse W. Melatonin treatment for sleep disorders in children with neurodevelopmental disorders: An observational study. *Dev Med Child Neurol* 44(5):339–344, 2002.

Schempp CM, Windeck T, Hezel S, et al. Topical treatment of atopic dermatitis with St. John's wort cream: A randomized, placebo controlled, double blind half-side comparison. *Phytomed* 10(Suppl 4):31–37, 2003.

Smits MG, Nagtegaal EE, van der Heijden J, et al. Melatonin for chronic sleep onset insomnia in children: A randomized placebo-controlled trial. *J Child Neurol* 16(2):86–92, 2001.

Smits MG, van Stel H, van der Heijden K, et al. Melatonin improves health status and sleep in children with idiopathic chronic sleep-onset insomnia: A randomized placebo-controlled trial. *J Am Acad Child Adolesc Psychiatry* 42(11):1286–1293, 2003.

Stevens LJ, Zentall SS, Abate ML, et al. Omega-3 fatty acids in boys with behavior, learning, and health problems. *Physiol Behav* 59:915–920, 1996.

Stevinson C, Ernst E. Valerian for insomnia: A systematic review of randomized clinical trials. *Sleep Med* 1:91–99, 2000.

Stoll AL, Severus WE, Freeman MP, et al. Omega 3 fatty acids in bipolar disorder: A preliminary double-blind, placebo-controlled trial. *Arch Gen Psychiatry* 56:407–412, 1999.

Voigt RG, Llorente AM, Jensen CL, et al. A randomized, double-blind, placebo-controlled trial of docosahexaenoic acid supplementation in children with attention deficit/hyperactivity disorder. *J Pediatr* 139(2):189–196, 2001.

Volz HP, Murck H, Kasper S, et al. St John's wort extract (LI 160) in somatoform disorders: Results of a placebo-controlled trial. *Psychopharmacol (Berl)* 164(3):294–300, 2002.

Yehuda S, Rabinovitz S, Mostofsky D. Effects of essential fatty acid preparation (SR-3) on brain lipids, biochemistry, and behavioural and cognitive functions. In:

Yehuda S, Mostofsky D (Eds.), *Handbook of Essential Fatty Acid Biology, Biochemistry, Physiology, and Behavioural Neurobiology.* Totowa, NJ: Humana Press, pp. 427–452, 1997.

ELECTROCONVULSIVE THERAPY IN ADOLESCENTS

American Academy of Child and Adolescent Psychiatry. Work Group on Quality Issues. Practice parameters for use of electroconvulsive therapy with adolescents. *J Am Acad Child Adolesc Psychiatry* 43(12):1521–1539, 2004.

American Psychiatric Association. *Electroconvulsive Therapy: Recommendations for Treatment, Training, and Privileging.* Washington, DC: Author, 1990.

Bloch Y, Levcovitch Y, Bloch AM, et al. Electroconvulsive therapy in adolescents: Similarities to and differences from adults. *J Am Acad Child Adolesc Psychiatry* 40(11):1332–1336, 2001.

Cohen D, Flament M, Taieb O, et al. Electroconvulsive therapy in adolescence. *Eur Child Adolesc Psychiatry* 9(1):1–6, 2000.

Cohen D, Paillere-Martinot ML, Basquin M. Use of electroconvulsant therapy in adolescents. *Convuls Ther* 13:25–31, 1997.

Cohen D, Taieb O, Flament M, et al. Absence of cognitive impairment at long-term follow-up in adolescents treated with ECT for severe mood disorder. *Am J Psychiatry* 157(3):460–462, 2000.

Freeman CP. ECT in those under 18 years old. In: Freeman CP (Ed.), *The ECT Handbook.* London: Royal College of Psychiatrists, pp. 18–21, 1995.

Ghaziuddin N, King CA, Naylor MW, et al. Electroconvulsive treatment in adolescents with pharmacotherapy-refractory depression. *J Child Adolesc Psychopharmacol* 6:259–271, 1996.

Ghaziuddin N, Laughrin D, Giordani B. Cognitive side effects of electroconvulsive therapy in adolescents. *J Child Adolesc Psychopharmacol* 10(4):269–276, 2000.

BIBLIOGRAPHY

Kutcher S, Robertson HA. Electroconvulsive therapy in treatment-resistant bipolar youth. *J Child Adolesc Psychopharmacol* 5:167–175, 1995.

Moise FN, Petrides G. Case study: Electroconvulsive therapy in adolescents. *J Am Acad Child Adolesc Psychiatry* 35:312–318, 1996.

Strober M, Rao U, DeAntonio M, et al. Effects of electroconvulsive therapy in adolescents with severe endogenous depression resistant to pharmacotherapy. *Biol Psychiatry* 43:335–338, 1998.

Taieb O, Flament MF, Chevret S, et al. Clinical relevance of electroconvulsive therapy (ECT) in adolescents with severe mood disorder: Evidence from a follow-up study. *Eur Psychiatry* 17(4):206–212, 2002.

Taieb O, Flament MF, Corcos M, et al. Electroconvulsive therapy in adolescents with mood disorder: Patients' and parents' attitudes. *Psychiatr Res* 104(2):183–190, 2001.

Walter G, Rey JM. Has the practice and outcome of ECT in adolescents changed? Findings from a whole-population study. *J ECT* 19(2):84–87, 2003.

Walter G, Rey JM, Ghaziuddin N. Electroconvulsive therapy and transcranial magnetic stimulation. In: Martin A, Scahill L, Charney DS, Leckman JF (Eds.), *Pediatric Psychopharmacology Principles and Practice.* New York: Oxford University Press, pp. 377–386, 2003.

Walter G, Rey JM. An epidemiological study of the use of ECT in adolescents. *J Am Acad Child Adolese Psychiatry* 36(6):809–815, 1997.

Walter G, Rey JM, Mitchell PB. Practitioner review: Electroconvulsive therapy in adolescents. *J Child Psychol Psychiatr* 40(3):325–334, 1999.

ATTENTION-DEFICIT HYPERACTIVITY DISORDER

Abikoff H, McGough J, Vitiello B, et al. Sequential pharmacotherapy for children with comorbid attention-deficit/hyperactivity and anxiety disorders. *J Am Acad Child Adolesc Psychiatry* 44(5):418–427, 2005.

American Academy of Child and Adolescent Psychiatry. Practice parameters for the assessment and treatment of children, adolescents, and adults with attention-deficit/hyperactivity disorder. *J Am Acad Child Adolesc Psychiatry* 36(10 Suppl): 85S–121S, 1997.

American Academy of Child and Adolescent Psychiatry. Practice parameters for the use of stimulant medications in the treatment of children, adolescents, and adults. *J Am Acad Child Adolese Psychiatry* 41:265–495, 2002.

American Academy of Pediatrics, Subcommittee on Attention-Deficit/Hyperactivity Disorder and Committee on Quality Improvement. Clinical practice guideline: treatment of the school-aged child with attention-deficit/hyperactivity disorder. *Pediatrics* 108(4):1033–1044, 2001.

Barkley RA, Fischer M, Smallish L, Fletcher K. Does the treatment of attention-deficit/hyperactivity disorder with stimulants contribute to drug use/abuse? A 13-year prospective study. *Pediatrics* 111(1):97–109, 2003.

Barrickman LL, Perry PJ, Allen AJ, et al. Bupropion versus methylphenidate in the treatment of attention-deficit hyperactivity disorder. *J Am Acad Child Adolesc Psychiatry* 34(5):649–657, 1995.

Biederman J, Baldessarini RJ, Wright V, et al. A double-blind placebo controlled study of desipramine in the treatment of ADD: I. Efficacy. *J Am Acad Child Adolesc Psychiatry* 28(5):777–784, 1989.

Biederman J, Lopez FA, Boellner SW, et al. A randomized, double-blind, placebo-controlled, parallel-group study of SLI381 (Adderall XR) in children with attention-deficit/hyperactivity disorder. *Pediatrics* 110(2 Pt 1): 258–266, 2002.

Brown TE. *Brown Attention-Deficit Disorder Scales for Children and Adolescents*. San Antonio, TX: Psychological Corporation, 2001.

Cantwell DP. Attention deficit disorder: A review of the past 10 years. *J Am Acad Child Adolesc Psychiatry* 35(8):978–987, 1996.

Collett BR, Ohan JL, Myers KM. Ten-year review of rating scales. V: Scales assessing attention-deficit/hyperactivity disorder. *J Am Acad Child Adolesc Psychiatry* 42(9):1015–1037, 2003.

Conners C. *Conners' Rating Scales—Revised Technical Manual*. North Tonawanda, NY: Multi-Health Systems, 1997.

Conners CK, Casat CD, Gualtieri CT, et al. Bupropion hydrochloride in attention deficit disorder with hyperactivity. *J Am Acad Child Adolesc Psychiatry* 35(10):1314–1321, 1996.

Connor DF. Preschool attention deficit hyperactivity disorder: A review of prevalence, diagnosis, neurobiology, and stimulant treatment. *Development Behav Peds* 23(1S): S1–S9, 2002.

Connor DF, Barkley RA, Davis HT. A pilot study of methylphenidate, clonidine, or the combination in ADHD comorbid with aggressive oppositional defiant or conduct disorder. *Clin Pediatr* 39:15–25, 2000.

DuPaul GJ, Power TJ, Anastopoulos AD, et al. *ADHD Rating Scale–IV: Checklist, Norms, and Clinical Interpretation*. New York: Guilford Press, 1998.

Gillberg C, Melander H, von Knorring AL, et al. Long-term stimulant treatment of children with attention-deficit hyperactivity disorder symptoms. A randomized, double-blind, placebo-controlled trial. *Arch Gen Psychiatry* 54(9):857–864, 1997.

Green WH. *Child and Adolescent Clinical Psychopharmacology* (3rd ed.). Philadelphia: Lippincott, Williams & Wilkins, pp. 32–33, 2001.

Greenhill LL, the Adolescent Study Group. Efficacy and safety of OROS® MPH in adolescents with ADHD. Poster presentation #4, 49th Annual Meeting of the American Academy of Child and Adolescent Psychiatry, October 22–27, 2002. San Francisco.

Greenhill LL, Findling RL, Swanson JM, et al. A double-blind, placebo-controlled study of modified-release methylphenidate in children with attention-deficit/hyperactivity disorder. *Pediatrics* 109(3):E39, 2002.

Handen BL, Johnson CR, Lubetsky M. Efficacy of methylphenidate among children with autism and symptoms of attention-deficit hyperactivity disorder. *J Autism Dev Disord* 30(3):245–255, 2000.

Hemmer SA, Pasternak JF, Zecker SG, Trommer BL. Stimulant therapy and seizure risk in children with ADHD. *Pediatr Neurol* 24(2):99–102, 2001.

Holland ML, Gimpel GA, Merrell KW. *ADHD Symptoms Rating Scale Manual*. Wilmington, DE: Wide Range, 2001.

Loney J, Milich R. Hyperactivity, inattention, and aggression in clinical practice. In: Wolraich M and Routh DK (Eds.), *Advances in Developmental and Behavioral Pediatrics*, (vol. 3, pp 113–147). Greenwich, CT: JAI Press, 1982.

McCarney SB. *The Attention Deficit Disorders Evaluation Scale, Home and School Versions, Technical Manuals*. Columbia, MO: Hawthorne Educational Service, 1989.

Michelson D, Adler L, Spencer T, et al. Atomoxetine in adults with ADHD: Two randomized, placebo-controlled studies. *Biol Psychiatry* 53(2):112–120, 2003.

Michelson D, Allen AJ, Busner J, et al. Once-daily atomoxetine treatment for children and adolescents with attention deficit hyperactivity disorder: A randomized, placebo-controlled study. *Am J Psychiatry* 159(11):1896–1901, 2002.

Michelson D, Faries D, Wernicke J, et al. Atomoxetine in the treatment of children and adolescents with attention-deficit/hyperactivity disorder: A randomized, placebo-controlled, dose-response study. *Pediatrics* 108(5):E83, 2001.

BIBLIOGRAPHY

Multimodal Treatment of ADHD Group (MTA Group). A 14-month randomized clinical trial of treatment strategies for attention-deficit/hyperactivity disorder. The MTA Cooperative Group. Multimodal treatment study of children with ADHD. *Arch Gen Psychiatry* 56(12):1073–1086, 1999.

Paterson R, Douglas C, Hallmayer J, et al. A randomized, double-blind, placebo-controlled trial of dexamphetamine in adults with attention deficit hyperactivity disorder. *Aust and New Zeal J Psychiatr* 33(4):494–502, 1999.

Pliszka SR. Comorbidity of attention-deficit/hyperactivity disorder with psychiatric disorders, An overview. *J Clin Psychiatry* 59(Suppl 7):50–58, 1998.

Pliszka SR, Greenhill LL, Crismon ML, et al. and the Texas Consensus Conference Panel on Medication Treatment of Childhood Attention-Deficit/Hyperactivity disorder. The Texas children's medication algorithm project: Report of the Texas Consensus Conference Panel on medication treatment of childhood attention-deficit/hyperactivity disorder. Part I. *J Am Acad Child Adolesc Psychiatry* 39:908–919, 2000.

Pliszka SR, Lopez M, Crismon ML, et al. A feasibility study of the children's medication algorithm project (CMAP) algorithm for the treatment of ADHD. *J Am Acad Child Adolesc Psychiatry* 42(3):279–287, 2003.

Prince JT, Wilens TE, Biederman J, et al. A controlled study of nortriptyline in children and adolescents with attention deficit hyperactivity disorder. *J Child Adolesc Psychopharmacol* 10(3):193–204, 2000.

Rugino TA, Copley TC. Effects of modafinil in children with attentiondeficit/hyperactivity disorder. *J Am Acad Child Adolesc Psychiatry* 40(2):230–235, 2001.

Scahill L, Chappell PB, Kim YS, et al. A placebo-controlled study of guanfacine in the treatment of children with tic disorders and attention deficit hyperactivity disorder. *Am J Psychiatry* 158(7):1067–1074, 2001.

Scheffer RE, Kowatch RA, Carmody T, et al. Randomized, placebo-controlled trial of mixed amphetamine salts for symptoms of comorbid ADHD in pediatric bipolan disorder after mood. Stabilization with divalproex sodium. *Am J Psychiatry* 162(1): 58–64, 2005.

Smith BH, Pelham WE, Gnagy E, et al. Equivalent effects of stimulant treatment for attention-deficit hyperactivity disorder during childhood and adolescence. *J Am Acad Child Adolesc Psychiatry* 37(3):314–321, 1998.

Spencer T, Biederman J, Wilens T, et al. Effectiveness and tolerability of tomoxetine in adults with attention deficit hyperactivity disorder. *Am J Psychiatry* 155(5):693–695, 1998.

Spencer T, Biederman J, Wilens T, et al. Efficacy of a mixed amphetamine salts compound in adults with attention-deficit/hyperactivity disorder. *Arch Gen Psychiatry* 58:775–782, 2001.

Spencer T, Wilens T, Biederman J, et al. A double-blind, crossover comparison of methylphenidate and placebo in adults with childhood-onset attention-deficit hyperactivity disorder. *Arch Gen Psychiatry* 52(6):434–443, 1995.

Swanson J. *School Based Assessments and Interventions for ADD Students.* Irvine, CA: K. C. Publishers, Irvine CA.

Taylor FB, Russo J. Efficacy of modafinil compared to dextroamphetamine for the treatment of attention deficit hyperactivity disorder in adults. *J Child Adolesc Psychopharmacol* 10(4):311–320, 2000.

Tourette's Syndrome Study Group. Treatment of ADHD in children with tics: A randomized controlled trial. *Neurology* 58(4):527–536, 2002.

Ullman RK, Sleator EK, Sprague RL. *ACTeRS Teacher and Parent Forms Manual.* Champaign, IL: Metri Tech, 2000.

Wilens TE, Biederman J, Prince J, et al. Six-week, double-blind, placebo-controlled study of desipramine for adult attention deficit hyperactivity disorder. *Am J Psychiatry* 153(9):1147–1153, 1996.

Wilens TE, Faraone SV, Biederman J, Gunawardene S. Does stimulant therapy of attention-deficit/hyperactivity disorder beget later substance abuse? A meta-analytic review of the literature. *Pediatrics* 111(1):179–185, 2003.

Wilens TE, Spencer TJ, Biederman J, et al. A controlled trial of bupropion for attention deficit hyperactivity disorder in adults. *Am J Psychiatry* 158(2):282–288, 2001.

Wolraich ML. *Vanderbilt ADHD Teacher Rating Scale (VADTRS) and the Vanderbilt ADHD Parent Rating Scale (VADPRS)*. Oklahoma City: University of Oklahoma Health Sciences Center, 2003

Wolraich ML, Greenhill LL, Pelham W, et al. Randomized, controlled trial of oros methylphenidate once a day in children with attention-deficit/hyperactivity disorder. *Pediatrics* 108(4):883–892, 2001.

TIC DISORDERS AND TOURETTE'S DISORDER

Allen AJ, Leonard HL, Swedo SE. Case study: A new infection-triggered, autoimmune subtype of pediatric OCD and Tourette's syndrome. *J Am Acad Child Adolesc Psychiatry* 34(3):307–311, 1995.

Bruggeman R, van der Linden C, Buitelaar JK, et al. Risperidone versus pimozide in Tourette's disorder: A comparative double-blind parallel-group study. *J Clin Psychiatry* 62(1):50–56, 2001.

Castellanos FX, Giedd JN, Elia J, et al. Controlled stimulant treatment of ADHD and comorbid Tourette's syndrome: Effects of stimulant and dose. *J Am Acad Child Adolesc Psychiatry* 36(5):589–596, 1997.

Coffey BJ, Biederman J, Geller DA, et al. The course of Tourette's disorder: A literature review. *Harv Rev Psychiatry* 8(4):192–198, 2000.

Coffey BJ, Biederman J, Smoller JW, et al. Anxiety disorders and tic severity in juveniles with Tourette's disorder. *J Am Acad Child Adolesc Psychiatry* 39(5):562–568, 2000.

Dion Y, Annable L, Sandor P, et al. Risperidone in the treatment of Tourette syndrome: A double-blind, placebo-controlled trial. *J Clin Psychopharmacol* 22(1):31–39, 2002.

Eapen V, Trimble MR, Robertson MM. The use of fluoxetine in Gilles de la Tourette's syndrome and obsessive compulsive behaviours: Preliminary clinical experience. *Prog Neuropsychopharmacol Biol Psychiatry* 20(4):737–743, 1996.

Feigin A, Kurlan R, McDermott MP, et al. A controlled trial of deprenyl in children with Tourette's syndrome and attention deficit hyperactivity disorder. *Neurology* 46(4):965–968, 1996.

Gadow KD, Nolan EE, Sverd J. Methylphenidate in hyperactive boys with comorbid tic disorder: II. Short-term behavioral effects in school settings. *J Am Acad Child Adolesc Psychiatry* 31(3):462–471, 1992.

Gadow KD, Sverd J, Sprafkin J, et al. Efficacy of methylphenidate for attention-deficit hyperactivity disorder in children with tic disorder. *Arch Gen Psychiatry* 52(6):444–455, 1995.

Gadow KD, Sverd J, Sprafkin J, et al. Long-term methylphenidate therapy in children with comorbid attention-deficit hyperactivity disorder and chronic multiple tic disorder. *Arch Gen Psychiatry* 56(4):330–336, 1999.

Gaffney GR, Perry PJ, Lund BC, et al. Risperidone versus clonidine in the treatment of children and adolescents with Tourette's syndrome. *J Am Acad Child Adolesc Psychiatry* 41(3):330–336, 2002.

Gilbert DL, Batterson JR, Sethuraman G, et al. Tic reduction with risperidone versus pimozide in a randomized, double-blind, crossover trial. *J Am Acad Child Adolesc Psychiatry* 43(2):206–214, 2004.

B
I
B
L
I
O
G
R
A
P
H
Y

Gilbert DL, Sethuraman G, Sine L, et al. Tourette's syndrome improvement with pergolide in a randomized, double-blind, crossover trial. *Neurology* 54(6):1310–1315, 2000.

Goetz CG, Kompoliti K. Rating scales and quantitative assessment of tics. *Adv Neurol* 85:31–42, 2001.

Hanna GL, Piacentini J, Cantwell DP, et al. Obsessive–compulsive disorder with and without tics in a clinical sample of children and adolescents. *Depress Anxiety* 16(2):59–63, 2002.

Himle JA, Fischer DJ, Van Etten ML, et al. Group behavioral therapy for adolescents with tic-related and non-tic-related obsessive–compulsive disorder. *Depress Anxiety* 17(2):73–77, 2003.

Khalifa N, von Knorring AL. Prevalence of tic disorders and Tourette syndrome in a Swedish school population. *Dev Med Child Neurol* 45(5):315–319, 2003.

King RA, Scahill L, Lombroso P, et al. Tourette's syndrome and other tic disorders. In: Martin A, Scahill L, Charney DS, Leckman JF (Eds.). *Pediatric Psychopharmacology Principles and Practice.* New York: Oxford University Press, pp. 526–542, 2003.

Kurlan R, Como PG, Deeley C, et al. A pilot controlled study of fluoxetine for obsessive–compulsive symptoms in children with Tourette's syndrome. *Clin Neuropharmacol* 16(2):167–172, 1993.

Kurlan R, Como PG, Miller B, et al. The behavioral spectrum of tic disorders: A community-based study. *Neurology* 59(3):414–420, 2002.

Law SF, Schachar RJ. Do typical doses of methylphenidate cause tics in children treated for attention-deficit hyperactivity disorder? *J Am Acad Child Adolesc Psychiatry* 38(8):944–951, 1999.

Leckman JF, Hardin MT, Riddle MA, et al. Clonidine treatment of Gilles de la Tourette's syndrome. *Arch Gen Psychiatry* 48(4):324–328, 1991.

Leckman JF, Pauls DL, Zhang H, et al. Obsessive–compulsive symptom dimensions in affected sibling pairs diagnosed with Gilles de la Tourette syndrome. *Am J Genet* 116B(1):60–68, 2003.

Leckman JF, Peterson BS, Cohen DJ. Tic disorders. In: Lewis M (Ed.), *Child and Adolescent Psychiatry: A Comprehensive Textbook* (3rd ed.). Philadelphia: Lippincott, Williams & Wilkins, pp. 734–744, 2002.

Leckman JF, Riddle MA, Hardin MT, et al. The Yale Global Tic Severity Scale: Initial testing of a clinician-rated scale of tic severity. *J Am Acad Child Adolesc Psychiatry* 28:566–573, 1989.

Leckman JF, Towbin KE, Ort SI, et al. Clinical assessment of tic disorder severity. In: Cohen DJ, Bruun R, Leckman JF (Eds.), *Tourette's Syndrome and Tic Disorders: Clinical Understanding and Treatment.* New York: Wiley, pp. 212–224, 1988.

McDougle CJ, Goodman WK, Leckman JF, et al. Haloperidol addition in fluvoxamine-refractory obsessive–compulsive disorder. A double-blind, placebo-controlled study in patients with and without tics. *Arch Gen Psychiatry* 51(4):302–308, 1994.

Niederhofer H, Staffen W, Mair A. A placebo-controlled study of lofexidine in the treatment of children with tic disorders and attention deficit hyperactivity disorder. *J Psychopharmacol* 17(1):113–119, 2003.

Nolan EE, Gadow KD, Sprafkin J. Stimulant medication withdrawal during long-term therapy in children with comorbid attention-deficit hyperactivity disorder and chronic multiple tic disorder. *Pediatrics* 103(4 Pt 1):730–737, 1999.

Peterson AL, Azrin NH. An evaluation of behavioral treatments for Tourette syndrome. *Behav Res Ther* 30(2):167–174, 1992.

Rugino TA, Copley TC. Effects of modafinil in children with attention-deficit/hyperactivity disorder: An open-label study. *J Am Acad Child Adolesc Psychiatry* 40(2):230–235, 2001.

Rugino TA, Samsock TC. Modafinil in children with attention-deficit hyperactivity disorder. *Pediatr Neurol* 29(2):136–142, 2003.

Sallee FR, Kurlan R, Goetz CG, et al. Ziprasidone treatment of children and adolescents with Tourette's syndrome: A pilot study. *J Am Acad Child Adolesc Psychiatry* 39(3): 292–299, 2000.

Sallee FR, Nesbitt L, Jackson C, et al. Relative efficacy of haloperidol and pimozide in children and adolescents with Tourette's disorder. *Am J Psychiatry* 154(8):1043–1045, 1997.

Scahill L, Chappell PB, Kim YS, et al. A placebo-controlled study of guanfacine in the treatment of children with tic disorders and attention deficit hyperactivity disorder. *Am J Psychiatry* 158(7):1067–1074, 2001.

Scahill L, Kano Y, King RA, et al. Influence of age and tic disorders on obsessive–compulsive disorder in a pediatric sample. *J Child Adolesc Psychopharmacol* 13(Suppl 1):S7–S17, 2003.

Scahill L, Leckman JF, Schultz RT, et al. A placebo-controlled trial of risperidone in Tourette syndrome. *Neurology* 60(7):1130–1135, 2003.

Scahill L, Riddle MA, King RA, et al. Fluoxetine has no marked effect on tic symptoms in patients with Tourette's syndrome: A double-blind, placebo-controlled study. *J Child Adolesc Psychopharmacol* 7(2):75–85, 1997.

Shapiro AK, Shapiro ES, Young JG, et al. Measurement in tic disorders. In: Shapiro AK, Shapiro ES, Young JG, et al. (Eds.), *Gilles de la Tourette Syndrome* (2nd ed.). New York: Raven Press, pp. 451–480, 1988.

Shapiro E, Shapiro AK, Fulop G, et al. Controlled study of haloperidol, pimozide and placebo for the treatment of Gilles de la Tourette's syndrome. *Arch Gen Psychiatry* 46(8):722–730, 1989.

Silver AA, Shytle D, Philipp MK, et al. Transdermal nicotine and haloperidol in Tourette's disorder: A double-blind placebo-controlled study. *J Clin Psychiatry* 62(9):707–714, 2001.

Silver AA, Shytle RD, Sheehan KH, et al. Multicenter, double-blind, placebo-controlled study of mecamylamine monotherapy for Tourette's disorder. *J Am Acad Child Adolesc Psychiatry* 40(9):1103–1110, 2001.

Singer HS, Brown J, Quaskey S, et al. The treatment of attention-deficit hyperactivity disorder in Tourette's syndrome: A double-blind placebo-controlled study with clonidine and desipramine. *Pediatrics* 95(1):74–81, 1995.

Singer HS, Wendlandt J, Krieger M, et al. Baclofen treatment in Tourette syndrome: A double-blind, placebo-controlled, crossover trial. *Neurology* 56(5):599–604, 2001.

Snider LA, Seligman LD, Ketchen BR, et al. Tics and problem behaviors in schoolchildren: Prevalence, characterization, and associations. *Pediatrics* 110(2 Pt 1):331–336, 2002.

Spencer T, Biederman M, Coffey B, et al. The 4-year course of tic disorders in boys with attention-deficit/hyperactivity disorder. *Arch Gen Psychiatry* 56(9):842–847, 1999.

Spencer T, Biederman J, Coffey B, et al. A double-blind comparison of desipramine and placebo in children and adolescents with chronic tic disorder and comorbid attention-deficit/hyperactivity disorder. *Arch Gen Psychiatry* 59(7):649–656, 2002.

Spencer T, Biederman J, Harding M, et al. The relationship between tic disorders and Tourette's syndrome revisited. *J Am Acad Child Adolesc Psychiatry* 34(9):1133–1139, 1995.

Steingard RJ, Goldberg M, Lee D, et al. Adjunctive clonazepam treatment of tic symptoms in children with comorbid tic disorders and ADHD. *J Am Acad Child Adolesc Psychiatry* 33(3):394–399, 1994.

Tourette's Syndrome Study Group. Treatment of ADHD in children with tics: A randomized controlled trial. *Neurology* 58(4):527–536, 2002.

BIBLIOGRAPHY

Walkup JT, Rosenberg LA, Brown J, et al. The validity of instruments measuring tic severity in Tourette's syndrome. *J Am Acad Child Adolesc Psychiatry* 31(3):472–477, 1992.

CONDUCT DISORDER, OPPOSITIONAL DEFIANT DISORDER, AND IMPULSIVE AGGRESSION

Aman MG, De Smedt G, Derivan A, et al. Double-blind, placebo-controlled study of risperidone for the treatment of disruptive behaviors in children with subaverage intelligence. *Am J Psychiatry* 159(8):1337–1346, 2002.

American Academy of Child and Adolescent Psychiatry. Practice parameters for the assessment and treatment of children and adolescents with conduct disorder. *J Am Acad Child Adolesc Psychiatry* 36(10 Suppl):122S–139S, 1997.

American Psychiatric Association. *Diagnostic and Statistical Manual of Mental Disorders* (4th ed., text rev.). Washingtom, DC: Author, 2000.

August GJ, Realmuto GM, Joyce T, et al. Persistence and desistance of oppositional defiant disorder in a community sample of children with ADHD. *J Am Acad Child Adolesc Psychiatry* 38(1):1262–1270, 1999.

Biederman J, Faraone SV, Milberger S, et al. Is childhood oppositional defiant disorder a precursor to adolescent conduct disorder? Findings from a four-year follow-up study of children with ADHD. *J Am Acad Child Adolesc Psychiatry* 35(9):1193–1204, 1996.

Brestan EV, Eyberg SM. Effective psychosocial treatments of conduct-disordered children and adolescents: 29 years, 82 studies, and 5,272 kids. *J Clin Child Psychol* 27(2):180–189, 1998.

Buss AH, Warren WL. *Aggression Questionnaire*. Los Angeles: Western Psychological Services, 2000.

Campbell M, Adams PB, Small AM, et al. Lithium in hospitalized aggressive children with conduct disorder: A double-blind and placebo-controlled study. *J Am Acad Child Adolesc Psychiatry* 24:445–453, 1995.

Campbell M, Small AM, Green WH, et al. Behavioral efficacy of haloperidol and lithium carbonate. A comparison in hospitalized aggressive children with conduct disorder. *Arch Gen Psychiatry* 41(7):650–656, 1984.

Caspi A, McClay J, Moffitt TE, et al. Role of genotype in the cycle of violence in maltreated children. *Science* 297:851–854, 2002.

Collett BR, Ohan JL, Myers KM. Ten-year review of rating scales. VI: Scales assessing externalizing behaviors. *J Am Acad Child Adolesc Psychiatry* 42(10):1143–1170, 2003.

Conners CK. *Conners Rating Scales—Revised, Technical Manual*. Toronto: Multi-Health Systems, 1997.

Connor DF. *Aggression and Antisocial Behavior in Children and Adolescents: Research and Treatment*. New York: Guilford Press, 2002.

Connor DF, Barkley RA, Davis HT. A pilot study of methylphenidate, clonidine, or the combination in ADHD comorbid with agressive oppositional defiant or conduct disorder. *Clin Pediatr* 39:15–25, 2000.

Connor DF, Boone RT, Steingard RJ, et al. Psychopharmacology and aggression: II. A meta-analysis of nonstimulant medication effects on overt aggression-related behaviors in youth with SED. *J Emotion Behav Dis* 11(3):157–168, 2003.

Connor DF, Glatt SJ, Lopez ID, et al. Psychopharmacology and aggression. I: A meta-analysis of stimulant effects on overt/covert aggression-related behaviors in ADHD. *J Am Acad Child Adolesc Psychiatry* 41(3):253–261, 2002.

Crick NR. *The Children's Social Behavior Scale*, 2003. Available from Nicki Crick, PhD, Crick Social Development Lab, 51 East River Road, Minneapolis, MN, 55455. Online: *crick001@umn.edu*

Cueva JE, Overall JE, Small AM, et al. Carbamazepine in aggressive children with conduct disorder: A double-blind and placebo-controlled study. *J Am Acad Child Adolesc Psychiatry* 35:480–490, 1996.

Davanzo PA. Anticonvulsants. In: Rosenberg DR, Davanzo PA, Gershon S (Eds.), *Pharmacotherapy for Child and Adolescent Psychiatric Disorders* (2nd ed.). New York: Marcel Dekker, pp. 453–488, 2002.

Davanzo PA, McCracken J. Mood stabilizers: Lithium and anticonvulsants. In: Martin A, Scahill L, Charney DS, Leckman JF (Eds.), *Pediatric Psychopharmacology Principals and Practice*. New York: Oxford University Press, pp. 309–327, 2003.

DelBello MP, Kowatch RA. Lithium. In: Rosenberg DR, Davanzo PA, Gershon S (Eds.), *Pharmacotherapy for Child and Adolescent Psychiatric Disorders* (2nd ed.). New York: Marcel Dekker, pp. 415–452, 2002.

Dodge KA. *The Proactive and Reactive Aggression Scale*, 2003. Available from Kenneth Dodge, PhD, Duke University, Center for Child and Family Policy, Box 90264, Durham, NC 27708. Online: *dodge@pps.duke.edu*

Donovan SJ, Stewart JW, Nunes EV, et al. Divalproex treatment for youth with explosive temper and mood lability: A double-blind, placebo-controlled crossover design. *Am J Psychiatry* 157:818–820, 2000.

Findling RL, McNamara NK, Branicky LA, et al. A double-blind pilot study of risperidone in the treatment of conduct disorder. *J Am Acad Child Adolesc Psychiatry* 39:509–561, 2000.

Foley DL, Eaves LJ, Wormley B, et al. Childhood adversity, monoamine oxidase A genotype, and risk for conduct disorder. *Arch Gen Psychiatry* 61:738–744, 2004.

Frazier JA. Agitation and aggression. In: Martin A, Scahill L, Charney DS, Leckman JF (Eds.), *Pediatric Psychopharmacology Principals and Practice*. New York: Oxford University Press, pp. 671–685, 2003.

Gordon CT, State RC, Nelson JE, et al. A double-blind comparison of clomipramine, desipramine, and placebo in the treatment of autistic disorder. *Arch Gen Psychiatry* 50:441–447, 1993.

Green WH. *Child and Adolescent Clinical Psychopharmacology* (3rd ed.), Philadelphia: Lippincott, Williams & Wilkins, pp. 238–268, 2001.

Greene RW, Biederman J, Zerwas S, et al. Psychiatric comorbidity, family dysfunction, and social impairment in referred youth with oppositional defiant disorder. *Am J Psychiatry* 159(7):1214–1224, 2002.

Halperin JM, MacKay KE, Grayson RH, et al. Reliability, validity, and preliminary normative data for the Children's Aggression Scale—Teacher Version. *J Am Acad Child Adolesc Psychiatry* 42(8):965–971, 2003.

Halperin JM, McKay KE, Newcorn JH. Development, reliability, and validity of the Children's Aggression Scale—Parent Version. *J Am Acad Child Adolesc Psychiatry* 41(3):245–252, 2002.

Hazell PL, Stuart JE. A randomized controlled trial of clonidine added to psychostimulant medication for hyperactive and aggressive children. *J Am Acad Child Adolesc Psychiatry* 42(8):886–894, 2003.

Hinshaw SP, Anderson CA. Conduct and oppositional disorders. In: Mash EJ, Barkley RA (Eds.), *Child Psychopathology*. New York: Guilford Press, pp. 113–149, 1996.

Kay SR, Wolkenfeld F, Murrill LM. Profiles of aggression among psychiatric patients: I. Nature and prevalence. *J Ner Men Dis* 176(9):539–546, 1988.

Klein RG. Preliminary results: Lithium effects in conduct disorders. CME Syllabus and Proceedings Summary presented at Annual Meeting of the American Psychiatric Association, New Orleans, LA, May 11–16, 1991.

Klein RG, Abikoff H, Klass E, et al. Clinical efficacy of methylphenidate in conduct disorder with and without attention deficit hyperactivity disorder. *Arch Gen Psychiatry* 54:1073–1080, 1997.

Kruese MJ, Stoewe J. Conduct disorder and sociopathy. In: Coffey CE, Brumback RA (Eds.), *Textbook of Pediatric Neuropsychiatry*. Washington, DC: American Psychiatric Press, pp. 527–545, 1998.

Malone RP, Delaney MA, Luebbert JF, et al. A double-blind placebo-controlled study of lithium in hospitalized aggressive children and adolescents with conduct disorder. *Arch Gen Psychiatry* 57:649–654, 2000.

McCracken JT, McGough J, Shah B, et al. Risperidone in children with autism and serious behavioral problems. *NEJM* 347(5):314–321, 2002.

Miller LS, Klein RG, Piacentini J, et al. The New York teacher rating scale for disruptive and antisocial behavior. *J Am Acad Child Adolesc Psychiatry* 34(3):359–370, 1995.

Moffitt TE. Life-course persistent and adolescence-limited antisocial behavior: A developmental taxonomy. *Psychol Rev* 100:674–701, 1993.

Newcorn JH, Spencer TJ, Biederman J, et al. Atomoxetive treatment in children and adolescents with attention-deficit/hyperactivity disorder and comorbid oppositional defiant disorder. *J Am Acad Child Adolesc Psychiatry* 44(3):240–248, 2005.

Pappadopulos E, MacIntyre II JC, Crismon ML, et al. Treatment recommendations for the use of antipsychotics for aggressive youth (TRAAY): Part II. *J Am Acad Child Adolesc Psychiatry* 42(2):145–161, 2003.

Patterson GR. *Coercive Family Process*. Eugene, OR: Castalia, 1982.

Patterson GR, Reid JB, Dishion TJ. *Antisocial Boys*. Eugene, OR: Castalia, 1992.

Pelham WE, Milich R, Murphy HA. Normative data on the IOWA Conners teacher rating scale. *J Clin Child Psychol* 18:259–262, 1989.

Rifkin A, Karajgi B, Dicker R, et al. Lithium treatment of conduct disorders in adolescents. *Am J Psychiatry* 154:554–555, 1997.

Schur SB, Sikich L, Findling RL, et al. Treatment recommendations for the use of antipsychotics for aggressive youth (TRAAY): Part I. A review. *J Am Acad Child Adolesc Psychiatry* 42(2):132–144, 2003.

Sorgi P, Ratey J, Knoedler DW, et al. Rating aggression in the clinical setting: A retrospective adaptation of the overt aggression scale. *J Neuropsychiatr Clin Neurosci* 3(2):S52–S56, 1991.

Steiner H, Petersen M, Saxena K, et al. A randomized clinical trial of divalproex sodium in conduct disorders. *J Clin Psychiatry*, 64(10):1183–1191, 2003.

Steiner H, Saxena K, Chang K. Psychopharmacologic strategies for the treatment of aggression in juveniles. *CNS Spectrums* 8(4):298–308, 2003.

Viesselman JO. Antidepressant and antimanic drugs. In: Werry JS, Aman MG (Eds.), *Practitioner's Guide to Psychoactive Drugs for Children and Adolescents* (2nd ed.). New York: Plenum Press, pp. 249–296, 1999.

Vitiello B, Behar D, Hunt J, et al. Subtyping aggression in children and adolescents. *J Neuropsychiatr Clin Neurosci* 2:189–192, 1990.

Weller EB, Weller RA, Fristad MA. Lithium dosage guide for prepubertal children: A preliminary report. *J Am Acad Child Adolesc Psychiatry* 25:92–95, 1986.

Yudofsky SC, Silver JM, Jackson W, et al. The overt aggression scale for the objective rating of verbal and physical aggression. *Am J Psychiatry* 143(1):35–39, 1986.

MOOD DISORDERS

Akiskal HS, Hantouche EG, Bourqeois ML et al. Gender, temperament, and the clinical picture in dysphoric mixed mania: Findings from a French national study (EPIMAN). *J Affect Disord* 50(2–3):175–186, 1998.

Alexopoulos GS, Abrams RC, Young RC, et al. Cornell Scale for Depression in Dementia. *Biol Psychiatry* 23:271–284, 1988.

Ambrosini PJ, Bianchi MD, Rabinovich H et al. Treatments in children and adolescents: I. Affective disorders. *J Am Acad Child Adolesc Psychiatry* 32(1):1–6, 1993.

American Academy of Child and Adolescent Psychiatry. 10/15/04 FDA launches a multi-pronged strategy to strengthen safeguards for children treated with antidepressant medication. Available at www.aacap.org.

American Academy of Child and Adolescent Psychiatry Work Group on Quality Issues. Practice parameters for the assessment and treatment of children and adolescents with depressive disorders. *J Am Acad Child Adolesc Psychiatry* 37(10 Suppl):63S–83S, 1998.

American Psychiatric Association. *Diagnostic and Statistical Manual of Mental Disorders* (4th ed., text rev.). Washington, DC: Author 2000.

Angst J. The emerging epidemiology of hypomania and bipolar II disorder. *J Affect Disord* 50(2–3):143–151, 1998.

Balon R, Yeragani VK, Pohl RB, et al. Lithium discontinuation: Withdrawal or relapse? *Compr Psychiatry* 29(3):330–334, 1988.

Bamber D, Tamplin A, Park RJ, et al. Development of a short Leyton obsessional inventory for children and adolescents. *J Am Acad Child Adolesc Psychiatry* 41(10): 1246–1252, 2002.

Beck AT. Beck depression inventory. Philadelphia, PA: Center for Cognitive Therapy, 1961.

Beck AT, Steer RA, Brown GK. BDI-II, Beck depression inventory: manual, 2nd edition. Boston: Harcourt Brace, 1996.

Beck AT, Guth D, Steer AA, et al. Screening for major depression disorders in medical inpatients with the Beck Depression inventory for primary Care. *Behav Res Ther* 35:785–791, 1997.

Biederman J, Mick E, Wozniak J, et al. Can a subtype of conduct disorder linked to bipolar disorder be identified? Integration of findings from the Massachusetts General Hospital Pediatric Psychopharmacology Research Program. *Biol Psychiatry* 53(11): 952–960, 2003.

Birmaher B, Bridge JA, Williamson DE, et al. Psychosocial functioning in youths at high risk to develop major depressive disorder. *J Am Acad Child Adolesc Psychiatry* 43(7):839–846, 2004.

Birmaher B, Ryan ND, Williamson DE, et al. Childhood and adolescent depression: A review of the past 10 years. Part I. *J Am Acad Child Adolesc Psychiatry* 35:1427–1439, 1996a.

Birmaher B, Ryan ND, Williamson DE, et al. Childhood and adolescent depression: A review of the past 10 years. Part II. *J Am Acad Child Adolesc Psychiatry* 35:1575–1583, 1996b.

Birmaher B, Waterman GS, Ryan ND, et al. Randomized, controlled trial of amitriptyline versus placebo for adolescents with treatment-resistant major depression. *J Am Acad Child Adolesc Psychiatry* 37(5):527–535, 1998.

Bowden CL, Brugger AM, Swann AC, et al. Efficacy of divalproex vs lithium and placebo in the treatment of mania. The Depakote Mania Study Group. *JAMA* 271(12):918–924, 1994.

Bowden CL, McElroy SL. History of the development of valproate for treatment of bipolar disorder *J Clin Psychiatry* 56(Suppl 3):3–5, 1995.

Braconnier A, Le Coent R, Cohen D, DEROXADO Study Group. Paroxetine versus clomipramine in adolescents with severe major depression: A double-blind, randomized, multicenter trial. *J Am Acad Child Adolesc Psychiatry* 42(1):22–29, 2003.

Burns JJ, Cottrell L, Perkins K, et al. Depressive symptoms and health risk among rural adolescents. *Pediatrics* 113(5):1313–1320, 2004.

Carlson GA, Jensen PS, Findling RL, et al. Methodological issues and controversies in clinical trials with child and adolescent patients with bipolar disorder: Report of a consensus conference. *J Child Adolesc Psychopharmacol* 13(1):13–27, 2003.

Carlson GA, Loney J, Salisbury H, et al. Stimulant treatment in young boys with symptoms suggesting childhood mania: A report from a longitudinal study. *J Child Adolesc Psychopharmacol* 10(3):175–184, 2000.

Carlson PJ, Merlock MC, Suppes T. Adjunctive stimulant use in patients with bipolar disorder: Treatment of residual depression and sedation. *Bipolar Disord* 6(5): 416–420, 2004.

Carlsten A, Waern M, Ekedahl A, et al. Antidepressant medication and suicide in Sweden. *Pharmacoepidemiol Drug Safety* 10(6):525–530, 2001.

Chang KD, Dienes K, Blasey C, et al. Divalproex monotherapy in the treatment of bipolar offspring with mood and behavioral disorders and at least mild affective symptoms. *J Clin Psychiatry* 64(8):936–942, 2003.

Charney DS, Manji HK. Life stress, genes, and depression: Multiple pathways lead to increased risk and new opportunities for intervention. *Sci STKE*(Mar 16): 225, 2004.

Costello EJ, Pine DS, Haminen G, et al. Development and natural history of mood disorders. *Biol Psychiatry* 52(6):529–542, 2002.

Cox JL, Chapman G, Murray D, et al. Validation of the Edinburgh Postratal Depression Scale (EPDS) in non-postnatal women. *J Affect Disord* 39:185–189, 1996.

Coyle JT, Pine DS, Charney DS, et al. Depression and bipolar support alliance consensus statement on the unmet needs in diagnosis and treatment of mood disorders in children and adolescents. *J Am Acad Child Adolesc Psychiatry* 42(12):1494–1503, 2003.

DelBello MP, Carlson GA, Tohen M, et al. Rates and predictors of developing a manic or hypomanic episode 1 to 2 years following a first hospitalization for major depression with psychotic features. *J Child Adolesc Psychopharmacol* 13(2):173–185, 2003.

DelBello MP, Schwiers ML, Rosenberg HL, et al. A double-blind, randomized, placebo-controlled study of quetiapine as adjunctive treatment for adolescent mania. *J Am Acad Child Adolesc Psychiatry* 41(10):1216–1223, 2002.

Eley TC, Liang H, Plomin R, et al. Parental familial vulnerability, family environment, and their interactions as predictors of depressive symptoms in adolescents. *J Am Acad Child Adolesc Psychiatry* 43(3):298–306, 2004.

Emslie GJ, Heilqenstein JH, Hoog SL, et al. Fluoxetine treatment for prevention of relapse of depression in children and adolescents: A double-blind, placebo-controlled study. *J Am Acad Child Adolesc Psychiatry* 43(11):1397–1405, 2004.

Emslie GJ, Heiligenstein JH, Hoog SL, et al. Fluoxetine treatment for prevention of relapse of depression in children and adolescents: A double-blind, placebo-controlled study. *J Am Acad Child Adolesc Psychiatry* 43(11):1397–1405, 2004.

Emslie GJ, Heilgienstein JH, Wagner KD, et al. Fluoxetine for acute treatment of depression in children and adolescents: A placebo-controlled, randomized clinical trial. *J Am Acad Child Adolesc Psychiatry* 41(10):1205–1215, 2002.

Emslie GJ, Rush AJ, Weinberg WA, et al. A double-blind, randomized, placebo-controlled trial of fluoxetine in children and adolescents with depression. *Arch Gen Psychiatry* 54(11):1031–1037, 1997.

Fendrich M, Weissman MM, Warner J. Screening for depressive disorder in children and adolescents. Validating the Center for Epidemiologic studies depression scale for children. *Am J Epidemiol* 131:538–551, 1990.

Findling RL, McNamara NK. Atypical antipsychotics in the treatment of children and adolescents: Clinical applications. *J Clin Psychiatry* 65(Suppl 6):30–44, 2004.

Findling RL, McNamara NK, Gracious BL, et al. Combination lithium and divalproex sodium in pediatric bipolarity. *J Am Acad Child Adolesc Psychiatry* 42(8): 895–901, 2003.

Findling RL, McNamara NK, Youngstrom EA, et al. Double-blind 18-month trial of lithium versus divalproex maintenance treatment in pediatric bipolar disorder. *J Am Acad Child Adolesc Psychiatry* 44(5):409–417, 2005.

Finn PR, Sharkansky EJ. The effects of familial risk, personality, and expectancies on alcohol use and abuse. *J Abnorm Psychol* 109(1):122–133, 2000.

Frazier JA, Biederman J, Tohen M, et al. A prospective open-label treatment trial of olanzapine monotherapy in children and adolescents with bipolar disorder. *J Child Adolesc Psychopharmacol* 11(3):239–250, 2001.

Fristad MA, Goldberg-Arnold JS, Gavazzi SM. Multifamily psychoeducation groups (MFPG) for families of children with bipolar disorder. *Bipolar Disord* 4(4):254–262, 2002.

Frye MA, Ketter TA, Kimbrell TA, et al. A placebo-controlled study of lamotrigine and gabapentin monotherapy in refractory mood disorders. *J Clin Psychopharmacol* 20(6):607–614, 2000.

Geller B, Cooper TB, McCombs HG, et al. Double-blind, placebo-controlled study of nortriptyline in depressed children using a "fixed plasma level" design. *Psychopharmacol Bull* 25(1):101–108, 1989.

Geller B, Tillman R, Craney JL, et al. Four-year prospective outcome and natural history of mania in children with a prepubertal and early adolescent bipolar disorder phenotype. *Arch Gen Psychiatry* 61(5):459–467, 2004.

Geller B, Zimerman MA, Williams M, et al. Phenomenology of prepubertal and early adolescent bipolar disorder: Examples of elated mood, grandiose behaviors, decreased need for sleep, racing thoughts, and hypersexuality. *J Child Adolesc Psychopharmacol* 12(1):3–9, 2002a.

Geller B, Zimerman MA, Williams M, et al. DSM-IV mania symptoms in a prepubertal and early adolescent bipolar disorder phenotype compared to attention-deficit hyperactive and normal controls. *J Child Adolesc Psychopharmacol* 12(1):11–25, 2002b.

Goodyer IM, Herbert J, Secher SM, et al. short term outcomes of major depression: I. Comorbidity and severity at presentation as predictors of persistent disorder. *J Am Acad Child Adolesc Psychiatry* 36:179–187, 1997.

Gracious BL, Youngstrom EA, Findling RL, et al. Discriminative validity of a parent version of the Young Mania Rating Scale. *J Am Acad Child Adolesc Psychiatry* 41(11):1350–1359, 2002.

Grunebaum MF, Ellis SP, Li S, et al. Antidepressants and suicide risk in the United States, 1985–1999. *J Clin Psychiatry* 65(11):1456–1462, 2004.

Hantouche EG, Akiskal HS, Lancrenov S, et al. Systematic clinical methodology for validating bipolar-II disorder: Data in mid-stream from a French national multi-site study (EPIDEP). *J Affect Disord* 50(2–3):163–173, 1998.

Harrington R, Myatt T. Is preadolescent mania the same condition as adult mania? A British perspective. *Biol Psychiatry* 53(11):961–969, 2003.

Hazell PL, Carr V, Lewin TJ, et al. Manic symptoms in young males with ADHD predict functioning but not diagnosis after 6 years. *J Am Acad Child Adolesc Psychiatry* 42(5):552–560, 2003.

Hirschfeld RM, Allen MH, McEvoy JP, et al. Safety and tolerability of oral loading divalproex sodium in acutely manic bipolar patients. *J Clin Psychiatry* 60(12):815–818, 1999.

Hirschfeld RM, Calabrese JR, Weissman MM, et al. Screening for bipolar disorder in the community. *J Clin Psychiatry* 64(1):53–59, 2003.

BIBLIOGRAPHY

Hirschfeld RM, Lewis L, Vornik LA. Perceptions and impact of bipolar disorder: How far have we really come? Results of the National Depressive and Manic–Depressive Association 2000 survey of individuals with bipolar disorder. *J Clin Psychiatry* 64(2): 161–174, 2003.

Holahan CJ, Moos RH, Holahan CK, et al. Unipolar depression, life context vulnerabilities, and drinking to cope. *J Consult Clin Psychol* 72(2):269–275, 2004.

Hughes CW, Preskorn SH, Wrona M, et al. Follow-up of adolescents initially treated for prepubertal-onset major depressive disorder with imipramine. *Psychopharmacol Bull* 26(2):244–248, 1990.

Judd LL, Schettler PJ, Akiskal HS. Prevalence, clinical relevance, and public health significance of subthreshold depressions. *Psychiatr Clin North Am* 25(4):685–698, 2002.

Kafantaris V, Coletti DJ, Dicker R, et al. Lithium treatment of acute mania in adolescents: A large open trial. *J Am Acad Child Adolesc Psychiatry* 42(9):1038–1045, 2003.

Kafantaris V, Coletti DJ, Dicker R, et al. Lithium treatment of acute mania in adolescents: A placebo-controlled discontinuation study. *J Am Acad Child Adolesc Psychiatry* 43(8):984–993, 2004.

Kahana SY, Youngstrom EA, Findling RL, et al. Employing parent, teacher, and youth self-report checklists in identifying pediatric bipolar spectrum disorders: An examination of diagnostic accuracy and clinical utility. *J Child Adolesc Psychopharmacol* 13(4):471–488, 2003.

Kashani JH, Shekim WO, Reid JC. Amitriptyline in children with major depressive disorder: A double-blind crossover pilot study. *J Am Acad Child Adolesc Psychiatry* 23(3):348–351, 1984.

Kaufman J. Depressive disorders in maltreated children. *J Am Acad Child Psychiatry* 30:257–265, 1991.

Kaufman J, Martin A, King RA, Charney D. Are child-, adolescent-, and adult-onset depression one and the same disorder? *Biol Psychiatry* 49:980–1001, 2001.

Keller MB, Ryan ND, Strober M, et al. Efficacy of paroxetine in the treatment of adolescent major depression: A randomized, controlled trial. *J Am Acad Child Adolesc Psychiatry* 40(7):762–772, 2001.

Khan A, Khan S, Kolts R, et al. Suicide rates in clinical trials of SSRIs, other antidepressants, and placebo: Analysis of FDA reports. *Am J Psychiatry* 160(4):790–792, 2003.

Kim EY, Miklowitz DJ. Childhood mania, attention deficit hyperactivity disorder and conduct disorder: A critical review of diagnostic dilemmas. *Bipolar Disor* 4(4):215–223, 2002.

Klein RG, Mannuzza S, Koplewicz HS, et al. Adolescent depression: Controlled desipramine treatment and atypical features. *Depress Anxiety* 7(1):15–31, 1998.

Kovacs M. Children's depression inventory. North Tonawanda, N. Y.: Multi-Health System, 1992.

Kovacs M, Akiskal HS, Gatsonis C, et al. Childhood-onset dysthymic disorder: Clinical features and prospective naturalistic outcome. *Arch Gen Psychiatry* 51(5):365–374, 1994.

Kovacs M, Gatsonis C. Secular trends in age at onset of major depressive disorder in a clinical sample of children. *J Psychiatr Res* 28(3):319–329, 1994.

Kovacs M, Goldston D. Cognitive and social cognitive development of depressed children and adolescents. *J Am Acad Child Adolesc Psychiatry* 30(3):388–392, 1991.

Kovacs M, Krol RS, Voti L. Early onset psychopathology and the risk for teenage pregnancy among clinically referred girls. *J Am Acad Child Adolesc Psychiatry* 33(1): 106–113, 1994.

Kowatch RA, Sethuraman G, Hume JH, et al. Combination pharmacotherapy in children and adolescents with bipolar disorder. *Biol Psychiatry* 53(11):978–984, 2003.

Kramer AD, Feiguine RJ. Clinical effects of amitriptyline in adolescent depression: A pilot study. *J Am Acad Child Psychiatry* 20(3):636–644, 1981.

Kupfer DJ, Frank E, Perel JM, et al. Five-year outcome for maintenance therapies in recurrent depression. *Arch Gen Psychiatry* 49(10):769–773, 1992.

Kutcher S, Boulos C, Ward B, et al. Response to desipramine treatment in adolescent depression: A fixed-dose, placebo-controlled trial. *J Am Acad Child Adolesc Psychiatry* 33(5):686–694, 1994.

Kye CH, Waterman GS, Ryan ND, et al. A randomized, controlled trial of amitriptyline in the acute treatment of adolescent major depression. *J Am Acad Child Adolesc Psychiatry* 35(9):1139–1144, 1996.

Leibenluft E, Charney DS, Towbin KE et al. Defining clinical phenotypes of juvenile mania. *Am J Psychiatry* 160(3):430–437, 2003.

Lizardi H, Klein DN, Shankman SA. Psychopathology in the adolescent and young adult offspring of parents with dysthymic disorder and major depressive disorder. *J Nerv Ment Dis* 192(3):193–199, 2004.

March J, Silva S, Petryckis et al. Fluoxetine, cognitive–behavioral therapy, and their combination for adolescents with depression: Treatment for Adolescents with Depression Study (TADS) randomized controlled trial. *JAMA* 292(7):807–820, 2004.

Marcotte D. Irrational beliefs and depression in adolescence. *Adolescence* 31(124): 935–954, 1996.

Maser JD, Akiskal HS. Spectrum concepts in major mental disorders. *Psychiatr Clin North Am* 25(4):xi–xiii, 2002.

Matthews JD, Bottonari KA, Polania LM, et al. An open study of olanzapine and fluoxetine for psychotic major depressive disorder: Interim analyses. *J Clin Psychiatry* 63(12):1164–1170, 2002.

McElroy SL, Keck PE, Stanton SP, et al. A randomized comparison of divalproex oral loading versus haloperidol in the initial treatment of acute psychotic mania. *J Clin Psychiatry* 57(4):142–146, 1996.

McLeer SV, Dixon JF, Henry D, et al. Psychopathology in non-clinically referred sexually abused children. *J Am Acad Child Adolesc Psychiatry* 37(12):1326–1333, 1998.

Miklowitz DJ, Simoneau TL, George EL, et al. Family-focused treatment of bipolar disorder: 1-year effects of a psychoeducational program in conjunction with pharmacotherapy. *Biol Psychiatry* 48(6):582–592, 2000.

Milin RP, Simeon J, Spenst WP. Paroxetine in the treatment of children and adolescents with major depression. Poster NR67:104-105, presented at the 46th annual meeting of the American Academy of Child and Adolescent Psychiatry, Chicago, October 19–21, 1999.

Moscovitch A, Blashko CA, Eagles JM, et al. A placebo-controlled study of sertraline in the treatment of outpatients with seasonal affective disorder. *Psychopharmacology (Berl)* 171(4):390–397, 2004.

Motavalli Mukaddes N, Abali O. Venlafaxine in children and adolescents with attention deficit hyperactivity disorder. *Psychiatry Clin Neurosci* 58(1):92–95, 2004.

Mufson L, Dorta KP, Wickramaratne P, et al. A randomized effectiveness trial of interpersonal psychotherapy for depressed adolescents. *Arch Gen Psychiatry* 61(6):577–584, 2004.

Oluboka OJ, Bird DC, Kutchers, et al. A pilot study of loading versus titration of valproate in the treatment of acute mania. *Bipolar Disord* 4(5):341–345, 2002.

Pande AC, Crockatt JG, Janney CA, et al. Gabapentin in bipolar disorder: A placebo-controlled trial of adjunctive therapy. Gabapentin Bipolar Disorder Study Group. *Bipolar Disord* 2(3 Pt 2):249–255, 2000.

Pavuluri MN, Birmaher B. A practical guide to using ratings of depression and anxiety in child psychiatric practice. *Curr Psychiatry Rep* 6(2):108–116, 2004.

Pavuluri MN, Graczyk PA, Henry DB, et al. Child- and family-focused cognitive–beahvioral therapy for pediatric bipolar disorder: Development and preliminary results. *J Am Acad Child Adolesc Psychiatry* 43(5):528–537, 2004.

Pavuluri MN, Henry DB, Devineni B, et al. A pharmacotherapy algorithm for stabilization and maintenance of pediatric bipolar disorder. *J Am Acad Child Adolesc Psychiatry* 43(7):859–867, 2004.

Perlis RH, Miyahara S, Marangell LB, et al. Long-term implications of early onset in bipolar disorder: Data from the first 1,000 participants in the systematic treatment enhancement program for bipolar disorder (STEP-BD). *Biol Psychiatry* 55(9): 875–881, 2004.

Petti TA, Law W III. Imipramine treatment of depressed children: A double-blind pilot study. *J Clin Psychopharmacol* 2(2):107–110, 1982.

Pine DS. Brain development and the onset of mood disorders. *Sem Clin Neuropsychiatry* 7(4):223–233, 2002.

Pine DS. Treating children and adolescents with selective serotonin reuptake inhibitors: How long is appropriate? *J Child Adolesc Psychopharmacol* 12(3):189–203, 2002.

Pine DS, Cohen P, Johnson JG, et al. Adolescent life events as predictors of adult depression. *J Affect Disord* 68(1):49–57, 2002.

Post RM, Chang KD, Findling RL, et al. Prepubertal bipolar I disorder and bipolar disorder NOS are separable from ADHD. *J Clin Psychiatry* 65(7):898–902, 2004.

Preskorn SH, Weller E, Hughes C, et al. Plasma monitoring of tricyclic antidepressants: Defining the therapeutic range for imipramine in depressed children. *Clin Neuropharmacol* 9(Suppl 4):265–267, 1986.

Preskorn SH, Weller EB, Wellev RA. Depression in children: Relationship between plasma imipramine levels and response. *J Clin Psychiatry* 43(11):450–453, 1982.

Puig-Antich J, Perel JM, Lupatkin W, et al. Imipramine in prepubertal major depressive disorders. *Arch Gen Psychiatry* 44(1):81–89, 1987.

Radloff LS. The CES-D Scale: A self-report depression scale for research in the general population. Applied Psychological Measurement 1:385–401, 1977.

Reinecke MA, Ryan NE, Lupatkin W, et al. Cognitive–behavioral therapy of depression and depressive symptoms during adolescence: A review and meta-analysis. *J Am Acad Child Adolesc Psychiatry* 37(1):26–34, 1998.

Reynolds WM. Reynolds child depression scale. Odessa, Fla.: Psychological Assessment Resources, 1989.

Reynolds WM. Reynolds adolescent depression scale. Odessa, Fla.: Psychological Assessment Resources, 1986.

Sallee FR, Gilbert DL, Vinks AA, et al. Pharmacodynamics of ziprasidone in children and adolescents: Impact on dopamine transmission. *J Am Acad Child Adolesc Psychiatry* 42(8):902–907, 2003.

Scheffer RE, Kowatch RA, Carmody T, et al. Randomized, placebo-controlled trial of mixed amphetamine salts for symptoms of comorbid ADHD in pediatric bipolar disorder after mood stabilization with divalproex sodium. *Am J Psychiatry* 162:58–64, 2005.

Sheikh JI, Yesavage JA. Geriatric depression scale (GDS): recent evidence and development of a shorter version. In: Brink TL (Ed.), Clinical gerontology: A guide to assessment and intervention. New York: Haworth, 1986.

Simeon JG, Dinicola VF, Ferguson HB, et al. Adolescent depression: A placebo-controlled fluoxetine treatment study and follow-up. *Prog Neuropsychopharmacol Biol Psychiatry* 14(5):791–795, 1990.

Strober M, Freeman R, Rigali J, et al. The pharacotherapy of depressive illness in adolescence: II. Effects of lithium augmentation in nonresponders to imipramine. *J Am Acad Child Adolesc Psychiatry* 31(1):16–20, 1992.

Strober M, Lampert C, Schmidt S, et al. The course of major depressive disorder in adolescents: I. Recovery and risk of manic switching in a follow-up of psychotic and nonpsychotic subtypes. *J Am Acad Child Adolesc Psychiatry* 32(1):34–42, 1993.

Strober M, Schmidt-Lackner S, Freeman R, Bower S, Lampert C, DeAntonio M. Recovery and relapse in adolescents with bipolar affective illness: A five-year naturalistic, prospective follow-up. *J Am Acad Child Adolesc Psychiatry* 34:724–731, 1995.

Swann AC, Bowden CL, Rush AJ, et al. Desipramine versus phenelzine in recurrent unipolar depression: Clinical characteristics and treatment response. *J Clin Psychopharmacol* 17(2):78–83, 1997.

Swann AC, Secunda SK, Katz MM, et al. Specificity of mixed affective states: Clinical comparison of dysphoric mania and agitated depression. *J Affect Disord* 28:81–89, 1993.

Thuppal M, Carlson GA, Sprafkin J, et al. Correspondence between adolescent report, parent report, and teacher report of manic symptoms. *J Child Adolesc Psychopharmacol* 12(1):27–35, 2002.

Wagner KD. Diagnosis and treatment of bipolar disorder in children and adolescents. *J Clin Psychiatry* 65(Suppl 15):30–34, 2004.

Wagner KD, Ambrosini P, Rynn M, et al. Efficacy of sertraline in the treatment of childen and adolescents with major depressive disorder: Two randomized controlled trials. *JAMA* 290(8):1033–1041, 2003.

Wagner KD, Robb AS, Findling RL, et al. A randomized, placebo-controlled trial of citalopram for the treatment of major depression in children and adolescents. *Am J Psychiatry* 161(6):1079–1083, 2004.

Wagner KD, Weller EB, Carlson GA, et al. An open-label trial of divalproex in children and adolescents with bipolar disorder. *J Am Acad Child Adolesc Psychiatry* 41(10):1224–1230, 2002.

Whittington CJ, Kendall T, Fongay P, et al. Selective serotonin reuptake inhibitors in childhood depression: Systematic review of published versus unpublished data. *Lancet* 363(9418):1341–1345, 2004.

Wileman SM, Eagles JM, Andrew JE, et al. Light therapy for seasonal affective disorder in primary care: Randomised controlled trial. *Br J Psychiatry* 178:311–316, 2001.

Wilens TE, Biederman J, Kwon A, et al. Risk of substance use disorders in adolescents with bipolar disorder. *J Am Acad Child Adolesc Psychiatry* 43(11):1380–1386, 2004.

Yerevanian BI, Koek RJ, Feusner JD, et al. Antidepressants and suicidal behaviour in unipolar depression. *Acta Psychiatr Scand* 110(6):452–458, 2004.

Yeung A, Chang D, Gresham RL Jr., et al. Illness beliefs of depressed Chinese American patients in primary care. *J Nerv Ment Dis* 192(4):324–327, 2004.

Yesavage JA, Brink TL, Rose TL, et al. Development and validation of a geriatric depression screening scale: A preliminary report. J Psychiatr Res 17:37–49, 1983.

Yorbik O, Birmaher B, Axelson D, et al. Clinical characteristics of depressive symptoms in children and adolescents with major depressive disorder. *J Clin Psychiatry* 65(12):1654–1659, 2004.

Zung WW. A Self-rating depression scale. Arch Gen Psychiatry 12:63–70, 1965.

B
I
B
L
I
O
G
R
A
P
H
Y

PSYCHOTIC DISORDERS

American Academy of Child and Adolescent Psychiatry. Work Group on Quality Issues. Practice parameters for the assessment and treatment of children and adolescents with schizophrenia. *J Am Acad Child Adolesc Psychiatry* 40(7 Suppl): 4S–23S, 2001.

Arboleda C, Holzman P. Thought disorder in children at risk for psychosis. *Arch Gen Psychiatry* 42:1004–1013, 1985.

Armenteros JL, Whitaker AH, Welikson M, et al. Risperidone in adolescents with schizophrenia: An open pilot study. *J Am Acad Child Adolesc Psychiatry* 36:694–700, 1997.

Arseneault L, Cannon M, Murray R, et al. Childhood origins of violent behaviour in adults with schizophreniform disorder. *Br J Psychiatry* 183(12):520–525, 2003.

Biederman J, Petty C, Faraone SV, et al. Phenomenology of childhood psychosis, findings from a large sample of psychiatrically referred youth. *J Nerv Ment Dis* 192(9): 607–614, 2004.

Calello DP, Osterhoudt KC. Acute psychosis associated with therapeutic use of dextroamphetamine. *Pediatrics* 113(5):1466, 2004.

Caplan R, Guthrie D, Tang B, et al. Thought disorder in childhood schizophrenia: Replication and update of concept. *J Am Acad Child Adolesc Psychiatry* 39(6):771–778, 2000.

Caplan R, Guthrie D, Tanguay P, et al. The Kiddie Formal Thought Disorder Scale (K-FTDS): Clinical assessment, reliability and validity. *J Am Acad Child Adolesc Psychiatry* 28:408–416, 1989.

Dawson KL, Carter ER. A steroid-induced acute psychosis in a child with asthma. *Pediatr Pulmonol* 26(5):362–364, 1998.

Devinsky O. Psychiatric comorbidity in patients with epilepsy: Implications for diagnosis and treatment. *Epilepsy Behav* Dec(4 Suppl):S2–S10, 2003.

El-Saadi O, Pedersen CB, McNeil TF, et al. Paternal and maternal age as risk factors for psychosis: Findings from Denmark, Sweden, and Australia. *Schizophr Res* 67(2–3): 227–236, 2004.

Fields J, Grochowski S, Linenmayer J, et al. Assessing positive and negative symptoms in children and adolescents. *Am J Psychiatry* 151:249–253, 1994.

Fish B. Children's Psychiatric Rating Scale. *Psychopharmacol Bull* 21:753–765, 1985.

Frazier JA, Gordon CT, McKenna K, et al. An open trial of clozapine in 11 adolescents with childhood-onset schizophrenia. *J Am Acad Child Adolesc Psychiatry* 33:658–663, 1994.

Fujii D, Ahmed I. Characteristics of psychotic disorder due to traumatic brain injury: An analysis of case studies in the literature. *J Neuropsychiatry Clin Neurosci* 14(2):130–140, 2002.

Haddad PM, Wieck A. Antipsychotic-induced hyperprolactinaemia: Mechanisms, clinical features, and management. *Drugs* 64(20):2291–2314, 2004.

Isohanni M, Isohanni I, Koponen H, et al. Developmental precursors of psychosis. *Curr Psychiatry Rep* 6(3):168–175, 2004.

Janssen I, Krabbendam L, Bak M, et al. Childhood abuse as a risk factor for psychotic experiences. *Acta Psychiatr Scand* 109(1):38–45, 2004.

Kanner AM. Recognition of the various expressions of anxiety, psychosis, and aggression in epilepsy. *Epilepsia* 45(Suppl 2):22–27, 2004.

Kumra S, Frazier JA, Jacobsen LK, et al. Childhood-onset schizophrenia: A double-blind clozapine–haloperidol comparison. *Arch Gen Psychiatry* 53:1090–1097, 1996.

Kumra S, Jacobsen LK, Lenane MC, et al. Childhood-onset schizophrenia: An open-label study of olanzapine in adolescents. *J Am Acad Child Adolesc Psychiatry* 37:377–385, 1998.

Mackinnon A, Copolov DL, Trauer T. Factors associated with compliance and resistance to command hallucinations. *J Nerv Ment Dis* 192(5):357–362, 2004.

Manchanda R, Malla A, Harricharan R, et al. EEG abnormalities and outcome in first-episode psychosis. *Can J Psychiatry* 48(11):722–726, 2003.

McClellan J, Prezbindowski A, Breiger D, et al. Neuropsychological functioning in early onset psychotic disorders. *Schizophr Res* 68(1):21–26, 2004.

McConville BJ, Arventis LA, Thyrum PT, et al. Pharmacokinetics, tolerability, and clinical effectiveness of quetiapine fumarate: An open-label trial in adolescents with psychotic disorders. *J Clin Psychiatry* 61:252–260, 2000.

Murphy KC, Owen MJ. Velo-cardio-facial syndrome: A model for understanding the genetics and pathogenesis of schizophrenia. *Br J Psychiatry* 179(11):397–402, 2001.

Nitin G, Giedd J, Rapoport JL. Brain development in healthy, hyperactive, and psychotic children. *Arch Neurol* 59(8):1244–1248, 2002.

Pavuluri MN, Herbener ES, Sweeney JA. Psychotic symptoms in pediatric bipolar disorder. *J Affect Disord* 80(1):19–28, 2004.

Raune D, Kuipers E, Bebbington PE. Expressed emotion at first-episode psychosis: Investigating a career appraisal model. *Br J Psychiatry* 184:321–326, 2004.

Reimherr JP, McClellan JM. Diagnostic challenges in children and adolescents with psychotic disorders. *J Clin Psychiatry* 65(Suppl 6):5–11, 2004.

Remschmidt H, Hebebrand J. Early-onset schizophrenia. In: Martin A, Scahill L, Charney DS, Leckman JF (Eds.), *Pediatric Psychopharmacology Principles and Practice.* New York: Oxford University Press, pp. 543–562, 2003.

Remschmidt H, Schulz E, Martin M. An open trial of clozapine in thirty-six adolescents with schizophrenia. *J Child Adolesc Psychopharmacol* 4:31–41, 1994.

Schultz SC, Finkling RL, Wise A, et al. Child and adolescent schizophrenia. *Psych Clin North Am* 21(1):43–56, 1998.

Semper TF, McClellan JM. The psychotic child. *Child Adolesc Psychiatr Clin North Am* 12(4):679–691, 2003.

Stayer C, Sporn A, Gogtay N, et al. Looking for childhood schizophrenia: Case series of false positives. *J Am Acad Child Adolesc Psychiatry* 43(8):1026–1029, 2004.

Tolbert HA. Psychoses in children and adolescents: A review. *J Clin Psychiatry* 57(Suppl 3):4–8, 1996.

Torrey EF. *Surviving Schizophrenia: A Manual for Families, Consumers and Providers* (3rd ed.). New York: Harper Collins, pp. 85–104, 1995.

Valkonen-Korhonen M, Tarvainen MP, Ranta-Aho P, et al. Heart rate variability in acute psychosis. *Psychophysiology* 40(5):716–726, 2003.

Volkmar FR. Childhood and adolescent psychosis: A review of the past 10 years. *J Am Acad Child Adolesc Psychiatry* 35(7):843–851, 1996.

Volkmar FR, Tsatsanis KD. Childhood schizophrenia. In: Lewis M (Ed.), *Child and Adolescent Psychiatry: A Comprehensive Textbook* (3rd ed.). Philadelphia: Lippincott, Williams & Wilkins, pp. 745–754, 2002.

Wheatley M, Plant J, Reader H, et al. Clozapine treatment of adolescents with posttraumatic stress disorder and psychotic symptoms. *J Clin Psychopharmacol* 24(2): 167–173, 2004.

EXTRAPYRAMIDAL SYNDROMES AND CENTRAL SEROTONIN SYNDROME

Armenteros JL, Adams PB, Campbell M, Eisenberg ZW. Haloperidol-related dyskinesias and pre- and perinatal complications in autistic children. *Psychopharmacol Bull* 31(2):363–369, 1995.

B
I
B
L
I
O
G
R
A
P
H
Y

Campbell M, Armenteros JL, Malone RP, et al. Neuroleptic-related dyskinesias in autistic children: A prospective longitudinal study. *J Am Acad Child Adolesc Psychiatry* 36(6):835–843, 1997.

Casey DE. Tardive dyskinesia: Psychopathology. In: Bloom FE, Kupfer DJ (Eds.), *Psychopharmacology: The Fourth Generation of Progress.* New York: Raven Press, pp. 1497–1502, 1995.

Connor DF, Benjamin S, Ozbayrak KR. Case study: Neuroleptic withdrawal dyskinesia exacerbated by ongoing stimulant treatment. *J Am Acad Child Adolesc Psychiatry* 37(3):247–248, 1998.

Connor DF, Fletcher KE, Wood JS. Neuroleptic-related dyskinesias in children and adolescents. *J Clin Psychiatry* 62(12):967–974, 2001.

Ener RA, Meglathery SB, Van Decker WA, et al. Serotonin syndrome and other serotonergic disorders. *Pain Med* 4(1):63–74, 2003.

Gardos G, Cole JO. The treatment of tardive dyskinesias. In: Bloom FE, Kupfer DJ (Eds.), *Psychopharmacology: The Fourth Generation of Progress.* New York: Raven Press, pp.1503–1511, 1995.

Glazer WM. Expected incidence of tardive dyskinesia associated with atypical antipsychotics. *J Clin Psychiatry* 61(Suppl 4):21–26, 2000.

Glazer WM. Extrapyramidal side effects, tardive dyskinesia, and the concept of atypicality. *J Clin Psychiatry* 61(Suppl 3):16–21, 2000.

Godinho EM, Thompson AE, Bramble DJ. Neuroleptic withdrawal versus serotonergic syndrome in an 8-year-old child. *J Child Adolesc Psychopharmacol* 12(3):265–270, 2002.

Green WH. *Child and Adolescent Clinical Psychopharmacology* (3rd ed.). Philadelphia: Lippincott, Williams & Wilkins, pp. 93–102, 2001.

Gualtieri CT, Quade D, Hicks RE, Mayo JP, Schroeder SR. Tardive dyskinesia and other clinical consequences of neuroleptic treatment in children and adolescents. *Am J Psychiatry* 141(1):20–23, 1984.

Kaminski CA, Robbins MS, Weibley RE. Sertraline intoxication in a child. *Ann Emerg Med* 23:1371–1374, 1994.

Keepers GA, Clappison VJ, Casey DE. Initial anticholinergic prophylaxis for neuroleptic-induced extrapyramidal syndromes. *Arch Gen Psychiatry* 40(10):1113–1117, 1983.

Kumra S, Jacobsen LK, Lenane M, et al. Case series: Spectrum of neuroleptic-induced movement disorders and extrapyramidal side effects in childhood-onset schizophrenia. *J Am Acad Child Adolesc Psychiatry* 37(2):221–227, 1998.

Lemmens P, Brecher M, Van Baelen B. A combined analysis of double-blind studies with risperidone vs. placebo and other antipsychotic agents: Factors associated with extrapyramidal symptoms. *Acta Psychiatr Scand* 99(3):160–170, 1999.

Lohr JB, Kuczenski R, Niculescu AB. Oxidative mechanisms and tardive dyskinesia. *CNS Drugs* 17(1):47–62, 2003.

Magulac M, Landsverk J, Golshan S, Jeste DV. Abnormal involuntary movements in neuroleptic-naive children and adolescents. *Can J Psychiatry* 44(4):368–373, 1999.

Mann SC, Caroff SN, Keck PE, Lazarus A. *Neuroleptic Malignant Syndrome and Related Conditions* (2nd ed.). Washington, DC: American Psychiatric Press, 2003.

Miller CH, Mohr F, Umbricht D, et al. The prevalence of acute extrapyramidal signs and symptoms in patients treated with clozapine, risperidone, and conventional antipsychotics. *J Clin Psychiatry* 59(2):69–75, 1998.

Munetz MR, Benjamin S. How to examine patients using the abnormal involuntary movement scale. *Hosp Com Psychiatry* 39(11):1172–1177, 1988.

Richardson MA, Haugland G. Typicality and atypicality in the development of neuroleptic side effects in child and adolescent psychiatric patients. In: Richardson MA, Haugland G (Eds.), *Use of Neuroleptics in Children: Clinical Practice, No. 37*. Washington, DC: American Psychiatric Association, pp. 43–66, 1996.

Schooler NR, Kane JM. Research diagnoses for tardive dyskinesia. *Arch Gen Psychiatry* 39:486–487, 1982.

Steingard R, Khan A, Gonzalez A, et al. Neuroleptic malignant syndrome: Review of experience with children and adolescence. *J Child Adolesc Psychopharmacol* 2(3):183–198, 1992.

Sternbach H. The serotonin syndrome. *Am J Psychiatry* 148:705–713, 1991.

Stigler KA, Potenza MN, McDougle CJ. Tolerability profile of atypical antipsychotics in children and adolescents. *Paediatr Drugs* 3(12):927–942, 2001.

Wolf DV, Wagner KD. Tardive dyskinesia, tardive dystonia, and tardive Tourette's syndrome in children and adolescents. *J Child Adolesc Psychopharmacol* 3(4): 175–198, 1993.

ANXIETY DISORDERS

Albano AM, Marten PA, Holt CS, et al. Cognitive–behavioral group treatment for social phobia in adolescents: a preliminary study. *J Nerv Ment Dis* 183:649–656, 1995.

American Academy of Child and Adolescent Psychiatry Work Group on Quality Issues. Practice parameters for the assessment and treatment of children and adolescents with anxiety disorders. *J Am Acad Child Adolesc Psychiatry* 36(10Suppl):69S–84S, 1997.

American Psychiatric Association. *Diagnostic and Statistical Manual of Mental Disorders* (4th ed., text rev.). Washington, DC: Author, 2000.

Barrett PM, Dadds MM, Rapee RM, et al. Family intervention for childhood anxiety. *J Consult Clin Psychol* 64:333–342, 1996.

Berney T, Kolvin I, Bhate RF, et al. School phobia: A therapeutic trial with clomipramine and short-term outcome. *Br J Psychiatry* 138:110–118, 1981.

Bernstein GA, Borchardt CM, Perwien AR. Anxiety disorders in children and adolescents: A review of the past 10 years. *J Am Acad Child Adolesc Psychiatry* 35(9):1110–1119, 1996.

Bernstein GA, Borchardt CM, Perwein AR, et al. Imipramine plus cognitive–behavioral therapy in the treatment of school refusal. *J Am Acad Child Adolesc Psychiatry* 39:276–283, 2000.

Bernstein GA, Garfinkel BD, Borchardt CM. Comparative studies of pharmacotherapy for school refusal. *J Am Acad Child Adolesc Psychiatry* 29:773–781, 1990.

Black B, Uhde TW. Treatment of elective mutism with fluoxetine: A double-blind, placebo-controlled study. *J Am Acad Child Adolesc Psychiatry* 33:1000–1006, 1994.

Brooks SJ, Kutcher S. Diagnosis and measurement of anxiety disorder in adolescents: A review of commonly used instruments. *J Child Adolesc Psychopharmacol* 13(3): 351–400, 2003.

Cobham VE, Dadds MR, Spence SH. The role of parental anxiety in the treatment of childhood anxiety. *J Consult Clin Psychol* 66:893–905, 1998.

Coyle JT. Drug treatment of anxiety disorders in children. *NEJM* 344:1326–1327, 2001.

Dummit ES III, Klein RG, Tancer NK, et al. Systematic assessment of 50 children with selective mutism. *J Am Acad Child Adolesc Psychiatry* 36:653–660, 1997.

Eisen AR, Dearney CA. *Practitioner's Guide to Treating Fear and Anxiety in Children and Adolescents: A Cognitive Behavioral Approach*. Northvale, NJ: Aronson, 1995.

BIBLIOGRAPHY

Flannery-Schroeder E, Kendall PC. Group and individual cognitive behavioral treatment for youth with anxiety disorders: A randomized trial. *Cognitive Ther Research* 24:251–278, 2000.

Freeman JB, Garcia AM, Leonard HL. Anxiety disorders. In: Lewis M (Ed.), *Child and Adolescent Psychiatry: A Comprehensive Textbook* (3rd ed.). Philadelphia: Lippincott, Williams & Wilkins, pp. 821–834, 2002.

Gittleman-Klein R, Klein D. Controlled imipramine treatment of school phobia. *Arch Gen Psychiatry* 25:204–207, 1971.

Graae F, Milner J, Rizzotto L, et al. Clonazepam in childhood anxiety disorders. *J Am Acad Child Adolesc Psychiatry* 33:372–376, 1994.

Greenhill LL, Pine D, March JS, et al. Assessment measures in anxiety disorders research. *Psychopharmacol Bull* 34:155–165, 1998.

Gullone E. The development of normal fear: A century of research. *Clin Psychol Rev* 20:429–451, 2000.

Hayward C, Killen JD, Taylor CB. Panic attacks in young adolescents. *Am J Psychiatry* 146:1061–1062, 1989.

Kashani JH, Orvaschel H. A community study of anxiety in children and adolescents. *Am J Psychiatry* 147:313–318, 1990.

Kearney CA, Albano AM, Eisen AR, et al. The phenomenology of panic disorder in youngsters: An empirical study of a clinical sample. *J Anxiety Disord* 11:49–62, 1997.

Kendall PC. Treating anxiety disorders in children: Results of a randomized clinical trial. *J Consult Clin Psychol* 62:200–210, 1994.

Kendall PC, Flannery-Schroeder E, Panichelli-Mindel SM, et al. Therapy for youths with anxiety disorders: A second randomized clinical trial. *J Consult Clin Psychol* 65:366–380, 1997.

Klein RG, Kopelwicz HS, Kanner A. Imipramine treatment in children with separation anxiety disorder. *J Am Acad Child Adolesc Psychiatry* 31:21–28, 1992.

Labellarte MJ, Ginsburg GS. Anxiety disorders. In: Martin A, Scahill L, Charney DS, Leckman JF (Eds.), *Pediatric Psychopharmacology Principles and Practice*. New York: Oxford University Press, pp. 497–510, 2003.

Last CG, Hansen C, Franco N. Cognitive–behavioral treatment of school phobia. *J Am Acad Child Adolesc Psychiatry* 37:404–411, 1998.

Last CG, Perrin S, Hersen M, et al. A prospective study of childhood anxiety disorders. *J Am Acad Child Adolesc Psychiatry* 35:1502–1510, 1996.

Research Units for Pediatric Psychopharmacology (RUPP) Anxiety Study Group. Fluvoxamine for the treatment of anxiety disorders in children and adolescents. *NEJM* 344:1279–1285, 2001.

Rynn MA, Siqueland L, Rickels K. Placebo-controlled trial of sertraline in the treatment of children with generalized anxiety disorder. *Am J Psychiatry* 158:2008–2014, 2001.

Silverman WK, Kurtines WM, Ginsburg GS, et al. Treating anxiety disorders in children with group cognitive behavior therapy: A randomized clinical trial. *J Consul Clin Psychol* 67:995–1003, 1999.

Simeon JG, Ferguson HB, Knott V, et al. Clinical, cognitive, and neurophysiological effects of alprazolam in children and adolescents with overanxious and avoidant disorders. *J Am Acad Child Adolesc Psychiatry* 31:29–33, 1992.

Simeon JG, Knott VJ, Dubois C, et al. Buspirone therapy of mixed anxiety disorders in childhood and adolescence: A pilot study. *J Child Adolesc Psychopharmacol* 4:159–170, 1994.

Spence SH, Donovan C, Brechman-Toussaint M. The treatment of childhood social phobia: The effectiveness of a social skills training-based, cognitive–behavioral intervention, with and without parental involvement. *J Child Psychol Psychiatry* 41:713–726, 2000.

Wagner KD, Berard R, Stein MB, et al. A multicenter, randomized, double-blind, placebo-controlled trial of paroxetine in children and adolescents with social anxiety disorder. *Arch Gen Psychiatry* 61:1153–1162, 2004.

Weisz JR, Weiss B, Alicke MD, et al. Effectiveness of psychotherapy with children and adolescents: A meta-analysis for clinicians. *J Consult Clin Psychol* 55:542–549, 1987.

OBSESSIVE–COMPULSIVE DISORDER

American Academy of Child and Adolescent Psychiatry Work Group on Quality Issues. Practice parameters for the assessment and treatment of children and adolescents with obsessive–compulsive disorder. *J Am Acad Child Adolesc Psychiatry* 37(10 Suppl):27S–45S, 1998.

Bamber D, Tamplin A, Park RJ, et al. Development of a short Leyton obsessional inventory for children and adolescents. *J Am Acad Child Adolesc Psychiatry* 41(10):1246–1252, 2002.

Barrett P, Healy-Farrell L, March JS. Cognitive–behavioral family treatment of childhood obsessive–compulsive disorder: A controlled trial. *J Am Acad Child Adolesc Psychiatry* 43(1):46–62, 2004.

Berg CA, Rapoport JL, Whitaker A, et al. Childhood obsessive–compulsive disorder: Two year prospective follow-up of a community sample. *J Am Acad Child Adolesc Psychiatry* 28:528–533, 1989.

Cook EH, Wagner KD, March JS, et al. Long-term sertraline treatment of children and adolescents with obsessive–compulsive disorder. *J Am Acad Child Adolesc Psychiatry* 40(10):1175–1181, 2001.

DeVeaugh-Geiss J, Moroz G, Biederman J, et al. Clomipramine hydrochloride in childhood and adolescent obsessive–compulsive disorder: A multicenter trial. *J Am Acad Child Adolesc Psychiatry* 31:45–49, 1992.

Figueroa Y, Fennig S, Pato M, et al. Combination treatment with clomipramine and selective serotonin reuptake inhibitors for obsessive–compulsive disorder in children and adolescents. *J Child Adolesc Psychopharmacol* 8:61–67, 1998.

Flament MF, Koby E, Rapoport J, et al. Childhood obsessive–compulsive disorder: A prospective follow-up study. *J Child Psychol Psychiatry* 31:363–380, 1990.

Flament MF, Whitaker A, Rapoport JL, et al. Obsessive compulsive disorder in adolescence: An epidemiologic study. *J Am Acad Child Adolesc Psychiatry* 27:764–772, 1988.

Geller DA, Biederman J, Jones J, et al. Is juvenile obsessive–compulsive disorder a developmental subtype of the disorder? A review of the pediatric literature. *J Am Acad Child Adolesc Psychiatry* 37:420–427, 1998.

Geller DA, Hoog SL, Heiligenstein JH, et al. Fluoxetine treatment for obsessive–compulsive disorder in children and adolescents: A placebo-controlled clinical trial. *J Am Acad Child Adolesc Psychiatry* 40(7):773–779, 2001.

Geller DA, Spencer T. Obsessive–compulsive disorder. In: Martin A, Scahill LS, Charney DS, and Leckman JF (Eds.), *Pediatric Psychopharmacology Principles and Practice.* New York: Oxford University Press, pp. 511–525, 2003.

Geller DA, Wagner KD, Emslie G, et al. paroxetine treatment of children and adolescents with obsessive–compulsive disorder: A randomized, multicenter, double–blind, placebo-controlled trial. *J Am Acad Child Adolesc Psychiatry* 43(11):1387–1396, 2004.

Giakas WJ. Risperidone treatment for a Tourette's disorder patient with comorbid obsessive–compulsive disorder. *Am J Psychiatry* 152:1097–1098, 1995.

Goodman WK, Price LH, Rasmussen SA, et al. The Yale–Brown obsessive–compulsive scale: I. Development, use, and reliability. *Arch Gen Psychiatry* 46(11):1006–1011, 1989a.

Goodman WK, Price LH, Rasmussen SA, et al. The Yale–Brown obsessive–compulsive scale: II. Validity. *Arch Gen Psychiatry* 46(11):1012–1016, 1989b.

Heyman I, Fombonne E, Simmons H, et al. Prevalence of obsessive compulsive disorder in the British nationwide survey of child mental health. *Br J Psychiatry* 179:324–329, 2001.

Leonard HL, Swedo SE, Lenane MC, et al. A double-blind desipramine substitution during long-term clomipramine treatment in children and adolescents with obsessive–compulsive disorder. *Arch Gen Psychiatry* 48(10):922–927, 1991.

Leonard HL, Topol D, Bukstein O, et al. Clonazepam as an augmenting agent in the treatment of childhood-onset obsessive–compulsive disorder. *J Am Acad Child Adolesc Psychiatry* 33:792–794, 1994.

Liebowitz MR, Turner SM, Piacentini J, et al. Fluoxetine in children and adolescents with OCD: A placebo-controlled trial. *J Am Acad Child Adolesc Psychiatry* 41(12): 1431–1438, 2002.

March JS, Biederman J, Wolkow R, et al. Sertraline in children and adolescents with obsessive–compulsive disorder. *JAMA* 280:1752–1756, 1998.

March JS, Frances A, Carpenter D, et al. The Expert Consensus Guideline Series: Treatment of obsessive–compulsive disorder. *J Clin Psychiatry* 58:5–72, 1997.

March JS, Leonard HL. Obsessive–compulsive disorder in children and adolescents: A review of the past 10 years. *J Am Acad Child Adolesc Psychiatry* 35:1265–1273, 1996.

March JS, Mulle K. *OCD in Children and Adolescents: A Cognitive–Behavioral Treatment Manual.* New York: Guilford Press, 1998.

March JS, the Pediatric OCD Treatment Study (POTS). Cognitive–behavior therapy, sertraline, and their combination for children and adolescents with obsessive–compulsive disorder. *JAMA* 292(16):1969–1976, 2004.

Nelson EC, Hanna GL, Hudziak JJ, et al. Obsessive–compulsive scale of the child behavior checklist: Specificity, sensitivity, and predictive power. *Pediatrics* 108(1):E14–25, 2001.

Noshirvani HF, Kasvikis Y, Marks IM, et al. Gender divergent aetiological factors in obsessive–compulsive disorder. *Br J Psychiatry* 158:260–263, 1991.

Riddle MA, Reeve EA, Yaryura-Tobias JA, et al. Fluvoxamine for children and adolescents with obsessive–compulsive disorder: A randomized, controlled, multicenter trial. *J Am Acad Child Adolesc Psychiatry* 40(2):222–229, 2001.

Riddle MA, Scahill L, King RA, et al. Double-blind, crossover trial of fluoxetine and placebo in children and adolescents with obsessive–compulsive disorder. *J Am Acad Child Adolesc Psychiatry* 31(6):1062–1069, 1992.

Scahill L, Riddle MA, McSwiggin-Hardin M, et al. Children's Yale–Brown Obsessive Compulsive Scale: Reliability and validity. *J Am Acad Child Adolesc Psychiatry* 36: 844–852, 1997.

Skoog G, Skoog I. A 40-year follow-up of patients with obsessive–compulsive disorder. *Arch Gen Psychiatry* 56:121–127, 1999.

Swedo SE, Leonard HL, Garvey M, et al. Pediatric autoimmune neuropsychiatric disorders associated with streptococcal infections: Clinical description of the first fifty cases. *Am J Psychiatry* 155:264–271, 1998.

Swedo SE, Leonard HL, Mittleman BB, et al. Identification of children with pediatric autoimmune neuropsychiatric disorders associated with streptococcal infections by a marker associated with rheumatic fever. *Am J Psychiatry* 154:110–112, 1997.

Thompson PH. Child and adolescent obsessive–compulsive disorder treated with citalopram: Findings from an open trial of 23 cases. *J Child Adolesc Psychopharmacol* 7:157–166, 1997.

Towbin KE, Riddle MA. Obsessive–compulsive disorder. In: Lewis M (Ed.), *Child and Adolescent Psychiatry: A Comprehensive Textbook* (3rd ed.). Philadelphia: Lippincott, Williams & Wilkins, pp. 834–847, 2002.

Zohar A, Ratzoni G, Pauls DL, et al. An epidemiologic study of obsessive compulsive disorder and related disorders in Israeli adolescents. *J Am Acad Child Adolesc Psychiatry* 31:1057–1061, 1992.

POSTTRAUMATIC STRESS DISORDER

American Academy of Child and Adolescent Psychiatry Work Group on Quality Issues. Practice parameters for the assessment and treatment of children and adolescents with posttraumatic stress disorder. *J Am Acad Child Adolesc Psychiatry* 37 (10 Suppl):4S–26S, 1998.

American Psychiatric Association. *Desk Reference to the Diagnostic Criteria from DSM-IV-TR.* Washington, DC: Author 2000.

Brady K, Pearlstein T, Asnis GM, et al. Efficacy and safety of sertraline treatment of posttraumatic stress disorder. *JAMA* 283:1837–1844, 2000.

Chemtob CM, Nakashima JP, Hamada RS. Psychosocial intervention for post disaster trauma symptoms in elementary school children: A controlled community field study. *Arch Pediatr Adolec Med* 156(3):211–216, 2002.

Domon SE, Anderson MS. Nefazodone for PTSD [letter]. *J Am Acad Child Adolesc Psychiatry* 39(8):942–943, 2000.

Donnelly CL. Post-traumatic stress disorder. In: Martin A, Scahill L, Charney DS, and Leckman JF (Eds.), *Pediatric Psychopharmacology Principles and Practice.* New York: Oxford University Press, pp. 580–591, 2003.

Eisen M. Posttraumatic symptom inventory for children. In: Carlson E (Ed.), *Trauma Assessments: A Clinician's Guide.* New York: Guilford Press, pp. 254–255, 1997.

Eth S, Pynoos R. Developmental perspectives on psychic trauma in childhood. In: Figley CR (Ed.), *Trauma and Its Wake.* New York: Brunner/Mazel, pp. 36–52, 1985.

Famularo R, Kinscherff R, Fenton T. Propranolol treatment for childhood post-traumatic stress disorder, acute type: A pilot study. *Am J Dis Child* 142:1244–1247, 1988.

Fletcher KE. When Bad Things Happen scale. In: Carson E. (Ed.), *Trauma Assessments: A Clinician's Guide.* New York: Guilford Press, pp. 257–258, 1997.

Fletcher KE. Childhood posttraumatic stress disorder. In: Mash EJ, Barkley RA (Eds.), *Child Psychopathology* (2nd ed.). New York: Guilford Press, pp. 330–371, 2003.

Ford JD, Thomas JE, Rogers KC, et al. Assessment of children's PTSD following abuse or accidental trauma. Presented at the Annual Meeting of the International Society for Traumatic Stress Studies, San Francisco, November 9–13, 1996.

Harmon RJ, Riggs PD. Clinical perspectives: Clonidine for posttraumatic stress disorder in preschool children. *J Am Acad Child Adolesc Psychiatry* 35:1247–1249, 1996.

Johnson KM, Foa EB, Jaycox LH, et al. A self-report diagnostic instrument for children with PTSD. Presented at the Annual Meeting of the International Society for Traumatic Stress Studies, San Francisco, November 9–13, 1996.

King NJ, Tonge BJ, Mullen P, et al. Treating sexually abused children with posttraumatic stress symptoms: A randomized clinical trial. *J Am Acad Child Adolesc Psychiatry* 39(11):1347–1355, 2000.

Loof D, Grimley P, Kuller F, et al. Carbamazepine for PTSD [letter]. *J Am Acad Child Adolesc Psychiatry* 34:703–704, 1995.

Marshall RD, Beebe KL, Oldham M, et al. Efficacy and safety of paroxetine treatment for chronic PTSD: A fixed-dose, placebo-controlled study. *Am J Psychiatry* 158:1928–1988, 2001.

Martenyi F, Brown EB, Zhang H, et al. Fluoxetine v. placebo in prevention of relapse in post-traumatic stress disorder. *Br J Psychiatry* 181:315–320, 2002.

Perry BD. Neurobiological sequelae of childhood trauma: PTSD in children. In: Murburg MM (Ed.), *Catecholamine Function in Post-Traumatic Stress Disorder: Emerging Concepts*. Washington, DC: American Psychiatric Press, pp. 233–255, 1994.

Pfefferbaum B. Posttraumatic stress disorder in children: A review of the past 10 years. *J Am Acad Child Adolesc Psychiatry* 36(11):1503–1511, 1997.

Pfefferbaum B. Posttraumatic stress disorder. In: Lewis M (Ed.), *Child and Adolescent Psychiatry: A Comprehensive Textbook* (3rd ed.). Philadelphia: Lippincott, Williams & Wilkins, pp. 912–925, 2002.

Pynoos RS, Frederick C, Nader K, et al. Life threat and posttraumatic stress in school-age children. *Arch Gen Psychiatry* 44:1057–1063, 1987.

Roberts R, Blakeney PE, Villarreal C, et al. Imipramine treatment in pediatric burn patients with symptoms of acute stress disorder: A pilot study. *J Am Acad Child Adolesc Psychiatry* 38:873–882, 1999.

Saigh P. The development and validation of the Children's Posttraumatic Stress Disorder Inventory. *Int J Spec Educ* 4:75–84, 1989.

Saigh P. The validity of the DSM-III posttraumatic stress disorder classification as applied to adolescents. *Prof Sch Psychol* 3:283–290, 1988.

Saxe GN, Stoddard FJ, Markey C, et al. The Child Stress Reaction Checklist: A measure of ADH and PTSD in children. Presented at the Annual Meeting of the International Society for Traumatic Stress Studies, San Francisco, November 9–13, 1996.

Scheeringa MS, Zeanah CH, Drell MJ, et al. Two approaches to diagnosing posttraumatic stress disorder in infancy and early childhood. *J Am Acad Child Adolesc Psychiatry* 34:191–200, 1995.

Seedat S, Stein DJ, Ziervogel C, et al. Comparison of response to a selective serotonin reuptake inhibitor in children, adolescents, and adults with posttraumatic stress disorder. *J Child Adolesc Psychopharmacol* 12(1):37–46, 2002.

Stein BD, Jaycox LH, Kataoka SH, et al. A mental health intervention for schoolchildren exposed to violence. *JAMA* 290:603–611, 2003.

MENTAL RETARDATION, AUTISM, AND OTHER PERVASIVE DEVELOPMENTAL DISORDERS

Agarwal V, Sitholey P, Kumar S, et al. Double-blind, placebo-controlled trial of clonidine in hyperactive children with mental retardation. *Ment Retard* 39(4):259–267, 2001.

Aman MG, De Smedt G, Derivan A, et al. Double-blind, placebo-controlled study of risperidone for the treatment of disruptive behaviors in children with subaverage intelligence. *Am J Psychiatry* 159:1337–1346, 2002.

Aman MG, Lindsay RL, Nash PL, et al. Individuals with mental retardation. In: Martin A, Scahill L, Charney DS, Leckman JF (Eds.), *Pediatric Psychopharmacology Principles and Practice*. New York: Oxford University Press, pp. 617–630, 2003.

Aman MG, Marks RE, Turbott SH, et al. Methylphenidate and thioridazine in the treatment of intellectually subaverage children: Effects on cognitive–motor performance. *J Am Acad Child Adolesc Psychiatry* 30(5):816–824, 1991.

Aman MG, Singh NN, Stewart AW, et al. The Aberrant Behavior Checklist: A behavior rating scale for the assessment of treatment effects. *Am J Ment Defic* 89:485–491, 1985.

Aman MG, Tasse MJ, Rojahn J, et al. The Nisonger CBRF: A Child Behavior Rating Form for children with developmental disabilities. *Res Dev Disabil* 17:41–57, 1996.

American Academy of Child and Adolescent Psychiatry Work Group on Quality Issues. Practice parameters for the assessment and treatment of children, adolescents, and adults with autism and other pervasive developmental disorders. *J Am Acad Child Adolesc Psychiatry* 38(12 Suppl):32S–54S, 1999a.

American Academy of Child and Adolescent Psychiatry Work Group on Quality Issues. Practice parameters for the assessment and treatment of children, adolescents, and adults with mental retardation and comorbid mental disorders. *J Am Acad Child Adolesc Psychiatry* 38(12 Suppl):5S–31S, 1999b.

American Association on Mental Retardation. *Mental Retardation: Definition, Classification, and Systems of Supports, Special 9th Edition.* Washington, DC: American Association on Mental Retardation, 1992.

Anderson LT, Campbell M, Adams P, et al. The effects of haloperidol on discrimination learning and behavioral symptoms in autistic children. *J Autism Dev Disord* 19(2):227–239, 1989.

Arnold LE, Aman MG, Martin A, et al. Assessment in multisite randomized clinical trials of patients with autistic disorder: The autism RUPP network. *J Autism Dev Disord* 30:99–111, 2000.

Belsito KM, Law PA, Kirk KS, et al. Lamotrigine therapy for autistic disorder: A randomized, double-blind, placebo-controlled trial. *J Autism Dev Disord* 31(2):175–181, 2001.

Buitelaar JK, van der Gaag RJ, Cohen-Kettenis P, et al. A randomized controlled trial of risperidone in the treatment of aggression in hospitalized adolescents with subaverage cognitive abilities. *J Clin Psychiatry* 62(4):239–248, 2001.

Campbell M, Anderson LT, Small AM, et al. Naltrexone in autistic children: Behavioral symptoms and attentional learning. *J Am Acad Child Adolesc Psychiatry* 32(6):1283–1291, 1993.

Caplan R, Arbelle S, Magharious W, et al. Psychopathology in pediatric complex partial and primary generalized epilepsy. *Dev Med Child Neurol* 40:805–811, 1998.

Chez MG, Buchanan CP, Aimonovitch MC, et al. Double–blind, placebo–controlled study of L–carnosine supplementation in children with autistic spectrum disorders. *J Child Neurol* 17(11):833–837, 2002.

Cohen IL. Criterion-related validity of the PDD Behavior Inventory. *J Autism Dev Disord* 33(1):47–53, 2003.

Connor DF, Posever TA. A brief review of atypical antipsychotics in individuals with developmental disability. *Men Health Aspect Dev Disabil* 1(4):93–102, 1998.

Connor DF, Ozbayrak KR, Benjamin S, et al. A pilot study of nadolol for overt aggression in developmentally delayed individuals. *J Am Acad Child Adolesc Psychiatry* 36(6):826–834, 1997.

Coplan J, Souders MC, Mulberg AE, et al. Children with autistic spectrum disorders. II: Parents are unable to distinguish secretin from placebo under double-blind conditions. *Arch Dis Child* 88:737–739, 2003.

Dykens EM. Measuring behavioral phenotypes: Provocations from the new genetics. *Am J Ment Retard* 99:522–532, 1995.

Dykens EM. Psychopathology in children with intellectual disabilities. *J Child Psychol Psychiatry* 41:407–417, 2000.

Fankhauser MP, Karumanchi VC, German ML, et al. A double-blind, placebo-controlled study of the efficacy of transdermal clonidine in autism. *J Clin Psychiatry* 53(3):77–82, 1992.

Feldman HM, Kolmen BK, Gonzaga AM. Naltrexone and communication skills in young children with autism. *J Am Acad Child Adolesc Psychiatry* 38(5):587–593, 1999.

Findling RL, Maxwell K, Scotese-Wojtila L, et al. High-dose pyridoxine and magnesium administration in children with autistic disorder: An absence of salutary effects in a double-blind, placebo-controlled study. *J Autism Dev Disord* 27(4):467–478, 1997.

Freeman BJ, Ritvo ER, Yokota A, et al. A scale for rating symptoms of patients with the syndrome of autism in real life settings. *J Am Acad Child Adolesc Psychiatry* 25(1):130–136, 1986.

BIBLIOGRAPHY

Gilliam JS. *Gilliam Autism Rating Scale.* Austin, TX: PRO-ED, 1995.

Gordon CT, State RC, Nelson JE, et al. A double-blind comparison of clomipramine, desipramine, and placebo in the treatment of autistic disorder. *Arch Gen Psychiatry* 50(6):441–447, 1993.

Goulden KK, Shinnar S, Koller K, et al. Epilepsy in children with mental retardation: A cohort study. *Epilepsia* 32:690–697, 1991.

Guy W. *ECDEU Assessment Manual for Psychopharmacology* (NIMH Publication No. 76-338). Washington, DC: U.S. Department of Health, Education, and Welfare, National Institute of Mental Health, 1976.

Handen BL, Janosky J, McAuliffe S, et al. Prediction of response to methylphenidate among children with ADHD and mental retardation. *J Am Acad Child Adolesc Psychiatry* 33(8):1185–1193, 1994.

Handen BL, Johnson CR, Lubetsky M. Efficacy of methylphenidate among children with autism and symptoms of attention-deficit hyperactivity disorder. *J Autism Dev Disord* 30(3):245–255, 2000.

Harris JC. *Developmental Neuropsychiatry,* Vols. 1 and 2. New York: Oxford University Press, 1995.

Jaselskis CA, Cook EH Jr, Fletcher KE, et al. Clonidine treatment of hyperactive and impulsive children with autistic disorder. *J Clin Psychopharmacol* 12(5):322–327, 1992.

King BH, State MW, Shah B, et al. Mental retardation: A review of the past 10 years. Part I. *J Am Acad Child Adolesc Psychiatry* 36(12):1656–1663, 1997.

King BH, Wright DM, Handen BL, et al. Double-blind, placebo-controlled study of amantadine hydrochloride in the treatment of children with autistic disorder. *J Am Acad Child Adolesc Psychiatry* 40(6):658–665, 2001.

Levy SE. Pediatric evaluation of the child with developmental delay. *Child Adolesc Psychiatr Clin North Am* 5:809–826, 1996.

Levy SE, Souders MC, Wray J, et al. Children with autistic spectrum disorders. I: Comparison of placebo and single dose of human synthetic secretin. *Arch Dis Child* 88:731–736, 2003.

Lord C, Rutter M, Le Couteur A. Autism Diagnostic Interview—Revised: A revised version of a diagnostic interview for caregivers of individuals with possible pervasive developmental disorders. *J Autism Dev Disord* 24:659–685, 1994.

McCracken JT, McGough J, Shah B, et al. Risperidone in children with autism and serious behavioral problems. *NEJM* 347(5):314–321, 2002.

McDougle CJ. Psychopharmacology. In: Cohen DJ, Volkmar FR (Eds.), *Handbook of Autism and Pervasive Developmental Disorders* (2nd ed.). New York: Wiley, pp. 707–729, 1997.

McDougle CJ, Naylor ST, Cohen DJ, et al. A double-blind, placebo-controlled study of fluvoxamine in adults with autistic disorder. *Arch Gen Psychiatry* 53(11):1001–1008, 1996.

McDougle CJ, Posey DJ. Autistic and other pervasive developmental disorders. In: Martin A, Scahill L, Charney DS, Leckman JF (Eds.). *Pediatric Psychopharmacology Principles and Practice.* New York: Oxford University Press, pp. 563–579, 2003.

Niederhofer H, Staffen W, Mair A, et al. Brief report: melatonin facilitates sleep in individuals with mental retardation and insomnia. *J Autism Dev Disord* 33(4):469–472, 2003.

Prizant B. Review of the Childhood Autism Rating Scale. In: Kramer JJ, Conoley JC, Murphy LL (Eds.), *The Eleventh Mental Measurements Yearbook.* Lincoln: University of Nebraska Press, pp. 170–171, 1992.

Quintana H, Birmaher B, Stedge D, et al. Use of methylphenidate in the treatment of children with autistic disorder. *J Autism Dev Disord* 25(3):283–294, 1995.

Reiss S. *Handbook of Challenging Behavior: Mental Health Aspects of Mental Retardation.* Worthington, OH: IDS Publishing, 1994.

Reiss S, Aman MG. *Psychotropic Medications and Developmental Disabilities: The International Consensus Handbook.* Columbus, OH: Ohio State University Nisonger Center UAP, 1998.

Reiss S, Valenti-Hein D. Development of a psychopathology rating scale for children with mental retardation. *J Consult Clin Psychol* 62:28–33, 1994.

Remington G, Sloman L, Konstantareas M, et al. Clomipramine versus haloperidol in the treatment of autistic disorder: A double-blind, placebo-controlled, crossover study. *J Clin Psychopharmacol* 21(4):440–444, 2001.

Richardson S, Koller H. Vulnerability and resilience of adults who were classified as mildly mentally handicapped in childhood. In: Tizard B, Varma V (Eds.), *Vulnerability and Resilience in Human Development.* London: Jessica Kingsley, pp. 102–119, 1992.

Rutter M, Tizard J, Yule W, et al. Research report: Isle of Wight studies. *Psychol Med* 6:313–332, 1976.

Saemundsen E, Magnusson P, Smari J, et al. Autism Diagnostic Interview—the Childhood Autism Rating Scale Revised: Convergence and discrepancy in diagnosing autism. *J Autism Dev Disord* 33(3):319–328, 2003.

Scahill L, Riddle MA, McSwiggin-Hardin M, et al. Children's Yale–Brown Obsessive–Compulsive Scale: Reliability and validity. *J Am Acad Child Adolesc Psychiatry* 36:844–852, 1997.

Snyder R, Turgay A, Aman M, et al. Effects of risperidone on conduct and disruptive behavior disorders in children with subaverage IQs. *J Am Acad Child Adolesc Psychiatry* 41(9):1026–1036, 2002.

Sparrow S, Balla D, Cicchetti D. *Vineland Adaptive Behavioral Scales.* Circle Pines, MN: American Guidance Service, 1994.

State MW, King BH, Dykens E. Mental retardation: A review of the past 10 years. Part II. *J Am Acad Child Adolesc Psychiatry* 36(12):1664–1671, 1997.

Steingard RJ, Zimnitzky B, DeMaso DR, et al. Sertraline treatment of transition-associated anxiety and agitation in children with autistic disorder. *J Child Adolesc Psychopharmacol* 7(1):9–15, 1997.

Szymanski LS, King BH, Goldberg B, et al. Diagnosis of mental disorders in people with mental retardation. In: Reiss S, Aman MG (Eds.), *Psychotropic Medications and Developmental Disabilities: The International Consensus Handbook.* Columbus, OH: Ohio State University Press, pp. 3–17, 1998.

Turgay A, Binder C, Snyder R, et al. Long-term safety and efficacy of risperidone for the treatment of disruptive behavior disorders in children with subaverage IQs. *Pediatrics* 110(3):E34–53, 2002.

Unis AS, Munson JA, Rogers SJ, et al. A randomized, double-blind, placebo-controlled trial of porcine versus synthetic secretin for reducing symptoms of autism. *J Am Acad Child Adolesc Psychiatry* 41(11):1315–1321, 2002.

Van Bellinghen M, de Troch C. Risperidone in the treatment of behavioral disturbances in children and adolescents with borderline intellectual functioning: A double-blind, placebo-controlled pilot trial. *J Child Adolesc Psychopharmacology* 11(1):5–13, 2001.

Volkmar FR, Dykens E. Mental retardation. In: Lewis M (Ed.), *Child and Adolescent Psychiatry: A Comprehensive Textbook* (3rd ed.). Philadelphia: Lippincott, Williams & Wilkins, pp. 603–611, 2002.

Volkmar FR, Lord C, Klin A, et al. Autism and the pervasive developmental disorders. In: Lewis M (Ed.), *Child and Adolescent Psychiatry: A Comprehensive Textbook* (3rd ed.). Philadelphia: Lippincott, Williams & Wilkins, pp. 587–597, 2002.

B
I
B
L
I
O
G
R
A
P
H
Y

Willemsen-Swinkels SH, Buitelaar JK, van Engeland H. The effects of chronic naltrexone treatment in young autistic children: A double-blind placebo-controlled crossover study. *Bio Psychiatry* 39(12):1023–1031, 1996.

EATING DISORDERS

Agras WS. *Eating Disorders: Management of Obesity, Bulimia and Anorexia Nervosa.* Oxford, UK: Pergamon Press, 1987.

Agras WS, Rossiter, EM, Arnow B, et al. Pharmacologic and cognitive–behavioral treatment for bulimia nervosa: A controlled comparison. *Am J Psychiatry* 149:82–87, 1992.

American Psychiatric Association. Practice guidelines for the treatment of patients with eating disorders (revision). *Am J Psychiatry* 157(1 Suppl):1–39, 2000.

Bergh C, Brodin U, Lindberg G, et al. Randomized controlled trial of a treatment for anorexia and bulimia nervosa. *Proc Natl Acad Sci USA* 99(14):9486–9491, 2002.

Carruba MO, Cuzzolaro M, Riva L, et al. Efficacy and tolerability of moclobemide in bulimia nervosa: A placebo-controlled trial. *Int Clin Psychopharmacol* 16(1):27–32, 2001.

Carter FA, McIntosh VVW, Joyce PR, et al. Role of exposure with response prevention in cognitive–behavioral therapy for bulimia nervosa: Three-year follow-up results. *Int J Eat Disord* 33:127–135, 2003.

Carter JC, Olmsted MP, Kaplan AS, et al. Self-help for bulimia nervosa: A randomized controlled trial. *Am J Psychiatry* 160(5):973–978, 2003.

Eisler I, Dare C, Hodes M, et al. Family therapy for adolescent anorexia nervosa: The results of a controlled comparison of two family interventions. *J Child Psychol Psychiatry* 41(6):727–736, 2000.

Eisler I, Dare C, Russell G, et al. Family and individual therapy in anorexia nervosa: A 5-year follow-up. *Arch Gen Psychiatry* 54:1025–1030, 1997.

Fairburn CG, Beglin SJ. The assessment of eating disorders: Interview or self-report questionnaire? *Int J Eat Disord* 16:363–370, 1994.

Fairburn CG, Cooper Z. The Eating Disorders Examination—12th Edition. In: Fairburn CG, Wilson GT (Eds.), *Binge Eating: Nature, Assessment and Treatment.* New York: Guilford Press, 1993.

Fassino S, Leombruni P, Daga GA, et al. Efficacy of citalopram in anorexia nervosa: A pilot study. *Eur Psychopharmacol* 12(5):453–459, 2002.

Garner DM. *The Eating Disorders Inventory–2 Professional Manual.* Odessa, FL: Psychological Assessment Resources, 1991.

Garner DM, Olmsted MP, Bohr Y, et al. The Eating Attitudes Test: Psychometric features and clinical correlates. *Psychol Med* 12:871–878, 1982.

Goldbloom DS, Olmsted M, Davis R, et al. A randomized controlled trial of fluoxetine and cognitive behavioral therapy for bulimia nervosa: Short-term outcome. *Behav Res Ther* 35:803–811, 1997.

Halmi KA. Anorexia nervosa and bulimia nervosa. In: Lewis M (Ed.), *Child and Adolescent Psychiatry: A Comprehensive Textbook* (3rd ed.). Philadelphia: Lippincott, Williams & Wilkins, pp. 692–700, 2002.

Halmi KA. Eating disorders. In: Martin A, Scahill L, Charney DS, Leckman JF (Eds.). *Pediatric Psychopharmacology Principles and Practice.* New York: Oxford University Press, pp. 592–602, 2003.

Halmi KA, Eckert E, LaDu TJ, et al. Anorexia nervosa: Treatment efficacy of cyproheptadine and amitriptyline. *Arch Gen Psychiatry* 43(2):177–181, 1986.

Hedges DW, Reimherr FW, Hoopes SP, et al. Treatment of bulimia nervosa with topiramate in a randomized, double-blind, placebo-controlled trial: Part 2. Improvement in psychiatric measures. *J Clin Psychiatry* 64(12): 1449–1454, 2003.

Hoek HW. The incidence and prevalence of anorexia nervosa and bulimia nervosa in primary care. *Psychol Med* 21:455–460, 1991.

Hoopes SP, Reimherr FW, Hedges DW, et al. Treatment of bulimia nervosa with topiramate in a randomized, double-blind, placebo-controlled trial: Part 1. Improvement in binge and purge measures. *J Clin Psychiatry* 64(11):1335–1341, 2003.

Hudson JI, McElroy SL, Raymond NC, et al. Fluvoxamine in the treatment of binge-eating disorder: A multicenter placebo-controlled, double-blind trial. *Am J Psychiatry* 155(12):1756–1762, 1998.

Johnson C. Diagnostic Survey for Eating Disorders (DSED). In: Johnson C, Connors M (Eds.), *The Etiology and Treatment of Bulimia Nervosa.* New York: Basic Books, 1987.

Kaye WH, Nagata T, Weltzin TE, et al. Double-blind placebo-controlled administration of fluoxetine in restricting- and restricting-purging-type anorexia nervosa. *Biol Psychiatry* 49(7):644–652, 2001.

Keel P, Mitchell JE. Outcome in anorexia nervosa. *Am J Psychiatry* 154:313–321, 1997.

Kleifield EI, Wagner W, Halmi KA. Cognitive–behavioral treatment of anorexia nervosa. *Psychiatr Clin North Am* 19:715–737, 1996.

Kotler LA, Devlin MJ, Davies M, et al. An open trial of fluoxetine for adolescents with bulimia nervosa. *J Child Adolesc Psychopharmacol* 13(3):329–335, 2003.

Lucas AR, Berd CM, O'Fallon WN, et al. 50 year trend in the incidence of anorexia nervosa in Rochester, Minn: A population-based study. *Am J Psychiatry* 148:917–922, 1991.

Malina A, Gaskill J, McConaha C, et al. Olanzapine treatment of anorexia nervosa: A retrospective study. *Int J Eat Disord* 33:234–237, 2003.

Mazure CM, Halmi KA, Sunday SR, et al. Yale–Brown–Cornell Eating Disorder Scale: Development, use, reliability and validity. *J Psychiatr Res* 28:425–445, 1994.

McElroy SL, Arnold LM, Shapira NA, et al. Topriamate in the treatment of binge eating disorder associated with obesity: A randomized, placebo-controlled trial. *Am J Psychiatry* 160(2):255–261, 2003.

McElroy SL, Casuto LS, Nelson EB, et al. Placebo-controlled trial of sertraline in the treatment of binge eating disorder. *Am J Psychiatry* 157(6):1004–1006, 2000.

McElroy SL, Hudson JI, Malhotra S, et al. Citalopram in the treatment of binge-eating disorder: A placebo-controlled trial. *J Clin Psychiatry* 64(7):807–813, 2003.

McElroy SL, Kotwal R, Hudson JI, et al. Zonisamide in the treatment of binge-eating disorder: An open-label, prospective trial. *J Clin Psychiatry* 65(1):50–56, 2004.

Mitchell JE, Hatsukami D, Eckert E, et al. The Eating Disorders Questionnaire. *Psychopharmacol Bull* 21:1025–1043, 1985.

Mitchell JE, Pyle R, Eckert ED, et al. A comparison study of antidepressants and structured intensive group psychotherapy in the treatment of bulimia nervosa. *Arch Gen Psychiatry* 47:149–157, 1990.

Nangle DW, Ghonson WG, Carr-Nangle RD, et al. Binge eating disorder and the proposed DSM-IV criteria: Psychometric analysis of the Questionnaire of Eating and Weight Patterns. *Int J Eat Disord* 16:147–157, 1993.

Pallanti S, Quercioli L, Ramacciotti A. Citalopram in anorexia nervosa. *Eat Weight Disord* 2(4):216–221, 1997.

Pike KM, Walsh BT, Vitousek K, et al. Cognitive behavior therapy in the posthospitalization treatment of anorexia nervosa. *Am J Psychiatry* 160(11):2046–2049, 2003.

Powers PS, Santana CA, Bannon YS. Olanzapine in the treatment of anorexia nervosa: An open label trial. *Int J Eat Disord* 32:146–154, 2002.

Robin AL, Siegel PT, Moye AW, et al. A controlled comparison of family versus individual therapy for adolescents with anorexia nervosa. *J Am Acad Child Adolesc Psychiatry* 38(12):1482–1489, 1999.

B
I
B
L
I
O
G
R
A
P
H
Y

Romano SJ, Halmi KA, Sarkar NP, et al. A placebo-controlled study of fluoxetine in continued treatment of bulimia nervosa after successful acute fluoxetine treatment. *Am J Psychiatry* 159(1):96–102, 2002.

Russell GFM, Szmukler GI, Dare C, et al. An evaluation of family therapy in anorexia nervosa and bulimia nervosa. *Arch Gen Psychiatry* 44:1047–1056, 1987.

Santonastaso P, Friederici S, Favaro A. Sertraline in the treatment of restricting anorexia nervosa: An open controlled trial. *J Child Adolesc Psychopharmacol* 11(2):143–150, 2001.

Soundy TJ, Lucas AR, Suman VJ, et al. Bulimia nervosa in Rochester, Minnesota, 1980–1990. *Psychol Med* 25:1065–1071, 1995.

Strober M, Patake C, Freeman R, et al. No effect of adjunctive fluoxetine on eating behavior or weight phobia during the inpatient treatment of anorexia nervosa: An historical case-control study. *J Child Adolesc Psychopharmacol* 9(3):195–201, 1999.

Walsh BT, Wilson GT, Loeb KL, et al. Medication and psychotherapy in the treatment of bulimia nervosa. *Am J Psychiatry* 154:523–531, 1997.

SLEEP DISORDERS

Adair R, Bauchner H, Philipp B, et al. Night waking during infancy: Role of parental presence at bedtime. *Pediatrics* 84:500–504, 1991.

American Sleep Disorders Association. *The International Classification of Sleep Disorders: Diagnostic and Coding Manual* (2nd ed.). Lawrence, KS: Allen Press, 1990.

Anders TF, Eiben LA. Pediatric sleep disorders: A review of the past 10 years. *J Am Acad Child Adolesc Psychiatry* 36(1):9–20, 1997.

Anders TF, Halpern L, Hua J. Sleeping through the night: A developmental perspective. *Pediatrics* 90:554–560, 1992.

Carno MA, Hoffman LA, Carcillo JA, et al. Developmental stages of sleep from birth to adolescence, common childhood sleep disorders: Overview and nursing implications. *J Pediatr Nurs* 18(4):274–283, 2003.

Carskadon MA. Patterns of sleep and sleepiness in adolescents. *Pediatrician* 17:5–12, 1990.

Dahl RE. Sleep and arousal: Development and psychopathology. *J Dev Psychopathol* 8:3–27, 1996.

Dahl RE. Sleep disorders. In: Coffey CE, Brumback RA (Eds.), *Textbook of Pediatric Neuropsychiatry*. Washington, DC: American Psychiatric Press, pp. 821–838, 1998.

Dahl RE, Holttum J, Trubnick L. A clinical picture of child and adolescent narcolepsy. *J Am Acad Child Adolesc Psychiatry* 33:834–841, 1994.

Ferber R. *Solve Your Child's Sleep Problems*. New York: Simon & Schuster, 1985.

Gau SF, Soong WT. The transition of sleep–wake patterns in early adolescence. *Sleep* 26(4):449–454, 2003.

Goodwin JL, Babar SI, Kaemingk KL, et al. Symptoms related to sleep-disordered breathing in white and Hispanic children: The Tucson assessment of sleep apnea study. *Chest:* 124(1):196–203, 2003.

Gottlieb DJ, Vezina RM, Chase C, et al. Symptoms of sleep-disordered breathing in 5-year-old children are associated with sleepiness and problem behaviors. *Pediatrics* 112(4):870–877, 2003.

Handford HA, Vgontzas N. Sleep disturbances and disorders. In: Lewis M (Ed.), *Child and Adolescent Psychiatry: A Comprehensive Textbook* (3rd ed.). Philadelphia: Lippincott, Williams & Willkins, pp. 876–889, 2002.

Jan J, Espeze L, Appleton R. The treatment of sleep disorders with melatonin. *Dev Med Child Neurol* 36:97–107, 1994.

Minde K, Popiel K, Leos N, et al. The evaluation and treatment of sleep disturbances in young children. *J Child Psychol Psychiatry* 34:521–533, 1993.

Mitler M, Nelson S, Hajdokovic R. Narcolepsy: Diagnosis, treatment and management. *Sleep Disord* 10(40):593, 1987.

Moffat MEK, Harlos S, Kirshen AJ, et al. Desmopressin acetate and nocturnal enuresis: How much do we know? *Pediatrics* 92:420–425, 1993.

Morrison D, McGee R, Stanton WR. Sleep problems in adolescence. *J Am Acad Child Adolesc Psychiatry* 31:94–99, 1992.

Niederhofer H, Staffen W, Mair A, et al. Brief report: Melatonin facilitates sleep in individuals with mental retardation and insomnia. *J Autism Dev Disord* 33(4):469–472, 2003.

Quan SF, Goodwin JL, Babar SI, et al. Sleep architecture in normal Caucasian and Hispanic children aged 6–11 years recorded during unattended home polysomnography: Experience from the Tucson children's assessment of sleep apnea study (TuCASA). *Sleep Med* 4(1):13–19, 2003.

Rapoport JL, Mikkelsen EJ, Zavadila A, et al. Childhood enuresis, II: Psychopathology, tricyclic concentration in plasma, and antienuretic effect. *Arch Gen Psychiatry* 37:1146–1152, 1980.

Schwartz JR, Feldman NT, Fry JM, et al. Efficacy and safety of modafinil for improving daytime wakefulness in patients treated previously with psychostimulants. *Sleep Med* 4(1):43–49, 2003.

Smits MG, van Stel HF, van der Heijden K, et al. Melatonin improves health status and sleep in children with idiopathic chronic sleep-onset insomnia: A randomized placebo-controlled trial. *J Am Acad Child Adolesc Psychiatry* 42(11):1286–1293, 2003.

Stores G. Children's sleep disorders: Modern approaches, developmental effects, and children at special risk. *Dev Med Child Neurol* 41(8):568–573, 1999.

Stores G. *A Clinical Guide to Sleep Disorders in Children and Adolescents.* New York: Cambridge University Press, 2001.

Stores G. Medication for sleep–wake disorders. *Arch Dis Child* 88:899–903, 2003.

U.S. Modafinil in Narcolepsy Multicenter Study Group. Randomized trial of modafinil for the treatment of pathological somnolence in narcolepsy. *Ann Neurol* 43(1):88–97, 1998.

Zuckerman B, Stevenson J, Baily V. Sleep problems in early childhood: Predictive factors and behavioral correlates. *Pediatrics* 80:664–671, 1987.

B
I
B
L
I
O
G
R
A
P
H
Y

OTHER IMPORTANT TOPICS IN PEDIATRIC PSYCHOPHARMACOLOGY

American Academy of Child and Adolescent Psychiatry Work Group on Quality Issues. Practice parameters for the assessment and treatment of children and adolescents with substance use disorders. *J Am Acad Child Adolesc Psychiatry* 36(10 Suppl):140S–155S, 1997.

Barkley RA, Fischer M, Smallish L, et al. Does the treatment of attention-deficit/hyperactivity disorder with stimulants contribute to drug use/abuse? A 13-year prospective study. *Pediatrics* 111(1):97–109, 2003.

Bhatara VS, Feil M, Hoagwood K, et al. Trends in combined pharmacotherapy with stimulants for children. *Psychiatr Serv* 53:244, 2002.

Brent DA, Baugher M, Bridge J, et al. Age- and sex-related risk factors for adolescent suicide. *J Am Acad Child Adolesc Psychiatry* 38:1497–1505, 1999.

Carlson GA, Rapport MD, Kelly KL, et al. Methylphenidate and desipramine in hospitalized children with comorbid behavior and mood disorders: Separate and combined effects on behavior and mood. *J Child Adolesc Psychopharmacol* 5:191–204, 1995.

Connor DF, Barkley RA, Davis HT. A pilot study of methylphenidate, clonidine, or the combination in ADHD comorbid with aggressive oppositional defiant or conduct disorder. *Clin Pediatr* 39:15–25, 2000.

Connor DF, Ozbayrak KR, Kusiak KA, et al. Combined pharmacotherapy in children and adolescents in a residential treatment center. *J Am Acad Child Adolesc Psychiatry* 36(2):248–254, 1997.

DeBattista C, Schatzberg AF. 2003 psychotropic dosing and monitoring guidelines. *Prim Psychiatry* 10(7):80–96, 2003.

DelBello MP, Schwiers ML, Rosenberg HL, et al. A double-blind, randomized, placebo-controlled study of quetiapine as adjunctive treatment for adolescent mania. *J Am Acad Child Adolesc Psychiatry* 41(10):1216–1223, 2002.

Federal Drug Administration, 2004. Antidepressant use in children, adolescents, and adults. *http://www.fda.gov/*

Geller B, Cooper T, Sun K, et al. Double-blind and placebo-controlled study of lithium for adolescent bipolar disorders with secondary substance dependency. *J Am Acad Child Adolesc Psychiatry* 37:171–178, 1998.

Gittelman-Klein R, Klein DF, Katz S, et al. Comparative effects of methylphenidate and thioridazine in hyperkinetic children: I. Clinical results. *Arch Gen Psychiatry* 33:1217–1231, 1976.

Hazell PL, Stuart JE. A randomized controlled trial of clonidine added to psychostimulant medication for hyperactive and aggressive children. *J Am Acad Child Adolesc Psychiatry* 42(8):886–894, 2003.

Kandel D, Johnson J, Bird H, et al. Psychiatric comorbidity among adolescents with substance use disorders: Findings from the MECA study. *J Am Acad Child Adolesc Psychiatry* 38:693–698, 1999.

Kurlan R (Tourette's Syndrome Study Group). Treatment of ADHD in children with tics. *Neurology* 58:527–536, 2002.

Morehead D. Exacerbation of hallucinogen-persisting perception disorder with risperidone. *J Clin Psychopharm* 17:327–328, 1997.

Olfson M, Marcus SC, Weissman MW, et al. National trends in the use of psychotropic medication by children. *J Am Acad Child Adolesc Psychiatry* 41:514–521, 2002.

Pfeffer CR. Suicidal behavior in children and adolescents: Causes and management. In: Lewis M (Ed.), *Child and Adolescent Psychiatry: A Comprehensive Textbook* (3rd ed.). Philadelphia: Lippincott, Williams & Wilkins, pp. 796–805, 2002.

Riggs P. Clinical approach to treatment of ADHD in adolescents with substance use disorders and conduct disorder. *J Am Acad Child Adolesc Psychiatry* 37:331–332, 1998.

Riggs P, Mikulich S, Coffman L, et al. Fluoxetine in drug-dependent delinquents with major depression: An open trial. *J Child Adolesc Psychopharmacol* 7:87–95, 1997.

Safer DJ, Zito JM, dosReis S. Concomitant psychotropic medication for youths. *Am J Psychiatry* 160(3):438–449, 2003.

Shader RI. Assessment and treatment of suicide risk. In: Shader RI. *Manual of Psychiatric Therapeutics* (3rd ed.). Philadelphia: Lippincott, Williams & Wilkins, pp. 229–239, 2003.

Venkatakrishnan K, Shader RI, von Moltke LL, et al. Drug interactions in psychopharmacology. In: Shader RI (Ed.), *Manual of Psychiatric Therapeutics* (3rd ed.). Philadelphia: Lippincott, Williams & Wilkins, pp. 441–469, 2003.

Waxmonsky JG, Wilens T. Substance-abusing youths. In: Martin A, Scahill L, Charney DS, Leckman JF (Eds.), *Pediatric Psychopharmacology Principles and Practice*. New York: Oxford University Press, pp. 605–616, 2003.

Wilens TE, Biederman J, Abrantes A, et al. Clinical characteristics of psychiatrically referred adolescent outpatients with substance use disorder. *J Am Acad Child Adolesc Psychiatry* 36:941–947, 1997.

Wilens TE, Faraone SV, Biederman J, et al. Does stimulant therapy of attention deficit/hyperactivity disorder beget later substance abuse? A meta-analytic review of the literature. *Pediatrics* 111(1):179–185, 2003.

Wilens TE, Spencer T, Biederman J, et al. Combined pharmacotherapy: An emerging trend in pediatric psychopharmacology. *J Am Acad Child Adolesc Psychiatry* 34(1):110–112, 1995.

Zito JM, Safer DJ, DosReis S, et al. Psychotropic practice patterns for youth: A 10-year perspective. *Arch Pediatr Adolesc Med* 157(1):17–25, 2003.

PEDIATRIC PSYCHOPHARMACOLOGY AND THE CARDIOVASCULAR SYSTEM

Gutgesell H, Atkins D, Barast R, et al. AHA scientific statement: Cardiovascular monitoring of children and adolescents receiving psychotropic drugs. *J Am Acad Child Adolesc Psychiatry* 38:1047–1050, 1999.

Report of the Task Force on Blood Pressure Control in Children, National Heart, Lung, and Blood Institute. *Pediatrics* (Suppl) 59:803, 1977.

Welch R, Chue P. Antipsychotic agents and QT changes. *J Psychiatry Neurosci* 25: 154–160, 2000.

B
I
B
L
I
O
G
R
A
P
H
Y

Index

Abnormal Involuntary Movement
Scale, 568–572
absorption, 16–17
acute dystonic reaction, 401–402
acute stress disorder, 440
AdderallXR®
adverse effects, 49
formulations, 42
indications, 46
ADHD. *see* attention-deficit/
hyperactivity disorder
adjustment disorder, 362
administration, drug, 16–17
adrenergic agents, 213
for aggression management, 331
contraindications, 450
for disruptive behavior in child with
mental retardation, 463
indications, 450
medical monitoring, 450
tic disorder treatment, 312–313
withdrawal, 451
see also beta-blockers; clonidine;
guanfacine
aggression
assessment, 599–601
in child with mental retardation,
463–465
classification, 325–326
clinical approach, 332–335
disorders of, 319
etiology, 319
management with antipsychotics,
145
prevalence, 319
treatment, 319–320, 326–332

see also conduct disorder;
oppositional defiant
disorder
agoraphobia, 416–417
akathisia, 146, 403
albumin, 18
algorithms, prescribing, 7
Allegra®. *see* fexofenadine
alpha-1-acid glycoprotein, 18
alpha-tocopherol. *see* Vitamin E
alprazolam, 186–187
amantadine
contraindications, 179
dosing, 179
drug interactions, 180
efficacy, 178
formulations, 178
indications, 177, 178
interference with laboratory tests,
180
pharmacology, 177
side effects, 179
Ambien®. *see* zolpidem
aminophylline, 506
amitriptyline
discontinuation, 100
dosing, 99, 358
indications, 99
pharmacology, 98–99
amphetamines
adverse effects, 49
dosing, 286
early research, 4
pharmacology, 43, 45, 238,
526
animal studies, 9

INDEX

671

I
N
D
E
X

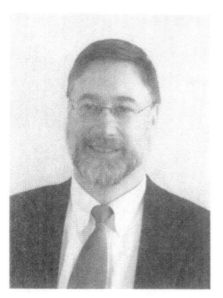 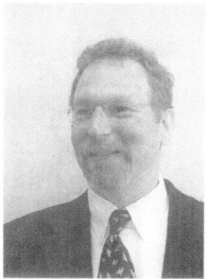

DANIEL F. CONNOR, M.D. (left), is the Lockean Distinguished Professor in Mental Health Education, Research, and Clinical Improvement, and Chief of Child and Adolescent Psychiatry in the Department of Psychiatry, University of Connecticut Health Center, Farmington, Connecticut. He was previously Professor of Psychiatry and Pediatrics, and Director of Pediatric Psychopharmacology and Ambulatory Child and Adolescent Psychiatry at the University of Massachusetts Medical School in Worcester, Massachusetts. Dr Connor has authored or co-authored over 80 journal articles, abstracts, and book chapters. He is the author of *Aggression and Antisocial Behaviors in Children and Adolescents: Research and Treatment.*

BRUCE M. MELTZER, M.D. (right), is Assistant Professor of Pediatrics and Child Psychiatry at the University of Massachusetts Medical School, Worcester. He attended Tufts University School of Medicine before completing residencies in Pediatrics at Mt. Sinai School of Medicine and Adult Psychiatry at Brown University. He completed fellowships in Child Psychiatry and Pediatric Mood Disorders, both at Brown University. Dr. Meltzer is currently the Medical Director of Adolescent Continuing Care Services at the University of Massachusetts Medical School.

CPSIA information can be obtained at www.ICGtesting.com
Printed in the USA
LVOW071715190912

299477LV00008B/9/P